UPDATE ON DEMENTIA

Edited by **Davide Vito Moretti**

Update on Dementia
http://dx.doi.org/10.5772/61983
Edited by Davide Vito Moretti

Contributors
Hitoshi Sohma, Yasuo Kokai, Alyssa Brewer, Brian Barton, Liqin Zhao, Sarah Woody, José M. Ramírez, Elena Salobrar-García, Ana I. Ramírez, Rosa De Hoz, Pilar Rojas, Juan J Salazar, Blanca Rojas, Pedro Gil, Raquel Yubero, Alberto Triviño, Rodrigo Quintanilla, María José Pérez, Claudia Jara, Ernesto Muñoz, Marco Meraz-Ríos, Perla Leal-Galicia, Teresa Juarez-Cedillo, Ging-Yuek Hsiung, Amir Ali Sepehry, B. Lynn Beattie, Claudia Jacova, Jorge Escobedo De La Peña, Ricardo B. Maccioni, Inelia Morales, Gonzalo Farias, Nicole Cortes, Robyn Gillespie, Pippa Burns, Judy Mullan, Lindsey Harrison, Amanda Baker, Khin Win, Victoria Traynor, Kendra Ray, Renita Davis, Jan Maier, Ayelet Dassa, Olayinka Ogunlade, Dongming Cai, Farida El Gaamouch, Gonzalo E. Aranda-Abreu, Sonia Lilia Mestizo Gutiérrez, María Elena Hernández Aguilar, Fausto Rojas Durán, J Arjuna Ratnayaka, Savannah A. Lynn, Rubesh Gooriah, Jolanta Dorszewska, Michal Prendecki, Jolanta Florczak-Wyspianska, Marta Kowalska, Margarita Lianeri, Wojciech Kozubski, Teresa Mayordomo Rodríguez, Siu Kwan Sze, Sunil S Adav, Daniele Sancarlo, Grazia D'Onofrio, Antonio Greco, Pablo Escribá, Manuel Torres, Xavier Busquets, Luis Fernando Hernandez-Zimbron, Hugo Quiroz-Mercado, Gohar Gevorkian-Markosian, Elisa Gorostieta-Salas, Roxanna Pérez-Garmendia, Mei-Li Díaz-Hung, Erika Maria Orta Salazar, Isaac Vargas-Rodríguez, Susana Angelica Castro-Chavira, Alfredo I Feria-Velasco, Sofia Diaz-Cintra

Published by InTech
Janeza Trdine 9, 51000 Rijeka, Croatia

Publishing Process Manager Romina Rovan
Technical Editor SPi Global
Cover InTech Design team

First published September, 2016
Printed in Croatia

Additional hard copies can be obtained from orders@intechopen.com

Update on Dementia, Edited by Davide Vito Moretti
p. cm.
Print ISBN 978-953-51-2654-6
Online ISBN 978-953-51-2655-3

For EU product safety concerns:
IN TECH d.o.o., Prolaz Marije Krucifikse Kozulić 3, 51000 Rijeka, Croatia,
info@intechopen.com or visit our website at intechopen.com.

Meet the editor

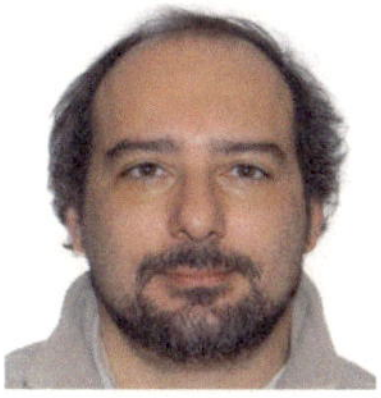

Dr. Davide Vito Moretti is a consultant neurologist and senior researcher at the National Institute of Research and Cure for Mental Disorders and Dementia, St. John of God Institute, Brescia, Italy. Since 2014, he is a professor of Neurophysiology at the UniLudes University in Lugano. He received his medical degree from the Catholic University in Rome and completed his residency in neurology and fellowship in movement disorders at the State University in Trieste. Moreover, he received his PhD in Neurophysiology at the Sapienza University of Rome. Dr. Moretti is currently involved in research and care of subjects with Alzheimer's disease and dementia in the Memory Clinic/Alzheimer Operative Unit of the St. John of God Institute. Moreover, he is the chief of the clinical neurophysiology unit and of the Alzheimer's disease rehabilitation operative unit. Since March 2015, he is also the head of the whole rehabilitation in dementia line research in the St. John of God Institute. His research is primarily concerned about Alzheimer's disease both in prodromic and in clinically evident phase of the disease, Parkinson's disease, movement disorders, and clinical neurophysiology.

Contents

Preface

The world's older population currently comprises almost 900 million men and women. Most of them are living in what are presently slightly poor countries. Mortality charges among older individuals are falling, and life expectancy from age 60 continues to increase in all world areas, without an upper limit in sight. As individuals live longer, chronic diseases end up more established, a trend exacerbated by changes in the direction of life and behaviors that predispose the development of the diseases.

About 47 million individuals at the moment are residing with dementia worldwide, with numbers projected to just about double each two decades, growing to 74.7 million by 2030 and 131.5 million by 2050. While dementia shortens the lives of those affected, the quality of life of both patients and their family and caregivers is heavily affected.

A growing evidence suggests that, among older humans, dementia has a bigger impact on disability than other physical and/or intellectual disorders, needing for care and attendant fees. In step with trending expenditure projections, the worldwide price of dementia will have reached US$1 trillion in 2018. Therefore, the scientific and social groups need a specific knowledge that dementia is a world difficulty and a better working out of the extent of the current therapy gap in terms of analysis, therapies, services, and help are needed.

While there has been a productive pipeline of promising new agents with plausible ambitions linked to Alzheimer's disease pathology, there have been a dispiritingly excessive percentage of failures in phase II human trials and phase III definitive randomized controlled clinical trials. This raises professional questions involving the validity of our current disease models and the experimental drug design method. Despite the fact that the course of dementia is not able to be altered, symptomatic cures and support are invaluable. Earlier analysis makes it possible for those affected to take part in evolved care planning while they nonetheless have the ability to take action. Education, coaching, and support for carers are important in lowering caregiver's pressure and psychological morbidity and in delaying or warding off transition into care houses.

Support groups for people with dementia, current pharmacological interventions, and cognitive stimulation to strengthen cognitive performance and behavioral interventions for fighting depression are all potent interventions in early-stage dementia. The common efforts and the final aim of the whole society will have to be the progress of a "dementia-constructive" procedure, enabling an actual social inclusion and no longer a simple support or even toleration of individuals with dementia. This book is a proposal of the major updates on dementia physiopathological mechanisms and possible treatment options.

Dr. Davide Vito Moretti
Rehabilitation in Alzheimer's Disease Operative Unit,
National Institute for Research and Cure in Dementia and Mental Health Fatebenefratelli,
St. John of God Hospital, Italy

Section 1

Experimental Section

Chapter 1

Alternative Splicing and Alzheimer's Disease

Gonzalo Emiliano Aranda Abreu,
Sonia Lilia Mestizo Gutiérrez,
María Elena Hernández Aguilar and
Fausto Rojas Durán

Additional information is available at the end of the chapter

http://dx.doi.org/10.5772/64513

Abstract

Alzheimer's disease is a neurodegenerative process whose origin is unknown. It has been associated with this process at least two important proteins: the first is the β-amyloid forming amyloid plaques and the second protein is Tau, which has been determined to precipitates inside the neuron because hyperphosphorylation, causing instability in the axon. Tau microtubule-associated protein (MAP) is essential for the development of neuronal cell polarity. Tau protein is preferentially localized in the axons, whereas MAP2, another neuronal specific microtubule-associated protein, is localized in the somatodendritic domain. Previous studies have demonstrated that the localization of these proteins depends, at least in part, on messenger RNA (mRNA) subcellular localization, that is, Tau mRNA into the axon and MAP2 mRNA into the dendrite. Tau protein has an essential role in the pathology of Alzheimer's disease, and hyperphosphorylated Tau promotes destabilization of microtubules. Tau alternative splicing generates six isoforms in the adult human brain due to the inclusion or exclusion of exons 2, 3, and 10. The failure in the splicing process of exon 10 generates a tauopathy, which can be carried out by the amyloid peptide; however, the splicing of other exons is less studied. The impact of amyloid peptide on the alternative splicing of exons 2, 3, and 6 caused formed cell processes to retract in differentiated cells and altered the expression of exons 2/3 in cell culture. Expression of exon 6 was repressed under β-amyloid treatment. The molecular mechanism for this amyloid-Tau interaction remains to be determined, but may have potential implications for the understanding of the underlying neuropathological processes in Alzheimer's disease.

Keywords: Alzheimer, Tau, APP, PSEN1, PSEN2, alternative splicing

1. Introduction

Alzheimer's disease (AD) is a neurodegenerative condition characterized by progressive loss of memory, orientation, sanity, and language. AD is a slow evolving disorder of multigenic nature with an average duration between 8 and 12 years. During the disease onset, symptoms are overlooked generally for the first 2 or 3 years. There are few hereditary cases (genetic or familial AD) resulting from autosomal dominant inheritance of chromosomal alterations. This condition is the most common type of dementia, and it is globally recognized as one of the leading causes of morbidity and mortality among the advanced age population. In 2004, approximately 44 million cases of dementia were diagnosed worldwide and the number of cases in 2050 is estimated to be 135 million [1].

In AD, there is neuron loss and two typical alterations appear: the neuritic plaque produced by the β-amyloid (Aβ) and the neurofibrillary tangle that contains the hyperphosphorylated Tau protein as the main component.

Neuritic plaques are sphere-like structures in which the major component is the β-amyloid (Aβ) protein. The latter is generated by proteolytic cleavage of a larger protein, βAPP (Aβ precursor protein), and the neurofibrillar tangle, an intracellular damage affecting pyramidal neurons [2].

When the disease is diagnosed, its pathology has progressed several years [3]. Cerebral changes underlying AD probably develop 20–30 years before the first symptoms appear.

AD diagnosis combines psychological and imaging tests as well as the exclusion of neurologic disorders [4].

The pathological processes frequently linked to AD are as follows: aging, amyloid deposition, neurofibrillar degeneration, synaptic loss, inflammation, loss of vascular integrity, and neuron loss [5].

The development of tangles and plaques leads to neuron death. Tangles are mainly located at the entorhinal cortex, hippocampus, parahippocampal gyrus, amygdala, and frontal, temporal, parietal, and occipital cortices and some subcortical nuclei projected toward these regions [6].

Tangles are composed by paired helical filaments (PHF), in which the latter are gathered in helixes. Neuritic plaques are microscopic foci of extracellular amyloid depositions associated with axon and neurite damage. They are found in large amounts at the limbic and association cortex [7].

At the neuritic plaques, it is observed an abnormal extracellular accumulation of the Aβ peptide, comprised by 40 or 42 amino acids (Aβ40 and Aβ42) [8]. Dystrophic neurites are located both within and surrounding the amyloid depositions, and they are distinguished by structural abnormalities including lysosomes, mitochondria, and PHF.

These plaques are associated with microglia either contiguous or within the amyloid nucleus. The period of time for neuritic plaque development is unknown. Most of the fibrillar Aβ located at the neuritic plaques is the species ending in the amino acid 42 (Aβ42), which is the slightly larger and hydrophobic form, prone to aggregation [9].

In AD, there is neurotransmitter deficiency at brain level. Dementia symptoms develop because the severe degeneration suffered by neurons that synthesize and liberate acetylcholine. The level and activities of the synthesizing and degrading enzymes, choline acetyltransferase and acetylcholinesterase, decrease at the limbic and cerebral cortex showing an associated loss of cholinergic cell bodies at the septal nucleus and the anterior forebrain cholinergic system [6].

Glutamatergic system is also deteriorated in AD. There are interactions between β-amyloid and glutamate at the synaptic function: the former has influence on the generation of the latter and glutamate levels may be modified by the peptide. Concentration changes of these two molecules may impact AD progression. Because hippocampus and cortex are fundamental for learning and memory, it is possible that glutamatergic neuron degeneration appears at early stages of AD [10].

The cerebral regions severely affected by AD are as follows: hippocampus, entorhinal cortex, amygdala, cerebral cortex, and some subcortical areas such as cholinergic neurons at the anterior forebrain, serotoninergic neurons at the dorsal raphe, and noradrenergic neurons at the locus coeruleus [11].

Four main genes have been associated to Alzheimer's disease; all of them are processed by ribonucleic acid (RNA) alternative splicing.

2. RNA splicing

Ribonucleic acid (RNA) splicing is a mechanism used by eukaryotic cells in order to eliminate introns. These introns are non-coding RNA sequences, and therefore, they need to be removed by a ribonucleoprotein-rich structure termed the spliceosome complex. Thus, exon sequences are joined, producing a mature transcript that is available for migrating from the cell nucleus to the cytoplasm in order to be translated into a protein.

Splicing mechanism must be very accurate, as at least 50% of human genetic diseases are associated with mutations occurring in consensus sequences of splicing sites. These sequences consist on GU at the 5′ intron and an AG sequence at 3′. Toward the 5′ end of the intron, there is a pyrimidine-rich region (C U).

In order to carry out the splicing, the spliceosome complex needs to be assembled. The consensus sequences located at the exon–intron boundary are essential to bind the 5 ribonucleoproteins (snRNP) U1, U2, U4, U5, and U6 in such sequences in order to form the spliceosome. Several protein complexes constitute the spliceosome: the complex E (U1 binds to the GU sequence at the 5′ site of an intron, SF1 binds to the intron branch point, U2AF1 binds to the 3′ splicing site, and U2F2 binds to the polypirimidine sequence), the complex A (U2 displaces SF1 and it binds to the branch point sequence), the complex B (U5, U4, and U6 form a trimer that bind to U2 along with U5). U1 is released, U5 shifts from exon to intron, and U6 binds to the 5′ splicing site). Complex C (U4 is released, and U6/U2 catalyze a transesterification to induce the binding of the 5′-end intron to the complex A, forming an intron lariat. U5 bind to the exon 3′ splicing site, which is cleaved). Afterward, U2, U5, and U6 remain bound to the lariat forms and the 3′ site is cleaved, whereas exons are ligated by means of ATP hydrolysis. Lariat forms are degraded, and the snRNP are recycled (**Figure 1**).

Alternative splicing generally is a mean by which a gene may generate a variety of messenger RNAs (mRNAs) with biological significance, that is coding for a protein. It has been estimated that at least 90% of all expressed genes are subjected to alternative splicing.

It has been identified at least six ways to generate alternative splicing: (a) exon exclusion or inclusion, (b) selecting one or more exons, (c) and (d) competition for the splicing site at a defined exon either in the 5′ or 3′ region, (e) retaining an intron, (f) multiple promoters, (g) multiple poly-A sites [12] (**Figure 2**). Exon and intron sequences may regulate the splicing site through enhancer or silencer sequences.

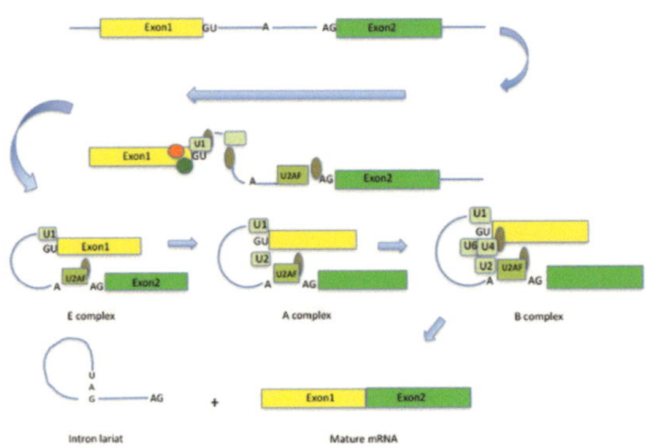

Figure 1. RNA splicing. Exon 1 flanked on its 3′ end by the GU sequence and exon 2 on its 5′ end by AG, with both target sites for the ribonucleoproteins and the assembled spliceosome complex. The spliceosome will cut the intron in the consensus sequences and will enable the joining of the exons, generating a mature RNA. Scheme taken from [49].

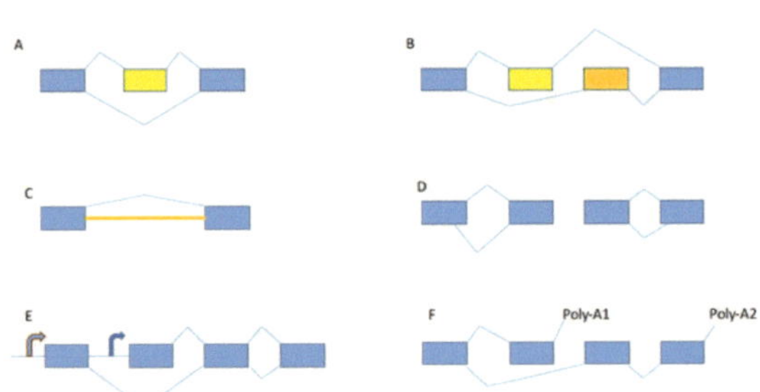

Figure 2. Forms of alternative splicing. (**A**) Exclusion or inclusion of exons, (**B**) selection of one or more exons, (**C**) intron retention, (**D**) competencies by the site of splicing in a particular exon in the region 5′ or 3′, (**E**) multiple promoters, (**F**) multiple poly-A sites.

http://dx.doi.org/10.5772/64513

3. The Tau gene and its alternative splicing

Tau is a cytoskeleton protein involved in neuron morphology and polarity. It posses the ability to bind to microtubules in order to provide stability, and it maintains the neuron phenotype at the axon level [13].

It has been determined that Tau is located at the axon hillock, the axon and the growth cone, as its mRNA is transported to its translation site by a protein complex involving kinesin-3 as transporter and the HuD protein as mRNA stabilizer [14–16]. This is possible because Tau mRNA posses in its 3′-UTR region a uracil-rich axon localization sequence [14, 17].

Tau protein is mainly constituted by two domains: the N-terminal whose function is to interact with the plasma membrane [18] and the C-terminal domain, in which the microtubule-binding region is coded [19].

The human Tau gene is located at chromosome 17 [20], it is formed by 16 exons, and it has a promoter region that confers it with neuron specificity [21].

This gene is transcribed into three RNAs of 2, 6, and 9 kb, which are differentially expressed in the central nervous system, depending on their maturity state and the neuron type [18]. Six Tau mRNA isoforms have been identified as consequence of alternative splicing, five of them in the adult central nervous system and one fetal isoform. These messenger RNAs code six proteins ranging from 352 to 441 amino acids (aa). The fetal isoform (352 aa) does not contain the exons 2, 3, and 10. The adult form of 383 aa lacks exons 2 and 3; however, it includes exon 10. The 381 aa isoform include exon 2 but not 10. The 412 aa isoform includes both exons 2 and 10; the 410 aa isoform includes exons 2 and 3, but not 10. The 441 aa isoform includes exons 2, 3, and 10 [22] (**Figure 3**).

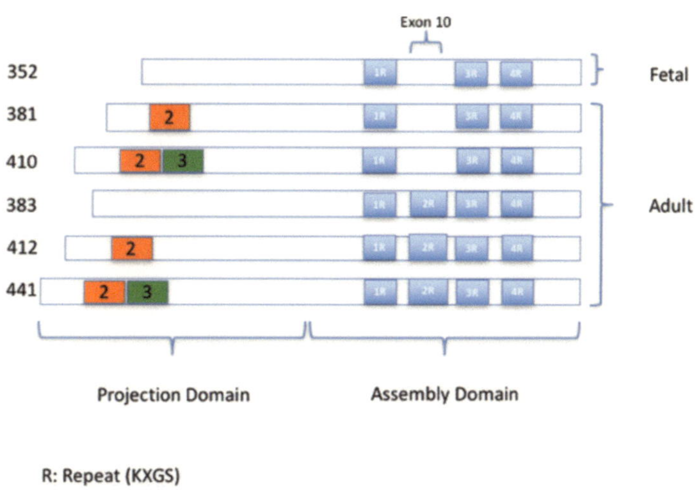

Figure 3. Tau isoforms, showing the different Tau proteins from the alternative splicing of exons 2, 3 and 10. Scheme taken from [49].

Tau alternative splicing occurs in exons 2, 3, and 10 and its form is of the (a) type that corresponds to exon exclusion or inclusion.

The studies conducted on Tau alternative splicing have been comprehensive, and most of them have been focused on exon 10.

Exon 10 displays a splicing pattern of inclusion and it is not present on fetal neurons. It is influenced by exon 9, which promotes its inclusion [18]. Exon 10 codes the second region of the (R) (KXGS) repeats in Tau. Alternative splicing generates Tau isoforms with 3 or 4 repeats that bind to microtubules. In mature brains, the level of 3R and 4R is similar. Exon 10 disruption is able and enough to cause neuron degeneration or taupathies [23].

Exon 10 is flanked by a long 13.6-kb intron and a short 3.8-kb intron, possessing a weak 5′ splicing site, which is similar to that in 3′. This would allow the inclusion or not of exon 10 in order to generate proteins with or without it [24, 25].

Exon 2 alternative splicing has been less studied. However, the studies conducted in our laboratory show that when PC12 cells (rat pheochromocytoma) cultures are exposed to the β1 → 42 amyloid peptide; alternative splicing of exons 2 and 3 is affected, as immature forms of Tau mRNA are transcribed in mature PC12 cells (phenotype differentiated into neuron). We observed that processes in these cells begin to retract. In spite the mechanism is still unknown, the effect produced in these cells indicate that immature Tau forms cease to stabilize microtubules in these cells processes [26] (**Figure 4**). The inclusion of exons 2 and 3 promotes the shift from immature Tau forms to their mature counterparts, stabilizing microtubules.

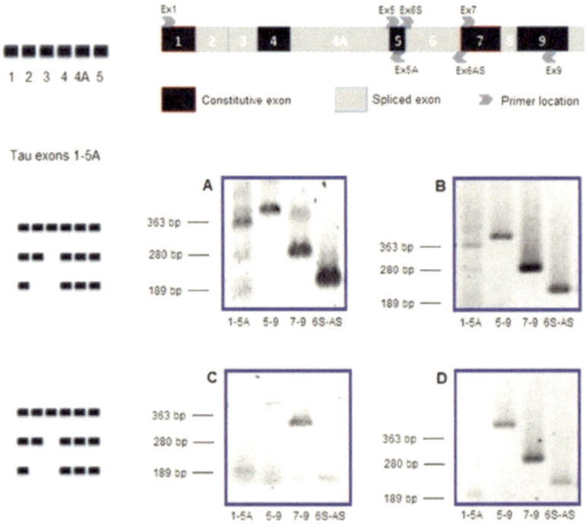

Figure 4. Tau exons 1–9 (modified from [50]), the primers Ex1 and Ex5A, amplify from exons 1 to 5. The exons 2 and 3 are amplified by (Ex1/Ex5A), the exon 6 is amplified by (Ex5/Ex9, Ex6S/Ex6AS) and exon 8 by (Ex7/Ex9). (**A**) Untreated undifferentiated cells and (**B**) NGF-induced differentiated PC12 cells; and from PC12 cells exposed to Aβ(1–42) peptide in (**C**) undifferentiated cells and (**D**) NGF-induced differentiated cells. Differentiation inhibits fetal tau expression. Aβ exposure promotes exclusion of exons 2/3 in undifferentiated and differentiated cells, and exclusion of exon 6 in undifferentiated cells. Scheme taken from [26].

It has been demonstrated that immature Tau forms are similar to those found on PHF [27], suggesting that exclusion of exons 2 and 3 induced by amyloid peptide in AD may destabilize neurites, and thus, the cells would lose their polarity.

Currently, splicing regulation has been studied with microRNAs (miRNAs), which are regulators of genetic expression [28]. miRNAs are short RNA molecules that bind to transcripts in order to repress and regulate expression. A miRNA deregulation was found on hippocampus and the prefrontal cortex. It was ascertained that miR-132-3-p was the most affected in this disease. miR-132-3-p downregulation in neurons was inversely proportional to the occurrence of hyperphosphorylated Tau [29], and it is linked to the splicing of exon 10 [30].

The inclusion of exon 10 is inhibited by the constitutive factors ASF/SF2, SRp55, SRp75, and SWAP [31].

Exon 2 regulation has been determined by inclusion and exclusion of exons 2 and 3, and it has been determined that exon 3 never appears without exon 2 [32].

4. Amyloid precursor protein (APP) gene

APP is one of the three members of a small gene family coding type I membrane proteins possessing an extracellular domain and a small cytoplasmic region. Only APP contains the sequence coding the Aβ domain. APP human gene is located at chromosome 21, which is involved in autosomal dominant inheritance in some families affected by early Alzheimer's disease. This gene contains 18 exons, and it is more than 170 kb long [33]. More than 25 mutations have been identified to cause the familial type of AD. All of these mutations substitute amino acids near or within the Aβ domain [34]. Aβ is derived from APP by proteolytic cleavage due to an alternative splicing process (generating three isoforms composed by 695, 751, and 770 residues, respectively) [35], of exons 7, 8, and 15 (**Figure 5**). The APP form without the residues coded by exon 15 is called L-APP, and this isoform is found in most tissues [36]. The APP695 isoform is predominantly expressed in neurons, whereas

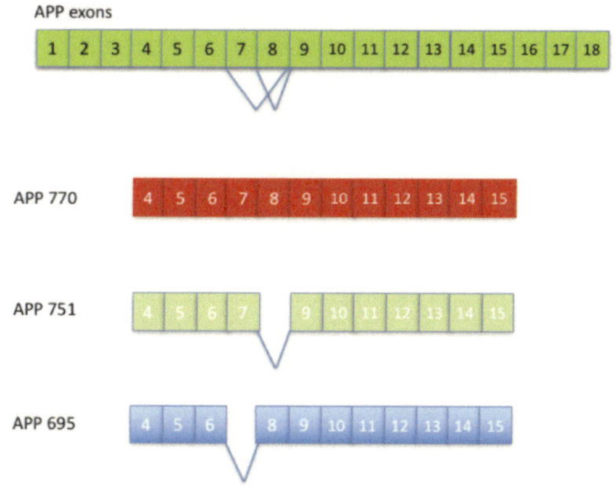

Figure 5. APP isoforms, showing the different APP proteins from alternative splicing of exons 7 and 8.

APP751 is expressed in all tissues and it includes exon 7, codifying a domain similar to that of the Kunitz protease inhibitor [37].

In neurons, APP is found on terminal vesicles in axons and it can be transported in an anterograde or retrograde manner [38]. Other brain cells also express APP and release variable amounts of Aβ, including astrocytes and microglia.

APP may be subjected to protelytic cleavage during and after its transit through the secretory pathway. The first of them is carried out by the α-secretase enzyme resulting in the release of a large and soluble ectodomain fragment (α-APP) [39] in the extracellular space, while retaining a 83-residue C-terminal fragment (CTF) in the membrane. Alternatively, some APP molecules that were not cleaved by α-secretase may be processed by the activity of an enzyme named β-secretase, generating a β-APP ectodomain that retains one residue from the 99 CTF [6].

The main β-secretase in neurons is a transmembrane aspartyl protease named BACE1, predominantly located at the transgolgi network (TGN) and also in endosomes [40]. The cleavage mediated by BACE1 generates the N-terminal fragment of Aβ. The high level of neuronal BACE1 expression preferably targets APP to the amyloidogenic processing pathway in the brain [34]. Aβ is constitutively released from cells expressing APP in normal conditions. The cleavage generated by β-secretase is followed by a constitutive trim at the C-terminal of the Aβ region, and it is carried out by the activity of γ-secretase. Simultaneously, a peptide fragment designated as p3 is produced from the sequential activity of both α- and γ-secretases [6]. A substantial amount of α-APP is generated by γ-secretase that acts on the inserted APP in plasma membrane.

The Aβ40 and Aβ42 fragments are generated to a large extent during APP internalization and endosomal processing. Most of the Aβ generated within the cell is destined for secretion.

APP has autocrine and paracrine functions during growth regulation. It has been best characterized as trophic as it has been demonstrated that it stimulates neurite growth. This phenotype is compatible with its increased expression during neuron maturation [41, 42].

5. PSEN 1 and PSEN 2

Presenilins (PSEN) are an important part of the γ-secretase enzyme activity, and they are responsible for the proteolytic cleavage of APP. γ-secretase is a multimeric complex of PSEN1 or PSEN2, nicastrin, and APH1. All mutations in PSEN1 increase APP cleaving activity by γ-secretase, which generates the Aβ42 fragment. The PSEN1 gene is located in chromosome 14 and that of PSEN2 in chromosome 1, both of them are approximately 60% similar [43]. Regarding the gene's structure, it has been demonstrated that the first 4 exons contain untranslated regions, and exons 1 and 2 possess alternative transcription sites. The function of these sites is still unclear. The first ATG is located in exon 4, and its 12 bp is used as an alternative splicing donor site. Exon 9 is subjected to alternative splicing in leukocytes but not in other tissues. Most of the expressed transcripts are polyadenylated after the TAG stop codon in exon 13 [44]. A PSEN 2 variant has been shown to lack exon 5, which has been detected on individuals with sporadic Alzheimer's disease [45].

Several mutations on the PSEN genes are responsible for early familial Alzheimer's disease. The loss of exons 3 and 4 of PSEN demonstrates that transcripts are efficiently translated as truncated proteins at their N-terminal; however, this does not affect their function as amyloid fragment generators [46].

A PSEN2 variant that does not possess exon 5 has been reported to increase the generation of the Aβ40 y 42 fragments [47].

6. Conclusion

Currently, there is no cure for Alzheimer's disease and the research conducted nowadays in order to fully understand this condition is relevant. Nevertheless, its underlying causes have not yet been determined.

The mechanism of the disease is not fully understood, and the conducted studies have shown that proteins such as Tau, APP, and both presenilins are highly important for developing the disease.

Through artificial intelligence studies, it has been demonstrated that more than 70 genes are associated to these proteins [48], rendering this disease extremely complex.

Alternative splicing is key in order to generate the appropriate proteins that do not affect neuron functioning; thus, the individual may carry a healthy life.

Final note

We seek the most current literature on the subject, and the database used was the PubMed for the development of this chapter.

Author details

Gonzalo Emiliano Aranda Abreu[1*], Sonia Lilia Mestizo Gutiérrez[2], María Elena Hernández Aguilar[1] and Fausto Rojas Durán[1]

*Address all correspondence to: garanda@uv.mx

1 Veracruzana University, Brain Research Center, Veracruz, Mexico

2 Faculty of Chemical Sciences, Xalapa, Veracruz, Mexico

References

[1] Brookmeyer, R., Johnson, E., Ziegler-Graham, K., & Arrighi, H. M. (2007). Forecasting the global burden of Alzheimer's disease. *Alzheimers Dement*, *3*, 186–191. doi:10.1016/j.jalz.2007.04.381

[2] Herrera-Rivero, M., Hernández-Aguilar, M. E., Manzo, J., & Aranda-Abreu, G. E. (2010). [Alzheimer's disease: immunity and diagnosis]. *Rev Neurol*, *51*(3), 153–164. Retrieved from http://www.ncbi.nlm.nih.gov/entrez/query.fcgi?cmd=Retrieve&db=PubMed&dopt=Citation&list_uids=20645266

[3] Ray, S., Britschgi, M., Herbert, C., Takeda-Uchimura, Y., Boxer, A., Blennow, K.,… Wyss-Coray, T. (2007). Classification and prediction of clinical Alzheimer's diagnosis based on plasma signaling proteins. *Nat Med*, *13*(11), 1359–1362. doi:10.1038/nm1653

[4] Baquero, M., Peset, V., Burguera, J. A., Salazar-Cifre, A., Boscá-Blasco, M. E., del Olmo-Rodríguez, A. (2009). [Quality of life in Alzheimer's disease]. *Rev Neurol*, *49*(7), 337–342. Retrieved from http://www.ncbi.nlm.nih.gov/entrez/query.fcgi?cmd=Retrieve&db=PubMed&dopt=Citation&list_uids=19774526

[5] Swaminathan, A., & Jicha, G. A. (2014). Nutrition and prevention of Alzheimer's dementia. *Front Aging Neurosci*, *6*, 282. doi:10.3389/fnagi.2014.00282

[6] Selkoe, D. J. (2001). Alzheimer's disease: genes, proteins, and therapy. *Physiol Rev*, *81*(2), 741–766. Retrieved from http://www.ncbi.nlm.nih.gov/entrez/query.fcgi?cmd=Retrieve&db=PubMed&dopt=Citation&list_uids=11274343

[7] Dickson, D. W. (1997). The pathogenesis of senile plaques. *J Neuropathol Exp Neurol*, *56*(4), 321–339. Retrieved from http://www.ncbi.nlm.nih.gov/entrez/query.fcgi?cmd=Retrieve&db=PubMed&dopt=Citation&list_uids=9100663

[8] Serrano-Pozo, A., Frosch, M. P., Masliah, E., & Hyman, B. T. (2011). Neuropathological alterations in Alzheimer disease. *Cold Spring Harb Perspect Med*, *1*, a006189. doi:10.1101/cshperspect.a006189

[9] Jarrett, J. T., Berger, E. P., & Lansbury, P. T. (1993). The carboxy terminus of the beta amyloid protein is critical for the seeding of amyloid formation: implications for the pathogenesis of Alzheimer's disease. *Biochemistry*, *32*(18), 4693–4697. Retrieved from http://www.ncbi.nlm.nih.gov/entrez/query.fcgi?cmd=Retrieve&db=PubMed&dopt=Citation&list_uids=8490014

[10] Revett, T. J., Baker, G. B., Jhamandas, J., & Kar, S. (2013). Glutamate system, amyloid ß peptides and tau protein: functional interrelationships and relevance to Alzheimer disease pathology. *J Psychiatry Neurosci*, *38*(1), 6–23. doi:10.1503/jpn.110190

[11] Selkoe, D. J., & Schenk, D. (2003). Alzheimer's disease: molecular understanding predicts amyloid-based therapeutics. *Annu Rev Pharmacol Toxicol*, *43*, 545–584. doi:10.1146/annurev.pharmtox.43.100901.140248

[12] Matlin, A. J., Clark, F., & Smith, C. W. (2005). Understanding alternative splicing: towards a cellular code. *Nat Rev Mol Cell Biol*, *6*(5), 386–398. doi:10.1038/nrm1645

[13] Littauer, U. Z., Giveon, D., Thierauf, M., Ginzburg, I., & Ponstingl, H. (1986). Common and distinct tubulin binding sites for microtubule-associated proteins. *Proc Natl Acad Sci USA*, *83*(19), 7162–7166. Retrieved from http://www.ncbi.nlm.nih.gov/entrez/query.fcgi?cmd=Retrieve&db=PubMed&dopt=Citation&list_uids=3463956

[14] Aranda-Abreu, G. E., Behar, L., Chung, S., Furneaux, H., & Ginzburg, I. (1999). Embryonic lethal abnormal vision-like RNA-binding proteins regulate neurite outgrowth and tau expression in PC12 cells. *J Neurosci*, *19*(16), 6907–6917. Retrieved from http://www.ncbi.nlm.nih.gov/entrez/query.fcgi?cmd=Retrieve&db=PubMed&dopt=Citation&list_uids=10436048

[15] Aronov, S., Aranda, G., Behar, L., & Ginzburg, I. (2001). Axonal tau mRNA localization coincides with tau protein in living neuronal cells and depends on axonal targeting signal. *J Neurosci*, *21*(17), 6577–6587. Retrieved from http://www.ncbi.nlm.nih.gov/entrez/query.fcgi?cmd=Retrieve&db=PubMed&dopt=Citation&list_uids=11517247

[16] Aronov, S., Aranda, G., Behar, L., & Ginzburg, I. (2002). Visualization of translated tau protein in the axons of neuronal P19 cells and characterization of tau RNP granules. *J Cell Sci*, *115*(Pt 19), 3817–3827. Retrieved from http://www.ncbi.nlm.nih.gov/entrez/query.fcgi?cmd=Retrieve&db=PubMed&dopt=Citation&list_uids=12235292

[17] Aranda-Abreu, G. E., Hernández, M. E., Soto, A., & Manzo, J. (2005). Possible Cis-acting signal that could be involved in the localization of different mRNAs in neuronal axons. *Theor Biol Med Model*, *2*, 33. doi:10.1186/1742-4682-2-33

[18] Andreadis, A. (2006). Misregulation of tau alternative splicing in neurodegeneration and dementia. *Prog Mol Subcell Biol*, *44*, 89–107. Retrieved from http://www.ncbi.nlm.nih.gov/entrez/query.fcgi?cmd=Retrieve&db=PubMed&dopt=Citation&list_uids=17076266

[19] Himmler, A., Drechsel, D., Kirschner, M. W., & Martin, D. W. (1989). Tau consists of a set of proteins with repeated C-terminal microtubule-binding domains and variable N-terminal domains. *Mol Cell Biol*, *9*(4), 1381–1388. Retrieved from http://www.ncbi.nlm.nih.gov/entrez/query.fcgi?cmd=Retrieve&db=PubMed&dopt=Citation&list_uids=2498649

[20] Neve, R. L., Harris, P., Kosik, K. S., Kurnit, D. M., & Donlon, T. A. (1986). Identification of cDNA clones for the human microtubule-associated protein tau and chromosomal localization of the genes for tau and microtubule-associated protein 2. *Brain Res*, *387*(3), 271–280. Retrieved from http://www.ncbi.nlm.nih.gov/entrez/query.fcgi?cmd=Retrieve&db=PubMed&dopt=Citation&list_uids=3103857

[21] Heicklen-Klein, A., & Ginzburg, I. (2000). Tau promoter confers neuronal specificity and binds Sp1 and AP-2. *J Neurochem*, *75*(4), 1408–1418. Retrieved from http://

www.ncbi.nlm.nih.gov/entrez/query.fcgi?cmd=Retrieve&db=PubMed&dopt=Citation&list_uids=10987820

[22] Buée, L., Bussière, T., Buée-Scherrer, V., Delacourte, A., & Hof, P. R. (2000). Tau protein isoforms, phosphorylation and role in neurodegenerative disorders. *Brain Res Rev, 33*(1), 95–130. Retrieved from http://www.ncbi.nlm.nih.gov/entrez/query.fcgi?cmd=Retrieve&db=PubMed&dopt=Citation&list_uids=10967355

[23] Adams, S. J., DeTure, M. A., McBride, M., Dickson, D. W., & Petrucelli, L. (2010). Three repeat isoforms of tau inhibit assembly of four repeat tau filaments. *PLoS One, 5*, e10810. doi:10.1371/journal.pone.0010810

[24] Schellenberg, G. D., D'Souza, I., & Poorkaj, P. (2000). The genetics of Alzheimer's disease. *Curr Psychiatry Rep, 2*, 158–164. Retrieved from http://www.ncbi.nlm.nih.gov/entrez/query.fcgi?cmd=Retrieve&db=PubMed&dopt=Citation&list_uids=11122949

[25] Qian, W., & Liu, F. (2014). Regulation of alternative splicing of tau exon 10. *Neurosci Bull, 30*(2), 367–377. doi:10.1007/s12264-013-1411-2

[26] Lagunes, T., Herrera-Rivero, M., Hernández-Aguilar, M. E., & Aranda-Abreu, G. E. (2014). Abeta(1–42) induces abnormal alternative splicing of tau exons 2/3 in NGF-induced PC12 cells. *An Acad Bras Cienc, 86*(4), 1927–1934. doi: 10.1590/0001-3765201420130333

[27] Smith, C. J., Anderton, B. H., Davis, D. R., & Gallo, J. M. (1995). Tau isoform expression and phosphorylation state during differentiation of cultured neuronal cells. *FEBS Lett, 375*(3), 243–248. Retrieved from http://www.ncbi.nlm.nih.gov/entrez/query.fcgi?cmd=Retrieve&db=PubMed&dopt=Citation&list_uids=7498509

[28] Roth, W., Hecker, D., & Fava, E. (2016). Systems biology approaches to the study of biological networks underlying Alzheimer's disease: role of miRNAs. *Methods Mol Biol, 1303*, 349–377. doi:10.1007/978-1-4939-2627-5_21

[29] Lau, P., Bossers, K., Janky, R., Salta, E., Frigerio, C. S., Barbash, S., …De Strooper, B. (2013). Alteration of the microRNA network during the progression of Alzheimer's disease. *EMBO Mol Med, 5*(10), 1613–1634. doi:10.1002/emmm.201201974

[30] Smith, P. Y., Delay, C., Girard, J., Papon, M. A., Planel, E., Sergeant, N., …Hébert, S. S. (2011). MicroRNA-132 loss is associated with tau exon 10 inclusion in progressive supranuclear palsy. *Hum Mol Genet, 20*, 4016–4024. doi:10.1093/hmg/ddr330

[31] Wang, J., Gao, Q. S., Wang, Y., Lafyatis, R., Stamm, S., & Andreadis, A. (2004). Tau exon 10, whose missplicing causes frontotemporal dementia, is regulated by an intricate interplay of cis elements and trans factors. *J Neurochem, 88*(5), 1078–1090. Retrieved from http://www.ncbi.nlm.nih.gov/entrez/query.fcgi?cmd=Retrieve&db=PubMed&dopt=Citation&list_uids=15009664

[32] Li, K., Arikan, M. C., & Andreadis, A. (2003). Modulation of the membrane-binding domain of tau protein: splicing regulation of exon 2. *Mol Brain Res, 116*(1–2), 94–105.

Retrieved from http://www.ncbi.nlm.nih.gov/entrez/query.fcgi?cmd=Retrieve&db=PubMed&dopt=Citation&list_uids=12941465

[33] Yoshikai, S., Sasaki, H., Doh-ura, K., Furuya, H., & Sakaki, Y. (1990). Genomic organization of the human amyloid beta-protein precursor gene. *Gene, 87*(2), 257–263. Retrieved from http://www.ncbi.nlm.nih.gov/entrez/query.fcgi?cmd=Retrieve&db=PubMed&dopt=Citation&list_uids=2110105

[34] Thinakaran, G., & Koo, E. H. (2008). Amyloid precursor protein trafficking, processing, and function. *J Biol Chem, 283*(44), 29615–29619. doi:10.1074/jbc.R800019200

[35] Tanaka, S., Nakamura, S., Ueda, K., Kameyama, M., Shiojiri, S., Takahashi, Y., …Ito, H. (1988). Three types of amyloid protein precursor mRNA in human brain: their differential expression in Alzheimer's disease. *Biochem Biophys Res Commun, 157*(2), 472–479. Retrieved from http://www.ncbi.nlm.nih.gov/entrez/query.fcgi?cmd=Retrieve&db=PubMed&dopt=Citation&list_uids=3144271

[36] Hartmann, T., Bergsdorf, C., Sandbrink, R., Tienari, P. J., Multhaup, G., Ida, N., … Beyreuther, K. (1996). Alzheimer's disease betaA4 protein release and amyloid precursor protein sorting are regulated by alternative splicing. *J Biol Chem, 271*(22), 13208–13214. Retrieved from http://www.ncbi.nlm.nih.gov/entrez/query.fcgi?cmd=Retrieve&db=PubMed&dopt=Citation&list_uids=8662794

[37] Sandbrink, R., Masters, C. L., & Beyreuther, K. (1996). APP gene family. Alternative splicing generates functionally related isoforms. *Ann N Y Acad Sci, 777*, 281–287. Retrieved from http://www.ncbi.nlm.nih.gov/entrez/query.fcgi?cmd=Retrieve&db=PubMed&dopt=Citation&list_uids=8624099

[38] Yamazaki, T., Selkoe, D. J., & Koo, E. H. (1995). Trafficking of cell surface beta-amyloid precursor protein: retrograde and transcytotic transport in cultured neurons. *J Cell Biol, 129*(2), 431–442. Retrieved from http://www.ncbi.nlm.nih.gov/entrez/query.fcgi?cmd=Retrieve&db=PubMed&dopt=Citation&list_uids=7721945

[39] Sisodia, S. S. (1992). Beta-amyloid precursor protein cleavage by a membrane-bound protease. *Proc Natl Acad Sci USA, 89*(13), 6075–6079. Retrieved from http://www.ncbi.nlm.nih.gov/entrez/query.fcgi?cmd=Retrieve&db=PubMed&dopt=Citation&list_uids=1631093

[40] Vassar, R. (2004). BACE1: the beta-secretase enzyme in Alzheimer's disease. *J Mol Neurosci, 23*(1–2), 105–114. doi:10.1385/JMN:23:1–2:105

[41] Hung, A. Y., Koo, E. H., Haass, C., & Selkoe, D. J. (1992). Increased expression of beta-amyloid precursor protein during neuronal differentiation is not accompanied by secretory cleavage. *Proc Natl Acad Sci USA, 89*(20), 9439–9443. Retrieved from http://www.ncbi.nlm.nih.gov/entrez/query.fcgi?cmd=Retrieve&db=PubMed&dopt=Citation&list_uids=1409654

[42] Muresan, V., Varvel, N. H., Lamb, B. T., & Muresan, Z. (2009). The cleavage products of amyloid-beta precursor protein are sorted to distinct carrier vesicles that are

independently transported within neurites. *J Neurosci, 29*(11), 3565–3578. doi:10.1523/JNEUROSCI.2558-08.2009

[43] Barber, R. C. (2012). The genetics of Alzheimer's disease. *Scientifica (Cairo), 2012*, 246210. doi:10.6064/2012/246210

[44] Rogaev, E. I., Sherrington, R., Wu, C., Levesque, G., Liang, Y., Rogaeva, E. A., …St George-Hyslop, P. (1997). Analysis of the 5′ sequence, genomic structure, and alternative splicing of the presenilin-1 gene (PSEN1) associated with early onset Alzheimer disease. *Genomics, 40*(3), 415–424. doi:10.1006/geno.1996.4523

[45] Sato, N., Hori, O., Yamaguchi, A., Lambert, J. C., Chartier-Harlin, M. C., Robinson, P. A., …Takagi, T. (1999). A novel presenilin-2 splice variant in human Alzheimer's disease brain tissue. *J Neurochem, 72*(6), 2498–2505. Retrieved from http://www.ncbi.nlm.nih.gov/entrez/query.fcgi?cmd=Retrieve&db=PubMed&dopt=Citation&list_uids=10349860

[46] Grünberg, J., Walter, J., Eckman, C., Capell, A., Schindzielorz, A., Younkin, S., …Haass, C. (1998). Truncated presenilin 2 derived from differentially spliced mRNA does not affect the ratio of amyloid beta-peptide 1-42/1-40. *Neuroreport, 9*(14), 3293–3299. Retrieved from http://www.ncbi.nlm.nih.gov/entrez/query.fcgi?cmd=Retrieve&db=PubMed&dopt=Citation&list_uids=9831466

[47] Sato, N., Imaizumi, K., Manabe, T., Taniguchi, M., Hitomi, J., Katayama, T., …Tohyama, M. (2001). Increased production of beta-amyloid and vulnerability to endoplasmic reticulum stress by an aberrant spliced form of presenilin 2. *J Biol Chem, 276*(3), 2108–2114. doi:10.1074/jbc.M006886200

[48] Mestizo Gutiérrez, S. L., Herrera Rivero, M., Cruz Ramírez, N., Hernández, E., & Aranda-Abreu, G. E. (2014). Decision trees for the analysis of genes involved in Alzheimer's disease pathology. *J Theor Biol, 357*, 21–25. doi:10.1016/j.jtbi.2014.05.002

[49] Aranda-Abreu, G. E., Hernández, M. E., Fausto Rojas Durán, A., Mestizo Gutierrez, S. L., & Denes, J. M. (2016). Tau alternative splicing in Alzheimer's disease. In: E. Massey (Ed.), Alternative Splicing and Disease. NOVA Science Publisher. https://www.novapublishers.com/catalog/product_info.php?products_id=56697&osCsid=b172d9ebb2bfdf1ed18a4f1ef5ac71b6.

[50] Vanier, M. T., Neuville, P., Michalik, L., & Launay, J. F. (1998). Expression of specific tau exons in normal and tumoral pancreatic acinar cells. *J Cell Sci, 111*(Pt 10), 1419–1432. Retrieved from http://www.ncbi.nlm.nih.gov/entrez/query.fcgi?cmd=Retrieve&db=PubMed&dopt=Citation&list_uids=9570759

Chapter 2

Neuroinflammation and Neurodegeneration

Inelia Morales, Gonzalo A. Farías, Nicole Cortes and
Ricardo B. Maccioni

Additional information is available at the end of the chapter

http://dx.doi.org/10.5772/64545

Abstract

Pathophysiological processes of neurodegenerative diseases are not clearly defined. However, an important body of evidence points toward the role of various inflammatory processes. The microglial cell is the main representative of the immune system in the central nervous system (CNS). This cell type can sense foreign or harmful pathogens and trigger its own activation and the generation of neuroinflammatory processes through phagocytosis and the release of cytokines, in order to maintain the cellular microenvironment. However, after maintaining a permanent state of activation due to sustained stimulation over time, microglial cells may generate a focus of persistent inflammation that in some cases precedes or enhances the neurodegenerative process. Thus, neuroinflammatory microenvironment becomes toxic and harmful for the neuronal cell, which degenerates and releases various factors that in turn activate the inflammatory response of microglia, potentiating the neurodegenerative cycle. In this chapter, we discuss the evidence on the role of microglial cell activation in neurodegenerative conditions and the association between neuroinflammatory processes and age-related neurological diseases. Finally, we outline how this new approach can help us to find new ways to understand neurodegenerative processes and to orientate the search for new therapies.

Keywords: neuroinflammation, neurodegeneration, Alzheimer disease, Parkinson disease, amyotrophic lateral sclerosis, microglia, neuroimmunomodulation hypothesis, inflammatory response

1. Introduction

Neurodegeneration is a degenerative process that occurs in the central nervous system (CNS), in which an injury or deleterious condition detonates progressive neuronal death, leading to the loss of cognitive and motor functions associated with the CNS. The causes that trigger this neuronal death are still unknown, but clinical evidence demonstrates that age is an important risk factor and that the number of people suffering from dementia and other neurodegenerative conditions will increase as a consequence of increased life expectancies [1]. The main diseases that are defined by neurodegenerative processes are: AD and PD, but this term also includes other conditions such as amyotrophic lateral sclerosis (ALS), multiple sclerosis and products of viral infections. These diseases have an impact not only on the individual suffering from the disease but also on their families, causing social isolation, family misunderstanding, and loss of friendships and social ties [2]. This is an important issue and should be further considered, especially because it is currently estimated that 94% of people living with dementia are cared for at home, generating an important amount of distress and economic burden on their closest relatives. This is particularly true for many low- and middle-income countries, where in many cases patients and caregivers have access only to limited support from the state and health providers.

According to epidemiological data from the "World Alzheimer Report 2015" [3], there are more than 46 million people with dementia worldwide, and it is estimated that this number will increase to 131.5 million by 2050. Moreover, it is also important to consider that this type of disease carries a huge economic impact. Currently, only AD monetarily translates in US $818 million per year globally and is estimated to be billions of dollars by 2018 [3]. This amount will certainly rise significantly if we consider other neurodegenerative diseases mentioned above. The reasons that trigger neurodegenerative processes in these diseases remain unclear, especially considering the many variables that are involved in their development. One of these variables, inflammation, became more relevant in recent years. One example is the evidence that exists today on neurodegeneration induced by viral infections [1, 4], as it involves the interaction of the CNS, environmental factors, and immune response. In parallel there are also studies that link the rising number of mild proinflammatory conditions described with major degenerative diseases of the elderly [5]. Thus, the major pathologies, associated with aging and increased physical frailty, are also associated with changes in body composition, energy imbalance, homeostatic dysregulation, and neurodegeneration. Chronic inflammation is strongly connected to each of these aging phenotypes [6].

The inflammatory response is triggered to fight and control an injury, infection or other stimulus and may involve many cell types. The impact of the response is dependent on the numerous factors secreted by these cells, and they have the ability to self-regulate their response in order to repair tissue damage and to eliminate pathogenic elements. But when the response is prolonged in time, it causes a chronic inflammatory environment that leads to progressive tissue damage [6]. One of the evidences that support the relation between inflammation and increasing age is given by the increase in inflammatory mediators IL-6 and IL-8 and the rise in C-reactive protein in men and women with age, and the fact that these values also increase in obesity and neurodegenerative diseases [7].

In this chapter, we present a complete summary of the neuroinflammatory process and we explain how it relates to the development of features of neurodegeneration and neuronal death as in dementia neuropathology. We describe the neuroinflammatory processes considering microglial cell as the main cell type involved in the development of the immune response in the CNS. Finally, we link the development of the immune response to long-term development of three of the most characteristic diseases related to neurodegenerative diseases: AD, PD and ALS.

2. Methodology

We performed a detailed assessment of current evidence about main and nascent topics in the area of "Neuroinflammation and Neurodegeneration." Additionally, we focused our search in the three prototypic neurodegenerative diseases, considering classical concepts on neuropathology and incorporating new evidence on the role of neuroinflammatory process.

The focus of this review is to show evidence on common pathological role of neuroinflammatory process and microglial cells in neurodegenerative diseases, proposing a new approach for research of these diseases, in order to give support for the development of innovative therapies.

We performed a systematic search in the main database of National Center for Biotechnology Information Database (PubMed). Key words were: *inflammatory response, neuroinflammation, neurodegeneration, neurodegenerative diseases, neuronal death, microglial cells, microgliosis, Parkinson disease, Alzheimer disease and Amyotrophic Lateral Sclerosis.*

3. Neuroinflammatory processes

Neuroinflammation is defined as the reactive response of CNS against elements that interfere with homeostasis, inside or outside the CNS, and this response is involved in all neurological diseases, including developmental, traumatic, ischemic, metabolic, infectious, toxic, neoplastic, and neurodegenerative diseases. Emerging evidence suggests that inflammation has a causal role in disease pathogenesis, and understanding and controlling interactions between the immune system and the nervous system might be key for the prevention or delay of most late onset CNS diseases.

The wide variety of cellular and molecular mechanisms of neuroinflammation, probably the same in aging and chronic metabolic diseases such as hypertension, diabetes, depression, dementia or traumatic brain injury, are currently considered as silent contributors to neuroinflammation [1]. In addition to these chronic diseases, another major risk factor that causes tissue destruction in CNS is stroke and atherosclerosis. This disease of brain arteries is characterized by vascular inflammation caused by monocyte infiltration in the injured vessel wall and increased interleukin (IL)-6 triggering significant damage in the area of the lesion [8]. Considering the current poor quality of life in many cities and unhealthy eating habits, we must know that this can lead to a number of disorders and diseases such as cardiovascular disease, stroke, hypertension, insulin resistance, and metabolic syndrome. Thus, lipid hormones, cytokines, and adipokines play an important role in inflammatory metabolic diseases through induction of adverse regulatory responses [1]. In other way, the chronic activation of proinflammatory signals in aging CNS may contribute to an increased vulnerability to neuropsychiatric disorders [9]. For example, the group of Dr. Ouchi linked obesity and inflammation, and they demonstrated that the inflammatory state was associated with a higher concentration of proinflammatory markers including IL-6, CRP, and adipokines [10]. All these proinflammatory markers are correlated positively with symptoms of depression and anxiety, and in agreement with those findings, metabolic diseases such as obesity, hypertension, and even senescence are prevalent risk factors for depression, cognitive dysfunction, and dementia [1] favoring the neurodegenerative process. On the other hand, the mechanism linking inflammation and depression involves oxidative stress and elevated levels of proinflammatory cytokines IL-6 and IL-8 among other factors. For example, major depressive disorder, a serious psychiatric illness, is associated with increased levels of peripheral inflammatory markers and to mortality due to depression and suicide [11, 12]. Therefore, inflammatory markers, identified in neurodegenerative diseases including psychiatric disorders, are related to increased processes of neuronal death.

It is important to consider that some biological mechanisms involved in neuroinflammatory processes, such as the participation of complement cascade and microglial cells in responses of pruning synapses, also occur in healthy brain development [13].

On the other hand, the inflammatory response in the CNS is also linked to various processes such as aging, systemic infection, metabolic syndrome, and intrinsic CNS disease. Activation of the immune system in the CNS may compromise the generation of neurotrophic factors and the secretion of cytotoxic factors from the microglial cell. In line with the hypothesis that proinflammatory molecules such as the IL-1β family of cytokines and factors that simulate Toll-like receptors (TLRs) can impair the clearance function of microglia, there are some findings showing that disrupting IRAK4, an essential kinase downstream of TLRs and receptors for IL-1β cytokines, shifts microglial cells from a proinflammatory phenotype toward an anti-inflammatory phenotype [14].

The main agent involved in neuroinflammation is the microglial cell, but other factors that are also present in the inflammatory response should be considered. In animal models of AD, it has been demonstrated in areas associated with amyloid plaques, infiltration of mononuclear cells into the CNS as part of an innate immune response, but the role and the participation of these cells is not very clear yet [15]. Evidence from a mouse model of AD showed that peripheral mononuclear phagocytes have an important role to reduce the buildup of amyloid-beta plaques, which improve local inflammatory response [16].

The astroglial cells are also involved in the inflammatory response. Astrocytes respond to all forms of CNS insults through a process referred to as reactive astrogliosis. This response is a complex, multistage and pathology-specific reaction. On the other hand, the response of astrocytes is generally aimed for neuroprotection and recovery of injured neural tissue [17]. Emerging evidence of sustained inflammatory response in the CNS supports the major contribution of microglia and astrocytes in the progression of a wide variety of diseases, suggesting an important role as effectors of neuroinflammation in neuronal dysfunction and death. Other cell types including neurons, astrocytes, endothelial cells, etc., also express

http://dx.doi.org/10.5772/64545

receptors for cytokines and other inflammatory mediators and can be activated by these signals and participate in the coordinated inflammatory response in the brain.

3.1. Microglia and neuroinflammation

Microglia is widely distributed throughout the brain and spinal cord but mainly in the hippocampus and the substantia nigra [18]. These cells are approximately 5–20% of the total population of glial cells in the CNS and are considered the representatives of the immune system in the central nervous system, since they have the ability to perform phagocytosis, release cytotoxic factors, and behave as antigen presenting cells [19, 20]. These cells are derived from macrophages produced by hematopoiesis in the primitive yolk sac [21], and they migrate to the developing neural tube, where they give rise to microglia [22].

This cellular type represents the major cellular component of the innate immune system of the brain. In normal conditions, microglia protects the brain environment by initiating a quick response to changes and effectively modulates inflammation.

Numerous signs that threaten homeostasis of the CNS, such as structures and/or residues from bacteria, viruses, and fungi; abnormal endogenous proteins; complement factors; antibodies; cytokines and chemokines, among others, are sensed by the microglia and consequently induce their activation [18]. Thus, there are two major functional aspects of the microglial cell: immune defense and maintenance of the CNS. Microglial cells function as immune cells acting as sentinels, detecting the first signs of invasion of pathogens or tissue damage. Furthermore, under inflammatory conditions produced by an active immune response, the microglia should moderate potential damage to the tissues that support, help to repair, and remodel CNS [22].

Microglial cells mediate immune and inflammatory responses in the CNS. These cells become functionally polarized to execute specific effector programs and thus, express specific functional reaction programs in response to diverse microenvironmental signals. Microglia have two functional states of polarization: one of them is phenotypically polarized to develop a classical proinflammatory or an alternative phenotype is anti-inflammatory and prohealing [23]. Thus, diverse pro- and anti-inflammatory cytokines, and others stimulus, can polarize microglia toward distinct functional phenotypes.

Microglial cells are characterized by the expression of distinct cell surface receptors and also by the release of numerous soluble factors. Activated cells with inflammatory phenotype are characterized by upregulation of CD16 Fc receptors, CD32, CD64, CD86, IL-1β, IL-6, IL-12, IL-23, tumor necrosis factor (TNF)-α, inducible nitric oxide synthase (iNOS), and chemokine, whereas microglial cells with anti-inflammatory phenotype display the upregulation of arginase (Arg)-1, mannose receptor (CD206), insulin-like growth factor (IGF)-1, triggering receptor expressed on myeloid cells 2 (TREM2), chitinase 3-like 3 (Ym-1), among others [23]. All these factors contribute to microglia activation that leads to further production of cytokines and other inflammatory mediators, which may contribute to the apoptotic cell death of neurons in multiple neurodegenerative diseases.

For these characteristics, microglia is considered the resident immune cells in the brain that are sensitive to even minor disturbances in homeostasis of the central nervous system (CNS) and become readily activated during most neuropathological conditions, including PD and AD [24].

But, which are the determinants that define whether the inflammatory response from microglial cells will result in a protective or neurodegenerative effect?

An important consideration, among other things, is the timing of the disease in which microglial activity begins. For example, in the case of AD, an increase in microglial activation at early stages has been observed [25]. This could be an indication that the microglia initially tries to eliminate harmful elements involved in disease such as amyloid-beta plaques. Thus, to assess whether microglial response is harmful or has a protective effect, we must distinguish between chronic and acute stimulation. An acute injury can cause oxidative and nitrosative stress, but it is usually short lived and unlikely to be detrimental to long-term neuronal survival. Therefore, it is believed that acute neuroinflammatory response is usually beneficial to the CNS, tends to minimize damage, and helps to repair damaged tissue. Moreover, microglial cells are capable of removing glutamate, a well-known neurotoxic substance that acts at NMDA receptors from neurons and can lead to neuronal death. In the case of AD, importance of glutamate and associated microglial function has been evidenced by the therapeutic effect of the drug memantine (an antagonist of NMDA receptors) that improves cognitive ability and everyday life functions in AD patients [26].

Oppositely, chronic microglia stimulation would trigger a chronic neuroinflammatory response, which is almost always harmful and damaging to nerve tissue. Thus, if neuroinflammation has beneficial or deleterious results in the brain, it depends primarily on the length of the inflammatory response given by the microglial cell. For example, in the initial phases of AD, the progressive deposition of amyloid-beta plaques could provide chronic stimulation for microglial cells [27]. The release of pathogenic tau protein (hyperphosphorylated and self-aggregated) from dying neurons would also cause a constant activation of microglia [28]. As for the relationship of the proinflammatory cytokine IL-1 and the anti-inflammatory cytokine IL-10, levels of IL-1 raises drastically in the serum of AD patients, giving these patients a defined proinflammatory long-term profile, indicating a chronic CNS neuroinflammatory state [29]. In addition, the loss of neurons that characterizes AD further contributes to the generation of waste that is liberated from degenerating neurons and maintains microglia indefinitely in a state of long-term activation. These data indicate that, in AD, inflammation may be more chronic and therefore contribute to disease progression [27].

It is important to consider that microglia can be stimulated with environmental toxins, or with endogenous proteins too, and in this way, the cell can enter an overactivated state and release reactive oxygen species (ROS) and also reactive nitrogen species (RNS), which cause environmental toxicity for surrounding neurons [30]. This information is of great interest because overactivated microglia can be detected using imaging techniques, and therefore this knowledge offers an opportunity for an early diagnosis, and eventually in the future, this could be a target for the development of targeted anti-inflammatory therapies that lead to diminish the progression of a disease or may support existing therapies.

Thus, chronic inflammation is characterized by the long-standing activation of microglia, produced by chronic stimuli, trauma, and even pathological aggregates of neuronal proteins such as tau and beta-amyloid. These stimuli induce sustained release of inflammatory mediators, leading to an increase in oxidative and nitrosative stress, which perpetuates the inflammatory cycle, causing a permanent and detrimental inflammatory state.

3.2. Astrocytes and neuroinflammation

These type of cells are the most abundant and heterogeneous type of glial cells in the CNS. Their morphology can change depending on their developmental stage, subtype, and localization [31]. For example, astrocytes of the gray matter are the protoplasmic ones; they exhibit short branches, whereas the fibrous astrocytes, present in the white matter, exhibit long unbranched processes [32].

The astrocytes are supportive for neuronal cell components in neural tissue and, as well as microglia, also respond to all forms of insults to the CNS through a process known as reactive astrogliosis, and this process is a reliable and sensitive marker of diseased tissue. These cells, which are responsible for a wide variety of complex and essential functions in healthy CNS, for example, are involved in primary roles in synaptic transmission and information processing by neural circuits [17], and they can contribute to synaptogenesis and dynamically modulate information processing and signal transmission, regulate neural and synaptic plasticity, and provide trophic and metabolic support for neurons [33, 34].

In effect, astrocytes are involved in very important processes such as controlling the environment by regulating pH, ion homeostasis, blood flow, and modulating oxidative stress [31], and they are also responsible for a massive number of homeostatic tasks in the CNS [35]. With all these capacities, astrocytes, together with microglia, act as the main effectors of the neuroinflammatory response. After suffering an injury, or detecting a damage signal, astrocytes rapidly act in response to pathology and undergo important changes in their morphology and functioning [17], as occurs with microglial cells. Thus the objective of the response is to control and to remove the brain insult, but this response may also have deleterious consequences. In fact, reactive gliosis is a self-perpetuating process, which, at the end, exacerbates the injury and, on the other hand, represents a nonphysiologic state in which astrocytes lose their helpful properties [31].

The mechanisms leading to the activation of these cells are actually unclear, and many factors that are involved in neurodegenerative diseases can trigger the response of these cells. In AD, for example, it has been demonstrated that the presence of amyloid activates astrocytes. As microglial cells, astrocytes also can phagocytose and degrade amyloid-beta, and to bring this capacity, astrocytes and microglia are activated through TLRs and RAGE receptors, thus causing local inflammation [36]. When the response of astrocytes is activated, they change their morphology and increase significantly the expression of the glial fibrillary acidic protein (GFAP), a recognized marker of astrocyte reactivity [37]. All these changes cause a disturbance of normal activities in astrocytes, which are essential for normal neuronal function.

Activation of astrocytes, internally, involves the activation of transcription factor NF-κB, which controls secretions of chemokine and adhesion molecules, and thus favors peripheral lymphocyte infiltration and increases inflammatory response, which leads to neurodegeneration [36]. It has been shown that blockage of NF-κB transcriptional activity in astrocytes can extensively reduce inflammation, thus suggesting that inhibition of NF-κB in astrocytes may be regarded as a potential therapy for diseases such as AD [38].

With this background, it is possible to say that activated astrocytes are able to cause neurodegeneration; moreover, when activated astrocytes express inflammation-associated factors, such as the peptide S100β, they represent a key factor for neuroinflammation. S100β is exclusively produced by astrocytes and, under physiological conditions, it is a neurotrophin responsible for survival, development, and function of neurons [39]. In neurodegenerative diseases such as AD and PD, among others, and also in subjects with severe brain trauma, the peptide S100β is overexpressed, and its levels correlate with the progression of the pathology [36, 40].

Another evidence linking astroglial activation with the development of neurodegenerative processes is proton resonance spectroscopy. Through this technique consistent evidence of significant increase of myoinositol (characteristic marker of astroglial cells) in neurodegenerative diseases has been obtained. This has been observed both in brains of patients with mild cognitive impairment (MCI) and AD patients, and according to some studies, it has been reported to correlate with progression of pathology [36, 41, 42].

4. Neuroinflammation in Alzheimer disease

AD is a neurodegenerative disease that affects more than 20 million people worldwide and is characterized by a progressive deterioration of cognitive functions, particularly memory [43].

Currently, it is the most common cause of dementia in older adults and accounts for 50–60% of cases [44]. This disease usually begins after 65 years of age with a gradual increase in oblivion accompanied with other cognitive impairments, such as problems with calculations, visuospatial orientation, and language [45, 46]. This disease is defined as a multifactorial disorder in which genetic and environmental factors combine, but that is mostly of sporadic origin; It is estimated that only 2–10% of cases are hereditary [47, 48]. However, experts agree that the development of AD would be the result of multiple converging factors in the same case with multiple pathophysiological mechanisms explaining the cognitive impairment that causes this disease.

AD is a neurodegenerative disorder, characterized by the formation of two types of protein aggregates in the brain: senile plaques and neurofibrillary tangles (NFTs) consisting of amyloid-beta and altered tau, respectively [49]. At present, it is also considered that astroglial and microglial activation is characteristic of the disease, which in interaction with abnormal protein aggregates ultimately leads to dysfunction and neuronal death [50]. Histological evidence suggests that NFTs formed by self-aggregation of hyperphosphorylated tau protein forming paired helical filaments (PHFs) are pathognomonic for the disease; the pathology of tau is directly correlated to clinical deterioration [48, 49]. There are numerous and diverse factors such as head injuries, high fat intake, B vitamin deficiency, recurrent infections, alterations in cholesterol homeostasis, obesity and poor eating habits, among others that are able to increase the risk of developing the disorder [1, 51–55]. However, none of these risk factors seems to act as the real cause of the disease, although all are involved in its development [56].

Furthermore, and looking for a common event in the existing hypotheses, neuroinflammation in the CNS appears as a key event in the pathophysiology of AD. Based on this, promising targets for AD treatment have emerged by regulating neuroinflammation and cross-talk mechanisms between microglia and neurons [57–59].

In this context, it becomes interesting to identify the levels of neuroinflammation and microglial activation, leading to the permanent release of cytokines, which have neurotoxic effects and are involved in the progression of this pathophysiological process [60].

In the case of AD, there is evidence to correlate high expression of inflammatory mediators in the vicinity of deposits of amyloid-beta peptide and neurofibrillary tangles, which in turn are associated with the development of neurodegeneration, exemplifying the relationship between neuroinflammation, neurodegeneration, and cell types involved [58].

As explained above, neuroinflammation is a key event in the development of AD, as it involves the different triggers of the disease. Based on this, it has been suggested that the use of anti-inflammatory drugs could be beneficial and could delay the onset or progression of AD. To continue, we must at least mention the role of the cyclooxygenase (COX) enzyme. COX is an enzyme that exhibits two catalytic activities: an activity of bis-oxygenase (catalyzes the formation of prostaglandins G_2 (PG) from arachidonic acid) and its second peroxidase activity (reduced PG G_2 to PG H_2) [61]. COX in its peroxidase activity also produces free radicals, which are partly used for the same enzyme [61]. With this information, the possible mechanism of NSAIDs in neurodegenerative diseases such as AD would be based on their inhibitory effect on brain COX. COX-1 and COX-2 enzymes are expressed in the CNS, but COX-2 plays a unique role in the brain compared to the periphery: COX-2 is expressed constitutively only in the brain, while elsewhere expression is activation dependent [27]. Although expression of this enzyme is related primarily to neurons, authors have already shown expression in astrocytes and microglia [62]. It has also been demonstrated that COX-inhibiting NSAIDs reduce microglial activation and, on the other hand, neuronal stress processes, such as ischemia and excitotoxicity, are associated with strong upregulation of neuronal COX-2 expression. This suggests that COX-2 is involved in neurotoxic mechanisms and could be an effective target for treatment [27].

NSAIDs have another non-COX-dependent mechanism that can decrease the inflammatory response through direct activation of the peroxisome proliferator-activated receptor gamma (PPARγ), a nuclear transcription factor, which acts to suppress the expression of a broad range of proinflammatory genes [63], even in the microglial cell. NSAIDs act as PPARγ agonists and bind to it directly giving a start to its transcriptional activity, thus inhibiting the expression of proinflammatory cytokines such as IL-6 and TNF-α secreted by microglia and astrocytes, avoiding proinflammatory activity of these cells [27, 64].

In clinical studies, comparative analyzes were performed in the brains of cognitively normal patients chronically using NSAIDs over age versus those not using NSAIDs that revealed no changes in the appearance of senile plaques, but there was a threefold decrease in the number of activated microglia in the brains of chronic users of NSAIDs [65]. AD patients who used NSAIDs compared with another group of patients who did not use NSAIDs showed a significantly slower progression of disease [66]. These findings are correlated with the above and suggest that the protection provided by the chronic use of NSAIDs in AD patients may be derived at least partially from the attenuation of microglial activation [58].

Despite all these favorable results, we cannot overlook the fact that clinical trials of NSAIDs for patients with cognitive impairment and AD did not show clear results, and the observed effects vary depending on the cognitive instrument that is used. For example, the results indicate that the NSAID naproxen reduced cognitive decline in some patients but caused acceleration in cognitive decline in other patients. Conversely, celecoxib (another NSAID) appears to have similar, but attenuated effects in AD patients [67]. Therefore, it is still premature to make clinical recommendations, despite the positive results. However, positive findings open new avenues of research with significant clinical potential in order to develop an effective treatment for AD and other diseases with neuroinflammatory components.

On the other hand, as a result of the lack of efficacy of current treatments for AD, and based on the positive results obtained in patients taking anti-inflammatory drugs, a new possibility has opened up the study of the association of inflammatory processes and pathophysiology of AD.

A new form of prevention against the neuroinflammatory process, and thus also an interesting way to prevent neurodegenerative brain damage, is based on changes in diet and the consumption of nutritional supplements, functional foods, and nutraceuticals.

An interesting example of such food supplements is a new naturally occurring compound with high concentrations of antioxidants and anti-inflammatory properties called Andean Compound (initially called as Shilajit Andino). The Andean Compound is a very complex mixture of humic substances, generated by the decomposition of ancient plant material; it is originated as an endemic natural product of the Andes Mountains. Its main active principle is fulvic acid [68]. According to studies by Cornejo et al., fulvic acid is able to block tau self-aggregation affecting the length and morphology of PHFs generated *in vitro*, projecting as a good support for the treatment of AD. Also, after exposure of preformed tau fibrils to fulvic acid, a decrease in the length of PHFs can be detected [69]. So, this compound emerge as a novel nutraceutical with potential uses against neurodegenerative brain disorders [69].

The formation of tangles has been identified as a key and convergent event among many of the factors involved in the neurodegenerative process. Our multidisciplinary research group is currently working on a new nutraceutical containing Andean Compound plus B vitamins (B6, B9, and B12 vitamins) named Brain-Up 10®. Patients who have participated in a pilot clinical trial showed a trend toward lower cognitive impairment, a reduction in neuropsychological symptoms, and less distress for the caregiver. The appearance of new compounds that can open the way to new treatments becomes a necessity. In this search, compounds such as Andean Compound, which, because of their natural origin and the lack of adverse effects, appears as a promising therapy against neurodegenerative diseases, can give strong evidence that their effects are mediated by disruption of the inflammatory response and self-aggregation of the tau protein [58].

5. ALS: neuroinflammation and neurodegeneration

ALS is another neurodegenerative disease whose hallmark is a combination of degeneration of upper motor neurons in the brain stem and motor cortex and lower motor neuron death from spinal cord. This causes progressive muscle atrophy and paralysis, leading to death of the patient 3–5 years after the diagnosis. Although there are some variations, it is considered a late-onset disease, because visible symptoms appear around 55–60 years, including weakness in hands or legs, speech difficulties, and dysphagia [70]. The global incidence of ALS is 2–3 per 100,000 people, affecting more men than women [71]. The primary mechanism of disease still remains unknown, although there is evidence of calcium deregulation, mitochondrial damage, RNA alterations, protein misfolding and aggregation, ROS imbalance, and inflammation, among others [72, 73].

There are two subtypes of ALS: sporadic (sALS) that represents between 90 and 95% of total cases and familial ALS (fALS) that represents the remaining percentage (10–5%). It has been reported that fALS can be triggered by mutations in more than 24 different genes, associated with very diverse cellular functions. Superoxide dismutase 1 (SOD1) has been the most characterized gene, accounting for ~20% of total of fALS cases with more than 150 different mutations associated with the disease [74, 75]. Transactive response DNA binding protein 43 (TDP-43) is another remarkable gene in the disease, affecting both fALS and sALS [76, 77]. This protein is also linked with the development of frontotemporal dementia (FTD), both diseases sharing the deposition of TDP-43. This protein was identified as a major component of the ubiquitinated neuronal cytoplasmic inclusions deposited in cortical neurons in FTD and in upper and lower motor neurons in ALS, coinciding with an overlap in clinical development of FTD with ALS. This kind of overlapping syndrome may be expected since both diseases affect neurons in frontal cortex [78, 79]. In recent years, there are many reports of hexanucleotide repeat expansions in the chromosome 9 open reading frame 72 gene (C9ORF72) that has also been associated with FTD and ALS, being present in around 30% of familial cases [80].

Recent evidence suggests that motor neuron degeneration in ALS is not an autonomous process; instead it includes astrocyte and microglia participation as discussed below. The observation that nonneuronal cells contribute to neuron death in transgenic model of mice carrying $SOD1^{G37R}$ mutation, was broadly supported by different groups that saw the same effect on *in vitro* studies observing that astrocytes from human ALS patients and transgenic $SOD1^{MUT}$ mice induce motor neuron death [81–84]. In addition to astrocytes, an active contribution of microglia expressing $SOD1^{MUT}$ was evidenced in motor neuron degeneration

[85] and recently was demonstrated that microglia rather than astrocytes induce neuronal death through NF-κB, major regulator of inflammation in $SOD1^{G93A}$ mouse model [86].

5.1. Inflammation and neuroimmunomodulation: microglial signs

A lot of evidence, from animal models as well as patients from familial and sporadic cases, has been observed related to microglia involvement in ALS pathogenesis. In the last time, the microglia role in ALS went from being considered as a consequence of the pathogenic process to being considered as a key factor in the progress of disease, existing two different stages associated to opposite functions of microglia: first in a protective mode in early stages of disease and a later stage with neurotoxic participation [87]. In lumbar spinal cord from 11 weeks old (disease onset) $SOD1^{G93A}$ mice, microglial cells show an M2 phenotype and improve motor neuron survival, while microglia from end stage $SOD1^{G93A}$ mice display an M1 phenotype producing motor neuron death [88, 89]. Anti-inflammatory profile in ALS is documented by release of cytokines such as interleukin 4 (IL-4) and neurotrophic factors such as insulin-like growth factor 1 (IGF-1) and significantly increased expression in microglia from spinal cord of presymptomatic $SOD1^{G93A}$ mice [90]. Recently, through a technique that allows the *in vivo* following of activated microglia in $SOD1^{G93A}$ and $SOD1^{G37R}$ ALS mice, the overexpression of IL-10, an important regulator that would control the anti-inflammatory profile in the pre-symptomatic stage of disease, was demonstrated [91]. On the other hand, proinflammatory phenotype in ALS is evidenced by the increased expression of interleukin-1 beta (IL-1β) and tumor necrosis factor α (TNF-α) in spinal cord of $SOD1^{G93A}$ of advanced stages of disease [92–94]. Another consequence of neuroinflammatory process is ROS release and, in microglia from spinal cord of $SOD1^{G93A}$ mice, is that genes of enzymes that regulate the nitric oxide production, Arg1 and iNOS, are upregulated [95] contributing with more evidence to support the neuro-inflammatory theory for ALS pathogenesis. Moreover, astrocytes from ALS murine models including $SOD1^{G37R}$ and $SOD1^{G93A}$ have shown an increase in the expression of proinflamma-tory genes too, as diverse interleukins (IL-1β; IL-18), prostaglandin E_2, interferon gamma (interferon-γ), and TNF-α, among others, which could also potentiate the activation of microglia, participating in a vicious circle [96–98].

Meanwhile, in ALS patients, microgliosis also has been seen in the ventral horn of spinal cord, together with T cells near to corticospinal tract, in CSF, and in other regions of central nervous system at autopsy [99]. In addition to that, through a new technology used in other neurode-generative diseases, such as AD or Huntington disease, which utilizes a specific ligand for positron emission tomography (PET) that detects only activated microglia, *in vivo* microgliosis was observed in diverse areas of the brain such as motor and dorsolateral prefrontal cortex and thalamus, in a heterogeneous population of ALS patients, existing a correlation between the intensity of microgliosis and disease progression [100–102].

In AD, it has been demonstrated that after neuronal death, aggregated tau can induce micro-glial activation and generate a neuroinflammatory cascade resulting in the expression of damage signals [28], surging the possibility that in ALS, SOD1 and TDP43 aggregates (hall-mark of disease) could have a similar effect on inflammatory process. However, recent evidence shows that, in fact, inflammatory process through LPS and TNF-α stimulation induces the formation of TDP43 aggregates and its mislocalization in a motor neuron cellular model and primary culture of microglia and astrocytes from hTDP43^{A315T} transgenic model, as in spinal cord from the same mice [103], presenting new data to this possible vicious cycle between neuroinflammation and aggregates in the disease.

5.2. Other microglial evidence

Other possible link between microglia, neuroinflammation and ALS corresponds to hemichannels. The communication between glial cells mainly occurs through gap junctions (GJ) [104]. These are intercellular channels that connect the cytoplasmic compartment of neighboring cells, allowing the pass of ions and small molecules up to 1000 Da [105, 106]. Every GJ is composed of two hemichannels, and each hemichannel is formed by six subunit proteins called connexins [107, 108]. In general, hemichannels are closed in physiologic states; however under pathologic conditions, they present a higher activity and opening, which could be triggered by metabolic inhibition, inflammatory mediators, or connexin mutations [109, 110]. In addition to that, it has been proposed that in pathologic environments, activated microglia is capable of releasing proinflammatory molecules that increment the opening of hemichannels, reducing the communication between astrocytes; depriving neurons of protective role of glia and reduce the neuronal viability [109]. Otherwise, different inflammatory treatments such as TNF-α and interferon-γ enhance connexin-43 (Cx43) expression in activated microglia, establishing a possible mechanism of activation after inflammatory stimulus in ALS [104].

In AD, it has been observed that exposition of amyloid-beta peptide increases the activity of hemichannels in astrocytes, microglia, and neurons and that hemichannel blockers prevent death of hippocampal neurons [111, 112]. It was also demonstrated that a hemichannel blocker, capable of crossing the blood-brain barrier, INI-0602, alleviates AD symptoms in a transgenic model of disease [112].

In ALS, although there are few antecedents about hemichannels and the disease, the same publication shows that SOD1^{G93A} transgenic mice treated with the INI-0602 blocker incremented the life span in comparison to the nontreated group, preventing axonal lost and diminishing the atrophy and improving muscular size [112].

6. Neuroinflammation in Parkinson disease

PD is the second most prevalent neurodegenerative disease after AD. These diseases are prototypic examples of the clinical manifestations of pathological brain aging and are characterized by cognitive deterioration—the first—and movement disorder—the latter. About 3% of the population over 65 years old will develop PD and these patients will be affected by a combination of movement disorders -i.e. parkinsonian sindrome- cognitive and neuropsychiatric symptoms, and autonomic function impairment [113]. Neuropathological studies on AD, ALS and PD brains have demonstrated the presence of protein aggregates that have been considered as a central part of neurodegenerative process.

In PD there is a specific damage to neurons in substantia nigra pars compacta in midbrain. Degeneration of nigrostriatal connections is responsible for motor, cognitive, and psychiatric symptoms.

There is a complex interaction between genetic susceptibility and external factors that determines damage to dopaminergic neurons of the substantia nigra that is responsible for PD development.

Increased permeability of blood-brain barrier and neurovascular dysfunction has been linked to the risk of PD as has been suggested by positron emission tomography (PET) and neuropathology studies. This may be related to increased leakage of systemic inflammatory molecules into the midbrain, activation of microglia, and death of dopaminergic neurons [114]. The role of systemic inflammatory response in PD is supported by increased activation of peripheral lymphocytes and increased levels of serum cytokines—that is, TNF-α, IL-2, IL-6, and regulated on activation, normal T cell expressed and secreted (RANTES) protein in PD patients [114].

A role of adaptive immune response is also supported by increase of MHC II in ventral midbrain astrocytes and microglia as an inflammatory response to MPTP in a murine PD model [115]. On the other hand, MHC II null mice showed less MPTP-induced neuronal death, reduced invasion of astrocytes and microglia, and no elevation in IFN-γ and TNF-α [115].

Since astrocytes constitute near half of central nervous system cells and they may perform a function as immunocompetent cells producing a variety of cytokines. Aquaporin-4 (AQP4) is upregulated in astrocytes in several inflammatory conditions including PD. Sun et al. have described that AQP4 knockout mice treated with MPTP showed increased basal and inducible expression of NF-κB and increased gliosis and they propose that AQP4 may modulate neuroinflammation via regulating release of proinflammatory cytokines and ATP by astrocytes which in turn further activates microglia [116].

There are some features that explain localized damage in substantia nigra pars compacta (SNpc); neurons in the area are particularly susceptible to oxidative damage as they operate under high oxidant conditions due to reduced levels of the anti-oxidant glutathione and increased iron content. On the other hand, there is a high density of microglia cells that mediates neuroinflammatory processes [114]. Oxidative stress induces the generation of ROS by microglia that become activated. DJ-1, the product of PARK 7 gene, is a gene associated with hereditary PD, works as a repressor of phosphatase and tensin homolog (PTEN)—a tumor suppressor gene—and has important functions in cellular antioxidant response. Since loss-of-function mutations of DJ-1 have been associated with PD, Meiser et al. described that loss of DJ-1 impairs antioxidant response and induces weak constitutive microglia activation in mouse microglia [117].

Microglia may become activated by a wide variety of damage signals that include toxins, pathogens, endogenous proteins or products generated by dying neurons. The constitutive expression of proinflammatory cytokines IL-1β, TNF-α, IL-2, IL-6, and IFN-γ has been demonstrated in PD patients in postmortem brain analyses as well as in serum and cerebrospinal fluid *in vivo* [114].

Activation of microglia by dying neurons may result in a vicious circle of neuroinflammation and neurodegeneration [114]. Some of these substances liberated by degenerating neurons include α-synuclein aggregates, neuromelanin, adenosine triphosphate (ATP), and matrix metalloproteinase-3 (MMP-3) [114].

Microglia can get activated by pathologically altered forms of α-synuclein in PD, but also in other synucleinopathies such as dementia with Lewy bodies and multiple systems atrophy. Microglia activation gives raise to a balance between clearance of α-synuclein by phagocytosis via TLR4 microglia and neuronal dysfunction and neurodegeneration via oxidative stress and proinflammatory cytokine production by microglia [113].

7. Substances that inhibit microglial activation and neuroinflammation are protective in neurodegenerative diseases

Many different substances that prevent the triggering of inflammation in neurons have been used against AD, PD and ALS on primary cell cultures, mice models, and humans.

Resveratrol (3,5,4′-trihydroxy-trans-stilbene) is a natural polyphenolic compound with antioxidant properties capable of penetrating the blood-brain barrier efficiently [118–120].

Regarding AD, it has been shown that resveratrol inhibits amyloid-beta aggregation *in vitro* [121] and that has neuroprotective properties in cell cultures and animal models [122, 123]. Moreover, a recent clinical study showed that resveratrol was safe and well tolerated in individuals with mild to moderate Alzheimer disease, and although some biomarker levels were altered, a larger research to determine whether resveratrol may be beneficial for AD patients is necessary [124].

In murine models of ALS, resveratrol ameliorated motor neuron loss and degeneration, delayed disease symptoms onset, improved locomotion impairment, and extended the lifespan in the $SOD1^{G93A}$ mice [125], and importantly, it was found that resveratrol administration reduces microglial immunoreactivity in the $SOD1^{G93A}$ mice spinal cord [125]. It has been amply described that one of the mechanisms by which resveratrol promotes neuroprotection is increasing Sirt1 activity, whose increase and activation were demonstrated in motor neuron from spinal cord of $SOD1^{G93A}$ mice [125], showing a crucial role of the antioxidant in the prevention of the neuroinflammation in the disease, specifically through the microglial activation and not astroglial activation. This is in concordance with another evidence that showed that despite that resveratrol was capable of preventing slowly the ROS increase, it could not improve motor neuron survival in a rat primary spinal cord culture after exposition to astrocyte conditioned media from transgenic $SOD1^{G93A}$ [126].

In PD resveratrol participation is still being studied, but it seems to have a protective effect against dopamine-induced cytotoxicity and certain toxins and can also attenuate the inflammatory response in activated microglia [127, 128].

In spite of the neuroprotective properties that characterize resveratrol, it has the drawback of its low bioavailability in the body, so there have been some important efforts to develop analogs with better bioavailability [121].

Another example of natural neuroprotective substances is curcumin. It is also a phenolic compound extracted from perennial herb *Curcuma longa* (turmeric), characterized for its anti-inflammatory and antioxidant properties [129, 130]. It is mainly known for helping to improve impaired cognitive functions in AD [131]. Among its properties, curcumin inhibits microglial proliferation and differentiation [132] and reduces the inflammation inhibiting amyloid-beta-induced expression of specific proteins in monocyte cells, decreasing the transcription of inflammatory cytokines, among others [133].

In transgenic AD mice tg2576, curcumin significantly reduced the levels of amyloid-beta and plaque burden in comparison to not treated tg2576 mice [134]. Finally, a preparation with a high bioavailability of curcumin called "*Longvida*" showed significant improvements in working memory and mood after 4 weeks treatment in a randomized, double-blind, placebo-controlled in a cohort of healthy, elderly subjects [135].

In ALS, in a motor neuron-like cellular model from TDP-43^{MUT}, curcumin abolished the excitability previously induced by the mutation, through the inhibition of the oxidative stress and mitochondrial dysfunction [136].

In another example, Riluzole [2-amino-6-(trifluoromethoxy) benzothiazole], which is the only approved disease-modifying drug for ALS, exhibited protective skills in different neurodegenerative alterations and disorders. It acts as a sodium channel blocker and protects neurons against glutamatergic toxic effects [137, 138] and its anti-inflammatory effects have been demonstrated. In ALS, Riluzole prevents hyperexcitability and motor neuron death in ventral spinal cord cell culture [82], it prolongs survival and delays muscle strength deterioration in a mice model of motor neuropathy (similar motor symptoms to ALS) [139], and it preserves motor neuron function in a transgenic model of ALS [140] but just extends the lifespan by a couple of months in patients [141].

In AD, due to a previous work indicating that the amyloid-beta peptide significantly alters the expression of glutamatergic transporter (GLUT1), which leads to increase of synaptic glutamate levels [142], it has been proposed that Riluzole could have potential benefits in the treatment of the disease. Nowadays, there is a phase 2 clinical trial in curse to test cognitive functional changes in mild AD patients [143].

In PD, Riluzole has shown neuroprotective properties reducing GFAP levels in the lesioned striatum in a rodent model [144].

At this point there is an important body of evidence that supports that neuroimmunomodulation/neuroinflammation has an active and potent role in many neurodegenerative diseases. Our three examples (AD, PD and ALS) show that instead of having different and specific targets, all of them share common pathways and participants that lead to activation of microglia and release of inflammatory factors that contribute to neuron death.

8. Conclusion

The increase in life expectancy and the associated increase in the elderly population have led to a rise in cases of age-associated diseases; thus neurodegenerative diseases, such as AD, ALS and PD, are transformed into global issues and hot points for research and development of new drugs, especially considering the lack of effective treatment. In fact, most of the currently existing treatments, which are designed on the basis of symptom control, are only palliative.

In this chapter, we have delivered some of the evidence linking the development of inflammatory responses in the central nervous system with neuroinflammatory processes, present in the three very characteristic neurodegenerative conditions such as AD, PD and ALS. As we have mentioned an approach that considers similarities in pathophysiologic aspects of these diseases in spite of the very different clinical spectrum of each of them. This integrative approach is a new alternative road to the study of these diseases. Thus, the elements that define prolonged neuroinflammatory processes in time could be important elements to be considered in the early stage and even during pre-clinical asymptomatic stages of disease. In this context,

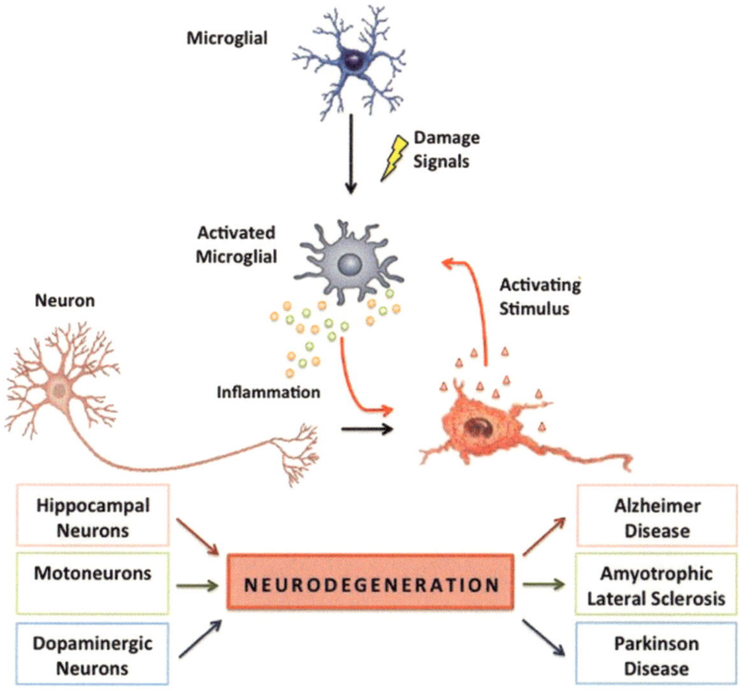

Figure 1. Model of neuroinflammation and neurodegeneration cycle. The microglial cell at rest is sensitive to different factors or signs of damage that lead to its activation. When these damage signals are maintained in time, the result is an altered response of activated microglial cells. This means that there will be a constant release of cytotoxic factors (mainly proinflammatory cytokines and ROS) that promote neuronal damage and/or lead to neurodegenerative processes. Hippocampal neurons, motor neurons, and dopaminergic neurons are susceptible to the action of overactive microglia, favoring neurodegeneration, which will trigger or will promote the development of AD, ALS and PD, respectively. In this model, once neurons degenerate, they release substances into the extra-cellular environment that are recognized by the microglia and act as a further sign of damage, promoting a neurodegenerative cycle.

the neuroimmunomodulation hypothesis [48, 58, 145–147] appears as a very plausible explanation for neurodegenerative stereotypical pathogenic process as well as a guide in the search for new therapeutic and new effective disease-modifying treatments.

We have also shown that microglial cell has an important role in the neuroinflammation and how this cell is linked with the neurodegenerative processes in these three diseases (**Figure 1**). That is, alterations in hippocampal neurons in AD, in motor neurons in ALS, and in dopaminergic neurons of substantia nigra in the PD are linked directly to the inflammatory response of the surrounding altered microglial cells, promoting the neurodegenerative process.

Another evidence of the effect and the importance of this negative neuroinflammatory-neurodegenerative cycle in the development of these diseases is the experimental response obtained after using compounds with anti-inflammatory properties in AD and ALS [131, 136], turning scientific interest in the development of future treatments that act on abnormal inflammatory response of microglial cell, so that might disrupt the neurodegenerative cycle.

Finally, it is of great interest to search for compounds that have fewer adverse effects and at the same time have a preventive action. In this context, the finding of anti-inflammatory and antioxidant properties in natural compounds opens new research possibilities, projecting a possible neuroprotective and anti-neuroinflammatory effects, which based on control of key elements of neuroimmunomodulation hypothesis could be a new tool for the treatment of these diseases.

Acknowledgements

This work was supported by CORFO INNOVA CHILE grants 14IEAT-28658.

Author details

Inelia Morales[1,2*], Gonzalo A. Farías[2,3], Nicole Cortes[1,2] and Ricardo B. Maccioni[1,2,4]

*Address all correspondence to: inelia.morales@gmail.com

1 Laboratory of Cellular and Molecular Neurosciences, Faculty of Sciences, University of Chile, Santiago, Chile

2 International Center for Biomedicine (ICC), Santiago, Chile

3 Department of Neurology and Neurosurgery, Faculty of Medicine, University of Chile, Santiago, Chile

4 Department of Neurological Sciences East, Faculty of Medicine, University of Chile, Santiago, Chile

References

[1] Chen WW, Zhang X, Huang WJ. Role of neuroinflammation in neurodegenerative diseases (Review). Mol Med Rep. 2016 Apr;13(4):3391-6. 10.3892/mmr.2016.4948.

[2] Batsch N, Mittelman M. World Alzheimer Report 2012—Overcoming the Stigma of Dementia. Published by Alzheimer's Disease International (ADI), London. September 2012. Copyright © Alzheimer's Disease International.

[3] Prince MJ, Wimo A, Guerchet MM, Ali GC, Wu Y-T, Prina M. World Alzheimer Report 2015—The Global Impact of Dementia: An Analysis of Prevalence, Incidence, Cost and Trends. London: Alzheimer's Disease International. 2015.

[4] Perry VH, Teeling J. Microglia and macrophages of the central nervous system: the contribution of microglia priming and systemic inflammation to chronic neurodegeneration. Semin Immunopathol. 2013 Sep;35(5):601-12. 10.1007/s00281-013-0382-8.

[5] Czirr E, Wyss-Coray T. The immunology of neurodegeneration. J Clin Invest. 2012 Apr;122(4):1156-63. 10.1172/jci58656.

[6] Howcroft TK, Campisi J, Louis GB, Smith MT, Wise B, Wyss-Coray T, Augustine AD, McElhaney JE, Kohanski R, Sierra F. The role of inflammation in age-related disease. Aging (Albany NY). 2013 Jan;5(1):84-93.

[7] Norden DM, Godbout JP. Review: microglia of the aged brain: primed to be activated and resistant to regulation. Neuropathol Appl Neurobiol. 2013 Feb;39(1):19-34. 10.1111/j.1365-2990.2012.01306.x.

[8] Tousoulis D. Inflammation in atherosclerosis: current therapeutic approaches. Curr Pharm Des. 2011 Dec;17(37):4087-8.

[9] Capuron L, Su S, Miller AH, Bremner JD, Goldberg J, Vogt GJ, Maisano C, Jones L, Murrah NV, Vaccarino V. Depressive symptoms and metabolic syndrome: is inflammation the underlying link? Biol Psychiatry. 2008 Nov 15;64(10):896-900. 10.1016/j.biopsych.2008.05.019.

[10] Ouchi N, Parker JL, Lugus JJ, Walsh K. Adipokines in inflammation and metabolic disease. Nat Rev Immunol. 2011 Feb;11(2):85-97. 10.1038/nri2921.

[11] Baune BT, Smith E, Reppermund S, Air T, Samaras K, Lux O, Brodaty H, Sachdev P, Trollor JN. Inflammatory biomarkers predict depressive, but not anxiety symptoms during aging: the prospective Sydney Memory and Aging Study. Psychoneuroendocrinology. 2012 Sep;37(9):1521-30. 10.1016/j.psyneuen.2012.02.006.

[12] Zunszain PA, Hepgul N, Pariante CM. Inflammation and depression. Curr Top Behav Neurosci. 2013;14:135-51. 10.1007/7854_2012_211.

[13] Ransohoff RM, Schafer D, Vincent A, Blachere NE, Bar-Or A. Neuroinflammation: ways in which the immune system affects the brain. Neurotherapeutics. 2015 Oct;12(4): 896-909. 10.1007/s13311-015-0385-3.

[14] Heneka MT, O'Banion MK. Inflammatory processes in Alzheimer's disease. J Neuroimmunol. 2007 Mar;184(1-2):69-91. 10.1016/j.jneuroim.2006.11.017.

[15] Heneka MT, Golenbock DT, Latz E. Innate immunity in Alzheimer's disease. Nat Immunol. 2015 Mar;16(3):229-36. 10.1038/ni.3102.

[16] Simard AR, Rivest S. Neuroprotective properties of the innate immune system and bone marrow stem cells in Alzheimer's disease. Mol Psychiatry. 2006 Apr;11(4):327-35. 10.1038/sj.mp.4001809.

[17] Sofroniew MV, Vinters HV. Astrocytes: biology and pathology. Acta Neuropathol. 2010 Jan;119(1):7-35. 10.1007/s00401-009-0619-8.

[18] Venneti S, Wiley CA, Kofler J. Imaging microglial activation during neuroinflammation and Alzheimer's disease. J Neuroimmune Pharmacol. 2009 Jun;4(2):227-43. 10.1007/s11481-008-9142-2.

[19] Perry VH. A revised view of the central nervous system microenvironment and major histocompatibility complex class II antigen presentation. J Neuroimmunol. 1998 Oct 1;90(2):113-21.

[20] Hanisch UK, Kettenmann H. Microglia: active sensor and versatile effector cells in the normal and pathologic brain. Nat Neurosci. 2007 Nov;10(11):1387-94. 10.1038/nn1997.

[21] Alliot F, Godin I, Pessac B. Microglia derive from progenitors, originating from the yolk sac, and which proliferate in the brain. Brain Res Dev Brain Res. 1999 Nov 18;117(2): 145-52.

[22] Ginhoux F, Lim S, Hoeffel G, Low D, Huber T. Origin and differentiation of microglia. Front Cell Neurosci. 2013;7:45. 10.3389/fncel.2013.00045.

[23] Jha MK, Lee WH, Suk K. Functional polarization of neuroglia: implications in neuroinflammation and neurological disorders. Biochem Pharmacol. 2016 Mar 1;103:1-16. 10.1016/j.bcp.2015.11.003.

[24] Zhang W, Wang T, Pei Z, Miller DS, Wu X, Block ML, Wilson B, Zhang W, Zhou Y, Hong JS, Zhang J. Aggregated alpha-synuclein activates microglia: a process leading to disease progression in Parkinson's disease. FASEB J. 2005 Apr;19(6):533-42. 10.1096/fj.04-2751com.

[25] Francis PT. The interplay of neurotransmitters in Alzheimer's disease. CNS Spectr. 2005 Nov;10(11 Suppl 18):6-9.

[26] Mrak RE. Microglia in Alzheimer brain: a neuropathological perspective. Int J Alzheimers Dis. 2012;2012:165021. 10.1155/2012/165021.

[27] Krause DL, Muller N. Neuroinflammation, microglia and implications for anti-inflammatory treatment in Alzheimer's disease. Int J Alzheimers Dis. 2010;2010. 10.4061/2010/732806.

[28] Morales I, Jimenez JM, Mancilla M, Maccioni RB. Tau oligomers and fibrils induce activation of microglial cells. J Alzheimers Dis. 2013;37(4):849-56. 10.3233/JAD-131843.

[29] Remarque EJ, Bollen EL, Weverling-Rijnsburger AW, Laterveer JC, Blauw GJ, Westendorp RG. Patients with Alzheimer's disease display a pro-inflammatory phenotype. Exp Gerontol. 2001 Jan;36(1):171-6.

[30] Innamorato NG, Lastres-Becker I, Cuadrado A. Role of microglial redox balance in modulation of neuroinflammation. Curr Opin Neurol. 2009 Jun;22(3):308-14. 10.1097/WCO.0b013e32832a3225.

[31] Steardo L, Jr., Bronzuoli MR, Iacomino A, Esposito G, Steardo L, Scuderi C. Does neuroinflammation turn on the flame in Alzheimer's disease? Focus on astrocytes. Front Neurosci. 2015;9:259. 10.3389/fnins.2015.00259.

[32] Verkhratsky A, Parpura V. Astrogliopathology in neurological, neurodevelopmental and psychiatric disorders. Neurobiol Dis. 2016 Jan;85:254-61. 10.1016/j.nbd.2015.03.025.

[33] Perea G, Navarrete M, Araque A. Tripartite synapses: astrocytes process and control synaptic information. Trends Neurosci. 2009 Aug;32(8):421-31. 10.1016/j.tins.2009.05.001.

[34] Sofroniew MV. Multiple roles for astrocytes as effectors of cytokines and inflammatory mediators. Neuroscientist. 2014 Apr;20(2):160-72. 10.1177/1073858413504466.

[35] Hertz L, editor. Book Review: 'Glial Physiology and Pathophysiology' by Alexei Verkhratsky and Arthur Butt, Wiley-Blackwell 2013. Front. Syst. Neurosci. 8:17, 2014.10.3389/fnsys.2014.00017.

[36] Meraz-Rios MA, Toral-Rios D, Franco-Bocanegra D, Villeda-Hernandez J, Campos-Pena V. Inflammatory process in Alzheimer's Disease. Front Integr Neurosci. 2013;7:59. 10.3389/fnint.2013.00059.

[37] Chow SK, Yu D, Macdonald CL, Buibas M, Silva GA. Amyloid beta-peptide directly induces spontaneous calcium transients, delayed intercellular calcium waves and gliosis in rat cortical astrocytes. ASN Neuro. 2010;2(1):e00026. 10.1042/AN20090035.

[38] Medeiros R, LaFerla FM. Astrocytes: conductors of the Alzheimer disease neuroinflammatory symphony. Exp Neurol. 2013 Jan;239:133-8. 10.1016/j.expneurol.2012.10.007.

[39] Donato R. Intracellular and extracellular roles of S100 proteins. Microsc Res Tech. 2003 Apr 15;60(6):540-51. 10.1002/jemt.10296.

[40] Mrak RE, Sheng JG, Griffin WS. Correlation of astrocytic S100 beta expression with dystrophic neurites in amyloid plaques of Alzheimer's disease. J Neuropathol Exp Neurol. 1996 Mar;55(3):273-9.

[41] Kantarci K, Knopman DS, Dickson DW, Parisi JE, Whitwell JL, Weigand SD, Josephs KA, Boeve BF, Petersen RC, Jack CR, Jr. Alzheimer disease: postmortem neuropathologic correlates of antemortem ^{1}H MR spectroscopy metabolite measurements. Radiology. 2008 Jul;248(1):210-20. 10.1148/radiol.2481071590.

[42] Tumati S, Martens S, Aleman A. Magnetic resonance spectroscopy in mild cognitive impairment: systematic review and meta-analysis. Neurosci Biobehav Rev. 2013 Dec; 37(10 Pt 2):2571-86. 10.1016/j.neubiorev.2013.08.004.

[43] Sillen A, Andrade J, Lilius L, Forsell C, Axelman K, Odeberg J, Winblad B, Graff C. Expanded high-resolution genetic study of 109 Swedish families with Alzheimer's disease. Eur J Hum Genet. 2008 Feb;16(2):202-8. 10.1038/sj.ejhg.5201946.

[44] Blennow K, de Leon MJ, Zetterberg H. Alzheimer's disease. Lancet. 2006 Jul 29;368(9533):387-403. 10.1016/S0140-6736(06)69113-7.

[45] Weiner HL, Frenkel D. Immunology and immunotherapy of Alzheimer's disease. Nat Rev Immunol. 2006 May;6(5):404-16. 10.1038/nri1843.

[46] McKhann GM, Knopman DS, Chertkow H, Hyman BT, Jack CR, Jr., Kawas CH, Klunk WE, Koroshetz WJ, Manly JJ, Mayeux R, Mohs RC, Morris JC, Rossor MN, Scheltens P, Carrillo MC, Thies B, Weintraub S, Phelps CH. The diagnosis of dementia due to Alzheimer's disease: recommendations from the National Institute on Aging-Alzheimer's Association workgroups on diagnostic guidelines for Alzheimer's disease. Alzheimers Dement. 2011 May;7(3):263-9. 10.1016/j.jalz.2011.03.005.

[47] Elbaz A, Dufouil C, Alperovitch A. Interaction between genes and environment in neurodegenerative diseases. C R Biol. 2007 Apr;330(4):318-28. 10.1016/j.crvi.2007.02.018.

[48] Maccioni RB, Rojo LE, Fernandez JA, Kuljis RO. The role of neuroimmunomodulation in Alzheimer's disease. Ann N Y Acad Sci. 2009 Feb;1153:240-6. 10.1111/j.1749-6632.2008.03972.x.

[49] Maccioni RB, Munoz JP, Barbeito L. The molecular bases of Alzheimer's disease and other neurodegenerative disorders. Arch Med Res. 2001 Sep-Oct;32(5):367-81.

[50] Venigalla M, Sonego S, Gyengesi E, Sharman MJ, Munch G. Novel promising therapeutics against chronic neuroinflammation and neurodegeneration in Alzheimer's disease. Neurochem Int. 2016 May;95:63-74. 10.1016/j.neuint.2015.10.011.

[51] Itzhaki RF, Wozniak MA, Appelt DM, Balin BJ. Infiltration of the brain by pathogens causes Alzheimer's disease. Neurobiol Aging. 2004 May-Jun;25(5):619-27. 10.1016/j.neurobiolaging.2003.12.021.

[52] Koseoglu E, Karaman Y. Relations between homocysteine, folate and vitamin B12 in vascular dementia and in Alzheimer disease. Clin Biochem. 2007 Aug;40(12):859-63. 10.1016/j.clinbiochem.2007.04.007.

[53] Lovati C, Galimberti D, Pomati S, Capiluppi E, Dolci A, Scapellato L, Rosa S, Mailland E, Suardelli M, Vanotti A, Clerici F, Santarato D, Panteghini M, Scarpini E, Mariani C, Bertora P. Serum folate concentrations in patients with cortical and subcortical dementias. Neurosci Lett. 2007 Jun 15;420(3):213-6. 10.1016/j.neulet.2007.04.060.

[54] Ostrowski SM, Wilkinson BL, Golde TE, Landreth G. Statins reduce amyloid-beta production through inhibition of protein isoprenylation. J Biol Chem. 2007 Sep 14;282(37):26832-44. 10.1074/jbc.M702640200.

[55] Rojo L, Sjoberg MK, Hernandez P, Zambrano C, Maccioni RB. Roles of cholesterol and lipids in the etiopathogenesis of Alzheimer's disease. J Biomed Biotechnol. 2006;2006(3): 73976. 10.1155/JBB/2006/73976.

[56] Fernandez JA, Rojo L, Kuljis RO, Maccioni RB. The damage signals hypothesis of Alzheimer's disease pathogenesis. J Alzheimers Dis. 2008 Jul;14(3):329-33.

[57] Maccioni RB. Tau protein in Alzheimer's disease. Curr Alzheimer Res. 2011 Sep;8(6): 607.

[58] Morales I, Guzman-Martinez L, Cerda-Troncoso C, Farias GA, Maccioni RB. Neuroinflammation in the pathogenesis of Alzheimer's disease. A rational framework for the search of novel therapeutic approaches. Front Cell Neurosci. 2014;8:112. 10.3389/fncel.2014.00112.

[59] Neumann K, Farias G, Slachevsky A, Perez P, Maccioni RB. Human platelets tau: a potential peripheral marker for Alzheimer's disease. J Alzheimers Dis. 2011;25(1):103-9. 10.3233/JAD-2011-101641.

[60] Frank-Cannon TC, Alto LT, McAlpine FE, Tansey MG. Does neuroinflammation fan the flame in neurodegenerative diseases? Mol Neurodegener. 2009;4:47. 10.1186/1750-1326-4-47.

[61] Smith WL, Garavito RM, DeWitt DL. Prostaglandin endoperoxide H synthases (cyclooxygenases)-1 and -2. J Biol Chem. 1996 Dec 27;271(52):33157-60.

[62] Hirst WD, Young KA, Newton R, Allport VC, Marriott DR, Wilkin GP. Expression of COX-2 by normal and reactive astrocytes in the adult rat central nervous system. Mol Cell Neurosci. 1999 Jan;13(1):57-68. 10.1006/mcne.1998.0731.

[63] Jiang C, Ting AT, Seed B. PPAR-gamma agonists inhibit production of monocyte inflammatory cytokines. Nature. 1998 Jan 1;391(6662):82-6. 10.1038/34184.

[64] Combs CK, Johnson DE, Karlo JC, Cannady SB, Landreth GE. Inflammatory mechanisms in Alzheimer's disease: inhibition of beta-amyloid-stimulated proinflammatory

responses and neurotoxicity by PPARgamma agonists. J Neurosci. 2000 Jan 15;20(2): 558-67.

[65] McGeer PL, McGeer EG. NSAIDs and Alzheimer disease: epidemiological, animal model and clinical studies. Neurobiol Aging. 2007 May;28(5):639-47. 10.1016/j.neurobiolaging.2006.03.013.

[66] Rich JB, Rasmusson DX, Folstein MF, Carson KA, Kawas C, Brandt J. Nonsteroidal anti-inflammatory drugs in Alzheimer's disease. Neurology. 1995 Jan;45(1):51-5.

[67] Leoutsakos JM, Han D, Mielke MM, Forrester SN, Tschanz JT, Corcoran CD, Green RC, Norton MC, Welsh-Bohmer KA, Lyketsos CG. Effects of general medical health on Alzheimer's progression: the Cache County Dementia Progression Study. Int Psychogeriatr. 2012 Oct;24(10):1561-70. 10.1017/S104161021200049X.

[68] Carrasco-Gallardo C, Farias GA, Fuentes P, Crespo F, Maccioni RB. Can nutraceuticals prevent Alzheimer's disease? Potential therapeutic role of a formulation containing shilajit and complex B vitamins. Arch Med Res. 2012 Nov;43(8):699-704. 10.1016/j.arcmed.2012.10.010.

[69] Cornejo A, Jimenez JM, Caballero L, Melo F, Maccioni RB. Fulvic acid inhibits aggregation and promotes disassembly of tau fibrils associated with Alzheimer's disease. J Alzheimers Dis. 2011;27(1):143-53. 10.3233/JAD-2011-110623.

[70] Rowland LP, Shneider NA. Amyotrophic lateral sclerosis. N Engl J Med. 2001 May 31;344(22):1688-700. 10.1056/NEJM200105313442207.

[71] Wood-Allum C, Shaw PJ. Motor neurone disease: a practical update on diagnosis and management. Clin Med (Lond). 2010 Jun;10(3):252-8.

[72] Cleveland DW, Rothstein JD. From Charcot to Lou Gehrig: deciphering selective motor neuron death in ALS. Nat Rev Neurosci. 2001 Nov;2(11):806-19. 10.1038/35097565.

[73] Pasinelli P, Brown RH. Molecular biology of amyotrophic lateral sclerosis: insights from genetics. Nat Rev Neurosci. 2006 Sep;7(9):710-23. 10.1038/nrn1971.

[74] Bento-Abreu A, Van Damme P, Van Den Bosch L, Robberecht W. The neurobiology of amyotrophic lateral sclerosis. Eur J Neurosci. 2010 Jun;31(12):2247-65. 10.1111/j.1460-9568.2010.07260.x.

[75] Ferraiuolo L, Kirby J, Grierson AJ, Sendtner M, Shaw PJ. Molecular pathways of motor neuron injury in amyotrophic lateral sclerosis. Nat Rev Neurol. 2011 Nov;7(11):616-30. 10.1038/nrneurol.2011.152.

[76] Chio A, Calvo A, Mazzini L, Cantello R, Mora G, Moglia C, Corrado L, D'Alfonso S, Majounie E, Renton A, Pisano F, Ossola I, Brunetti M, Traynor BJ, Restagno G, Parals. Extensive genetics of ALS: a population-based study in Italy. Neurology. 2012 Nov 6;79(19):1983-9. 10.1212/WNL.0b013e3182735d36.

[77] Mackenzie IR, Rademakers R, Neumann M. TDP-43 and FUS in amyotrophic lateral sclerosis and frontotemporal dementia. Lancet Neurol. 2010 Oct;9(10):995-1007. 10.1016/S1474-4422(10)70195-2.

[78] Arai T, Hasegawa M, Akiyama H, Ikeda K, Nonaka T, Mori H, Mann D, Tsuchiya K, Yoshida M, Hashizume Y, Oda T. TDP-43 is a component of ubiquitin-positive tau-negative inclusions in frontotemporal lobar degeneration and amyotrophic lateral sclerosis. Biochem Biophys Res Commun. 2006 Dec 22;351(3):602-11. 10.1016/j.bbrc.2006.10.093.

[79] Neumann M, Sampathu DM, Kwong LK, Truax AC, Micsenyi MC, Chou TT, Bruce J, Schuck T, Grossman M, Clark CM, McCluskey LF, Miller BL, Masliah E, Mackenzie IR, Feldman H, Feiden W, Kretzschmar HA, Trojanowski JQ, Lee VM. Ubiquitinated TDP-43 in frontotemporal lobar degeneration and amyotrophic lateral sclerosis. Science. 2006 Oct 6;314(5796):130-3. 10.1126/science.1134108.

[80] Renton AE, Chio A, Traynor BJ. State of play in amyotrophic lateral sclerosis genetics. Nat Neurosci. 2014 Jan;17(1):17-23. 10.1038/nn.3584.

[81] Di Giorgio FP, Carrasco MA, Siao MC, Maniatis T, Eggan K. Non-cell autonomous effect of glia on motor neurons in an embryonic stem cell-based ALS model. Nat Neurosci. 2007 May;10(5):608-14. 10.1038/nn1885.

[82] Fritz E, Izaurieta P, Weiss A, Mir FR, Rojas P, Gonzalez D, Rojas F, Brown RH, Jr., Madrid R, van Zundert B. Mutant SOD1-expressing astrocytes release toxic factors that trigger motoneuron death by inducing hyperexcitability. J Neurophysiol. 2013 Jun;109(11):2803-14. 10.1152/jn.00500.2012.

[83] Haidet-Phillips AM, Hester ME, Miranda CJ, Meyer K, Braun L, Frakes A, Song S, Likhite S, Murtha MJ, Foust KD, Rao M, Eagle A, Kammesheidt A, Christensen A, Mendell JR, Burghes AH, Kaspar BK. Astrocytes from familial and sporadic ALS patients are toxic to motor neurons. Nat Biotechnol. 2011 Sep;29(9):824-8. 10.1038/nbt.1957.

[84] Nagai M, Re DB, Nagata T, Chalazonitis A, Jessell TM, Wichterle H, Przedborski S. Astrocytes expressing ALS-linked mutated SOD1 release factors selectively toxic to motor neurons. Nat Neurosci. 2007 May;10(5):615-22. 10.1038/nn1876.

[85] Boillee S, Yamanaka K, Lobsiger CS, Copeland NG, Jenkins NA, Kassiotis G, Kollias G, Cleveland DW. Onset and progression in inherited ALS determined by motor neurons and microglia. Science. 2006 Jun 2;312(5778):1389-92. 10.1126/science.1123511.

[86] Frakes AE, Ferraiuolo L, Haidet-Phillips AM, Schmelzer L, Braun L, Miranda CJ, Ladner KJ, Bevan AK, Foust KD, Godbout JP, Popovich PG, Guttridge DC, Kaspar BK. Microglia induce motor neuron death via the classical NF-kappaB pathway in amyotrophic lateral sclerosis. Neuron. 2014 Mar 5;81(5):1009-23. 10.1016/j.neuron.2014.01.013.

[87] Hooten KG, Beers DR, Zhao W, Appel SH. Protective and toxic neuroinflammation in amyotrophic lateral sclerosis. Neurotherapeutics. 2015 Apr;12(2):364-75. 10.1007/s13311-014-0329-3.

[88] Liao B, Zhao W, Beers DR, Henkel JS, Appel SH. Transformation from a neuroprotective to a neurotoxic microglial phenotype in a mouse model of ALS. Exp Neurol. 2012 Sep; 237(1):147-52. 10.1016/j.expneurol.2012.06.011.

[89] Zhao W, Beers DR, Appel SH. Immune-mediated mechanisms in the pathoprogression of amyotrophic lateral sclerosis. J Neuroimmune Pharmacol. 2013 Sep;8(4):888-99. 10.1007/s11481-013-9489-x.

[90] Chiu IM, Chen A, Zheng Y, Kosaras B, Tsiftsoglou SA, Vartanian TK, Brown RH, Jr., Carroll MC. T lymphocytes potentiate endogenous neuroprotective inflammation in a mouse model of ALS. Proc Natl Acad Sci U S A. 2008 Nov 18;105(46):17913-8. 10.1073/pnas.0804610105.

[91] Gravel M, Beland LC, Soucy G, Abdelhamid E, Rahimian R, Gravel C, Kriz J. IL-10 controls early microglial phenotypes and disease onset in ALS caused by misfolded superoxide dismutase 1. J Neurosci. 2016 Jan 20;36(3):1031-48. 10.1523/JNEUROSCI.0854-15.2016.

[92] Appel SH, Beers DR, Henkel JS. T cell-microglial dialogue in Parkinson's disease and amyotrophic lateral sclerosis: are we listening? Trends Immunol. 2010 Jan;31(1):7-17. 10.1016/j.it.2009.09.003.

[93] Beers DR, Zhao W, Liao B, Kano O, Wang J, Huang A, Appel SH, Henkel JS. Neuroinflammation modulates distinct regional and temporal clinical responses in ALS mice. Brain Behav Immun. 2011 Jul;25(5):1025-35. 10.1016/j.bbi.2010.12.008.

[94] Lewis CA, Manning J, Rossi F, Krieger C. The neuroinflammatory response in ALS: the roles of microglia and T cells. Neurol Res Int. 2012;2012:803701. 10.1155/2012/803701.

[95] Lewis KE, Rasmussen AL, Bennett W, King A, West AK, Chung RS, Chuah MI. Microglia and motor neurons during disease progression in the SOD1G93A mouse model of amyotrophic lateral sclerosis: changes in arginase1 and inducible nitric oxide synthase. J Neuroinflammation. 2014;11:55. 10.1186/1742-2094-11-55.

[96] Barbeito AG, Mesci P, Boillee S. Motor neuron-immune interactions: the vicious circle of ALS. J Neural Transm (Vienna). 2010 Aug;117(8):981-1000. 10.1007/s00702-010-0429-0.

[97] Bowerman M, Vincent T, Scamps F, Perrin FE, Camu W, Raoul C. Neuroimmunity dynamics and the development of therapeutic strategies for amyotrophic lateral sclerosis. Front Cell Neurosci. 2013 Nov 19;7:214. 10.3389/fncel.2013.00214.

[98] Hensley K, Mhatre M, Mou S, Pye QN, Stewart C, West M, Williamson KS. On the relation of oxidative stress to neuroinflammation: lessons learned from the G93A-SOD1

mouse model of amyotrophic lateral sclerosis. Antioxid Redox Signal. 2006 Nov-Dec; 8(11–12):2075-87. 10.1089/ars.2006.8.2075.

[99] Banati RB, Gehrmann J, Kellner M, Holsboer F. Antibodies against microglia/brain macrophages in the cerebrospinal fluid of a patient with acute amyotrophic lateral sclerosis and presenile dementia. Clin Neuropathol. 1995 Jul–Aug;14(4):197-200.

[100] Brettschneider J, Toledo JB, Van Deerlin VM, Elman L, McCluskey L, Lee VM, Trojanowski JQ. Microglial activation correlates with disease progression and upper motor neuron clinical symptoms in amyotrophic lateral sclerosis. PLoS One. 2012;7(6):e39216. 10.1371/journal.pone.0039216.

[101] Turner MR, Cagnin A, Turkheimer FE, Miller CC, Shaw CE, Brooks DJ, Leigh PN, Banati RB. Evidence of widespread cerebral microglial activation in amyotrophic lateral sclerosis: an [^{11}C](R)-PK11195 positron emission tomography study. Neurobiol Dis. 2004 Apr;15(3):601-9. 10.1016/j.nbd.2003.12.012.

[102] Zurcher NR, Loggia ML, Lawson R, Chonde DB, Izquierdo-Garcia D, Yasek JE, Akeju O, Catana C, Rosen BR, Cudkowicz ME, Hooker JM, Atassi N. Increased in vivo glial activation in patients with amyotrophic lateral sclerosis: assessed with [(^{11})C]-PBR28. Neuroimage Clin. 2015;7:409-14. 10.1016/j.nicl.2015.01.009.

[103] Correia AS, Patel P, Dutta K, Julien JP. Inflammation induces TDP-43 mislocalization and aggregation. PLoS One. 2015;10(10):e0140248. 10.1371/journal.pone.0140248.

[104] Giaume C, Naus CC. Connexins, gap junctions, and glia. WIREs Membr Transp Signal. 2013;2(4):133-42. 10.1002/wmts.87.

[105] Goldberg GS, Valiunas V, Brink PR. Selective permeability of gap junction channels. Biochim Biophys Acta. 2004 Mar 23;1662(1-2):96-101. 10.1016/j.bbamem.2003.11.022.

[106] Yeager M, Harris AL. Gap junction channel structure in the early 21st century: facts and fantasies. Curr Opin Cell Biol. 2007 Oct;19(5):521-8. 10.1016/j.ceb.2007.09.001.

[107] Laird DW. Life cycle of connexins in health and disease. Biochem J. 2006 Mar 15;394(Pt 3):527-43. 10.1042/BJ20051922.

[108] Willecke K, Eiberger J, Degen J, Eckardt D, Romualdi A, Guldenagel M, Deutsch U, Sohl G. Structural and functional diversity of connexin genes in the mouse and human genome. Biol Chem. 2002 May;383(5):725-37. 10.1515/BC.2002.076.

[109] Orellana JA, Saez PJ, Shoji KF, Schalper KA, Palacios-Prado N, Velarde V, Giaume C, Bennett MV, Saez JC. Modulation of brain hemichannels and gap junction channels by pro-inflammatory agents and their possible role in neurodegeneration. Antioxid Redox Signal. 2009 Feb;11(2):369-99. 10.1089/ars.2008.2130.

[110] Schalper KA, Palacios-Prado N, Retamal MA, Shoji KF, Martinez AD, Saez JC. Connexin hemichannel composition determines the FGF-1-induced membrane permeabil-

ity and free [Ca^{2+}]i responses. Mol Biol Cell. 2008 Aug;19(8):3501-13. 10.1091/mbc.E07-12-1240.

[111] Bosch M, Kielian T. Hemichannels in neurodegenerative diseases: is there a link to pathology? Front Cell Neurosci. 2014;8:242. 10.3389/fncel.2014.00242.

[112] Takeuchi H, Mizoguchi H, Doi Y, Jin S, Noda M, Liang J, Li H, Zhou Y, Mori R, Yasuoka S, Li E, Parajuli B, Kawanokuchi J, Sonobe Y, Sato J, Yamanaka K, Sobue G, Mizuno T, Suzumura A. Blockade of gap junction hemichannel suppresses disease progression in mouse models of amyotrophic lateral sclerosis and Alzheimer's disease. PLoS One. 2011;6(6):e21108. 10.1371/journal.pone.0021108.

[113] Bruck D, Wenning GK, Stefanova N, Fellner L. Glia and alpha-synuclein in neurodegeneration: a complex interaction. Neurobiol Dis. 2016 Jan;85:262-74. 10.1016/j.nbd.2015.03.003.

[114] Collins LM, Toulouse A, Connor TJ, Nolan YM. Contributions of central and systemic inflammation to the pathophysiology of Parkinson's disease. Neuropharmacology. 2012 Jun;62(7):2154-68. 10.1016/j.neuropharm.2012.01.028.

[115] Martin HL, Santoro M, Mustafa S, Riedel G, Forrester JV, Teismann P. Evidence for a role of adaptive immune response in the disease pathogenesis of the MPTP mouse model of Parkinson's disease. Glia. 2016 Mar;64(3):386-95. 10.1002/glia.22935.

[116] Sun H, Liang R, Yang B, Zhou Y, Liu M, Fang F, Ding J, Fan Y, Hu G. Aquaporin-4 mediates communication between astrocyte and microglia: implications of neuroinflammation in experimental Parkinson's disease. Neuroscience. 2016 Mar 11;317:65-75. 10.1016/j.neuroscience.2016.01.003.

[117] Meiser J, Delcambre S, Wegner A, Jager C, Ghelfi J, d'Herouel AF, Dong X, Weindl D, Stautner C, Nonnenmacher Y, Michelucci A, Popp O, Giesert F, Schildknecht S, Kramer L, Schneider JG, Woitalla D, Wurst W, Skupin A, Weisenhorn DM, Kruger R, Leist M, Hiller K. Loss of DJ-1 impairs antioxidant response by altered glutamine and serine metabolism. Neurobiol Dis. 2016 May;89:112-25. 10.1016/j.nbd.2016.01.019.

[118] Barber SC, Higginbottom A, Mead RJ, Barber S, Shaw PJ. An in vitro screening cascade to identify neuroprotective antioxidants in ALS. Free Radic Biol Med. 2009 Apr 15;46(8):1127-38. 10.1016/j.freeradbiomed.2009.01.019.

[119] Lin Y, Chen F, Zhang J, Wang T, Wei X, Wu J, Feng Y, Dai Z, Wu Q. Neuroprotective effect of resveratrol on ischemia/reperfusion injury in rats through TRPC6/CREB pathways. J Mol Neurosci. 2013 Jul;50(3):504-13. 10.1007/s12031-013-9977-8.

[120] Singh N, Agrawal M, Dore S. Neuroprotective properties and mechanisms of resveratrol in in vitro and in vivo experimental cerebral stroke models. ACS Chem Neurosci. 2013 Aug 21;4(8):1151-62. 10.1021/cn400094w.

[121] Lu C, Guo Y, Yan J, Luo Z, Luo HB, Yan M, Huang L, Li X. Design, synthesis, and evaluation of multitarget-directed resveratrol derivatives for the treatment of Alzheimer's disease. J Med Chem. 2013 Jul 25;56(14):5843-59. 10.1021/jm400567s.

[122] Ma T, Tan MS, Yu JT, Tan L. Resveratrol as a therapeutic agent for Alzheimer's disease. Biomed Res Int. 2014;2014:350516. 10.1155/2014/350516.

[123] Rege SD, Geetha T, Griffin GD, Broderick TL, Babu JR. Neuroprotective effects of resveratrol in Alzheimer disease pathology. Front Aging Neurosci. 2014;6:218. 10.3389/fnagi.2014.00218.

[124] Turner RS, Thomas RG, Craft S, van Dyck CH, Mintzer J, Reynolds BA, Brewer JB, Rissman RA, Raman R, Aisen PS, Alzheimer's Disease Cooperative S. A randomized, double-blind, placebo-controlled trial of resveratrol for Alzheimer disease. Neurology. 2015 Oct 20;85(16):1383-91. 10.1212/WNL.0000000000002035.

[125] Mancuso R, del Valle J, Modol L, Martinez A, Granado-Serrano AB, Ramirez-Nunez O, Pallas M, Portero-Otin M, Osta R, Navarro X. Resveratrol improves motoneuron function and extends survival in SOD1(G93A) ALS mice. Neurotherapeutics. 2014 Apr; 11(2):419-32. 10.1007/s13311-013-0253-y.

[126] Rojas F, Cortes N, Abarzua S, Dyrda A, van Zundert B. Astrocytes expressing mutant SOD1 and TDP43 trigger motoneuron death that is mediated via sodium channels and nitroxidative stress. Front Cell Neurosci. 2014;8:24. 10.3389/fncel.2014.00024.

[127] Ferretta A, Gaballo A, Tanzarella P, Piccoli C, Capitanio N, Nico B, Annese T, Di Paola M, Dell'aquila C, De Mari M, Ferranini E, Bonifati V, Pacelli C, Cocco T. Effect of resveratrol on mitochondrial function: implications in parkin-associated familiar Parkinson's disease. Biochim Biophys Acta. 2014 Jul;1842(7):902-15. 10.1016/j.bbadis. 2014.02.010.

[128] Gordon BS, Delgado Diaz DC, Kostek MC. Resveratrol decreases inflammation and increases utrophin gene expression in the mdx mouse model of Duchenne muscular dystrophy. Clin Nutr. 2013 Feb;32(1):104-11. 10.1016/j.clnu.2012.06.003.

[129] Aggarwal BB, Harikumar KB. Potential therapeutic effects of curcumin, the anti-inflammatory agent, against neurodegenerative, cardiovascular, pulmonary, metabolic, autoimmune and neoplastic diseases. Int J Biochem Cell Biol. 2009 Jan;41(1):40-59. 10.1016/j.biocel.2008.06.010.

[130] Lu Z, Shen Y, Wang T, Cui M, Wang Z, Zhao H, Dong Q. Curcumin promotes neurite outgrowth via reggie-1/flotillin-2 in cortical neurons. Neurosci Lett. 2014 Jan 24;559:7-12. 10.1016/j.neulet.2013.11.029.

[131] Mishra S, Palanivelu K. The effect of curcumin (turmeric) on Alzheimer's disease: an overview. Ann Indian Acad Neurol. 2008 Jan;11(1):13-9. 10.4103/0972-2327.40220.

[132] Ambegaokar SS, Wu L, Alamshahi K, Lau J, Jazayeri L, Chan S, Khanna P, Hsieh E, Timiras PS. Curcumin inhibits dose-dependently and time-dependently neuroglial cell proliferation and growth. Neuro Endocrinol Lett. 2003 Dec;24(6):469-73.

[133] Giri RK, Rajagopal V, Kalra VK. Curcumin, the active constituent of turmeric, inhibits amyloid peptide-induced cytochemokine gene expression and CCR5-mediated chemotaxis of THP-1 monocytes by modulating early growth response-1 transcription factor. J Neurochem. 2004 Dec;91(5):1199-210. 10.1111/j.1471-4159.2004.02800.x.

[134] Yang F, Lim GP, Begum AN, Ubeda OJ, Simmons MR, Ambegaokar SS, Chen PP, Kayed R, Glabe CG, Frautschy SA, Cole GM. Curcumin inhibits formation of amyloid beta oligomers and fibrils, binds plaques, and reduces amyloid in vivo. J Biol Chem. 2005 Feb 18;280(7):5892-901. 10.1074/jbc.M404751200.

[135] Cox KH, Pipingas A, Scholey AB. Investigation of the effects of solid lipid curcumin on cognition and mood in a healthy older population. J Psychopharmacol. 2015 May;29(5): 642-51. 10.1177/0269881114552744.

[136] Dong H, Xu L, Wu L, Wang X, Duan W, Li H, Li C. Curcumin abolishes mutant TDP-43 induced excitability in a motoneuron-like cellular model of ALS. Neuroscience. 2014 Jul 11;272:141-53. 10.1016/j.neuroscience.2014.04.032.

[137] Fumagalli E, Funicello M, Rauen T, Gobbi M, Mennini T. Riluzole enhances the activity of glutamate transporters GLAST, GLT1 and EAAC1. Eur J Pharmacol. 2008 Jan 14;578(2-3):171-6. 10.1016/j.ejphar.2007.10.023.

[138] Grant P, Song JY, Swedo SE. Review of the use of the glutamate antagonist riluzole in psychiatric disorders and a description of recent use in childhood obsessive-compulsive disorder. J Child Adolesc Psychopharmacol. 2010 Aug;20(4):309-15. 10.1089/cap. 2010.0009.

[139] Kennel P, Revah F, Bohme GA, Bejuit R, Gallix P, Stutzmann JM, Imperato A, Pratt J. Riluzole prolongs survival and delays muscle strength deterioration in mice with progressive motor neuronopathy (pmn). J Neurol Sci. 2000 Nov 1;180(1-2):55-61.

[140] Gurney ME, Fleck TJ, Himes CS, Hall ED. Riluzole preserves motor function in a transgenic model of familial amyotrophic lateral sclerosis. Neurology. 1998 Jan;50(1): 62-6.

[141] Miller RG, Mitchell JD, Lyon M, Moore DH. Riluzole for amyotrophic lateral sclerosis (ALS)/motor neuron disease (MND). Cochrane Database Syst Rev. 2007 (1):CD001447. 10.1002/14651858.CD001447.pub2.

[142] Scimemi A, Meabon JS, Woltjer RL, Sullivan JM, Diamond JS, Cook DG. Amyloid-beta1-42 slows clearance of synaptically released glutamate by mislocalizing astrocytic GLT-1. J Neurosci. 2013 Mar 20;33(12):5312-8. 10.1523/JNEUROSCI.5274-12.2013.

[143] Pereira A. Glutamatergic Dysfunction in Cognitive Aging: Riluzole in Mild Alzheimer's Disease. Phase 2, Clinical Study, 2016. Available from: https://clinicaltrials.gov/ct/show/NCT01703117.

[144] Carbone M, Duty S, Rattray M. Riluzole neuroprotection in a Parkinson's disease model involves suppression of reactive astrocytosis but not GLT-1 regulation. BMC Neurosci. 2012;13:38. 10.1186/1471-2202-13-38.

[145] Maccioni RB, Farias G, Morales I, Navarrete L. The revitalized tau hypothesis on Alzheimer's disease. Arch Med Res. 2010 Apr;41(3):226-31. 10.1016/j.arcmed.2010.03.007.

[146] Morales I, Farias G, Maccioni RB. Neuroimmunomodulation in the pathogenesis of Alzheimer's disease. Neuroimmunomodulation. 2010;17(3):202-4. 10.1159/000258724.

[147] Rojo LE, Fernandez JA, Maccioni AA, Jimenez JM, Maccioni RB. Neuroinflammation: implications for the pathogenesis and molecular diagnosis of Alzheimer's disease. Arch Med Res. 2008 Jan;39(1):1-16. 10.1016/j.arcmed.2007.10.001.

Chapter 3

High-Fat and Cholesterol Intake Affects Brain Homeostasis and Could Accelerate the Development of Dementia: A Systemic View

Marco Antonio Meraz-Ríos and Perla Leal-Galicia

Additional information is available at the end of the chapter

http://dx.doi.org/10.5772/64357

Abstract

Alzheimer's disease is the most common type of dementia in occidental countries. The majority of the cases develop the disease for no genetic reasons; therefore, it is crucial to establish which environmental factors trigger the development of the disease. It has been proposed that nutritional habits, especially main components of Western countries' diet such as saturated fat or cholesterol, increase the risk for development of Alzheimer's disease (AD) and/or accelerate the onset of the disease, which is a big concern in countries where obesity is a public health problem. It is crucial to understand the links between alimentary habits and the development of AD and other types of dementia. A possible mechanism is the disruption of blood–brain barrier (BBB), which is the protection of the brain from circulating blood. Such disruptions can result from consuming high-fat diet (HFD) or high-cholesterol diet (HCD) and inflammation produced by alteration in brain vasculature resulted for chronic consumption of such type of diets. What has named a "Systemic view" comprises the idea that; what happens outside of the brain environment does affect brain functioning and the modifications experienced in the brain environment resulted from the influence of external factors will affect the entire body. In the current chapter, we will review the state of the art in the studies of the impact of a diet rich in fat or cholesterol on the brain and how the alterations induced in other organs can impact brain functioning increasing the susceptibility of development of dementia.

Keywords: high-fat diet, high-cholesterol diet, Alzheimer's disease, blood–brain barrier, brain plasticity, cognition

1. Introduction

In the recent decades, the population in the industrialized Western countries has become remarkable sedentary and have had a considerable increase in the intake of what has been called "fast food," meals that are rich in fat and carbohydrates and contain elevate levels of cholesterol as well. The elevated consumption of fast food has had a strong impact on public health, which has important repercussions in several levels including an economic impact due to the elevated cost of a chronic use of specialized health services and a detrimental effect in both, life quality and expectancy for the patients. Among the adverse health effects of this type of diet, we can mention obesity, vascular diseases, and metabolic syndrome, and it has been recently proposed that it can increase the risk of developing Alzheimer's disease (AD), which is the most common type of dementia in elderly people. It is considered that a particular type of diet could accelerate the progress of the disease for a not yet well-known mechanism [1]. It is a revolutionary idea, since we have had for several years the conception that brain is actually protected by the blood–brain barrier (BBB); however, experimental evidence suggests that the consumption of diets rich in fat can disrupt the permeability of BBB, making it vulnerable to systemic molecules that could trigger degenerative processes [1, 2].

In the current chapter, we will review the state of the art related to the impact of diets rich in fat or cholesterol on the brain, and how the alterations induced in other organs can impact brain functioning and could increase the susceptibility to develop dementia. The bibliographic revision was carried out running an exhaustive search on the research articles related to the topic employing the database of the US National Library of Medicine, National Institutes of Health, PubMed.gov. Firstly, reviewing the most recent papers and those with the most relevant information. Thereafter, we carefully followed the references cited by the reviewed articles in order to study the grounding data on the subject and which direction it followed until our days in order to document the accuracy and evolution of the data.

2. Findings on amyloid-β production induced by saturated fat diet in noncerebral tissue

One of the histopathological hallmarks of AD is the extracellular deposition of amyloid-β peptide (Aβ) in the brain. It is widely accepted that Aβ deposition occurs when the neuronal synthesis of the peptide exceeds the clearance capacity [3, 4]. However, some decades ago, the idea was proposed that Aβ generated systemically could pass the BBB and be deposited in the brain, since Aβ was detected in noncerebral biological fluids. Such idea raised from grounding data of Seubert et al. [5], who demonstrated that Aβ fragment comprising the amino acids 13–28 can be detected in cerebrospinal fluid and plasma of several species including human as well as in conditioned media from human brain cell cultures. It originated the idea that cerebral Aβ deposits could be generated systemically and for unknown mechanism, accumulate in the brain where they affect the capacity, to be clear, increasing the amount of the peptide and eventually form the extracellular deposits. A good amount of data has focused on this idea since then. An interesting line of study has focus on the production of Aβ by noncerebral tissue induced by consumption of diets rich in fat. One of the physiological functions of Aβ is relate to lipids metabolism and many Aβ transport proteins have been associated with lipids *in vivo* [6]. The association of the Aβ soluble fraction with high-density lipoproteins from healthy human plasma and cerebrospinal fluid was reported as well [7, 8]. The association between lipids and Aβ was demonstrated in a very elegant study where Aβ activity was followed labeling it with radioactivity, and it was found that the peptide is expressed in tissues rich in fat, such as spleen, marrow, liver, adipose tissue, brain, kidney, lung, and skeletal muscle. It was shown that the expression of Aβ is associated with postprandial lipoproteins such as chylomicrons, lipoproteins that are in charge to move dietary fat from intestine to the target organs. These associations remain during lipolysis and tissue uptaking processes [9]. Therefore, it can be proposed that an increased plasmatic amount of such proteins containing Aβ could produce an imbalance and could even be delivered in brain contributing to cerebral amyloidosis, one of the responsible events related to Alzheimer's disease [9, 10]. The natural question is: how can we increase the amount of Aβ associated to postprandial lipids? One answer is the intake of diets rich in fat or cholesterol because they could break the balance of lipids content, but by which way? An interesting direction has been to study the expression of Aβ in organs rich in lipids and if such expression is regulated by fat or cholesterol diets.

Koudinov et al. [11] reported that hepatocytes secrete amyloid-β as a lipoprotein complex. Another organ where it has been documented that Aβ is produced is the small intestine. Given the evidence that Aβ is associated to postprandial lipoproteins, chylomicrons, Galloway et al. [10] followed this line of evidence and studied small intestinal epithelial cells (where the chylomicrons are produced). They fed wild-type mice with low- or high-fat diet. After six months of treatment they determinate by immunohistochemistry, the expression of the amyloid precursor protein in absorptive cells in the small intestine and observed a greater expression of this molecule in small intestinal epithelial cells of high-fat fed animals, whereas animals fasting 65 h did not show any expression. There is another study where the group of John CL Mamo evaluated the expression of Aβ in enterocytes after a low- or high-fat diet with 1% cholesterol in apoliprotein E (apo E) (-/-) knockout mice. Apoliprotein E is a lipoprotein that modulates Aβ biogenesis [12–14]. After six months of dietary treatment, the small intestine of apo E (-/-) KO mice fed with low-fat diet showed the same levels of expression of Aβ as the wild-type animals detected by immunohistochemistry. On the other hand, both groups of animals, wild-type and apo E (-/-) KO mice fed with high-fat diet, showed an increased expression of Aβ in enterocytes being higher in the KO animals. Also in these study, the group evaluates villi length between the groups treated, finding that the high-fat diet did not affect villi length in apo E(-/-) KO mice, but interestingly there is an increase in villi length of KO mice treated with low-fat diet when compared with wild-type mice under the same dietary conditions [15]. These groups also carried out a very elegant study to corroborate the association of Aβ production with recently generated lipoproteins, employing three-dimensional immunofluorescence microscopy and determinated that Aβ produced by enterocytes certainly has a clear colocalization with chylomicrons in small intestine enterocyte after three months of dietary treatment (free of cholesterol). They found that the amount of Aβ colocalizing with chylomicrons reaches the double [16]. These data together confirms the presence of Aβ in lipoproteins generated in small intestine and that a diet rich in fat could increase the production of transport lipoproteins. However, the open question stills remains: how this Aβ produced systemically reaches the brain? **(Figure 1)**. Further studies are necessary to establish if indeed an imbalance in lipids production induced by diet can promote the delivery of these systemic Aβ to brain and induce cerebral amyloidosis.

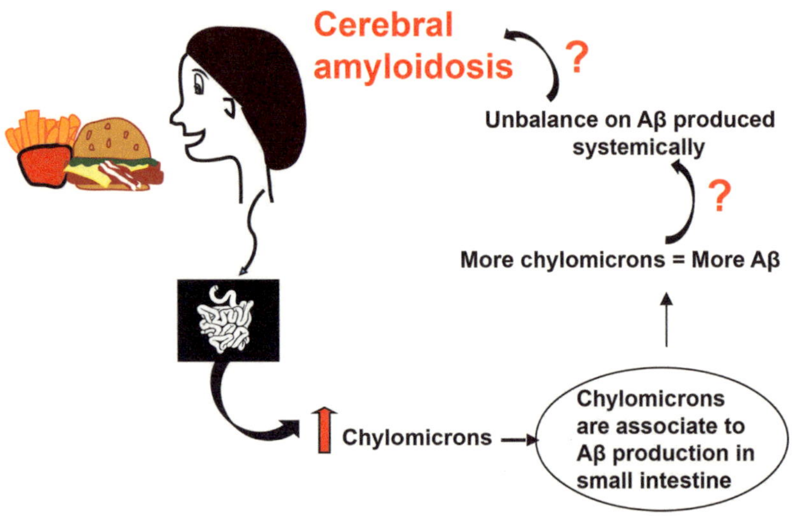

Figure 1. The ingestion of food rich on fat and cholesterol can increase the amount of postprandial lipoproteins chylomicrons. An increased production of chylomicrons can lead to an overproduction of *Aβ* and potentially produce an unbalance on *Aβ* processing and lead to cerebral amyloidosis.

3. Effect on vascularity and BBB integrity

The brain is a very well-protected organ with two barrier systems. One is a highly specialized microvascular endothelial system known as blood brain barrier (BBB), its function is to protect the brain from the entry of damaging substances and at the same time, allows the entry of nutrients as well as endocrine signals by means of an active transport and a passive diffusion system. The second is the choroid plexus, whose function is to prevent the entry of blood in the cerebrospinal circulation [17]. An unbalance in such systems could lead to disease conditions regarding the entrance of damaging molecules or disrupting the entrance of proper nutrients or endocrine signals. A good body of data has focused in study; how dietary habits can trigger BBB disruption? A longitudinal study, carried out in Sweden, evaluated the integrity of BBB *in vivo* in 81 women with a wide range of body size, who acceded to receive a lumbar puncture in order to obtain cerebrospinal fluid and compared the index of albumin content. Albumin is a constitutive protein that is absent in the brain, since its access is stopped by the BBB; therefore its presence in cerebrospinal fluid is a sign of disruption of the protection systems. Among these large group studied, the obese and overweight women between 70 and

84 years had the highest amount of albumin reported as the ratio of albumin in cerebrospinal fluid/Serum albumin (CSF/S albumin). Interestingly, they found a correlation between low levels of sex hormone binding globulin (SHBG) in the same group of women when they were younger [18]. It is known that SHBG decreases with overweight in both, male and female [19–21]. In the Swedish longitudinal study, SHBG was employed as measure of endocrine signal in the same group of females when they were in there middle forties, and decades later when they were analyzed for several parameters besides the CSF/S albumin ratio, such measures included behavioral evaluations finding that they had cognitive alterations [18]. It strongly suggests that since youth, these group of obese and overweighting women had less content of SHBG accompanied in elderly years by BBB disruption and cognitive decline. These data suggest that an unbalance between the selective entrance and exit of molecules and signaling drived by a failed BBB filtering can lead to development of dementia, but more experimental data is needed in order to elucidate the mechanism behind this effect. One way to explain the cognitive detriment found in these patients could be the diminishment of factors that have been shown to be protective for the brain, such as SHBG. High levels of SHBG have been associated with neuroprotection in stroke, vascular and cardiovascular diseases, diabetes [21–25], and an increased amount of molecules potentially damaging for the brain, such as Aβ [26–28]. Such idea can be supported by the fact that it was found in the obese and overweight women, a higher ratio of CSF/S albumin has been observed in subjects with AD as well [29, 30]. In this study, the CSF/S albumin content was measured in 118 patients diagnosed with AD and clinical data of vascular alterations was registered as well. The AD subjects were compared with individuals without dementia of the same age, finding a higher albumin ratio in those with both AD and vascular factors. There was not significant BBB disruption in the patients without vascular alterations; additionally, there is no correlation with BBB disturbances and age in the control group, which strongly suggests a relationship with the vascular alterations, BBB disruption, and AD [29]. Controversially in a study, albumin content as well as IgG in serum and cerebrospinal fluid in several groups of patients with different dementias such as early-progression familial AD, the senile dementia of Alzheimer type (Late Onset Alzherimer's Disease LOAD), and two types of vascular dementia: a group diagnose with vascular dementia and others with multiinfarct, were measured. The multiinfarct group was reported with the highest significant alteration of the BBB but not in AD group. All these data supports the idea that vascular factors associated to BBB disruption are in relationship with the development of many dementia syndromes and are not restricted to AD [31]. That controversial information can be clarified with animal experimental data, where several variables can be controlled. The very first experimental evidence that the Aβ peptide can actually cross BBB and be deposited in the brain parenchyma was done in 1993 by Zlokovic et al. [32]. The researchers injected synthetic forms of Aβ peptide: 1–28 and 1–40, which were labeled with a radioactive marker in order to follow it after carrying out an injection in the neck vessel of the guinea pigs. The research group found a specific deposition of both synthetic peptides in the BBB microvasculature, initiating in the luminal side and transcellular transport into the brain parenchyma. This study strongly supports the idea that the Aβ produced systemically can cross the BBB. However, the mechanism remains unclear so far.

Although there is evidence that BBB can be disrupted in patients with dementia, it is possible that the development on AD can be due to systemically produced Aβ that can cross the BBB and form the deposits in the brain, but how does this happen? As we reviewed, obese patients apparently have a disrupted BBB permeability, although, what triggers that? Are the intake habits involved in such phenomenon? There is experimental evidence that suggest that components of Western diet, such as cholesterol and saturated fat, can contribute to that phenomenon. Studies with rabbits fed with a diet containing 2% cholesterol for 8 weeks, have demonstrated that such type of diet disrupts BBB permeability, alters vascularity, and induce vessels inflammation and Aβ peptide accumulation in parenchyma [26–28]; and this accumulation is similar to that observed in brains of AD patients [33]. This body of data, mainly generated by D.L. Sparks and collaborators, strongly supports the idea that high cholesterol consumption, importantly, contributes to the development of AD onset by the accumulation of Aβ, vascular alterations, as well as BBB selective permeability disruption.

The contribution of BBB disruption of a high energetic diet (HE) (approximately 40% Kcal of fat versus 13% of standard laboratory rodent diet) based on high saturated fat and glucose was evaluated in 60-days-old 32 male rats that were fed for 90 days with this type of diet. The researchers evaluated the BBB integrity, measuring by ELISA, the content of sodium fluorescein (NaFl) injected throughout the femoral artery in the prefrontal cortex, striatum, and hippocampus of the treated rats. They found a significant increased amount of NaFl in the hippocampus of the treated rats compared with the control but not in prefrontal cortex or in striatum. They also measured the mRNA expression of tight junction proteins by RT-PCR in choroid plexus and BBB capillaries. Thigh junction proteins are critical components for maintenance of selective BBB permeability, its diminishment can alter the BBB function. They found a decrease expression of the thigh junction proteins and alterations in behavioral task directly associated with hippocampal function [1]. A further study was carried out by Davidson et al. [34], where they fed 24 male rats with a high energy diet as well as high saturated fat and glucose and following for different time points (7, 14, 21 and 28 days), evaluated BBB integrity by injecting NaFl following the same procedure reported by Kanoski et al. [1]. They found that the hippocampus was the brain structure that exhibit the highest concentration of the dye compared with prefrontal cortex and striatum. In this study, the researchers evaluate the differences between those animals, under HE diet, that show what they called *obesity resistant* versus those that developed obesity. The obesity resistant group was the one that consumed the HE diet but gained the least weight and body fat. The animals included in the obesity group were those that gained the most bodyweight and fat. It was this last group that showed the major BBB permeability and had the highest deposit of NaFl in the hippocampus. Interestingly, they found that those animals, in the HE diet, had the lowest bodyweight and the lowest amount of fat, and did not show difference in the behavioral performance compared with the control group. However, those rats that developed obesity and had the higher deposit of dye in the hippocampus, showed alterations in the performance of the hippocampal-dependent tasks [34]. These evidences directly shows a relationship between diets rich in fat, obesity development, and hippocampal-related cognitive alterations. We will discuss in the next section, the relevance of the hippocampal structure, cognitive performance, and its detriment.

From the information reviewed in this section, we can conclude that BBB alteration is a feature that takes part of dementia onset in both, AD and vascular dementia. Obesity can contribute to this phenomenon and, although the mechanism is not well known, a particular factor that can participate in this process is the intake of diets rich in cholesterol or fat, as well as glucose, those known components of a typical Western diet **(Figure 2)**.

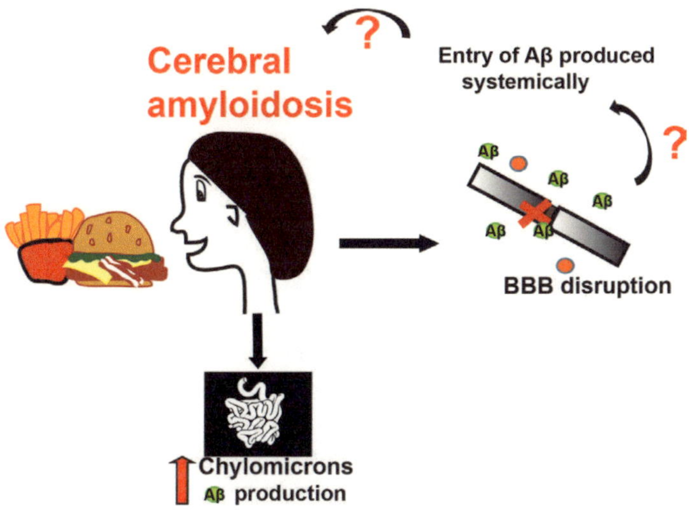

Figure 2. The overproduction of systemic Aβ, produced by consume diets rich on fat or cholesterol, can promote and alter the selective permeability of BBB, allowing the passage of molecules to the brain, such as systemic Aβ that was not clear and lead to cerebral amyloidosis and brain inflammation.

4. Impact of a diet rich in cholesterol or fat on the development of AD onset

The hippocampus is a brain structure considered as a part of the allocortex, which is one of the oldest brain areas from the phylogenetical point of view. It has a high capacity of plasticity; it is directly involved in learning and memory process and, interestingly, is very susceptible to damage and has attracted the research focus for several years since it is one of the first brain structures that degenerate during the AD process [35]. As we reviewed in the last section, the hippocampus seems to be very susceptible to the effect of consumed diets rich in fat or cholesterol, but can this actually drive the brain into a degenerative process? Can it contribute to the development of dementia? We will discuss this idea in the current section. First, we will review how the diet high in cholesterol or fat can contribute to the development of features associated with AD, particularly with amyloidosis.

Diets rich in cholesterol, as we have reviewed, can induce vascular inflammation, BBB, and promotes Aβ peptide accumulation in the brain parenchyma in an animal model of rabbit fed with high-cholesterol diet [26–28]. Supporting the association of elevated concentrations of cholesterol and AD detriment in a very recent *in vitro* study carried out by Avila-Muñoz and

Arias [36] in isolated astrocytes obtained from brain cortex of 1- to 3-day-old Wistar rats, they found astrocyte activation, An increase on the expression of amyloid precursor protein (APP), and promoted its amyloidogenic processing, and an increase in reactive species oxygen (ROS), a marker of oxidative stress, after treating the culture for 48 h with cholesterol concentrated at 25 or 50 μM. All these parameters measured, including glia activation, resemble features that have been found in postmortem brain tissues obtained from AD patients [37–39], but how the consumption of a diet high in cholesterol can contribute to the development of AD? *In vivo* studies can answer this question. Transgenic mice Tg2576 (which express the human APP695 carrying the Swedish double mutation at codons 595 and 596, Hsiao et al. [40]), were fed with a 5% cholesterol diet for 6 weeks. They found an increase of the APP cytosolic fragment but apparently the hypocholesteremia induced by the diet does not deregulates Aβ metabolism (George et al, 2004).

In a further work, carried out by Refolo et al [41], with 5-months-old double-mutant for presenilin (PS) and amyloid precursor protein (PSAPP) mice, which express familial mutant PS1M146V and the APP695 mutations [42], evaluated the effect of a combined diet with 5% cholesterol and 10% fat for 7 weeks. They found that the dietary treatment induced elevated levels of cholesterol in both, plasma and brain, which is an important data since it showed that brain cholesterol is produced *in situ,* and this data demonstrates that brain cholesterol is increased by diet. This increase in brain cholesterol correlates with an increase of total Aβ in brain. In addition, there was an enhanced amount of Aβ, particularly not in Aβ 1–40 and 1–42, but in 1–30 and 1–34 as well. This was accompanied with an increase in the number of Aβ deposits as well as an increase in the plaque area in the hypercholesteremic transgenic mice. Interestingly, there were no changes found in presenilin 1 (PS1) processing. These data strongly supported the hypothesis that a diet high in fat and cholesterol can contribute to the development of amyloidosis, one of the main conditions to develop AD.

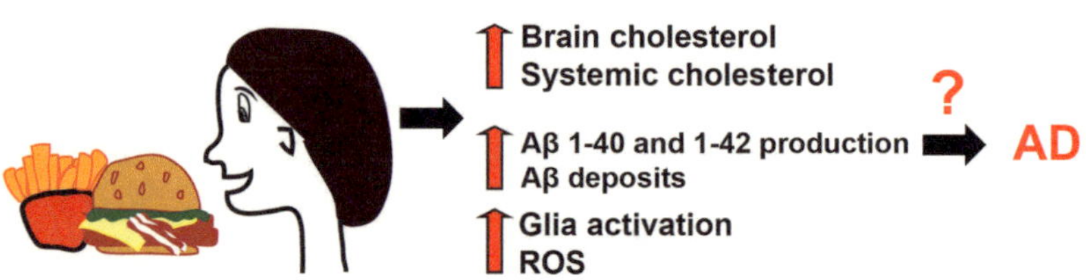

Figure 3. As result of consume diets high on fat and cholesterol there is an increase levels of brain cholesterol and systemic cholesterol. Also elevates Aβ production in brain and its deposit and increases as well the glia activation and production of ROS in brain. All these together can lead to AD onset.

All these data shows experimental evidence linking the consumption of diets rich in fat and/or cholesterol with the development of amyloidosis. Nevertheless, dementia is a more complex syndrome, comprised of many other features such as cognitive decline and neuronal lost. Particularly in the hippocampus, which is as we mentioned before, one of the first areas affected during the neurodegenerative process, its susceptibility to suffer alterations resulted from consuming diets high in fat or cholesterol appears crucial as one of the possible mechanism involved in the development of AD **(Figure 3)**. We will discuss that idea in the section below.

5. Impact on brain morphology, plasticity, and cognition

In the last sections, we have discussed how the consumption of diets rich in fat or cholesterol can contribute to the production of Aβ peptide in noncerebral tissue. The impact that this could have in the BBB selective permeability and its participation in brain amyloidosis conditions that can contribute to the dementia onset but, besides these alterations, one of the main conditions found in dementia patients is brain atrophy and behavioral alterations. Is brain functionality affected by the components typically found in the Western diet? Could diet composition affect brain architecture and plasticity? Moreover, is cognition affected the consumption of diets rich in fat or cholesterol? We will review such ideas in the current section.

A link between cognitive decline and dietary habits has been proposed. There is an epidemiological study carried out with Japanese men living in Hawaii compared with age-matched men living in Japan that evaluated the prevalence of dementia employing the Diagnostic and Statistical Manual of Mental Disorders. The results found that those subjects living in the USA have a higher prevalence of dementia: 9.3% for all type dementia, 5.4% for Alzheimer's disease, and 4.2% for vascular [43]. Continuing in this line of evidence, there is another study that was carried out with people from same ethnic background living in their natal land or in a foreign country (USA). They found in concordance with the study cited before, that those individual living in Indiana (where the study was carried out on) had a higher prevalence of dementia compared with age-matched individuals living in Nigeria or Ibadan [44]. This data strongly suggests that there are some stimuli in this Western country, which contribute to the development of several types of dementia, and the question is: what are these stimuli? A good candidate are the nutritional habits. In Western countries, especially countries such as the USA or Mexico, people consume food with high amounts of saturated fat and cholesterol and show the highest rates of obesity worldwide. The brain is an organ rich in lipids and essential fatty acids that are mainly obtained from food and have a crucial participation on brain functioning [45]. So, to think that lipids elevation induced by diet could be in detriment of the brain, which is a logical assumption, but what are the cellular mechanisms involved in the possible detrimental effect of food components such as fat and cholesterol? Well, experimental work has demonstrated evidence of the interplay between obesity, brain alteration, and cognitive decline, more especially with hippocampal-related cognitive processes. Seminal works in this area were carried out in the University of Toronto by Greenwood and Winocur [46]. They fed 1-month-old Long-Evans rats with two types of high-fat diets containing 40% of calories: a saturated fatty acids (lard-based) or a polyunsaturated fatty acids (soybean oil-based) and compared with a standard laboratory diet containing 4.5% of fat. They tested learning and memory abilities in the rats after 3 months of dietary treatment with the radial arm maze test, the variable-interval delayed alternation task, and the Hebb-Williams maze series. These tests evaluate spatial learning and memory performance and report failures in working or reference memories. They found that those animals fed with the lard-based diet showed impairment in all the tests. Following this line of evidence, they analyzed further with different types of saturated fatty acid diets: monounsaturated (MUFA) and polyunsaturated (PUFA) fatty acids, finding a direct relationship between the 3 months consumption of saturated fatty acids and failures in basic alternation rule, and remembering trial-specific information over time in the variable-interval delayed alternation task. Interestingly, they found alterations in brain's phosphatidylcholine fatty acid profile. However, the changes in the membrane did not correlate with cognitive alterations [47]. It suggested there is another mechanism elucidating the cognitive impairment related to consumption of diets rich in fat; a good candidate is brain inflammation. Chronic inflammation is one of the principal altered events associated with AD [48], and it has been linked to obesity and has been reported that there is a correlation between both, obesity and AD [49, 50]. Middle-aged C57BL6 male mice were fed for 21 weeks with chow equivalent to Western diet containing 41% fat or a high-fat lard diet containing 60% fat for 16 weeks. They showed an alteration on learning acquisition measured by the Stone T-maze and it is accompanied by microglial activation, increase expression of cytokines like TNFα, IL-6, and MCP-1, and a decrease on brain-derivated neurotrophic factor (BNDF) [51]. Interestingly, there was not any detrimental effect observed in those animals that consumed the like-Western diet. These data agree with results from Greenwood and Winocur and propose a possible way underlying the effect diet, which is an inflammation process, and the decrease on neural factors crucial for learning processes. The results demonstrate that diet can interfere with learning abilities, but is it everything behind the diet effect on cognitive decline? There is a report with 344 white middle-aged male Fischer rats. The researchers evaluate the effect of a diet high in cholesterol and fat (diet containing 2% cholesterol and 10% hydrogenated coconut oil). The results showed a failure in working memory, here evaluated with the water radial arm maze as well as elevated lipids profile and reduce expression of Map-2 as an indicator of alteration of dendritic integrity, which correlates with memory mistakes measured in the test, and increase in inflammation markers such as microglia activation [52]. In a study carried out with Sprague-Dawley rats, which were fed for 7 days with high fat and fructose, several hippocampal alterations, such as decreased insulin signaling, were reported. In addition, they found that treated animals had a decrease in hippocampus total weight in addition with some other morphological alterations such as a diminishment on the number of dendritic spines and a reduction in the complexity of the hippocampal dendritic arborization. Moreover, there was a decrease in the expression of the microtubule-associated protein 2 (MAP-2) and in the content of synaptophysin in the CA1 region concomitant with an increased phosphorylation of tau protein, and in the presence of reactive astrocyte associated [53]. It directly demonstrates alterations in hippocampal cytoarchitecture that definitively have a strong impact on brain functionality, especially in hippocampal-related learning and memory processes.

Another feature which affected by consuming diets rich in fat is adult hippocampal neurogenesis (AHN). Adult neurogenesis is a highly specialized plasticity phenomenon that, under basal conditions, occurs in two restricted brain areas: a) the subventricular zone and b) the hippocampal dentate gyrus [54, 55]. Hippocampus is a crucial area for memory processes, since its decrease is associated to memory failures, especially in short-term memory, spatial memory, and learning flexibility [56–59]. The AHN is a complex process that comprises several developmental steps starting from the division of an endogenous neural precursor cell followed by its expansion, differentiation, and fully integration to the hippocampal network [60]. These steps are reported as number of proliferative cells measured by markers of cell division; cell fate decision with the marker of early differentiation, the cytoeskeleton protein doublecortin (DCX) that is expressed in newly differentiated cells, and with NeuN, a nuclear marker of granular cells when the cell is fully differentiated. It has been recently documented that there are some food components which can regulate the neurogenic process (for a review [61]). The hippocampal neurogenesis has captured the attention since it was described in 1965 by Dass and Altman [62] due, as we already mentioned, the hippocampus is closely related to memory as well as neurodegenerative processes. Juvenile male and female Sprague-Dawley rats under a dietary regimen of high- (42% coconut butter and corn oil fat) or low-fat diet (10% fat by energy) or standard laboratory chow for 4 weeks, was found that males under high-fat diet show less cell proliferation than females and reported elevated levels of corticosterone, a stress hormone [63]. Differences in AHN were studied in mice susceptible to develop obesity (C57BL/6N) and obesity resistant (C3H/HeN). They were fed with high- and low-fat diet finding that those animals that developed obesity and consumed the high-fat diet had much lower number of proliferative cells and cells committed to neural linage (DCX positive cells), which establish a clear link between obesity and AHN diminishment [64]. In our laboratory, we have observed that 8 weeks of diet rich in fat (60%) or high in cholesterol (1.4%) in 5-months-old male Wistar rats has an impact on AHN in both, cell proliferation and more especially in the morphology of DCX cells. These cell populations have less processes and a poor complexity than animals under normal laboratory diet, and we found alterations in short-term memory (Leal-Galicia and Meraz-Ríos data *not yet published*). All these data together strongly suggest a detrimental effect on diets rich in fat or cholesterol in cognitive components such as navigation memory, working memory, acquisition learning, and short-term memory suggesting as mediators, alterations in brain cytoarchitecture and AHN, and associates obesity with such cognitive alterations strongly supporting the hypothesis that obesity can lead to development of dementia **(Figure 4)**.

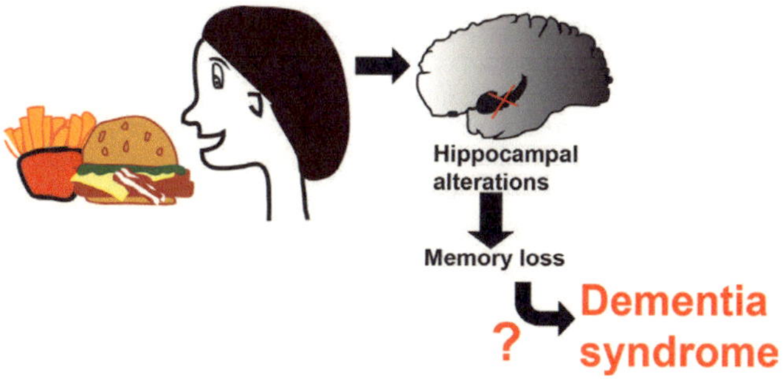

Figure 4. The intake of food with high amounts of fat or cholesterol produces alteration in the hippocampus such as: reduced expression of Map-2, reduction on the number of dendritic spines and in the complexity of the dendritic tree and a decrease on neurogenesis. Consume diets with these components has also a functional impact in short-term memory, working memory and learning flexibility, that could contribute to the detriment observed in the dementia syndrome.

6. Conclusion

The consumption of diets rich in cholesterol, fat, as well as another components (carbohydrates) of the so called "Western diet" can contribute to increase the production of the peptide Aβ. This could contribute to brain amyloidosis by means of alteration of the selective permeability of the BBB, since BBB alterations are induced for these type of diets. In addition, it has been shown in the brain of transgenic animals that the amyloidosis can be accelerated by the intake of fat or cholesterol, which can lead to accumulation of Aβ in the brain. Besides that, the intake of fat or cholesterol can induce alterations in brain morphology and plasticity accompanied by a detrimental in cognitive abilities in animal models that resemble those alterations in cognitive abilities reported in AD patients, such as short-term memory, working memory, and learning flexibility. These evidences strongly suggest an association with the dietary habits and the possible development of AD in both cases, Early Onset Alzheimer's Disease or Late Onset Alzheimer's Disease, and a connection with systemic disruptions and brain functions **(Figure 5)**.

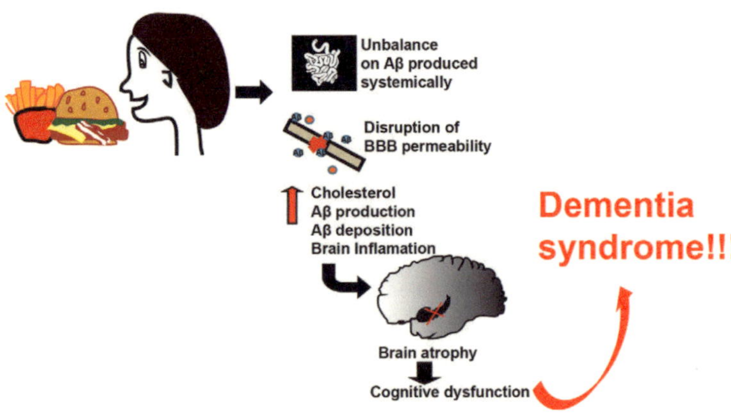

Figure 5. Diets rich on fat or cholesterol that are widely consume in Western countries can lead to develop dementia onset for several ways. One is the overproduction of systemic *Aβ* that can reach the brain due the chronic consume of these food components can affect the selective permeability of BBB. It can facilitate the pass of systemic *Aβ* as well as another molecules producing brain inflammation and *Aβ* deposits. It is accompanied for alterations in hippocampal plasticity and its cytoarchitecture. That can have an impact on brain functionality observed as memory failures. All these together can contribute to the development of dementia.

Author details

Marco Antonio Meraz-Ríos* and Perla Leal-Galicia

*Address all correspondence to: mmeraz@cinvestav.mx

Molecular Biomedicine Department, Center for Research and Advanced Studies of the National Polytechnic Institute, Mexico City, Mexico

References

[1] Kanoski SE, Zhang Y, Zheng W, Davidson TL. The effects of a high-energy diet on hippocampal function and blood-brain barrier integrity in the rat. J Alzheimers Dis. 2010;21:207–219. DOI: 10.3233/JAD-2010-091414

[2] Hsu TM, Kanoski SE. Blood-brain barrier disruption: mechanistic links between Western diet consumption and dementia. Front Aging Neurosci. 2014;9(6):88. DOI: 10.3389/fnagi.2014.00088

[3] Goldgaber D, Schwarzman AI, Bhasin R, Gregori L, Schmechel D, Saunders AM, et al. Sequestration of amyloid beta-peptide. Ann N Y Acad Sci. 1993;695:139–143.

[4] Wisniewski T, Ghiso J, Frangione B. Alzheimer's disease and soluble A beta. Neurobiol Aging. 1994;15:143–152.

[5] Seubert P, Vigo-Pelfrey C, Esch F, Lee M, Dovey H, Davis D, et al. Isolation and quantification of soluble Alzheimer's beta-peptide from biological fluids. Nature. 1992;359:325–327.

[6] Biere AL, Ostaszewski B, Stimson ER, Hyman BT, Maggio JE, Selkoe DJ. Amyloid beta-peptide is transported on lipoproteins and albumin in human plasma. J Biol Chem. 1996;271:32916–32922.

[7] Koudinov A, Matsubara E, Frangione B, Ghiso J. The soluble form of Alzheimer's amyloid beta protein is complexed to high density lipoprotein and very high density lipoprotein in normal human plasma. Biochem Biophys Res Commun. 1994;205:1164–1171.

[8] Koudinov AR, Berezov TT, Kumar A, Koudinova NV. Alzheimer's amyloid b interaction with normal human plasma high density lipoprotein: association with apolipoprotein and lipids. Clin Chim Acta. 1998;23:75–84.

[9] James AP, Pal S, Gennat HC, Vine DF, Mamo JC. The incorporation and metabolism of amyloid-beta into chylomicron-like lipid emulsions. J Alzheimer's Dis. 2003;5:179–188.

[10] Galloway S, Jian L, Johnsen R, Chew S, Mamo JC. Beta-amyloid or its precursor protein is found in epithelial cells of the small intestine and is stimulated by high-fat feeding. J Nutr Biochem. 2007;18:279–284.

[11] Koudinov AR, Koudinova NV. Alzheimer's soluble amyloid beta protein is secreted by HepG2 cells as an apolipoprotein. Cell Biol Int. 1997;21:265–271.

[12] Strittmatter WJ, Weisgraber KH, Huang DY, Dong LM, Salvesen GS, Pericak-Vance M, Schmechel D, Saunders AM, Goldgaber D, Roses AD. Binding of human apolipoprotein E to synthetic amyloid beta peptide: isoform-specific effects and implications for late-onset Alzheimer disease. Proc Natl Acad Sci U S A. 1993;90:8098–8102.

[13] LaDu MJ, Lukens JR, Reardon CA, Getz GS. Association of human, rat, and rabbit apolipoprotein E with beta-amyloid. J Neurosci Res. 1997;49:9–18.

[14] Ye S, Huang Y, Mullendorff K, Dong L, Giedt G, Meng EC, Cohen FE, Kuntz ID, Weisgraber KH, Mahley RW. Apolipoprotein (apo) E4 enhances amyloid beta peptide production in cultured neuronal cells: apoE structure as a potential therapeutic target. Proc Natl Acad Sci U S A. 2005;102:18700–18705.

[15] Galloway S, Pallebage-Gamarallage MM, Takechi R, Jian L, Johnsen RD, Dhaliwal SS, Mamo JC. Synergistic effects of high fat feeding and apolipoprotein E deletion on enterocytic amyloid-beta abundance. Lipids Health Dis. 2008;22:15. DOI: 10.1186/1476-511X-7-15

[16] Galloway S, Takechi R, Pallebage-Gamarallage MM, Dhaliwal SS, Mamo JC. Amyloid-beta co-localizes with apolipoprotein B in absorptive cells of the small intestine. Lipids Health Dis. 2009;22:8–46. DOI: 10.1186/1476-511X-8-46

[17] Saunders NR, Habgood MD, Møllgård K, Dziegielewska KM. The biological significance of brain barrier mechanisms: help or hindrance in drug delivery to the central nervous system? F1000Research 2016, 5(F1000 Faculty Rev):313. DOI: 10.12688/f1000research.7378.1

[18] Gustafson DR, Karlsson C, Skoog I, Rosengren L, Lissner L, Blennow K. Mid-life adiposity factors relate to blood-brain barrier integrity in late life. J Intern Med. 2007;262:643–650.

[19] Heiss CJ, Sanborn CF, Nichols DL, Bonnick SL, Alford BB. Associations of body fat distribution, circulating sex hormones, and bone density in postmenopausal women. J Clin Endocrinol Metab. 1995;80:1591–1596.

[20] Tchernof A, Després JP, Bélanger A, Dupont A, Prud'homme D, Moorjani S, Lupien PJ, Labrie F. Reduced testosterone and adrenal C19 steroid levels in obese men. Metabolism. 1995;44:513–519.

[21] Kalish GM, Barrett-Connor E, Laughlin GA, Gulanski BI. Association of endogenous sex hormones and insulin resistance among postmenopausal women: results from the postmenopausal estrogen/progestin intervention trial. J Clin Endocrinol Metab. 2003;88:1646–1652.

[22] Henderson VW, St John JA, Hodis HN, McCleary CA, Stanczyk FZ, Karim R, Shoupe D, Kono N, Dustin L, Allayee H, Mack WJ. Cognition, mood, and physiological concentrations of sex hormones in the early and late postmenopause. Proc Natl Acad Sci U S A. 2013;10:20290–20295. DOI: 10.1073/pnas.1312353110

[23] Ding EL, Song Y, Malik VS, Liu S. Sex differences of endogenous sex hormones and risk of type 2 diabetes: a systematic review and meta-analysis. JAMA. 2006;295:1288–1299.

[24] Lindstedt G, Lundberg PA, Lapidus L, Lundgren H, Bengtsson C, Bjorntorp P. Low sex-hormone-binding globulin concentration as independent risk factor for develop-

ment of NIDDM. 12-yr follow-up of population study of women in Gothenburg, Sweden. Diabetes. 1991;40:123–128.

[25] Lapidus L, Lindstedt G, Lundberg PA, Bengtsson C, Gredmark T. Concentrations of sex-hormone binding globulin and corticosteroid binding globulin in serum in relation to cardiovascular risk factors and to 12-year incidence of cardiovascular disease and overall mortality in postmenopausal women. Clin Chem. 1986;32:146–152.

[26] Sparks DL, Scheff SW, Hunsaker JC 3rd, Liu H, Landers T, Gross DR. Induction of Alzheimer-like β-amyloid immunoreactivity in the brains of rabbits with dietary cholesterol. Exp Neurol. 1994;126:88–94.

[27] Sparks, DL. Dietary cholesterol induces Alzheimer-like β-amyloid immunoreactivity in rabbit brain. Nutr Metab Cardiovasc. 1997;7:255–266.

[28] Sparks DL, Kuo YM, Roher A, Martin T, Lukas RJ. Alterations of Alzheimer's disease in the cholesterol-fed rabbit, including vascular inflammation. Preliminary observations. Ann N Y Acad Sci. 2000;903:335–344.

[29] Blennow K, Wallin A, Fredman P, Karlsson I, Gottfries CG, Svennerholm L. Blood–brain barrier disturbance in patients with Alzheimer's disease is related to vascular factors. Acta Neurol Scand. 1990;81:323–326.

[30] Skoog I, Wallin A, Fredman P, Hesse C, Aevarsson O, Karlsson I, Gottfries CG, Blennow K. A population study on blood–brain barrier function in 85-year-olds: relation to Alzheimer's disease and vascular dementia. Neurology. 1998;50:966–971.

[31] Mecocci P, Parnetti L, Reboldi GP, Santucci C, Gaiti A, Ferri C, Gernini I, Romagnoli M, Cadini D, Senin U. Blood-brain-barrier in a geriatric population: barrier function in degenerative and vascular dementias. Acta Neurol Scand. 1991;84:210–213.

[32] Zlokovic BV, Ghiso J, Mackic JB, McComb JG, Weiss MH, Frangione B. Blood-brain barrier transport of amyloid beta peptides in efflux pump knock-out animals evaluated by in vivo optical imaging . Biochem Biophys Res Commun. 1993;30:1034–1040.

[33] Sparks DL. Neuropathologic links between Alzheimer's disease and vascular disease. In: Iqbal K, Swaab DF, Winblad B, Wisniewski HM, editors. Alzheimer's Disease and Related Disorders. New York: John Wiley & Sons Ltd.; 1999, Vol 6, pp. 153–163.

[34] Davidson TL, Monnot A, Neal AU, Martin AA, Horton JJ, Zheng W. The effects of a high-energy diet on hippocampal-dependent discrimination performance and blood–brain barrier integrity differ for diet-induced obese and diet-resistant rats. Physiol Behav. 2012;20:26–33. DOI: 10.1016/j.physbeh.2012.05.015

[35] Arendt T. Alzheimer's disease as a loss of differentiation control in a subset of neurons that retain immature features in the adult brain. Neurobiol Aging. 2000;21:783–796.

[36] Avila-Muñoz E, Arias C. Cholesterol-induced astrocyte activation is associated with increased amyloid precursor protein expression and processing. GLIA 2015;63:2010–2022. DOI: 10.1002/glia.22874.

[37] Sidoryk-Wegrzynowicz M, Wegrzynowicz M, Lee E, Bowman AB, Aschner M. Role of astrocytes in brain function and disease. Toxicol Pathol. 2011;39:115–123.

[38] Wharton SB, O'Callaghan JP, Savva GM, Nicoll JA, Matthews F, Simpson JE, Forster G, Shaw PJ, Brayne C, Ince PG; MRC Cognitive Function and Ageing Neuropathology Study Group. 2009. Population variation in glial fibrillary acidic protein levels in brain ageing: relationship to Alzheimer type pathology and dementia. Dement Geriatr Cogn Disord. 2009;27:465–473.

[39] George AJ, Holsinger RM, McLean CA, Laughton KM, Beyreuther K, Evin G, Masters CL, Li QX. APP intracellular domain is increased and soluble AB is reduced with diet-induced hypercholesterolemia in a transgenic mouse model of Alzheimer disease. Neurobiol Dis. 2004;16:124–132.

[40] Hsiao K, Chapman P, Nilsen S, Eckman C, Harigaya Y, Younkin S, Yang F, Cole G. Correlative memory deficits, Abeta elevation, and amyloid plaques in transgenic mice. Science. 1996;274:99–102.

[41] Refolo LM, Malester B, LaFrancois J, Bryant-Thomas T, Wang R, Tint GS, Sambamurti K, Duff K, Pappolla MA. Hypercholesterolemia accelerates the Alzheimer's amyloid pathology in a transgenic mouse model. Neurobiol Dis. 2000;7:321–331. DOI: 10.1006/nbdi.2000.0304

[42] McGowan E, Sanders S, Iwatsubo T, Takeuchi A, Saido T, Zehr C, Yu X, Uljon S, Wang R, Mann D, Dickson D, Duff K. Amyloid phenotype characterization of transgenic mice overexpressing both mutant amyloid precursor protein and mutant presenilin 1 transgenes. Neurobiol Dis. 1999;6:231–244.

[43] White L, Petrovitch H, Ross GW, Masaki KH, Abbott RD, Teng EL, Rodriguez BL, Blanchette PL, Havlik RJ, Wergowske G, Chiu D, Foley DJ, Murdaugh C, Curb JD. Prevalence of dementia in older Japanese-American men in Hawaii. JAMA. 1996;276:955–960.

[44] Hendrie HC, Osuntokun BO, Hall KS, Ogunniyi AO, Hui SL, Unverzagt FW, Gureje O, Rodenberg CA, Baiyewu O, Musick BS. Prevalence of Alzheimer's disease and dementia in two communities: Nigerian Africans and African Americans. Am J Psychiatry. 1995;152:1485–1492.

[45] Vance JE, Karten B, Hayashi H. Lipid dynamics in neurons. Biochem Soc Trans. 2006;34:399–403.

[46] Greenwood CE, Winocur G. Learning and memory impairment in rats fed a high saturated fat diet. Behav Neural Biol. 1990;53:74–87.

[47] Greenwood CE, Winocur G . Cognitive impairment in rats fed high-fat diets: a specific effect of saturated fatty-acid intake. Behav Neurosci. 1996;110:451–459. DOI: 10.1037/0735-7044.110.3.451

[48] Combs CK. Inflammation and microglia actions in Alzheimer's disease. J Neuroimmune Pharmacol. 2009;4:380–388.

[49] Chandalia M, Abate N. Metabolic complications of obesity: inflated or inflamed? J Diabetes Complicat. 2007;21:128–138.

[50] Rader DJ. Inflammatory markers of coronary risk. N Engl J Med. 2000;343:1179–1182.

[51] Pistell PJ, Morrison CD, Gupta S, Knight AG, Keller JN, Ingram DK, Bruce-Keller AJ. Cognitive impairment following high fat diet consumption is associated with brain inflammation. J Neuroimmunol. 2010;219:25–32. DOI: 10.1016/j.jneuroim.2009.11.010

[52] Granholm AC, Bimonte-Nelson HA, Moore AB, Nelson ME, Freeman LR, Sambamurti K. Effects of a saturated fat and high cholesterol diet on memory and hippocampal morphology in the middle-aged rat. J Alzheimer's Dis. 2008;14:133–145.

[53] Calvo-Ochoa E, Hernández-Ortega K, Ferrera P, Morimoto S, Arias C. Short-term high-fat-and-fructose feeding produces insulin signaling alterations accompanied by neurite and synaptic reduction and astroglial activation in the rat hippocampus. J Cereb Blood Flow Metab. 2014;34:1001–1008. DOI: 10.1038/jcbfm

[54] Alvarez-Buylla A, Seri B, Doetsch F. Identification of neural stem cells in the adult vertebrate brain. Brain Res Bull. 2002;57:751–758.

[55] Kempermann G. Why new neurons? Possible functions for adult hippocampal neurogenesis. J Neurosci. 2002;22:635–638.

[56] Kempermann G, Kuhn HG, Gage FH. More hippocampal neurons in adult mice living in an enriched environment. Nature. 1997;3:493–495.

[57] Leal-Galicia P, Castañeda-Bueno M, Quiroz-Baez R, Arias C. Long-term exposure to environmental enrichment since youth prevents recognition memory decline and increases synaptic plasticity markers in aging. Neurobiol Learn Mem. 2008;90:511–518. DOI: 10.1016/j.nlm.2008.07.005

[58] Garthe A, Huang Z, Kaczmarek L, Filipkowski RK, Kempermann G. Not all water mazes are created equal: cyclin D2 knockout mice with constitutively suppressed adult hippocampal neurogenesis do show specific spatial learning deficits. Genes Brain Behav. 2014;13:357–364. DOI: 10.1111/gbb.12130

[59] Garthe A, Roeder I, Kempermann G. Mice in an enriched environment learn more flexibly because of adult hippocampal neurogenesis. Hippocampus. 2016;26:261–271. DOI: 10.1002/hipo.22520

[60] Kempermann G, Jessberger S, Steiner B, Kronenberg G. Milestones of neuronal development in the adult hippocampus. Trends Neurosci. 2004;27:447–452.

[61] Zainuddin MS, Thuret S. Nutrition, adult hippocampal neurogenesis and mental health. Br Med Bull. 2012;103:89–114. DOI: 10.1093/bmb/lds021

[62] Altman J, Das GD. Autoradiographic and histological evidence of postnatal hippocampal neurogenesis in rats. J Comp Neurol. 1965;124:319–335.

[63] Lindqvist A, Mohapel P, Bouter B, Frielingsdorf H, Pizzo D, Brundin P, Erlanson-Albertsson C. High-fat diet impairs hippocampal neurogenesis in male rats. Eur J Neurol. 2006;13:1385–1388.

[64] Hwang IK, Kim IY, Kim DW, Yoo KY, Kim YN, Yi SS, Won MH, Lee IS, Yoon YS, Seong JK. Strain-specific differences in cell proliferation and differentiation in the dentate gyrus of C57BL/6N and C3H/HeN mice fed a high fat diet. Brain Res. 2008;19:1–6. DOI: 10.1016/j.brainres

Chapter 4

Plasma Biomarkers in Alzheimer's Disease

Hitoshi Sohma and Yasuo Kokai

Additional information is available at the end of the chapter

http://dx.doi.org/10.5772/64512

Abstract

Biomarker study on dementia has developed widely. In applying biomarkers, there seems to be several utilizations such as presymptomatic- and early-stage detection, differential diagnosis, and evaluation of treatment effect. Currently, most reliable fluid markers are amyloid peptide (Aβ) with microtubule-associated protein tau (TAU) and phosphorylated TAU (P-TAU) detected in cerebrospinal fluid (CSF). $A\beta_{42}$ correlates with plaque pathology, TAU reflects the intensity of neuroaxonal degeneration, and P-TAU may correlate with neurofibrillary tangle (NFT) pathology. An attenuation of the level of $A\beta_{42}$ and elevation in the ratio of $A\beta_{42}$ relative to the shorter major species of $A\beta_{42}$ peptide with 40 amino acid residues ($A\beta_{40}$) has been identified as significant events in the early stage of Alzheimer's disease (AD) pathology. In addition, there is great interest in blood-based markers of AD since blood extraction is much less invasive. Moreover, plasma biomarkers can be measured at relatively low expense once a standard system of measurement is established. Although there is not yet an established or validated diagnostic test for plasma biomarkers, there is great interest in blood-based markers. We will summarize reported biomarkers, describe our novel potential plasma biomarker for AD (annexin A5), offering a strategy for selecting candidates, and show our results and evaluation.

Keywords: plasma biomarker, Alzheimer's disease, annexin A5, $A\beta_{42}$, Ca^{2+}-stress

1. Introduction

The augmented number of dementia patients has been dramatic due to the aging of society in advanced countries. Alzheimer's disease (AD) is the most common type of dementia and accounts for more than half (50–70% depending on the reports) of all dementia. AD is characterized by a gradual onset by developing neuronal damage and continuing cognitive decline related to stress-induced cell damage in the patient's brain [1], which ultimately causes significant impairment to social and occupational functions. The mean duration from the onset of clinical symptoms to the death of the patient has been reported to be approximately 8.5 years [2].

AD is defined by the presence of plaques and tangles in the brain, thus the gold standard for the diagnosis of Alzheimer's disease (AD) is set by means of the histological examination of brain tissue at autopsy, which is usually done after a patient has died, or, rarely, following brain biopsy. On the other hand, clinical diagnosis of AD during life has been performed with a sensitivity ranging from 70.9% to 87.3% and specificity from 44.3% to 70.8% [3]. It was also reported that dementia is often overlooked in community care settings [4].

For objective diagnostic analysis, several biomarkers are available. The reliable biomarker candidates for AD include brain imaging studies using magnetic resonance imaging (MRI) or positron emission tomography (PET), and proteins in cerebrospinal fluid (CSF). MRI is utilized for structural imaging, PET for molecular imaging of amyloid deposition and fluoro-deoxy-D-glucose (FDG)-PET for metabolic imaging, while measurements of amyloid peptide (Aβ) and TAU protein in cerebrospinal fluid (CSF) are used for quantitative analysis. However, structural changes measured by MRI only become apparent in the late stage of AD. Moreover, structural MRI and FDG-PET images are not direct measures of the core pathological hallmarks of AD. PET imaging is relatively expensive and limited in availability. CSF Aβ and TAU might be nonspecific for AD depending on each case [5]. At present, it can be stated that the most well-characterized and validated biomarkers are Aβ and TAU in CSF: the decrease in Aβ with 42 amino acid residues ($A\beta_{42}$) and increase in TAU and phosphorylated TAU (P-TAU) has been observed in AD patients in several of studies [6].

An alternative method to the invasive CSF collection and expensive specialized facilities for diagnostic imaging is most desirable. Thus, plasma biomarkers have raised expectations because blood sampling is a much less invasive procedure. Blood-based biomarkers have the potential to overcome access and cost barriers and greatly facilitate advanced neuroimaging and cerebrospinal fluid biomarker approaches. Due to the fact that preanalytical processing shows the largest variation in laboratory testing, there are currently no available standardized preanalytical guidelines. In this review, the primary focus is on the fluid biomarkers, especially blood plasma protein biomarkers, as indicators of AD development together with our study on results of a specific blood plasma candidate.

2. CSF markers

Diagnostic markers are anticipated to be present in secreted proteins followed by a result of cell damage in pathological states. Although CSF sampling by lumbar puncture definitely is known to be an invasive procedure, at present CSF is probably the most informative fluid in biomarker detection for neurodegenerative disease prognosis [7]. CSF has direct contact with the brain, and it does not easily escape from the brain owing to the fact that the blood-brain barrier (BBB) is tightly regulated. In general, if a biomarker candidate is identified in CSF, its possibility as a true biomarker for brain-specific activities, as well as disease pathology, would be considered to be more promising compared with any other body fluid biomarker candidate.

It has been demonstrated that senile plaque formation and neuronal loss precede clinical onset of Alzheimer's disease [8]. Senile plaques are polymorphous and comprise Amyloid β peptide (Aβ), a proteolytic product of amyloid precursor protein (APP) that accumulates in the brains of AD patients. Several species of Aβ peptide depending on the cleavage sites on APP have been identified in the body fluid. APP processing consists of initially proteolysis by β-secretase and then by β-secretase, which leads to the formation of Aβ peptides with 38–43 residues [9]. Of these, $A\beta_{42}$ with 42 amino acid residues is the most remarkably focused due to its toxic effect. $A\beta_{42}$ is highly hydrophobic and forms oligomers and fibrils that accumulate as extracellular plaques, which correlates inversely with plaque pathology [1, 10]. Attenuated activity of Aβ-degrading catabolic enzymes including neprilysin and insulin-degrading enzymes with age or abnormal production of Aβ due to gene mutation(s) of related proteins such as on APP have been identified, which in turn leads to the accumulation of $A\beta_{42}$ in the brain tissue [11].

On the other hand, TAU that is an intracellular protein, is believed to be involved in filament stabilization, and has been shown to aggregate to form filaments in neurons. In normal individuals, only a low concentration of TAU is present in CSF. The function of TAU is tightly regulated by a number of posttranslational modifications possibly due to phosphorylation at serine and threonine residues. Several studies have suggested that hyperphosphorylation and formation of neurofibrillary tangles (NFTs) is the pathophysiological phenomenon of the development of AD [12]. It is remarkable that functional loss of TAU following hyperphosphorylation, the dissociation of TAU from microtubule and subsequent polymerization into insoluble paired helical filaments (PHF) could result in the loss of axonal integrity in the neuronal cells [13, 14]. NFT formation and neuronal degradation is an essential part of AD pathology.

Due to significant disruption of the neuronal architecture, the TAU and its hyperphosphorylated form (P-TAU) could appear in CSF [15]. Therefore, the phenomenon of increased levels of TAU and P-TAU in CSF represents well with the onset of neurodegeneration in AD. The total TAU (t-TAU) concentration in CSF has been measured by the method of ELISA using monoclonal antibodies against all TAU isoforms. Several groups have indicated that t-TAU concentration in CSF of AD patients is significantly higher than control [15, 16]. On the other hand, the attenuation of the amount of $A\beta_{42}$ in CSF has been noted due to accumulation in the brain [17]. Thus, decrease in level of $A\beta_{42}$, increase in t-TAU and P-TAU have been utilized as CSF biomarkers contributing to the diagnosis of AD [18]. In addition, the development of imaging biomarkers has provided evidence of an ongoing AD pathophysiological process.

The Aβ ratio ($A\beta_{40}$ to $A\beta_{42}$) in the AD group was significantly increased compared with that in the normal control group, the non-AD type dementia group, and the other neuronal disease group [19]. For the enhancement of the diagnostic relevance of AD, AD index that is calculated by multiplying TAU level by the Aβ ratio was shown to be useful for discrimination of AD patients from healthy controls with good sensitivity and specificity [19].

It was reported that low CSF level of $A\beta_{42}$ appeared to predict conversion of mild cognitive impairment (MCI) to AD, while a decrease in $A\beta_{42}$ level has also been observed in other neurodegenerative disorders [20]. Furthermore, it was shown that levels of TAU and P-TAU at Ser181 (P-TAU181) in CSF, but not $A\beta_{42}$, correlated oppositely with whole brain volume in the early stage of AD, whereas levels of CSF Aβ_{42}, but not TAU or P-TAU181, was positively correlated with whole brain volume in nondemented controls [17].

It is thought that the production and accumulation of unfavorable Aβ species proceeds over time as the disease progresses. Abnormal activity by the Aβ species is initiated before pathological change and reaches a plateau before the clinical symptoms appear. Thereafter, elevation of TAU and P-TAU that are the biomarkers for neuronal injury, dysfunction, and degeneration, become apparent in the later stage of the disease and correlate with clinical symptom severity [8]. On the other hand, MRI imaging is valuable as it is the last biomarker to show abnormality. As such, MRI retains a closer relationship with cognitive performance later on in the disease compared with other biomarkers. Moreover, none of the biomarkers is stable; that is, the rate of change for each biomarker is not linear over time [8].

The revised guideline for AD diagnosis was released by a working group from the National Institute of Aging in 2011, in which both CSF and imaging biomarkers have been implemented. The new guideline provides evidence of an ongoing AD pathophysiological process, and it is also possible to make a preclinical diagnosis of MCI due to AD [21–23]. AD is classified into three separate stages: preclinical AD, MCI due to AD, and AD with dementia.

Since fluid biomarkers of either CSF or blood plasma can serve as objective criteria for dementia diagnosis, this guideline is aiming at early and reliable diagnosis. However, it is clear that at present no single biomarker plays a sufficient discriminatory role in screening for future development of late-onset AD or dementia.

3. Plasma markers

Compared with CSF, blood sampling is a less invasive procedure, more easily accessible, and cost reductive, thus the finding of reliable blood biomarkers for AD is being given the highest priority. There has been an increasing research effort to examine the potential biomarkers of AD in blood plasma. However, for blood-based biomarkers, it has to be noted that blood plasma contains several tens of thousands of different proteins. In addition, the range of protein concentrations are extremely varied (attaining to 12 orders of magnitude), and the lower the concentration, the greater the diversity of proteins [24, 25]. Moreover, none of the current methods allows us to directly detect components in the low concentration region [25]. These conditions make it extremely challenging or almost impossible to directly analyze blood, even though possible biomarker candidates are more likely to be present in the areas of low concentration. The change in concentration of the blood components may often be on a very small scale and cover a wide range of both peripheral and central processes. Additionally, the less abundant proteins may be masked by highly abundant plasma proteins such as albumin and immunoglobulin. Therefore, focusing on concentration change of a particular AD-specific marker, which may be in low concentration, can be the most challenging to discover [26, 27].

It was reported that the BBB is disrupted resulting in increased permeability with aging and in AD [28, 29]. It is also thought that this event occurs in the relatively early stage of the aging brain, which is related to increased cognitive impairment. Although the relationship between an analyte found as a biomarker candidate in blood plasma and the behavioral changes in the brain is not easily demonstrated, there is the possibility of a connection due to BBB disruption during the early stage. This might lead one to expect the possible appearance of a brain component in the peripheral blood stream.

The widely accepted CSF biomarker, Aβ peptides, have also been examined in blood, but its concentration in blood plasma is considerably lower than reported in CSF by about 100-fold [30]. Elevated plasma level of either $A\beta_{40}$ [31, 32] or $A\beta_{42}$ [33, 34] levels was used as an indicator for the development of AD, while the opposite results [35] or no association at all between plasma Aβ level and AD development [36, 37] were reported. Thus, results based on plasma Aβ as a biomarker have been inconsistent. A low plasma $A\beta_{42}$ to $A\beta_{40}$ ratio was utilized for the prediction of future AD [32, 38, 39], while contrary results, reporting a higher ratio [31, 33] in the nascent AD stage patients than the subjects who did not develop AD, and no significant differences were also shown [36].

Another promising candidate of a plasma protein biomarker was identified by means of the proteomic approach. The protein clusterin/apolipoprotein J, which is involved in the clearance of cellular debris and apoptosis, was associated with both hippocampal atrophy and clinical progression [40]. Increased plasma concentration of clusterin indicated the prediction of greater fibrillary amyloid-β burden in the medial temporal lobe and AD patients had increased clusterin messenger RNA in blood. Moreover, in the transgenic AD mouse model (APP/PS1), increased plasma clusterin level, age-dependent increase in brain clusterin, as well as amyloid and clusterin colocalization in plaques were shown [40, 41]. The recent finding is that increased plasma clusterin levels have been associated with increased risk of conversion to AD and the rate of cognitive decline [42]. Clusterin may have a role in Aβ aggregation and clearance [43, 44], and at high concentrations, clusterin may prevent Aβ aggregation through its binding to Aβ. Furthermore, clusterin possesses neurotoxic properties by involvement in noncanonical wnt signaling, which mediates Aβ toxicity [45]. Therefore, clusterin might fulfill different roles. Other plasma biomarker candidates have been reported, such as desmosterol [46], transthyretin [47], chitinase 3-like 1 protein [48], and matrix metalloproteinase 2 [49], which may be associated with AD. Using protein array technology, Ray et al. found 18 signaling proteins in blood plasma that can discriminate AD samples from control subjects with approximately 90% accuracy [50].

4. Another plasma biomarker study

The brain-derived proteins present in blood plasma are limited compared with those in CSF due to the presence of the BBB. It is also likely that if potential brain-derived proteins are present in blood plasma, it is conceivable they are considerably diluted in the large volume of plasma and underwent proteolysis and excretion. These possible events make the study more challenging. As mentioned previously, in plasma, there are several tens of thousands of different proteins present at concentrations in the millimolar to femtomolar or lower range.

This extremely varied range of protein concentrations in plasma makes it almost impossible to directly analyze low concentration components.

Therefore, in our study, instead of direct examination of plasma, we initially utilized a cell culture model, mouse primary culture neuron. After Aβ-treatment, we identified proteins present outside of the cells (culture supernatant), in which Aβ-dependent secreted proteins are expected to be present, using a proteomic approach, and focused on the proteins that were increased by Aβ-treatment, and discovered a biomarker candidate. Ultimately, we verified the potential candidate with animal model (transgenic mice) and human plasma samples (**Figure 1**).

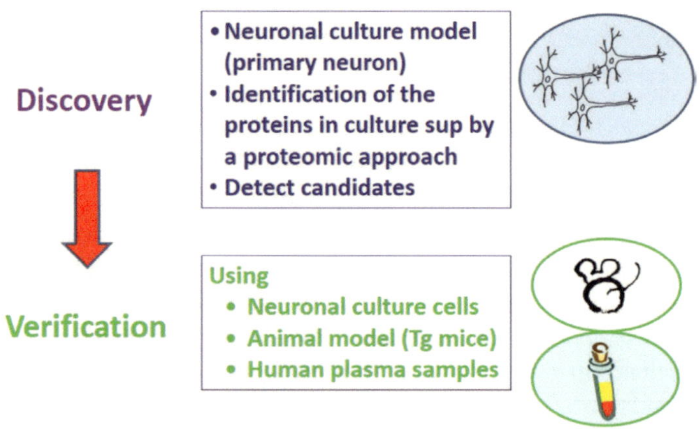

Figure 1. Process of biomarker identification (our study).

The cytotoxicity due to $A\beta_{42}$ is thought to be directly linked to neural cell death [1]. Amyloid-dependent neurotoxicity is known to perturb Ca^{2+} homeostasis in neuronal cells [51]. Possibly, Aβ impairs membrane Ca^{2+} pumps and enhances Ca^{2+} influx through voltage-dependent channels and ionotropic glutamate receptors (**Figure 2**).

By focusing on this mechanism, we identified the Ca^{2+}-related protein as a potential biomarker for AD using primary neurons as a cell culture model [52]. Since phosphatidylserine (PS) is flip-flopped and appears in the outer layer of the plasma membrane during the apoptotic process, we focused on PS-binding proteins in the culture supernatant and used a unique method to identify a potential biomarker candidate.

Thermoresponsive magnetic nanoparticles disperse well in an aqueous solution at a temperature below 10°C and are aggregated and become responsive to magnets at 20°C or higher. In this study, we coated magnetic beads with thermoresponsive polymers (polyethyleneimine) together with myristate and then coated them with PS [52]. We mixed these particles with a culture supernatant in the presence of Ca^{2+} and collected the PS binding fraction with ethylene glycol-bis(β-aminoethyl ether)-N,N,N',N'-tetraacetic acid (EGTA). After running SDS-PAGE, we performed in-gel digestion with trypsin and analyzed the tryptic peptides by reverse-phase liquid chromatography coupled with MALDI TOF/TOF MS spectrometry and performed database analysis for peptide sequencing. From this proteomic approach, about 240 types of proteins were indicated to be increased in the $A\beta_{42}$-treated sample, compared with the control, suggesting that they were upregulated by $A\beta_{42}$. From among these proteins, we focused on annexin A5, one of the annexin family proteins that commonly bind Ca^{2+} and phospholipid. It was shown that annexin A5 was augmented in both the brain and blood plasma in an AD-model mouse (Tg2576 transgenic mice), overexpressing mutant human APP [52]. Technetium-labeled annexin A5 was detectable in the brain after intravenous injection in humans, showing that annexin A5 crosses the BBB [53].

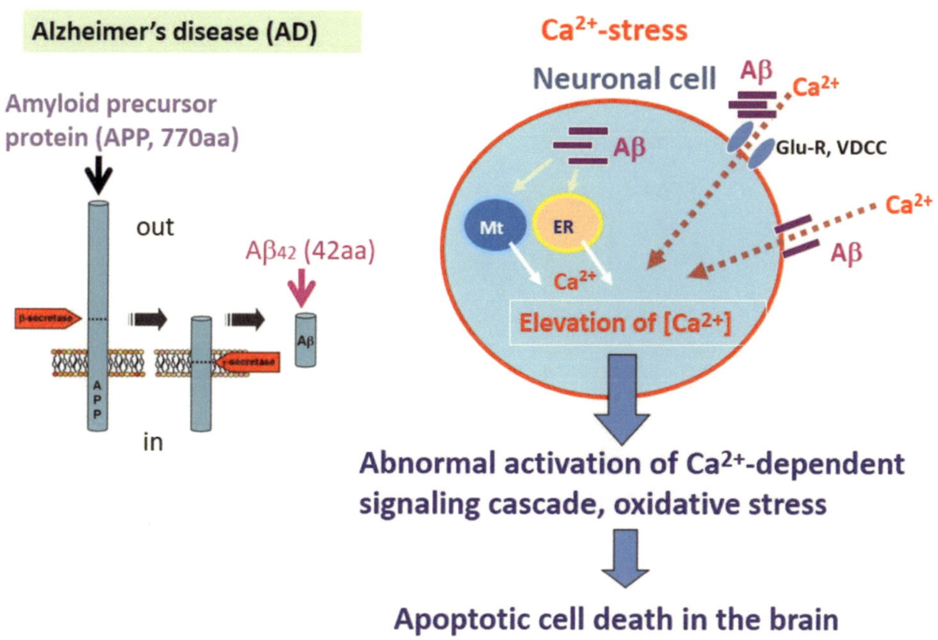

Figure 2. Aβ-dependent perturbation of calcium homeostasis in AD.

4.1. Methods

To quantify plasma annexin A5, we previously established the chemiluminescent enzyme immunoassay (CLEIA) system with two clones of monoclonal antibodies against human annexin A5: one clone was conjugated to a glass bead and used for trapping annexin A5 present in the blood plasma; the other clone was labeled with horseradish peroxidase (HRP) and used for quantification of the trapped annexin A5 [52]. The HRP catalyzes the oxidation of a luminol solution that includes a phenol-derivative acting as an enhancer, and produces light. This system was useful to quantify plasma annexin A5 in the range from 0.16 to 20.0 ng/ml [52]. We obtained blood samples from 150 AD, 50 DLB, 14 mild cognitive impairment (MCI), and six depression patients, and 298 healthy elderly individuals from the senior citizen's clubs. AD patients met NINCDS-ADRDA [54] and DLB patients diagnosed as probable DLB according to the latest consensus diagnostic criteria [55]. Statistical analysis was done using JMP version 9.0.0 (SAS Institute Inc., Cary, NC, USA). The mean response of each experimental group was compared with its simultaneous control by unpaired Student's *t*-test, setting a significant difference at $P < 0.05$. To examine the plasma annexin A5 levels in diagnoses of AD, DLB, and MCI, logistic regression modeling was employed to construct receiver operator (ROC) curves.

The plasma level of annexin A5 was significantly increased in AD patients compared to that of a control group (P-value < 0.0001 in the logistic regression analysis), suggesting that annexin A5 is a potentially positive biomarker for AD (**Figure 3**) [52].

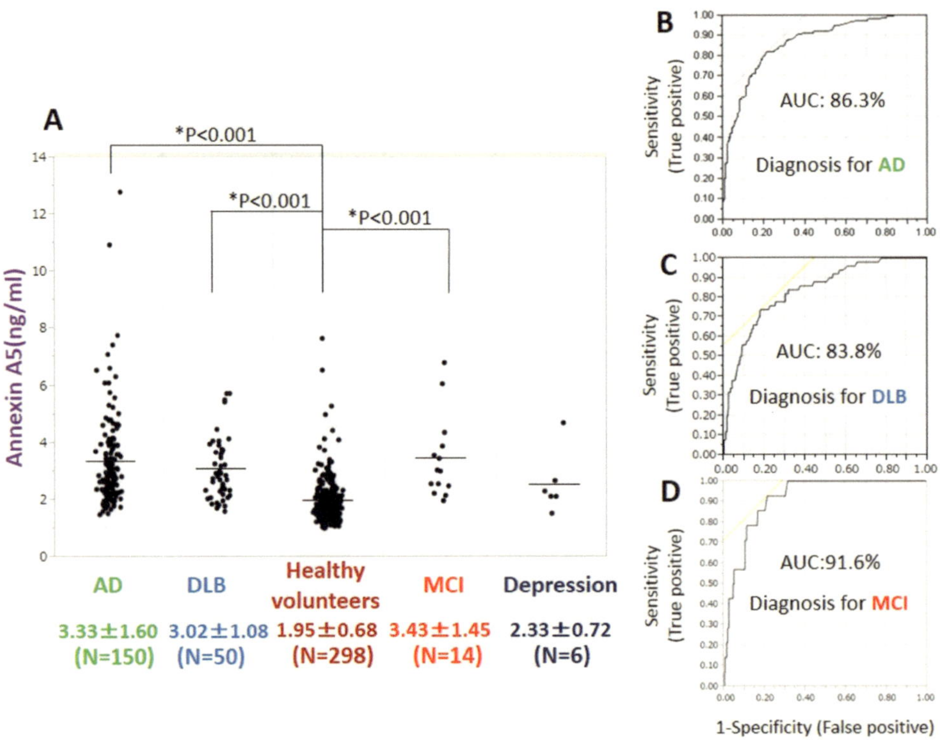

Figure 3. Comparison of plasma levels of annexin A5 in AD, DLB, MCI, depression, and age-matched healthy control.

For quantification of plasma annexin A5, we used a previously established chemiluminescent enzyme immunoassay system with monoclonal antibodies against human annexin A5 [52] (see Section 4.1). Individual plasma annexin A5 concentration is plotted in (A). The probability of either AD, DLB, or MCI can be predicted by a logistic regression model with the plasma level of annexin A5. Receiver operating characteristic (ROC) curves are shown in (B)–(D). The areas under the curve are 86.3%, 83.8%, and 91.6% for AD (B), DLB (C), and MCI (D), respectively. AD, Alzheimer's disease; DLB, dementia with Lewy bodies; MCI, mild cognitive impairment.

As annexin A5 binds not only phospholipids but also Ca^{2+}, it might have a role in protecting against Ca^{2+}-induced damage by chelating elevated intracellular Ca^{2+}. A defensive role against apoptosis induced by the participation of annexin A5 was also reported, in that annexin A5 plays a role in reducing the toxicity of the amyloidogenic proteins through interaction with them, such as amyloid polypeptides and α-synuclein [56].

On the other hand, dementia with Lewy bodies (DLB) shares clinical and pathological features with other dementia subtypes such as AD, vascular dementia, and Parkinson's disease (PD), which makes it difficult to distinguish in clinical practice. Lewy bodies are often found in the brains of AD patients. Also, the lack of valid and reliable methods for assessing the core clinical symptoms of both AD and DLB makes its identification even more difficult. We analyzed plasma level of annexin A5 in DLB. When average concentrations of plasma annexin A5 are compared among AD, DLB, and control groups, the values of AD and DLB were significantly higher than healthy control subjects (**Figure 3A**). Moreover, the ROC analyses showed good separation of patients with either AD or DLB from the control group (healthy volunteers) (**Figure 3B** and **C**) [57]. These suggest that annexin A5 is a potential biomarker for both AD and DLB. There is a similarity between AD and DLB. Lewy bodies are often found in the brains of AD patients. The therapeutic agent, acetylcholinesterase inhibitor, is effective not only in AD but also in DLB. From these results, annexin A5 reflects the above-mentioned similarity of AD and DLB.

To examine when annexin A5 becomes elevated during the course of disease development, we analyzed plasma samples from MCI patients (early stage of dementia). Average concentration was significantly higher than for the control group and the level was comparable with that of AD (**Figure 3A**). The areas under the ROC curve was 91.6% ($P < 0.001$) (**Figure 3D**), suggesting that annexin A5 is also a potential biomarker for MCI. Therefore, it is presumable that elevation of annexin A5 is likely to take place from the early developmental stage of AD. Although a sample number is very limited, plasma annexin A5 level in depression was comparable with the control (**Figure 3A**).

We next tracked plasma level of annexin A5 over a 3-year period in late stage AD patients. The plasma level of annexin A5 tended to be unchanged or slightly decreased, which indicates that biosynthesis of annexin A5 might be downregulated during the late stage, due to the progression of neuronal cell damage (data not shown).

5. Issues on blood sample

Since annexin A5 is also expressed in peripheral blood lymphocytes [58, 59], the effect of physical stress (such as osmotic pressure and temperature changes) upon blood cells may induce leakage of annexin A5. In fact, if a prolonged period of time passes (such as 12 h) after collecting blood, prior to centrifugation, the amount of plasma annexin A5 increases compared with a shorter period (such as within 6 h) (data not shown). Therefore, blood samples should be centrifuged within a specified period of time after collection. In our study, we did this within 6 h after blood collection. However, the lack of consistent technical standard for blood sampling in plasma biomarker studies may induce complicated and inconsistent observations depending on the study groups [60]. With respect to some conditions, such as anticoagulant reagent (EDTA or others), needle gauge, and 6-h fasting, standards should be proposed. For plasma preparation, a time limit until plasma separation after blood sampling may be critical to avoid induction of unwanted component leakage. Centrifugation speed (gravity force), duration, temperature, and number of spins, sample storage conditions may also require specification, though most common plasma samples are stored immediately at a temperature of –80°C for long-term storage. There will also be a number of factors that apply to subjects (patients and other participants involved): such as demographics (age, sex, and race/ethnicity), life style, overall health conditions (chronic drug administration, dietary supplements), smoking, and alcohol consumption.

6. AD risk factors

Several risk factors for AD have been indicated. Genetic factors are increasingly recognized as major risk factors for dementia. The most remarkable factor for AD from numerous studies is the ApoE gene on chromosome 19. ApoE, which is a major component of lipoproteins with 299 amino acid residues, plays a role in the metabolism and redistribution of cholesterol [61]. ApoE constitutes three major common isoforms, designated ApoE2, ApoE3, and ApoE4. ApoE isoforms interact differently with Aβ isoform-specific effects on Aβ-clearance. In ApoE4, domain interaction occurs as a result of a putative salt bridge, leading to tight structural formation. This interaction is unlikely to take place with ApoE2 and ApoE3 [62, 63]. ApoE4 is associated with an increased risk for AD along with early onset of the disease [64]. It was reported that ApoE4 carrier frequency was the highest in AD among AD, DLB, and control groups, and it was also higher in DLB than in the control groups [65]. Other findings have shown that ApoE4 carrier and allelic frequencies were comparable for those with AD and DLB with respect to Japanese subjects [57, 66].

Recently, a single nucleotide polymorphism in triggering receptor expressed on myeloid cells 2 (TREM2), an innate immune receptor expressed on the surface of microglia, were associated with both reduced hippocampal volume in healthy older adults and MCI [67, 68]. It was also shown that increased CSF sTREM2 levels were associated with higher CSF total TAU and phospho-TAU181P [69].

7. Future prospect

Biomarkers are usually employed as an indicator of processes related to the onset of a disease, specific disease conditions or response to therapeutic interventions [70]. However, it is clear that at present no single biomarker plays a sufficient discrimination role in screening for future development of late-onset AD or dementia. During development of the disease, the time when each unique biomarker becomes elevated will vary. Therefore, it is imperative to be able to determine when specific biomarkers need to be measured in order to provide timely therapeutic intervention.

http://dx.doi.org/10.5772/64512

Blood testing for measuring biomarkers will be easy and widely accepted due to the ease of collection and low cost. Moreover, the increasing availability of large sample sets obtained from a variety of technologies might contribute to diagnosis, prediction, and monitoring the progression of AD [71]. If a standardization of sample collection, standard operating procedures, comprehensive data management, and exchange of scientific findings is established, and if collaborative studies continue to progress, these should lead to a reduction in the variability and fragmentation of data. It is very likely that we may see plasma biomarkers become a reliable indicator for diagnosing AD.

Biomarkers of disease presence, subtypes (i.e., endophenotypes), treatment response, and progression are needed to advance therapeutic and preventative opportunities for this rapidly growing health care crisis.

8. Conclusions

In spite of the fact that reliable biomarkers have been established in CSF, no blood-based biomarker has been fully validated or qualified, even though an increasing number of plasma biomarker candidates have been reported. However, promising candidates have been emerging due to the progress in the field. Longitudinal studies from collaborative research and from the use of a variety of technologies and study designs are expected.

Acknowledgements

We are indebted to Kenneth E. Hartmann for critical reading of the manuscript. This study was supported in part by grant from the Ministry of Health, Labour and Welfare of Japan and from the Ministry of Education, Culture, Sports, Science and Technology of Japan (Grant number 24591686). All authors are free of any conflicts of interest.

Author details

Hitoshi Sohma[1,2*] and Yasuo Kokai[2]

*Address all correspondence to: sohma@sapmed.ac.jp

1 Department of Educational Development, Sapporo Medical University Center for Medical Education, Sapporo, Japan

2 Department of Biomedical Engineering, Sapporo Medical University School of Medicine, Sapporo, Japan

References

[1] Mattson MP: Pathways towards and away from Alzheimer's disease. Nature 2004, 430:631–639.

[2] Francis PT, Palmer AM, Snape M, Wilcock GK: The cholinergic hypothesis of Alzheimer's disease: a review of progress. J Neurol Neurosurg Psychiatry 1999, 66:137–147.

[3] Beach TG, Monsell SE, Phillips LE, Kukull W: Accuracy of the clinical diagnosis of Alzheimer disease at National Institute on Aging Alzheimer's Disease Centers, 2005–2010. J Neuropathol Exp Neurol 2012, 71(4):266–273.

[4] Ganguli M, Rodriguez E, Mulsant B, Richards S, Pandav R, Bilt JV, Dodge HH, Stoehr GP, Saxton J, Morycz RK et al.: Detection and management of cognitive impairment in primary care: The Steel Valley Seniors Survey. J Am Geriatr Soc 2004, 52(10):1668–1675.

[5] Hesse C, Rosengren L, Andreasen N, Davidsson P, Vanderstichele H, Vanmechelen E, Blennow K: Transient increase in total tau but not phospho-tau in human cerebrospinal fluid after acute stroke. Neurosci Lett 2001, 297:187–190.

[6] Blennow K, Vanmechelen E, Hampel H: CSF total tau, Abeta42 and phosphorylated tau protein as biomarkers for Alzheimer's disease. Mol Neurobiol 2001, 24:87–97.

[7] Blennow K, Hampel H, Weiner M, Zetterberg H: Cerebrospinal fluid and plasma biomarkers in Alzheimer disease. Nat Rev Neurol 2010, 6:131–144.

[8] Jack Jr CR, Knopman DS, Jagust WJ, Shaw LM, Aisen PS, Weiner MW, Petersen RC, Trojanowski JQ: Hypothetical model of dynamic biomarkers of the Alzheimer's pathological cascade. Lancet Neurol 2010, 9:119–128.

[9] Mao P, Reddy PH: Aging and amyloid beta-induced oxidative DNA damage and mitochondrial dysfunction in Alzheimer's disease: implications for early intervention and therapeutics. Biochim Biophys Acta 2011, 1812(11):1359–1370.

[10] Hardy J, Selkoe DJ: The amyloid hypothesis of Alzheimer's disease: progress and problems on the road to therapeutics. Science 2002, 297:353–356.

[11] Gouras GK, Tsai J, Naslund J, Vincent B, Edgar M, Checler F, Greenfiel JP, Haroutunian V, Buxbaum JD, Xu H et al.: Intraneuronal $A\beta_{42}$ accumulation in human brain. Am J Pathol 2000, 156(1):15–20.

[12] Lewis J, Dickson DW, Lin WL, Chisholm L, Corral A, Jones G, Yen SH, Sahara N, Skipper L, Yager D et al.: Enhanced neurofibrillary degeneration in transgenic mice expressing mutant tau and APP. Science 2001, 293(5534):1487–1491.

[13] Mandelkow EM, Mandelkow E: Tau in Alzheimer's disease. Trends Cell Biol 1998, 8(11):425–427.

[14] Goedert M: Tau protein and the neurofibrillary pathology of Alzheimer's disease. Trends Neurosci 1993, 16(11):460–465.

[15] Formichi P, Battisti C, Radi E, Federico A: Cerebrospinal fluid tau, A beta, and phosphorylated tau protein for the diagnosis of Alzheimer's disease. J Cell Physiol 2006, 208(1):39–46.

[16] Vandermeeren M, Mercken M, Vanmechelen E, Six J, van de Voorde A, Martin JJ, Cras P: Detection of tau proteins in normal and Alzheimer's disease cerebrospinal fluid with a sensitive sandwich enzyme-linked immunosorbent assay. J Neurochem 1993, 61(5): 1828–1834.

[17] Serot J-M, Peltier J, Fichten A, Ledeme N, Bourgeois A-M, Jouanny P, Toussaint P, Legars D, Godefroy O, Mazière J-C: Reduced CSF turnover and decreased ventricular $A\beta_{42}$ levels are related. BMC Neurosci 2011, 12:42.

[18] Ringman JM, Coppola G, Elashoff D, Rodriguez-Agudelo Y, Medina LD, Gylys K, Cummings JL, Cole GM: Cerebrospinal fluid biomarkers and proximity to diagnosis in preclinical familial Alzheimer's disease. Dement Geriatr Cogn Disord 2012, 33(1):1–5.

[19] Kanai M, Matsubara E, Isoe K, Urakami K, Nakashima K, Arai H, Sasaki H, Abe K, Iwatsubo T, Kosaka T et al.: Longitudinal study of cerebrospinal fluid levels of tau, Aβ1–40, and Aβ1–42(43) in Alzheimer's disease: a study in Japan. Ann Neurol 1998, 44:17–26.

[20] Bateman RJ, Wen G, Morris JC, Holtzman DM: Fluctuations of CSF amyloid-beta levels: implications for a diagnostic and therapeutic biomarker. Neurology 2007, 68(9):666–669.

[21] Hyman BT, Phelps CH, Beach TG, Bigio EH, Cairns NJ, Carrillo MC, Dickson DW, Duyckaerts C, Frosch MP, Masliah E et al.: National Institute on Aging-Alzheimer's Association guidelines for the neuropathologic assessment of Alzheimer's disease. Alzheimers Dement 2012, 8(1):1–13.

[22] Montine TJ, Phelps CH, Beach TG, Bigio EH, Cairns NJ, Dickson DW, Duyckaerts C, Frosch MP, Masliah E, Mirra SS et al.: National Institute on Aging-Alzheimer's Association guidelines for the neuropathologic assessment of Alzheimer's disease: a practical approach. Acta Neuropathol 2012, 123(1):1–11.

[23] Sperling RA, Aisen PS, Beckett LA, Bennett DA, Craft S, Fagan AM, Iwatsubo T, Jack Jr CR, Kaye J, Montine TJ et al.: Toward defining the preclinical stages of Alzheimer's disease: recommendations from the National Institute on Aging-Alzheimer's Association workgroups on diagnostic guidelines for Alzheimer's disease. Alzheimers Dement 2011, 7(3):280–292.

[24] Andree BA, Reutelingsperger CPM, Hauptmann R, Hemker HC, Hermens WH, Willems GM: Binding of vascular anticoagulant α (VACα) to planar phospholipid bilayers. J Biol Chem 1990, 265:4923–4928.

[25] Archakov AI, Ivanov YD, Lisitsa AV, Zogoda VG: AMF fishing nanotechnology is the way to reverse the Avogadro number in proteomics. Proteomics 2007, 7:4–9.

[26] Baird AL, Westwood S, Lovestone S: Blood-based proteomic biomarkers of Alzheimer's disease pathology. Front Neurol 2015, 6:article 236.

[27] Rosén C, Hansson O, Blennow K, Zetterberg H: Fluid biomarkers in Alzheimer's disease—current concepts. Mol Neurodegener 2013, 8:20.

[28] Iadecola C: Dangerous leaks: blood-brain barrier woes in the aging hippocampus. Neuron 2015, 85(2):231–233.

[29] Montagne A, Barnes SR, Sweeney MD, Halliday MR, Sagare AP, Zhao Z, Toga AW, Jacobs RE, Liu CY, Amezcua L et al.: Blood-brain barrier breakdown in the aging human hippocampus. Neuron 2015, 85:296–302.

[30] Lewczuk P, Esselmann H, Bibl M, Paul M, Svitek J, Miertscischk J, Meyrer R, Smirnov A, Mler JM, Klein C et al.: Electrophoretic separation of amyloid beta peptides in plasma. Electrophoresis 2004, 25(20):3336–3343.

[31] Mayeux R, Honig LS, Tang MX, Manly J, Stern Y, Schupf N, Mehta PD: Plasma $A\beta_{40}$ and $A\beta_{42}$ and Alzheimer's disease: relation to age, mortality, and risk. Neurology 2003, 61(9):1185–1190.

[32] van Oijen M, Hofman A, Soares HD, Koudstaal PJ, Breteler MM: Plasma $A\beta_{1-40}$ and $A\beta_{1-42}$ and the risk of dementia: a prospective case-cohort study. Lancet Neurol 2006, 8:655–660.

[33] Mayeux R, Tang MX, Jacobs DM, Manly J, Bell K, Merchant C, Small SA, Stern Y, Wisniewski HM, Mehta PD: Plasma amyloid beta-peptide 1–42 and incipient Alzheimer's disease. Ann Neurol 1999, 46(3):412–416.

[34] Schupf N, Tang MX, Fukuyama H, Manly J, Andrews H, Mehta P, Ravetch J, Mayeux R: Peripheral Abeta subspecies as risk biomarkers of Alzheimer's disease. Proc Natl Acad Sci USA 2008, 105:14052–14057.

[35] Sundelöf J, Giedraitis V, Irizarry MC, Sundström J, Ingelsson E, Rönnemaa E, Arnlöv J, Gunnarsson MD, Hyman BT, Basun H et al.: Plasma beta amyloid and the risk of Alzheimer disease and dementia in elderly men: a prospective, population-based cohort study. Arch Neurol 2008, 65(2):256–263.

[36] Hansson O, Zetterberg H, Vanmechelen E, Vanderstichele H, Andreasson U, Londos E, Wallin A, Minthon L, Blennow K: Evaluation of plasma $A\beta_{40}$ and $A\beta_{42}$ as predictors of conversion to Alzheimer's disease in patients with mild cognitive impairment. Neurobiol Aging 2010, 31(3):357–367.

[37] Lopez OL, Kuller LH, Mehta PD, Becker JT, Gach HM, Sweet RA, Chang YF, Tracy R, DeKosky ST: Plasma amyloid levels and the risk of AD in normal subjects in the Cardiovascular Health Study. Neurology 2008, 70:1664–1671.

[38] Graff-Radford NR, Crook JE, Lucas J, Boeve BF, Knopman DS, Ivnik RJ, Smith GE, Younkin LH, Petersen RC, Younkin SG: Association of low plasma $A\beta_{42}/A\beta_{40}$ ratios with increased imminent risk for mild cognitive impairment and Alzheimer disease. Arch Neurol 64:354–362.

[39] Yaffe K, Weston A, Graff-Radford NR, Satterfield S, Simonsick EM, Younkin SG, Younkin LH, Kuller L, Ayonayon HN, Ding J et al.: Association of plasma beta-amyloid level and cognitive reserve with subsequent cognitive decline. JAMA 2011, 305(261–266).

[40] Thambisetty M, Simmons A, Velayudhan L, Hye A, Campbell J, Zhang Y, Wahlund LO, Westman E, Kinsey A, Güntert A et al.: Association of plasma clusterin concentration with severity, pathology, and progression in Alzheimer disease. Arch Gen Psychiatry 2010, 67:739–748.

[41] Thambisetty M, An Y, Kinsey A, Koka D, Saleem M, Guntert A, Kraut M, Ferrucci L, Davatzikos C, Lovestone S et al.: Plasma clusterin concentration is associated with longitudinal brain atrophy in mild cognitive impairment. NeuroImage 2012, 59:212–217.

[42] Jongbloed W, van Dijk KD, Mulder SD, van de Berg WD, Blankenstein MA, van der Flier W, Veerhuis R: Clusterin levels in plasma predict cognitive decline and progression to Alzheimer's disease. J Alzheimers Dis 2015, 46(4):1103–1110.

[43] Li X, Ma Y, Wei X, Li Y, Wu H, Zhuang J, Zhao Z: Clusterin in Alzheimer's disease: a player in the biological behavior of amyloid-beta. Neurosci Bull 2014, 30(1):162–168.

[44] Wilson MR, Yerbury JJ, Poon S: Potential roles of abundant extracellular chaperones in the control of amyloid formation and toxicity. Mol Biosyst 2008, 4:42–52.

[45] Killick R, Ribe EM, Al-Shawi R, Malik B, Hooper C, Fernandes C, Dobson R, Nolan PM, Lourdusamy A, Furney S et al.: Clusterin regulatesβ-amyloid toxicity via Dickkopf-1-driven induction of the wnt-PCP-JNK pathway. Mol Psychiatry 2014, 19:88–98.

[46] Sato Y, Suzuki I, Nakamura T, Bernier F, Aoshima K, Oda Y: Identification of a new plasma biomarker of Alzheimer's disease using metabolomics technology. J Lipid Res 2012, 53:567–576.

[47] Velayudhan L, Killick R, Hye A, Kinsey A, Guntert A, Lynham S, Ward M, Leung R, Lourdusamy A, To AWM et al.: Plasma transthyretin as a candidate marker for Alzheimer's disease. J Alzheimer's Dis 2012, 28:369–375.

[48] Choi J, Lee HW, Suk K: Plasma level of chitinase 3-like 1 protein increases in patients with early Alzheimer's disease. J Neurol 2011, 258:2181–2185.

[49] Lim NK, Villemagne VL, Soon CP, Laughton KM, Rowe CC, McLean CA, Masters CL, Evin G, Li QX: Investigation of matrix metalloproteinases, MMP-2 and MMP-9, in plasma reveals a decrease of MMP-2 in Alzheimer's disease. J Alzheimer's Dis 2011, 26:779–786.

[50] Ray S, Britschgi M, Herbert C, Takeda-Uchimura Y, Boxer A, Blennow K, Friedman LF, Galasko DR, Jutel M, Karydas A et al.: Classification and prediction of clinical Alzheimer's disease based on plasma signaling proteins. Nat Med 2007, 13(11):1359–1562.

[51] LaFerla FM: Calcium dyshomeostasis and intracellular signalling in Alzheimer's disease. Nat Rev Neurosci 2002, 3:862–872.

[52] Yamaguchi M, Kokai Y, Imai S, Utsumi K, Matsumoto K, Honda H, Mizue Y, Momma M, Maeda T, Toyomasu Set al.: Investigation of annexin A5 as a biomarker for Alzheimer's disease using neuronal cell culture and mouse model. J Neurosci Res 2010, 88:2682–2692.

[53] Lampl Y, Lorberboym M, Blankenberg FG, Sadeh M, Gilad R: Annexin V SPECT imaging of phosphatidylserine expression in patients with dementia. Neurology 2006, 66:1253–1254.

[54] McKhann, G., Drachman, D., Folstein, M., Katzman, R., Price, D., Stadlan, E. M. Clinical diagnosis of Alzheimer's disease: report of the NINCDS-ADRDA work group under the auspices of department of health and human services task force on Alzheimer's disease. Neurology 1984, 34:939–944.

[55] McKeith IG, Dickson DW, Lowe J, Emre M, O'Brien JT, Feldman H, et al.: Diagnosis and management of dementia with Lewy bodies: third report of the DLB Consortium. Neurology 2005, 65:1863–1872.

[56] Bedrood S, Jayasinghe S, Sieburth D, Chen M, Erbel S, Butler PC, Langen R, Ritzel RA: Annexin A5 directly interacts with amyloidogenic proteins and reduces their toxicity. Biochemistry 2009, 48:10568–10576.

[57] Sohma H, Imai S, Takei N, Honda H, Matsumoto K, Utsumi K, Matsuki K, Hashimoto E, Saito T, Kokai Y: Evaluation of annexin A5 as a biomarker for Alzheimer's disease and dementia with Lewy bodies. Front Aging Neurosci 2013, 5:1–7.

[58] Masuda J, Takayama E, Satoh A, Ida M, Shinohara T, Kojima-Aikawa K, Ohsuzu F, Nakanishi K, Kuroda K, Murakami M et al.: Levels of annexin IV and V in the plasma of pregnant and postpartum women. Thromb Haemost 2004, 91:1129–1136.

[59] Cornelissen M, Philippé J, De Sitter S, De Ridder L: Annexin V expression in apoptotic peripheral blood lymphocytes: an electron microscopic evaluation. Apoptosis 2002, 7(1):41–47.

[60] O'Bryant SE, Gupta V, Henriksen K, Edwards M, Jeromin A, Lista S, Bazenet C, Soares H, Lovestone S, Hampel H et al.: Guidelines for the standardization of preanalytic

variables for blood-based biomarker studies in Alzheimer's disease research. Alzheimer's Dement 2015, 11(5):549–560.

[61] Hatters DM, Peters-Libeu CA, Weisgraber KH: Apolipoprotein E structure: insights into function. Trends Biochem Sci 2006, 31:445–454.

[62] Dong L-M, Weisgraber KH: Human apolipoprotein E4 domain interaction. Arginine 61 and glutamic acid 255 interact to direct the preference for very low density lipoproteins. J Biol Chem 1996, 271:19053–19057.

[63] Dong L-M, Wilson C, Wardell MR, Simmons T, Mahley RW, Weisgraber KH, Agard DA: Human apolipoprotein E. Role of arginine 61 in mediating the lipoprotein preferences of the E3 and E4 isoforms. J Biol Chem 1994, 269:22358–22365.

[64] Kim J, Basak JM, Holtzman DM: The role of apolipoprotein E in Alzheimer's disease. Neuron 2009, 63:287–303.

[65] Carrillo Garcia F, Gil Neciga E, Alberca R, Garcia-Solis D, Millan J, Rodriguez Uranga JJ, Franco E, Mir P, Suarez A, Garcia R et al.: Apolipoprotein E4 in dementia with Lewy bodies. Neurologia 2008, 23:152–156.

[66] Kobayashi S, Tateno M, Park TW, Utsumi K, Sohma H, Ito YM, Kokai Y, Saito T: Apolipoprotein E4 frequencies in a Japanese population with Alzheimer's disease and dementia with Lewy bodies. PLoS ONE 2011, 6(4):e18569.

[67] Lupton MK, Strike L, Hansell NK, Wen W, Mather KA, Armstrong NJ, Thalamuthu A, McMahon KL, de Zubicaray GI, Assareh AA et al.: The effect of increased genetic risk for Alzheimer's disease on hippocampal and amygdala volume. Neurobiol Aging 2016, 40:68–77.

[68] Suárez-Calvet M, Kleinberger G, Araque Caballero MÁ, Brendel M, Rominger A, Alcolea D, Fortea J, Lleó A, Blesa R, Gispert JD et al.: sTREM2 cerebrospinal fluid levels are a potential biomarker for microglia activity in early-stage Alzheimer's disease and associate with neuronal injury markers. EMBO Mol Med 2016, e201506123.

[69] Colonna M, Wang Y: TREM2 variants: new keys to decipher Alzheimer disease pathogenesis. Nat Rev Neurosci 2016, 17:201-207

[70] Wright CF, Hall A, Matthews FE, Brayne C: Biomarkers, dementia, and public health. Ann NY Acad Sci 2009, 1180:11–19.

[71] Thambisetty M, Lovestone S: Blood-based biomarkers of Alzheimer's disease: challenging but feasible. Biomark Med 2010, 4(1):65–79.

Chapter 5

Alzheimer's-Related Amyloid Beta Peptide Aggregates in the Ageing Retina: Implications for Sight Loss and Dementia

J. Arjuna Ratnayaka and Savannah Lynn

Additional information is available at the end of the chapter

http://dx.doi.org/10.5772/64790

Abstract

Although visual problems are reported by patients with Alzheimer's disease and dementia, studies into this particular aspect of neuropathology are scarce. The growing awareness of complex pathological processes in the ageing retina and brain, however, enables us to consider this from a new perspective. Here we discuss the latest findings on the wide-ranging visual defects experienced by those suffering from Alzheimer's disease and dementia. We propose that events leading to chronic degeneration of the retina and the brain in fact share many striking similarities. In particular, we discuss the role of the Alzheimer's-related amyloid beta (Aβ) group of peptides that has been shown to accumulate in senescent retinas, correlated with increased risk of retinal degeneration. The high photo-oxidative retinal environment creates ideal conditions for Aβ aggregation, evidenced by high Aβ loads reported in aged and donor eyes from patients with age-related macular degeneration. Consequently, longitudinal and non-invasive retinal assessments may provide invaluable information on incipient pathology and disease progression in the retina as well as the senescent brain. Such insights may not only lead to identifying new pathogenic mechanisms in the retina with implications for understanding Alzheimer's disease but reveal the underlying causes of visual abnormalities reported in patients with dementia.

Keywords: amyloid beta, retina, degeneration, Alzheimer's, age-related macular degeneration

1. Introduction

Dementia poses a significant risk to those over the age of 65, affecting up to 46.8 million individuals globally, a number that is expected to increase to approximately 131 million by 2050 [https://www.alz.co.uk/research/WorldAlzheimerReport2015.pdf]. Currently, no reliable treatments exist, although it has been estimated that slowing disease progression by just 5 years would reduce the number of dementia-related deaths by almost half [https://www.alzheimers.org.uk]. Alzheimer's disease (AD) is an age-related neurodegenerative disorder of the brain, and the most common cause of dementia amongst the elderly [1]. AD is typified by progressive memory loss and significant cognitive decline amongst other complications that ultimately leads to death [2].

A major pathological feature of AD is misfolding and aggregation of the naturally occurring amyloid beta (Aβ) family of proteins. A variety of different Aβ peptides are generated by successive proteolytic cleavage of the amyloid precursor protein (APP). These accumulate as large insoluble aggregates in AD brains and are referred to as 'senile plaques'. The amyloid cascade hypothesis proposes that Aβ plays a central role in AD [2]. However, AD and dementia are complex diseases, and the role of Aβ and other disease factors are still incompletely understood. Studies are also hampered by the brain's relative inaccessibility, and clinical diagnosis typically occurs many years after disease onset [3]. Consequently, there is considerable impetus towards developing non-invasive, reliable and cost-effective diagnostic methods so those at risk may be identified at relatively early stages to maximise the chances of clinical intervention. Most studies into AD and dementia are primarily focused on memory loss and cognitive decline [4, 5]. However, many AD patients are also reported to suffer from a variety of visual complications, which by contrast has received comparatively little attention. The recent discovery that Aβ deposits in the ageing human retina correlate with complex retinopathies such as age-related macular degeneration (AMD) has given support to the hypothesis that shared pathologies may exist between the brain and senescent retina.

In this chapter, we provide a comprehensive review of the latest findings reporting visual abnormalities in patients with AD and dementia. The methodology for this review is based on searches conducted in the NCBI PubMed (http://www.ncbi.nlm.nih.gov/pubmed) database using keywords 'dementia and retina' (396 articles) and 'AD and retina' (457 articles) in June 2016. These numbers contrast starkly with larger numbers of studies in areas related to memory loss and cognitive decline. For example, use of keywords 'dementia and memory loss' (12,383 articles) or 'AD and cognitive impairment' (19,883 articles) yield many more citations; highlighting the as yet limited interest in systematically reporting visual abnormalities in AD and dementia patients. Additionally, we used keywords such as 'retina and Aβ' (111 articles) and 'retinal pigment epithelium (RPE) and amyloid' (59 citations) to include specific articles related to ophthalmology and dementia, and to describe studies in ex vivo and animal models that provide insights into Aβ-mediated pathogenesis. Centring on these articles, specific information in hyperlinks, as well as insights from our own work, we discuss the role of Aβ in driving retinal degeneration and neurodegeneration, and propose that the eye may provide a powerful model to study Aβ pathology. We suggest that the retina may act as an anatomical window into the Alzheimer's brain through which early stages of neurodegeneration could non-invasively be identified.

2. The ageing brain and retina: intimate connections

The neuroretina and the central nervous system (CNS) share common origins as both derive from the developing neural ectoderm and maintain a direct and permanent connection via the optic nerve [6]. The neuroretina may therefore be considered an extension of the brain that resides within a discrete compartment—the eye. In addition to this anatomical link, both the retina and tissues of the CNS exhibit similar structural and functional arrangements. These include specialised structural adaptations such as surface infolds, postmitotic neuronal and epithelial cells, immunologically privileged compartmentalisation via a blood-brain/retinal barrier, as well as more importantly, similar patterns of damage with increasing age [7]. It is therefore possible that common disease mechanisms may also be involved in diseases of the ageing eye and brain.

Gathering of visual information first occurs when light enters the eye's anterior pole and is projected to the neuroretina. Here, incident light is converted by specialised photoreceptors in the neuroretina into electrical impulses which are subsequently relayed to second- and third-order neurons [8] (**Figure 1**). Axons of retinal ganglion cells (RGCs) then convey these signals to the brain. The synaptic arrangement in the neuroretina comprises of three sequential neuronal layers: photoreceptors, bipolar, and RGCs (referred to as the three neuron links) [9]. Neuronal cell bodies and processes exist in alternate layers giving rise to the laminated structure of the retina where cell bodies typically exist within the inner and outer nuclear layers, whereas processes and synapses of retinal neurons reside within the inner and outer plexiform layers [10]. In addition to these cell types, specialised neurons referred to as amacrine and horizontal cells facilitate the parallel processing of information [9]. Furthermore, a highly specialised monolayer of epithelial cells which originates from the neuroectoderm referred to as the RPE forms the margins of the outer retina and the interface with the outer vasculature (**Figure 1**) [11]. Here, within this strategic position, the RPE performs many critical metabolic and supportive functions for the overlying neuroretina. These include the absorption of stray light, phagocytosis of shed photoreceptor outer segments (POS) as part of the daily visual cycle, maintenance of the blood-retinal barrier (BRB), ion homeostasis as well as playing a role in retinal adhesion [11, 12]. The normal function of the RPE monolayer is therefore critical to maintain healthy vision in old age.

The arrangement of the mammalian retina is such that light must first traverse the entire length of the retina before reaching the photoreceptors. Two distinct types of photoreceptors exist which may be categorised according to histological morphology and which are each specialised for a specific function. Rod photoreceptors constitute 95% of all photoreceptors, express the photopigment rhodopsin and are responsible for scotopic (low light) visual processes [13]. Cone photoreceptors on the other hand encompass a highly invaginated membrane to provide an optimal surface area for phototransduction and are responsible for photopic (normal/high light) visual processes, the perception of colour and visual acuity. Colour vision is achieved through expression of the photopigment opsin, which, depending on the structure of the molecule, confers sensitivity to varying wavelengths of light [9]. Cone photoreceptors typically concentrate within the fovea—an area corresponding to 1.5 mm in diameter at the centre of the human retina where light from the central visual field is focused and which is responsible for high visual acuity and detailed image perception [14]. Within this area, the retina is devoid of the inner retinal layers and retinal vasculature, which ensures minimal interference to focused light when creating a clear foveal image [9]. The region peripheral to the fovea is termed the macula which has a high proportion of cones that extends to a radius of 5.5 mm in diameter [14].

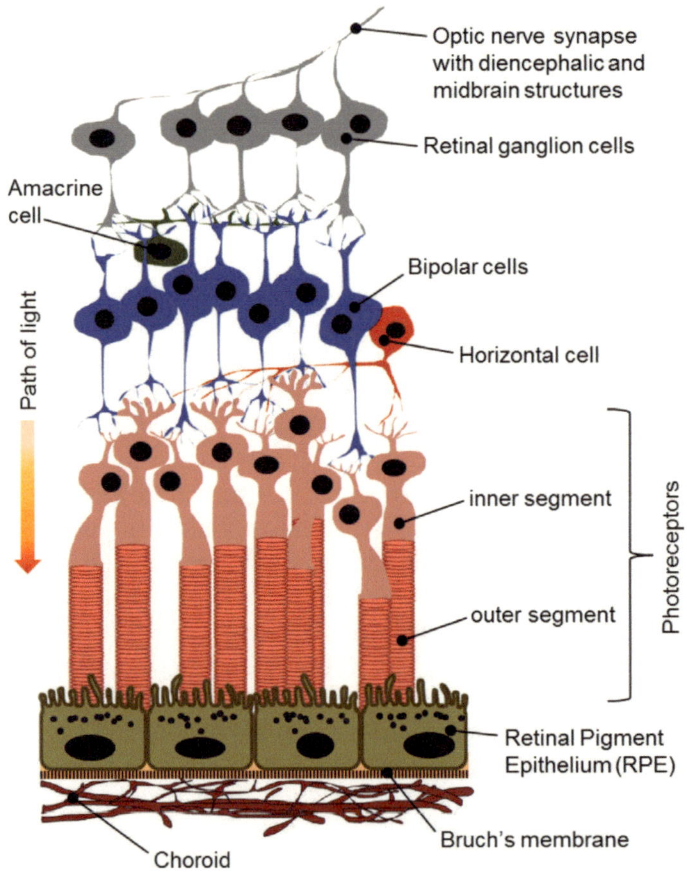

Figure 1. Synaptic arrangement of the neuroretina and associated layers. Diagram illustrating the inverted arrangement of the human neuroretina with light-sensitive photoreceptors forming intimate associations with the underlying retinal pigment epithelium (RPE).

The axons of the RGCs converge at the centre of the retina where they exit the eye through the optic disc and maintain a permanent connection with the brain via the optic nerves (**Figure 2**) [15]. The optic nerve (also referred to as the second cranial nerve) enters the cranial cavity via the optic canal where it runs parallel to the middle cranial fossa in close proximity to the pituitary gland. Anterior to the stalk of the pituitary gland, an anatomical crossroad exists known as the optic chiasm, where optic nerves unite and axons from RGCs that reside within the nasal side of both left and right retinas connect with the opposing hemisphere of the brain (**Figure 2**). Conversely, temporal RGC axons project to its corresponding cerebral hemisphere. Soon after exiting the optic chiasm, the RGC axons converge to form the optic tract which predominantly synapses with the lateral geniculate nucleus (LGN), a relay centre for the visual pathway that resides within the thalamus. The internal structure of the LGN comprises several layers which function as maps of visual space and which segregate information according to axonal origin. As the LGN receives information from the right and left visual fields, visual input from the opposing hemisphere is kept separate from that of the corresponding eye. This information is then passed to the visual cortex within the posterior brain for processing via optic radiations formed by the axons of the LGN neurons (**Figure 2**). Here, segregation of visual information is maintained according to the location in the retina from which information was perceived. For example, information derived from the fovea occupies a significant area of the posterior visual cortex, whereas progressively more anterior regions of the visual cortex represent visual perceptions from the periphery of the retina. Several other regions of the brain are innervated from the visual cortex including the occipital, parietal and temporal lobes. These areas are linked with visuoperceptual and visuospatial aspects of vision, as well as visual acuity and the recognition of familiar objects [16, 17].

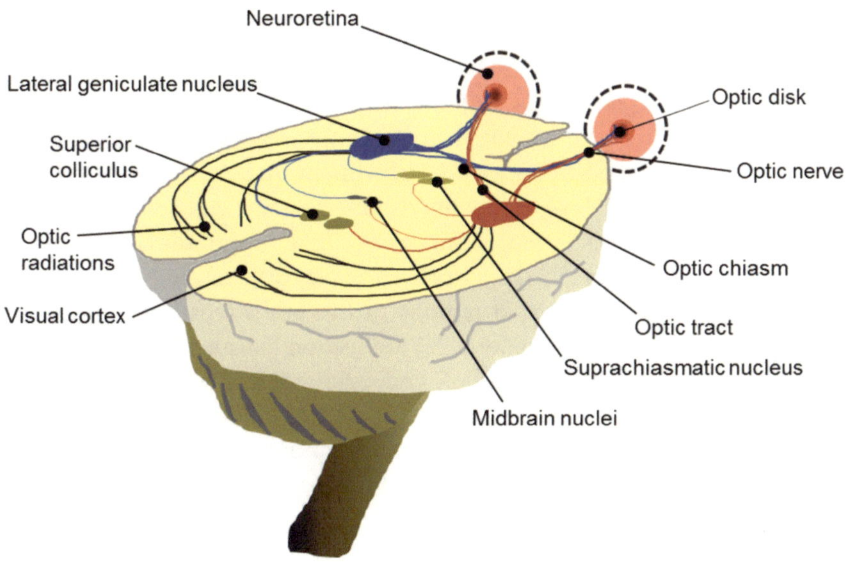

Figure 2. Synaptic terminals of the optic nerve and visual pathway in the brain.

RGC axons within the optic tracts also connect with several diencephalic and midbrain structures. These include the superior colliculi (SC), also termed the optic tectum which is situated on the roof of the midbrain and is involved in controlling eye movement; the suprachiasmatic nucleus (SCN) which is a small, wing-shaped structure within the hypothalamus located directly above the optic chiasm that is involved in circadian rhythm; and nuclei within the midbrain that are implicated in controlling pupil diameter (**Figure 2**). Of note, several of these aforementioned visual centres have been associated with AD pathology. For instance, the SC has been shown to progressively accumulate both Alzheimer-associated senile plaques as well as neurofibrillary tangles (NFT). AD-linked changes have also been reported in the SCN including a reduction in the size, cell number and accumulation of NFTs, which may collectively contribute to the wide range of visual complications reported in these patients [15, 17].

3. Visual abnormalities in Alzheimer's disease and in patients with dementia

A variety of visual abnormalities have been reported in patients with AD ranging from visuo-constructional and visuo-perceptual dysfunctions, object agnosia, prosopagnosia to visual hallucinations as well as simultanagnosia [5, 18, 19]. Patients with posterior cortical atrophy (PCA), which is associated with degeneration of the posterior cortex, also report particular difficulties with visual tasks often presenting with visual agnosia, visual neglect and visual hallucinations [20, 21]. However, compared to memory loss, visual deficits have received little attention and are thus poorly understood. Patients in the spectrum of, and leading to, clinical AD show marked reductions in the number of RGC [22], narrowing of venous blood column diameter and reduced venous blood flow rates [23], as well as optic nerve abnormalities such as loss of axonal densities [24], RGCs [25] and increased receptor expression for advances glycation end products [26]. Abnormalities are also observed in regions of AD brains that synapse with the optic nerve and/or are associated with the visual processing pathway (**Figure 2**). Some examples include the loss of myelin, diminished nucleolar volume in the LGN, as well as accumulation of lipofuscin (autofluorescent pigment granules) [27]. AD brains also show the presence of NFT in the SC [28] (which receives ~10% of the RGC axons), as well as the presence of Aβ/neuritic plaques in regions of the brain that are implicated in visual attention and the control of eye movement. Aβ deposition has also been reported in the lens of AD patients [29]. Additionally, histopathological evidence from post-mortem brains reveals significant pathological changes in the visual processing regions of the brain including the loss of pyramidal cells and reduced myelin in the outer laminae of the visual cortex [30–33]. A comprehensive list of such neurological changes in areas of the brain associated with vision has been described by Armstrong (2009) indicating the extensive nature of psyco-visual abnormalities in patients with AD and dementia [29].

Not surprisingly, a large number of AD transgenic animal models also develop visual deficits and have therefore been used to investigate retinal pathologies. These include, but are not limited to, the Tg2576 [34], APPswe/$PS1_{M146L}$ and APPswe/PSΔE9 [35], 5xFAD [36, 37], and P301S [38] mice. A wide range of retinal changes have been documented in these animals, including an age-dependent increase in APP/Aβ immunoreactivity in the neuroretina and associated vasculature, the accumulation of Aβ plaques/ hyperphosphorylated tau in the nerve fibre layer (NFL) and RGC, thinning of the RGC, as well as glial cell-derived neuro-inflammatory responses within the retina [4]. Of importance, a number of these changes are common to well-established animal models of retinal degeneration that are widely used to study AMD [39, 40].

4. The degenerating retina: sight loss in old age

Despite the growing number of Alzheimer's patients reporting visual complications, this has received comparatively little attention. This may be due to several reasons including incomplete diagnosis, associated complications, old age and cognitive impairment of patients as well as lack of medical devices or tools to obtain a clear clinical diagnosis. Consequently, the breadth and diversity of visual abnormalities in AD and dementia patients is yet to be fully recognised. For example, analysis of published literature in NCBI PubMed using keywords such as 'vision and dementia' (without the inclusion of any further search parameters) yielded only 447 citations in a 10-year period (between 2006 and June 2016), which is surprisingly few given the frequency of visual abnormalities reported in these patients. In contrast, search terms such as 'memory loss and cognitive decline' yield 3062 citations over a similar period. Understanding how the ageing retina becomes susceptible to degeneration and how it may affect the visual pathway and/or perception by the brain could provide insights into the molecular and cellular basis underlying visual abnormalities in AD. Here then is an opportunity to gain further insights into how the world may be perceived by those suffering from AD and dementia. Patients with retinopathies not only have damaged retinal tissues but also show impairments in how visual information is relayed to and processed by the brain. For instance, visual hallucinations classified under the term Charles Bonnet syndrome have been reported in patients with late-onset visual disorders such as AMD [41]. Indeed, almost half of AMD patients experience visual hallucinations, whilst a third report hallucinations that are distressing, intrusive and interfere with daily activities [41, 42]. AMD affects approximately 50 million individuals globally [8, 43]. Unlike rare diseases caused by single-gene mutations, AMD is a complex multifactorial disease which in many ways shows striking parallels with AD [4, 44, 45].

AMD exhibits an age-dependent prevalence with one in three individuals exhibiting some sign of early disease by their seventh decade [43]. Currently, there are over half million AMD patients in the United Kingdom (source: Macular Society), with comparable incidence rates in Europe and other Western populations as reported by the European Eye Study (EUREYE) [46]. This puts a significant strain on national healthcare budgets with the direct annual cost of AMD exceeding US$254 billion globally [14]. This figure is predicted to rise three-fold over the next 20 years as a result of increased life expectancy and reduced mortality rates [43]. This common, irreversible blinding condition derives its name from the macula; the anatomical region affected in disease. This specialised region, which we have introduced earlier, resides at the centre of the retina, temporal to the optic disk and is responsible for visual acuity and image resolution (mediating focused central vision). Patients with AMD therefore suffer loss of centrally mediated sight [45]. As the majority of patients are typically in the latter stages of life, this has a disproportionate social impact, similar to some social issues encountered by patients with AD and dementia [43].

The early stage of AMD is typically asymptomatic, and like AD, can remain so for many years before clinical diagnosis. Hence, most patients with early AMD exhibit few or no obvious visual symptoms [47], although a recent study found indications of early macular pathology even in those aged between 35 and 44 [48]. A major pathological hallmark of early AMD is the focal deposition of lipid-rich extracellular aggregates between the RPE and Bruch's membrane (**Figure 1**) [49]. With increasing age, such aggregates termed 'drusen' become common within the periphery of normal healthy retinas as hard structures with well-defined borders [50]. In contrast, patients with larger, soft drusen showing ill-defined borders (~125 μM) in the macula region are considered to be at a higher risk of developing AMD [51]. Late AMD presents as two distinct phenotypes; classified as geographic atrophy (dry) and neovascular (wet) AMD. If early stages of the disease are excluded, the numbers of dry and wet AMD patients are broadly similar [52]. Dry AMD is typified by gradual impairment of macular RPE cells and death of overlying photoreceptors. By contrast, wet AMD is characterised by growth of new leaky blood vessels from the underlying choroid (**Figure 1**). This results in accumulation of fluid/sub-retinal swelling and scaring of the macula due to disruption of the outer BRB [45]. The growth of new vessels in wet AMD may be managed in most cases through monthly intravitreal injections of vascular endothelial growth factor (VEGF) inhibitors. In contrast, dry AMD which affects the majority of AMD patients currently has no effective treatment [8]. Significant advances have been made in recent years to identify the genetic landscape of AMD and related retinopathies [45]. However, this new knowledge has yet to provide insights into key disease mechanisms, or translate into effective treatments against advancing blindness. It is therefore vital to gain a better understanding of disease processes in the ageing retina before effective AMD treatments can be developed. The recent discovery of the Alzheimer's-associated Aβ peptide, a well-known neurodegenerative agent associated in key stages of AMD, has opened up the possibilities of studying sight loss from a novel perspective. Such studies in a highly accessible tissue such as the retina could lead to a better understanding of Aβ mechanisms as well as new insights into AD and dementia.

5. Age-related macular degeneration and Aβ

The healthy retina is constitutively exposed to Aβ. In fact, recent findings demonstrate that Aβ synthesis occurs at local sites within the retinal environment including the RPE and RGCs [53, 54]. The RPE is considered to be the principal source of Aβ in the posterior eye; a tissue which also expresses APP [55]. The RPE also expresses the necessary factors for regulating Aβ synthesis including β- and γ-secretase, as well as the Aβ-degrading enzyme neprilysin [56,

57]. Furthermore, studies of mouse and bovine ocular fluids show the presence of Aβ in picomolar to nanomolar quantities within both aqueous and vitreous humours [58].

The retina is a particularly useful tissue to study Aβ pathology as it is continuously exposed to high photo-oxidative stresses throughout life, an ideal environment for Aβ accumulation [44, 59, 60]. Hence, it is not surprising that the Aβ burden in the retina increases with advancing age. To date, age-dependent accumulation of Aβ has been shown in multiple retinal locations including photoreceptors, RPE, Bruch's membrane and within the inner and outer retinal vasculature [39, 55, 61, 62]. This pattern of Aβ accumulation has been reported both in rodent models and in donor human eyes. For instance, Aβ deposits on photoreceptor were shown to be abundant on mature POS or outer tips which are phagocytosed by RPE cells as part of the daily visual cycle. Studies in wild-type mice show such Aβ-enriched outer tips of photoreceptors to be enlarged, possibly due to impaired internalisation of POS by senescent RPE [39]. The use of antibodies that recognise Aβ as well as APP also show immunoreactivity within the cytoplasm of RPE cells that are adjacent to drusen [55]. Numerous studies also reveal the presence of Aβ within drusen, which links a key clinical hallmark of AMD with Aβ [44, 55, 61–63]. Aβ within drusen have been shown organised into assemblies of approximately 2–10 μm in diameter. These spheres referred to as 'amyloid vesicles' were shown to have a concentric ring-like interior, permeated with Aβ immunoreactivity [55].

Interestingly, studies of post-mortem tissues show that the ageing human retina plays host to a variety of Aβ assemblies. The use of various antibodies including 4G8, 6E10, WO1, WO2, OC, A11 and 82E1 has revealed the presence of non-fibrillar oligomers, protofibrils and mature amyloid fibrils [55, 61, 62]. Furthermore, different Aβ structures were evident in different locations within amyloid vesicles. For example, in studies using 4G8, 6E10, WO1 and WO2 (which specifically recognise mature Aβ assemblies including protofibrils and mature fibrils), immunoreactivity was typically observed within the outer shell of amyloid vesicles [55, 61, 63]. Conversely, studies investigating Aβ oligomers (antibodies A11 and M204) showed preferential accumulation at the centre of drusen in close proximity to the inner collagenous layer of Bruch's membrane. Here, Aβ oligomers constituted the most abundant Aβ assembly within drusen [39, 62]. Moreover, the presence of Aβ within drusen appeared to correlate with drusen load as well as increasing age [63]. One study using a small number of patient samples found that Aβ deposition were only present within drusen of AMD patients; supporting the likelihood that Aβ accumulation is associated with more advanced forms of AMD [64].

As the RPE monolayer, which is strategically juxtaposed between the neuroretina and the outer retinal vasculature (**Figure 1**), appears to be the main focus of Aβ deposition, it is not surprising that Aβ has profound effects on its function. Of critical importance is the role of the RPE in maintaining the immune-privileged state of the retina via the outer BRB. Oligomeric $A\beta_{1-42}$ has been shown to impair both early zonular occludens (ZO-1) and mid-to-late occludin tight junctions in the RPE as well as induce actin cytoskeletal disorganisation. This suggests that Aβ may compromise BRB integrity [65]. This is comparable to Aβ's mode of action in the AD brain which results in blood-brain barrier (BBB) disruption, increased BBB permeability and endothelial cell dysfunction [66]. In fact recent studies have also shown a downregulation of both ZO-1 and occludin upon application of Aβ to human cerebral microvascular endothelial cells. Such insights reveal striking parallels between neurodegenerative processes between the ageing retina and brain, and how Aβ may play a key role in both pathologies [7, 66]. Similarly, oligomeric Aβ exposure causes an upregulation of VEGF in both the brain and retina which has been linked with AD and AMD. VEGF is essential in maintaining hippocampal plasticity as well as cognitive function. However, VEGF upregulation is correlated with $A\beta_{1-42}$ accumulation in AD brains resulting in neuronal cell death and BBB dysfunction [67]. In the eye, VEGF is primarily secreted by the RPE; the increased levels of which are correlated with the neovascular form of AMD [8]. Anti-VEGF inhibitors consequently form the current the mainstay of wet AMD treatments. Exposure of RPE cells to Aβ was shown to profoundly increase VEGF secretion, which may contribute to such an undesirable pro-angiogenic retinal environment [57].

Aβ also appears to play a central role in chronic inflammation of the ageing retina. Such pathology is similar to inflammatory conditions found in AD brains [68]. For example, transcriptome studies show enhanced complement gene expression in AD brains, particularly those of complement C1q and C3 proteins [69, 70]. AMD involves a similar chronic inflammatory response that is as yet incompletely understood. Here, compliment associated proteins deposit within drusen alongside Aβ including compliment factor C3, compliment factor H and the membrane attack complex, including its constituents C5, C6, C7 and C9 [55, 71]. Consequently, Aβ is thought to promote a pro-inflammatory retinal microenvironment where it co-localises with complement factor H (CFH) and iC3b to induce compliment activation. Studies have also shown the elevation of pro-inflammatory IL-1β, IL-6, IL-8, TNF-α and caspase-1 upon intravitreal Aβ injection in C57BL/6 J mice, as well as an increase in IL-8 and MMP-9 secretion levels by RPE upon exposure to $A\beta_{1-42}$ [72, 73]. Microglial activation and engulfment of Aβ have also been observed co-localised with retinal Aβ [39]. Similar pathology is also reported in the brains of patients with AD [68].

Unsurprisingly, key features of AMD observed in human donor eyes can be recapitulated by experimentally elevating retinal Aβ levels in wild-type mice. Our studies show that subretinal injection of human recombinant $A\beta_{1-42}$ at physiological doses (nM range) in C57BL/6 mice induces RPE pigment abnormalities, RPE plasticity as well as photoreceptor outer segment loss, hallmarks of AMD (**Figure 3**). Critically, using the 82E1 antibody specific to human Aβ, we found experimentally introduced Aβ to co-localise to multiple retinal locations corresponding to points of Aβ immunoreactivity reported in eyes of both AD [74, 75] and AMD patients/mouse models [55, 61–63]. Hence, Aβ was shown to localise to RGC, the outer nuclear layer, photoreceptors as well as the RPE-Bruch's membrane interface [39]. Attempts by others to elevate $A\beta_{1-42}$ levels in the rodent vitreous resulted in apoptotic cells in photoreceptor and nuclear layers as well as a significant reduction in RGC [76, 77]. However, our method of elevating the retinal Aβ load via subretinal injection appears to mimic the senescent eye more accurately (**Figure 3**), as the resulting phenotype certainly bears closer resemblance to human AMD [55, 63, 64]. Additional evidence for ocular Aβ pathology comes from studies implicating Aβ in other eye diseases such as supranuclear cataracts and glaucoma of which the latter is common amongst AD patients [4].

6. Similarities between AD and AMD

Degenerative processes in the ageing retina and brain share many common features. A major pathological hallmark common to both AD and AMD is the formation of insoluble extracellular aggregates that share several histochemical and compositional properties. Proteomic analyses of the molecular components of senile plaques and drusen, for instance, has revealed common proteins including tau, clusterin, vitronectin, apolipoprotein E (ApoE), serum amyloid P (SAP), Aβ, metal ions, as well as pro-inflammatory factors and components of the compliment cascade [4, 44, 78]. Histochemically, such deposits also stain with thioflavin T and Congo red which confirms the presence of misfolded or amyloid proteins. However, there appears to be differences between Aβ structures found in senile plaques and drusen. For instance, whilst

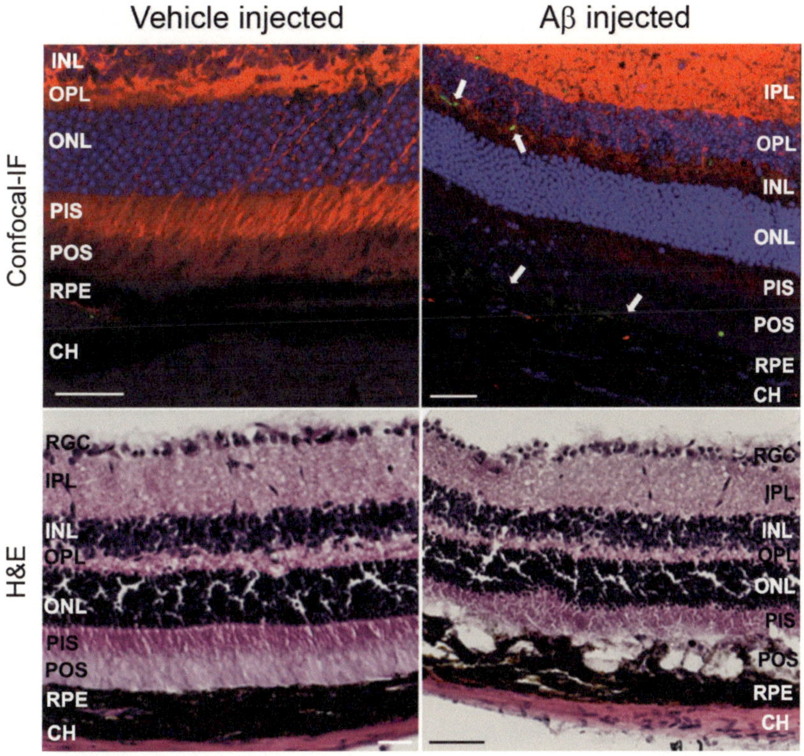

Figure 3. Subretinally injected Aβ in our mouse model recapitulates key aspects of retinal degeneration observed in age-related macular degeneration (AMD). Wild-type C57BL/6 mice injected with nM concentrations of recombinant human $A\beta_{1-42}$ recapitulated key features of AMD. At 8 days post-injection, retinas contained RPE pigment abnormalities, RPE hypertrophy as well as photoreceptor outer segment loss, in contrast to healthy retinas of vehicle injected mice. Confocal-immunofluorescence using the human Aβ-specific antibody 82E1 revealed focal Aβ deposits (green) in the inner nuclear layer and in the RPE-Bruch's membrane interface (arrows) corresponding to areas of Aβ synthesis/accumulation reports in aged human retinas. RGC, retinal ganglion cells; IPL, inner plexiform layer; INL, inner nuclear layer; OPL, outer plexiform layer; ONL, outer nuclear layer; PIS, photoreceptor inner layer; POS, photoreceptor outer segments; RPE, retinal pigment epithelium; BM, Bruch's membrane; CH, choroid. DAPI (blue). Scale bar corresponds to 100 μm.

both types of extracellular protein deposits stain for Congo red, only senile plaques are positive for the apple green birefringence dye specific for anti-parallel β-pleated sheets [49, 63].

Commonalities between AD and AMD are also observed in the manner in which highly localised and significant damage occurs to lysosomes and mitochondria. In AD brains, these include substantial increases in the size/number of endosomes, autophagosomes and lysosomes; accumulation of lysosomal dense bodies in dystrophic neurites, as well as changes in expression of lysosomal hydrolases such as cathepsins [2, 79]. Our studies as well as those of others have shown selective permeabilisation of lysosomal membranes and release of lytic content into the cytosol as a precursor to neuronal death, indicating a mechanism of early cellular compromise correlated with a specific vulnerability in certain neurons [2, 79, 80]. Analysis of fixed tissues from AMD patients show extrudes of senescent RPE cytoplasm with reactive lysosomes into the underlying Bruch's membrane, and the accumulation of incompletely digested POS from overlying photoreceptors as lipofuscin within lysosomes [14]. Senescent postmitotic RPE cells with lipofuscin-filled lysosomes are a characteristic feature of the ageing retina, and it accounts for as much as 20% of the cytoplasmic volume by the age of 80. Experiments using cell lines show the toxic nature of lipofuscin and its derivative N-retinylidene–N-retinylethanolamine (A2E) that disrupts the phagocytic mechanisms of RPE cells, impairs lysosomal proteases, inhibits the lysosomal ATPase proton pump and causes leakage of lysosomal contents into the cytosol [81]. Dysfunctional lysosomes with lipofuscin/A2E also generates reactive oxygen species (ROS), modify lipid peroxidation and forms high molecular weight components that are stable within lysosomes. Moreover, A2E causes detergent-like membrane disruption and inhibits lytic function. Healthy macula RPE cells contain high levels of lysosomal enzymes acid phosphatase and cathepsin D, relative to lysosomes from RPE cells in the nasal/mid-zone and peripheral retina [82]. Lysosomal enzyme activity decreases by up to 50% when exposed to lipofuscin [83], indicating the regional vulnerability of the macula in early AMD. Lysosomal damage may be further exacerbated by the highly photoxidative RPE environment, providing ideal conditions for ROS generation [84].

Mitochondria also show early damage in AD. Hence, post-mortem AD brains show significantly fewer mitochondria, abnormally enlarged as well as exceptionally small mitochondria, damaged cristae, changes to organelle physiology, fission/fusion rates and transport defects [85]. Mitochondrial abnormalities have also been linked to AMD primarily using studies of cell lines showing a decrease in the number/area of RPE mitochondria, changes in redox components and proteins involved in mitochondrial trafficking, increase in mitochondrial DNA repair and decreased RPE mitochondrial respiration. A2E specifically damages mitochondria inducing RPE apoptosis [60]. Our previous studies of a variant form of cystatin C associated with AMD revealed a striking endoplasmic reticulum (ER)/Golgi to mitochondria mis-localisation, which may have long-term consequences for RPE mitochondria [86, 87]. Recently, a strong association between the mitochondrial ARMS2 variant protein and AMD was reported which appeared to drive AMD towards a neovascular phenotype [8].

Genetic risk factors between AMD and AD also indicate evidence of a shared aetiology. For instance, studies have revealed a substantial link between allelic variants encoding components of the alternative compliment cascade and the risk of developing AMD including factor H, factor B and C3 [88–91]. Evidence for a similar genetic predisposition in AD has been reported where polymorphisms within the CFH allele have been linked with an increased risk of AD [92]. The large number of compliment cascade components that have been reported within drusen and senile plaques, as well as the fact that chronic inflammation is a key driver in both AD and AMD indicates that similar inflammatory responses may be involved in the aetiologies of both AD and AMD. A strong genetic link has also been associated with ApoE, a polymorphic gene encoding proteins ApoE2, ApoE3 and ApoE4 involved in lipid metabolism. Amongst these, ApoE4 is somewhat confusingly associated with a lower risk of developing AMD, whilst conferring an increased susceptibility to AD. Although the reason for this is not clear, the positively charged nature of ApoE4 is speculated to interact somewhat differently with Bruch's membrane in the outer retina compared to its behaviour in the brain [93, 94]. The opposite holds true with regard to ApoE2, which is protective in AD but is associated with a higher risk of developing AMD. The reason for this also remains elusive [4]. Collectively, it appears that ApoE dysregulation may affect Aβ metabolism/clearance in the retina and brain in somewhat different ways, but which nonetheless triggers or drives pathology in these respective tissues [93, 95, 96]. Several environmental factors are also shared between AD and AMD that are thought confer increased susceptibility. These include cigarette smoking and diet, as well as conditions such as high blood pressure, heart disease, stroke, diabetes, high cholesterol levels and obesity [97–99]. In fact, a recent study conducted by the World Health Organisation (WHO) revealed that smoking, which is the most prominent environmental risk factor for AMD, almost doubled the risk of developing dementia [http://www.who.int/tobacco/publications/en/]. The growing awareness of these shared pathologies in the senescent brain and retina as well as the increasing sophistication of detection methods are beginning to uncover closer links between AD and AMD. For instance, a recent study revealed the increased risk of AMD amongst AD patients [100].

Collectively, this body of evidence strongly suggests a significant overlap between the aetiologies of AMD and AD. This is not surprising, given the extensive visual complications being reported in patients with AD and dementia. Initial detection typically relies on self-diagnosis and/or observations by friends and family and is therefore often inconsistent, adding to the potential delay in recognising these neuropathological conditions in a timely manner. Hence, ocular studies have been proposed alongside studies to identify common biomarkers so that those at greater risks may be identified relatively early before progressing to more advanced stages.

7. Conclusions: amyloid beta and the retina as a biomarker for Alzheimer's disease

With increased sophistication of new imaging methods and related technologies, there is a growing interest in developing reliable and cost-effective methods of identifying those at greater risk of developing AD. These advances are welcome as current diagnostic techniques such as magnetic resonance imaging (MRI) do not always provide sufficient image resolution to detect incipient brain pathology, whilst positron emission tomography (PET) is prohibitively expensive and is not widely available [4]. Consequently, the most conclusive diagnosis of AD is only made following a brain autopsy, which is of little use as a predictor of disease. Various studies have explored the possibility of measuring peripheral Aβ in the blood or cerebrospinal fluid (CSF) as prognostic markers of disease. CSF as a biomarker has consistently been shown to provide an accurate indication of underlying AD pathology but is an invasive and costly procedure [4]. In contrast, plasma Aβ presents a more cost-effective and a less invasive method of diagnosis, but has proved less successful in identifying those at higher risk [101]. Interestingly, a recent study revealed that plasma Aβ levels accurately correlated across progressive stages of AMD [102]. Nonetheless, inconclusive data from other studies, as well as evidence from AD patients, suggest that such approaches require a more rigorous level of standardisation and further fine-tuning before clinical application [101].

In summary, we propose that the eye is not only a useful organ to study Aβ pathology but that a better understanding of retinal dystrophies may reveal insights into AD and dementia. The eye is amiable to manipulation and study in a way that the brain is not, thus providing a powerful diagnostic tool or an anatomical window to detect potential brain pathology. Consequently, non-invasive retinal imaging techniques may be exploited to measure the retinal Aβ burden and thus identify potential individuals at risk of developing AD. Such methods have already been demonstrated by those using retinal photography, scanning laser ophthalmoscopy (SLO), Doppler blood flowmetry and optical coherence tomography (OCT) to assess retinas of AD and dementia patients [23, 103, 104]. For example, funduscopy is widely used to assess the retina, which often detects the first clinical signs of AMD such as macular drusen. Using such an apparatus, a pilot study found a significant correlation between the appearance of peripheral retinal drusen and AD [103]. Furthermore, Doppler blood flowmetry has been used to measure retinal blood vessel diameters in AD patients. These studies show that decreased vessel diameter correlated with disease progression alongside impaired retinal blood-flow and circulation abnormalities [23]. Advances in OCT were also used to demonstrate NFL abnormalities in patients with open-angle glaucoma [104]. However, this may be of limited value as an early-disease indicator since NFL thinning only becomes apparent in advanced AD [23]. SLO, another non-invasive approach, is used to reliably assess optic nerve-head damage and optic disc topography in glaucoma patients [105], pathologies that are also evident in some AD patients [24]. Finally, trials have been undertaken in AD rodent models using systemic injections of the naturally occurring food ingredient curcumin, which fluoresces when bound to retinal Aβ [74]. Use of this compound has the added advantage of being able to traverse the BRB and BBB, demonstrating successfully use of a non-invasive retinal imaging in AD-Tg mice which correlated the extent of retinal Aβ with plaque load and disease. Curcumin labelling of retinal Aβ deposits in these mice was detected as early as 2.5 months, whereas Aβ deposition in the brain was only apparent after 5 months [74] supporting the idea that the aged eye may function as an early warning system for incipient brain pathology. As curcumin has also been shown to reliably label Aβ deposits/structures in post-mortem human retinas [74], its use could easily be extended to non-invasively detecting retinal Aβ in AD clinics. Hence, there is considerable interest in the pharmaceuticals industry to identify both

http://dx.doi.org/10.5772/64790

natural compounds as well as synthetic agents capable of reliably binding Aβ [106, 107]. Such studies will be highly informative in providing further insights into the role of Aβ in the ageing retina and brain, and help extend current understanding of shared pathologies in these intimately linked tissues.

Acknowledgements

We thank Mr Thomas Freeman and Ms Rosie Munday for their work on the Aβ-induced retinal degeneration mouse model, and Dr David A Johnston (Biomedical Imaging Unit, University of Southampton) for his expertise in imaging. We would also like to thank Dr Helen S.K Ratnayaka (Sussex Community NHS Foundation Trust) for reading the manuscript. SAL is funded by the National Centre for the Replacement Refinement & Reduction of Animals in Research (NC3R: grant # NC/L001152/1). This work was also supported by Fight for Sight (grant # 1485), the Gift of Sight Appeal and the Hampshire and Isle of Wight Community Foundation.

Author details

J. Arjuna Ratnayaka* and Savannah Lynn

*Address all correspondence to: J.Ratnayaka@soton.ac.uk

Clinical and Experimental Sciences, Faculty of Medicine, University of Southampton, SGH, Southampton, UK

References

[1] Castellano JM, Kim J, Stewart FR, Jiang H, DeMattos RB, Patterson BW, et al. Human apoE isoforms differentially regulate brain amyloid-beta peptide clearance. Science Translational Medicine. 2011;3(89):89ra57.

[2] De Strooper B. Proteases and proteolysis in Alzheimer disease: a multifactorial view on the disease process. Physiological Reviews. 2010;90(2):465–94.

[3] Bradford, A, Kunik ME, Schulz P, Williams SP, Singh H. Missed and delayed diagnosis of dementia in primary care: prevalence and contributing factors. Alzheimer Disease and Associated Disorders. 2009;23(4):306–14.

[4] Sivak JM. The aging eye: common degenerative mechanisms between the Alzheimer's brain and retinal disease. Investigative Ophthalmology & Visual Science. 2013;54(1): 871–80.

[5] Kirby E, Bandelow S, Hogervorst E. Visual impairment in Alzheimer's disease: a critical review. Journal of Alzheimer's Disease. 2010;21(1):15–34.

[6] Gilbert SF. Developmental Biology. 6th ed. Sunderland, MA: Sinauer Associates, Inc.; 2000.

[7] Nag S, Walker JM, editors. The Blood-Brain and Other Neural Barriers: Reviews and Protocols. Toronto, ON: Springer; 2011.

[8] Fritsche LG, Fariss RN, Stambolian D, Abecasis GR, Curcio CA, Swaroop A. Age-related macular degeneration: genetics and biology coming together. Annual Review of Genomics and Human Genetics. 2014;15:151–71.

[9] Purves D, Augustine, GJ Fitzpatrick D, Hall WC, LaMantia AS, McNamara JO, White LE. Vision: The Eye. Neuroscience. 4th ed. Sunderland, MA: Sinauer Associates, Inc.; 2008. p. 253–88.

[10] Sanes JR, Zipursky SL. Design principles of insect and vertebrate visual systems. Neuron. 2010;66(1):15–36.

[11] Strauss O. The retinal pigment epithelium in visual function. Physiological Reviews. 2005;85(3):845–81.

[12] Rizzolo LJ. Barrier properties of cultured retinal pigment epithelium. Experimental Eye Research. 2014;126:16–26.

[13] Saade CJ, Alvarez-Delfin K, Fadool JM. Rod photoreceptors protect from cone degeneration-induced retinal remodeling and restore visual responses in zebrafish. Journal of Neuroscience. 2013;33(5):1804–14.

[14] Khandhadia S, Cherry J, Lotery AJ. Age-related macular degeneration. Advances in Experimental Medicine and Biology. 2012;724:15–36.

[15] Besharse JC, Bok D. Information Processing: Ganglion Cells. The Retina and It's Disorders. Oxford, UK: Elsevier; 2011.

[16] Snell RS, Lemp MA. Clinical Anatomy of the Eye. 2nd ed. Oxford, UK: Wiley; 1998. p. 379–412.

[17] Purves D, Augustine GJ, Fitzpatrick D, Hall WC, LaMantia AS, McNamara JO, White LE. Central Visual Pathways. Neuroscience. 4th ed. Sunderland, MA: Sinauer Associates, Inc.; 2008. p. 289–311.

[18] Tzekov R, Mullan M. Vision function abnormalities in Alzheimer disease. Survey of Ophthalmology. 2014;59(4):414–33.

[19] Valenti DA. Alzheimer's disease: visual system review. Optometry (St Louis, MO). 2010;81(1):12–21.

[20] Kirshner HS, Lavin PJM. Posterior cortical atrophy: a brief review. Current Neurology and Neuroscience Reports. 2006;6:477–80.

[21] Josephs KA, Whitwell JL, Boeve BF, Knopman DS, Tang-Wai DF, Drubach DA, Jack CR Jr, Petersen RC. Visual hallucinations in posterior cortical atrophy. Archives of Neurology. 2006;63:1427–32.

[22] Blanks JC, Torigoe Y, Hinton DR, Blanks RH. Retinal pathology in Alzheimer's disease. I. Ganglion cell loss in foveal/parafoveal retina. Neurobiology of Aging. 1996;17(3):377–84.

[23] Berisha F, Feke GT, Trempe CL, McMeel JW, Schepens CL. Retinal abnormalities in early Alzheimer's disease. Investigative Ophthalmology & Visual Science. 2007;48(5): 2285–9.

[24] Sadun AA, Bassi CJ. Optic nerve damage in Alzheimer's disease. Ophthalmology. 1990;97(1):9–17.

[25] Syed AB, Armstrong RA, Smith CU. A quantitative analysis of optic nerve axons in elderly control subjects and patients with Alzheimer's disease. Folia Neuropathologica/ Association of Polish Neuropathologists and Medical Research Centre, Polish Academy of Sciences. 2005;43(1):1–6.

[26] Wang MY, Ross-Cisneros FN, Aggarwal D, Liang CY, Sadun AA. Receptor for advanced glycation end products is upregulated in optic neuropathy of Alzheimer's disease. Acta Neuropathology. 2009;118:381–9.

[27] Scholtz CL, Swettenham K, Brown A, Mann DM. A histoquantitative study of the striate cortex and lateral geniculate body in normal, blind and demented subjects. Neuropathology and Applied Neurobiology. 1981;7:103–14.

[28] Parvizi J, Van Hoesen GW, Damasio A. The selective vulnerability of brainstem nuclei to Alzheimer's disease. Annals of Neurology. 2001;49:53–66.

[29] Armstrong RA. Alzheimer's disease and the eye. Journal of Optometry. 2009;2(3):103–11.

[30] Hof PR, Morrison JH. Quantitative analysis of a vulnerable subset of pyramidal neurons in Alzheimer's disease: II. Primary and secondary visual cortex. The Journal of Comparative Neurology. 1990;301(1):56–64.

[31] Armstrong RA, Nochlin D, Sumi SM, Alvord EC. Neuropathological changes in the visual cortex in Alzheimer's disease. Neuroscience Research Communication. 1990;6:163–71.

[32] Armstrong R. Visual field defects in Alzheimer's disease patients may reflect differential pathology in the primary visual cortex. Optometry and Vision Science. 1996;73:677–82.

[33] Baker DR, Mendez MF, Townsend JC, Ilsen PF, Bright DC. Optometric management of patients with Alzheimer's disease. Journal of the American Optometric Association. 1997;68:483–94.

[34] Liu B, Rasool S, Yang Z, Glabe CG, Schreiber SS, Ge J, et al. Amyloid-peptide vaccinations reduce {beta}-amyloid plaques but exacerbate vascular deposition and inflammation in the retina of Alzheimer's transgenic mice. The American Journal of Pathology. 2009;175(5):2099–110.

[35] Ning A, Cui J, To E, Ashe KH, Matsubara J. Amyloid-beta deposits lead to retinal degeneration in a mouse model of Alzheimer disease. Investigative Ophthalmology & Visual Science. 2008;49(11):5136–43.

[36] Park SW, Kim JH, Mook-Jung I, Kim KW, Park WJ, Park KH, et al. Intracellular amyloid beta alters the tight junction of retinal pigment epithelium in 5XFAD mice. Neurobiology of Aging. 2014;35(9):2013–20.

[37] Oakley H, Cole SL, Logan S, Maus E, Shao P, Craft J, et al. Intraneuronal beta-amyloid aggregates, neurodegeneration, and neuron loss in transgenic mice with five familial Alzheimer's disease mutations: potential factors in amyloid plaque formation. The Journal of Neuroscience: The Official Journal of the Society for Neuroscience. 2006;26(40):10129–40.

[38] Gasparini L, Crowther RA, Martin KR, Berg N, Coleman M, Goedert M, et al. Tau inclusions in retinal ganglion cells of human P301S tau transgenic mice: effects on axonal viability. Neurobiology of Aging. 2011;32(3):419–33.

[39] Hoh Kam J, Lenassi E, Jeffery G. Viewing ageing eyes: diverse sites of amyloid Beta accumulation in the ageing mouse retina and the up-regulation of macrophages. PloS One. 2010;5(10):1–12.

[40] Pennesi ME, Neuringer M, Courtney RJ. Animal models of age related macular degeneration. Molecular Aspects of Medicine. 2012;33(4):487–509.

[41] Vojnikovic B, Radeljak S, Dessardo S, Zarkovic-Palijan T, Bajek G, Linsak Z. What associates Charles Bonnet syndrome with age-related macular degeneration? Collegium Antropologicum. 2010;34(Suppl. 2):45–8.

[42] Cox TM, Ffytche D. Negative outcome Charles Bonnet syndrome. British Journal of Ophthalmology. 2014;98(9):1236–9.

[43] Gehrs KM, Anderson DH, Johnson LV, Hageman GS. Age-related macular degeneration—emerging pathogenetic and therapeutic concepts. Annals of Medicine. 2006;38(7):450–71.

[44] Ohno-Matsui K. Parallel findings in age-related macular degeneration and Alzheimer's disease. Progress in Retinal and Eye Research. 2011;30(4):217–38.

[45] Lotery A, Trump D. Progress in defining the molecular biology of age related macular degeneration. Human Genetics. 2007;122(3–4):219–36.

[46] Augood CA, Vingerling JR, de Jong PT, Chakravarthy U, Seland J, Soubrane G, et al. Prevalence of age-related maculopathy in older Europeans: the European Eye Study (EUREYE). Archives of Ophthalmology (Chicago, IL: 1960). 2006;124(4):529–35.

[47] Khandhadia S, Cipriani V, Yates JR, Lotery AJ. Age-related macular degeneration and the complement system. Immunobiology. 2012;217(2):127–46.

[48] Korb CA, Kottler UB, Wolfram C, Hoehn R, Schulz A, Zwiener I, et al. Prevalence of age-related macular degeneration in a large European cohort: results from the population-based Gutenberg Health Study. Graefe's Archive for Clinical and Experimental Ophthalmology. 2014;252(9):1403–11.

[49] Mullins RF, Russell SR, Anderson DH, Hageman GS. Drusen associated with aging and age-related macular degeneration contain proteins common to extracellular deposits associated with atherosclerosis, elastosis, amyloidosis, and dense deposit disease. FASEB Journal: Official Publication of the Federation of American Societies for Experimental Biology. 2000;14(7):835–46.

[50] Bonilha VL. Age and disease-related structural changes in the retinal pigment epithelium. Clinical Ophthalmology (Auckland, NZ). 2008;2(2):413–24.

[51] Klein R, Klein BE, Linton KL. Prevalence of age-related maculopathy. The Beaver Dam Eye Study. Ophthalmology. 1992;99(6):933–43.

[52] Owen CG, Jarrar Z, Wormald R, Cook DG, Fletcher AE, Rudnicka AR. The estimated prevalence and incidence of late stage age related macular degeneration in the UK. British Journal of Ophthalmology. 2012;96(5):752–6.

[53] Wang J, Ohno-Matsui K, Morita I. Elevated amyloid beta production in senescent retinal pigment epithelium, a possible mechanism of subretinal deposition of amyloid beta in age-related macular degeneration. Biochemical and Biophysical Research Communications. 2012;423(1):73–8.

[54] Dutescu RM, Li QX, Crowston J, Masters CL, Baird PN, Culvenor JG. Amyloid precursor protein processing and retinal pathology in mouse models of Alzheimer's disease. Graefe's Archive for Clinical and Experimental Ophthalmology. 2009;247(9): 1213–21.

[55] Johnson LV, Leitner WP, Rivest AJ, Staples MK, Radeke MJ, Anderson DH. The Alzheimer's A beta—peptide is deposited at sites of complement activation in pathologic deposits associated with aging and age-related macular degeneration. Proceedings of the National Academy of Sciences of the United States of America. 2002;99(18): 11830–5.

[56] Ratnayaka JA, Serpell LC, Lotery AJ. Dementia of the eye: the role of amyloid beta in retinal degeneration. Eye (London, England). 2015;29(8):1013–26.

[57] Yoshida T, Ohno-Matsui K, Ichinose S, Sato T, Iwata N, Saido TC, et al. The potential role of amyloid beta in the pathogenesis of age-related macular degeneration. The Journal of Clinical Investigation. 2005;115(10):2793–800.

[58] Prakasam A, Muthuswamy A, Ablonczy Z, Greig NH, Fauq A, Rao KJ, et al. Differential accumulation of secreted AbetaPP metabolites in ocular fluids. Journal of Alzheimer's Disease. 2010;20(4):1243–53.

[59] Kaarniranta K, Hyttinen J, Ryhanen T, Viiri J, Paimela T, Toropainen E, et al. Mechanisms of protein aggregation in the retinal pigment epithelial cells. Frontiers in Bioscience (Elite edition). 2010;2:1374–84.

[60] Jarrett SG, Lin H, Godley BF, Boulton ME. Mitochondrial DNA damage and its potential role in retinal degeneration. Progress in Retinal and Eye Research. 2008;27(6):596–607.

[61] Luibl V, Isas JM, Kayed R, Glabe CG, Langen R, Chen J. Drusen deposits associated with aging and age-related macular degeneration contain nonfibrillar amyloid oligomers. The Journal of Clinical Investigation. 2006;116(2):378–85.

[62] Isas JM, Luibl V, Johnson LV, Kayed R, Wetzel R, Glabe CG, et al. Soluble and mature amyloid fibrils in drusen deposits. Investigative Ophthalmology & Visual Science. 2010;51(3):1304–10.

[63] Anderson DH, Talaga KC, Rivest AJ, Barron E, Hageman GS, Johnson LV. Characterization of β amyloid assemblies in drusen: the deposits associated with aging and age-related macular degeneration. Experimental Eye Research. 2004;78(2):243–56.

[64] Dentchev T, Milam AH, Lee VMY, Trojanowski JQ, Dunaief JL. Amyloid-β is found in drusen from some age-related macular degeneration retinas, but not in drusen from normal retinas. Molecular Vision. 2003;9:184–90.

[65] Bruban J, Glotin AL, Dinet V, Chalour N, Sennlaub F, Jonet L, et al. Amyloid-β (1-42) alters structure and function of retinal pigmented epithelial cells. Aging Cell. 2009;8:162–77.

[66] Liu W, Cai H, Lin M, Zhu L, Gao L, Zhong R, et al. MicroRNA-107 prevents amyloid-beta induced blood-brain barrier disruption and endothelial cell dysfunction by targeting endophilin-1. Experimental Cell Research. 2016;343(2):248–57.

[67] Dal Pra I, Armato U, Chioffi F, Pacchiana R, Whitfield JF, Chakravarthy B, et al. The Abeta peptides-activated calcium-sensing receptor stimulates the production and secretion of vascular endothelial growth factor-A by normoxic adult human cortical astrocytes. Neuromolecular Medicine. 2014;16(4):645–57.

[68] Wyss-Coray T, Rogers J. Inflammation in Alzheimer disease—a brief review of the basic science and clinical literature. Cold Spring Harbor Perspectives in Medicine. 2012;2(1); 1–23.

[69] Blalock EM, Geddes JW, Chen KC, Porter NM, Markesbery WR, Landfield PW. Incipient Alzheimer's disease: microarray correlation analyses reveal major transcrip-

tional and tumor suppressor responses. Proceedings of the National Academy of Sciences of the United States of America. 2004;101(7):2173–8.

[70] Katsel P, Tan W, Haroutunian V. Gain in brain immunity in the oldest-old differentiates cognitively normal from demented individuals. PloS One. 2009;4(10):e7642.

[71] Johnson LV, Leitner WP, Staples MK, Anderson DH. Complement activation and inflammatory processes in drusen formation and age related macular degeneration. Experimental Eye Research. 2001;73(6):887–96.

[72] Liu RT, Gao J, Cao S, Sandhu N, Cui JZ, Chou CL, et al. Inflammatory mediators induced by amyloid-beta in the retina and RPE in vivo: implications for inflammasome activation in age-related macular degeneration. Investigative Ophthalmology & Visual Science. 2013;54(3):2225–37.

[73] Cao L, Wang H, Wang F, Xu D, Liu F, Liu C. Aβ-Induced senescent retinal pigment epithelial cells create a proinflammatory microenvironment in AMD. Investigative Ophthalmology & Visual Science. 2013;54(5):3738–50.

[74] Koronyo-Hamaoui M, Koronyo Y, Ljubimov AV, Miller CA, Ko MK, Black KL, et al. Identification of amyloid plaques in retinas from Alzheimer's patients and noninvasive in vivo optical imaging of retinal plaques in a mouse model. NeuroImage. 2011;54(Suppl. 1):S204–17.

[75] Guo L, Salt TE, Luong V, Wood N, Cheung W, Maass A, et al. Targeting amyloid-beta in glaucoma treatment. Proceedings of the National Academy of Sciences of the United States of America. 2007;104(33):13444–9.

[76] Walsh DT, Montero RM, Bresciani LG, Jen AY, Leclercq PD, Saunders D, et al. Amyloid-beta peptide is toxic to neurons in vivo via indirect mechanisms. Neurobiology of Disease. 2002;10(1):20–7.

[77] Walsh DT, Bresciani L, Saunders D, Manca MF, Jen A, Gentleman SM, et al. Amyloid beta peptide causes chronic glial cell activation and neuro-degeneration after intravitreal injection. Neuropathology and Applied Neurobiology. 2005;31(5):491–502.

[78] Catchpole I, Germaschewski V, Hoh Kam J, Lundh von Leithner P, Ford S, Gough G, et al. Systemic administration of Abeta mAb reduces retinal deposition of Abeta and activated complement C3 in age-related macular degeneration mouse model. PLoS One. 2013;8(6):e65518.

[79] Nixon RA, Cataldo AM, Mathews PM. The endosomal-lysosomal system of neurons in Alzheimer's disease pathogenesis: a review. Neurochemical Research. 2000;25(9–10): 1161–72.

[80] Soura V, Stewart-Parker M, Williams TL, Ratnayaka A, Atherton J, Gorringe K, et al. Visualization of co-localization in Abeta42-administered neuroblastoma cells reveals lysosome damage and autophagosome accumulation related to cell death. The Biochemical Journal. 2012;441(2):579–90.

[81] Sundelin S, Wihlmark U, Nilsson SE, Brunk UT. Lipofuscin accumulation in cultured retinal pigment epithelial cells reduces their phagocytic capacity. Current Eye Research. 1998;17(8):851–7.

[82] Boulton M, Moriarty P, Jarvis-Evans J, Marcyniuk B. Regional variation and age-related changes of lysosomal enzymes in the human retinal pigment epithelium. The British Journal of Ophthalmology. 1994;78(2):125–9.

[83] Shamsi FA, Boulton M. Inhibition of RPE lysosomal and antioxidant activity by the age pigment lipofuscin. Investigative Ophthalmology & Visual Science. 2001;42(12):3041–6.

[84] Khandhadia S, Lotery A. Oxidation and age-related macular degeneration: insights from molecular biology. Expert Reviews in Molecular Medicine. 2010;12:e34.

[85] Silva DF, Selfridge JE, Lu J, Lezi E, Cardoso SM, Swerdlow RH. Mitochondrial abnormalities in Alzheimer's disease: possible targets for therapeutic intervention. Advances in Pharmacology (San Diego, Calif). 2012;64:83–126.

[86] Ratnayaka A, Paraoan L, Spiller DG, Hiscott P, Nelson G, White MR, et al. A dual Golgi- and mitochondria-localised Ala25Ser precursor cystatin C: an additional tool for characterising intracellular mis-localisation leading to increased AMD susceptibility. Experimental Eye Research. 2007;84(6):1135–9.

[87] Paraoan L, Ratnayaka A, Spiller DG, Hiscott P, White MR, Grierson I. Unexpected intracellular localization of the AMD-associated cystatin C variant. Traffic (Copenhagen, Denmark). 2004;5(11):884–95.

[88] Edwards AO, Malek G. Molecular genetics of AMD and current animal models. Angiogenesis. 2007;10(2):119–32.

[89] Spencer KL, Olson LM, Anderson BM, Schnetz-Boutaud N, Scott WK, Gallins P, et al. C3 R102G polymorphism increases risk of age-related macular degeneration. Human Molecular Genetics. 2008;17(12):1821–4.

[90] Yates JR, Sepp T, Matharu BK, Khan JC, Thurlby DA, Shahid H, et al. Complement C3 variant and the risk of age-related macular degeneration. The New England Journal of Medicine. 2007;357(6):553–61.

[91] Liao X, Lan CJ, Cheuk IW, Tan QQ. Four complement factor H gene polymorphisms in association with AMD: a meta-analysis. Archives of Gerontology and Geriatrics. 2016;64:123–9.

[92] Zetterberg M, Landgren S, Andersson ME, Palmer MS, Gustafson DR, Skoog I, et al. Association of complement factor H Y402H gene polymorphism with Alzheimer's disease. American Journal of Medical Genetics Part B, Neuropsychiatric Genetics: The Official Publication of the International Society of Psychiatric Genetics. 2008;147b(6):720–6.

[93] Holz FG, Pauleikhoff D, Spaide RF, Bird AC. Age-related Macular Degeneration.2nd ed. Heidelberg, Germany:Springer;2013

[94] Giau VV, Bagyinszky E, An SSA, Kim SY. Role of apolipoprotein E in neurodegenerative diseases. Neuropsychiatric Disease and Treatment. 2015;11:1723–37.

[95] Ricciarelli R, Canepa E, Marengo B, Marinari UM, Poli G, Pronzato MA, et al. Cholesterol and Alzheimer's disease: a still poorly understood correlation. IUBMB Life. 2012;64(12):931–5.

[96] Pikuleva IA, Curcio CA. Cholesterol in the retina: the best is yet to come. Progress in Retinal and Eye Research. 2014;41:64–89.

[97] Panpalli Ates M, Karaman Y, Guntekin S, Ergun MA. Analysis of genetics and risk factors of Alzheimer's disease. Neuroscience. 2016;325:124–31.

[98] Klein R, Cruickshanks KJ, Nash SD, Krantz EM, Nieto FJ, Huang GH, et al. The prevalence of age-related macular degeneration and associated risk factors. Archives of Ophthalmology (Chicago, IL: 1960). 2010;128(6):750–8.

[99] Hogg RE, Woodside JV, Gilchrist SE, Graydon R, Fletcher AE, Chan W, et al. Cardiovascular disease and hypertension are strong risk factors for choroidal neovascularization. Ophthalmology. 2008;115(6):1046–52.e2.

[100] Frost S, Guymer RH, Aung KZ, Macaulay SL, Sohrabi HR, Bourgeat P, et al. Alzheimer's disease and the early signs of age-related macular degeneration. Current Alzheimer Research. 2016[Epub ahead of print].

[101] Toledo JB, Shaw LM, Trojanowski JQ. Plasma amyloid beta measurements—a desired but elusive Alzheimer's disease biomarker. Alzheimer's Research & Therapy. 2013;5(2): 8.

[102] Guymer R, Cipriani T, Rittenhouse KD, Lim L, Robman LD, Li W, et al. Plasma levels of amyloid beta and other proinflammatory mediators in patients with age-related macular degeneration. Graefe's Archive for Clinical and Experimental Ophthalmology. 2015;253(8):1347–54.

[103] Aslam A, Peto T, Barzegar-Befroei N, Gregory S, Morrison G, Ritchie C, Lengyel I, editors Assessing Peripheral Retinal Drusen Progression in Alzheimer's Dementia: A Pilot Study Using Ultra-Wide Field Imaging. The Association for Research in Vision in Opthalmology. Orlando, FA: IOVS; 2014.

[104] Moschos MM, Georgopolous G, Chatziralli IP, Koutsandrea C. Multifocal VEP and OCT findings in patients with primary open angle glaucoma: a cross-sectional study. BMC Opthalmology. 2012;12(34):1–5.

[105] Danesh-Meyer HV, Gaskin BJ, Jayusundera T, Donaldson M, Gamble GD. Comparison of disc damage likelihood scale, cup to disc ratio, and Heidelberg retina tomograph in the diagnosis of glaucoma. British Journal of Opthalmology. 2006;90(4):437–41.

[106] Koronyo Y, Salumbides, BC, Black KL, Koronyo-Hamaoui M. Alzheimer's disease in the retina: imaging retinal aβ plaques for early diagnosis and therapy assessment. Neurodegeneration Diseases. 2012;10(1–4):285–93.

[107] Park YD, Park JH, Hur MG, Kim SW, Min JJ, Park SH, et al. Fluorescent 2-styrylpyridazin-3(2H)-one derivatives as probes targeting amyloid-beta plaques in Alzheimer's disease. Bioorganic & Medicinal Chemistry Letters. 2012;22(12):4106–10.

Chapter 6

Proteomic Study of Degenerative Protein Modifications in the Molecular Pathology of Neurodegeneration and Dementia

Sunil S. Adav and Siu Kwan Sze

Additional information is available at the end of the chapter

http://dx.doi.org/10.5772/64693

Abstract

Dementia is a major public health burden, and the World Health Organization has identified this disorder as a major public health priority. There are limited treatment options due to poor understanding of key mechanism of dementia pathogenesis. Dementia has been regarded as a proteinopathy in which alterations of brain protein structure and function are the key features of the disorder. Proteinopathy can be triggered by degenerative protein modifications (DPMs), misfolding, aggregation, and deposition of the malformed proteins. Despite the clinical significance of alteration in protein abundances, DPMs, protein misfolding, and aggregation, the molecular mechanism that promotes these changes remains inadequately understood, mostly due to technical challenges. Proteomic is a powerful, sensitive, and advanced tool to study the progressive brain tissue damage that critically dysregulates key enzymes, accumulates modified proteins, and causes protein misfolding and aggregation, resulting in cognitive decline and dementia. The proteomic profiling of protein abundances and correlating DPMs with protein misfolding and aggregation have potential to elucidate underlying molecular mechanism of the disease. This chapter summarizes the recent proteomic developments for studying brain proteome, DPMs, and protein aggregation mechanism that may lead to dementia. We attempted to correlate DPMs and its impact on protein aggregation and deposition in brain tissues.

Keywords: dementia, Alzheimer's disease, vascular dementia, neurodegenerative disease, proteomics, degenerative protein modifications (DPMs), deamidation, citrullination, amyloid

1. Introduction

Dementia is progressively more common disease in aging population. Worldwide, in 2015 about 46.8 million people were affected by dementia and projected to increase to about 74.7 million by 2030 [1]. The increase in dementia patients is in part due to the aging society, lack of effective prevention strategies, and curative treatments. Due to this exponential increase in dementia population, the social and economic cost of this disorder is surpassing those attributed to cancer and heart diseases [1, 2]. High global prevalence, impact of this disorder on families, caregivers, and communities have posed significant public health challenge [3] forcing the global health community to recognize the need for action and to place dementia on the public health agenda. Recently, the World Health Organization (WHO) has identified dementia as a major public health priority [3]. Unfortunately, dementia research has not been given priority as well as funding share, which could be another reason for significant increase in dementia population. For example, in the UK, only 11% of research funding has been allocated for dementia research while 64% was spent on cancer research in 2012.

The most common forms of dementia are Alzheimer's disease (AD) and vascular dementia (VaD), with respective frequencies of 70 and 15% of all dementias [4]. However, the boundaries between the subtypes are sometimes not clear and mixed forms often coexist [5]. In past decades, research in different subtypes of dementia has failed to improve our understanding of dementia pathogenesis and to develop effective treatments or interventions for this disorder [6, 7]. The major mystery is the lack of information on the main causes of the disorder. This remains the main obstacle in developing a cure for the disorder. Therefore, an urgent intervention is needed to identify the key molecular mechanism that promotes dementia pathogenesis. Several theories have been put forward and only few have survived the test of time. Induction of dementia by ischemic cerebral vascular diseases or stroke was first described in clinics a century ago. However, the later discovery of aggregated β-amyloid and *tau* proteins in the brain tissues of dementia patients diverted the majority of subsequent research toward the study of these two molecules. Accordingly, it was hypothesized that this disorder is triggered by the toxicity of oligomerized protein that forms senile plaque including amyloid-beta (Aβ) and *tau* proteins [8]. However, this hypothesis failed to answer several questions regarding pathogenesis and further development in therapeutics. Although Aβ-deposition has been considered as the main cause of AD, the degree of its deposition in the brain does not correlate with dementia severity [9]. According to Arriagada et al. [10], patients without dementia have the same density of senile plaques as patients with AD. Amyloidal hypothesis could not answer questions such as why healthy elderly people have abundant senile plaques in their brains but no signs of AD [11].

The burden of senile plaques does not correlate with cognitive dysfunction in dementia indicating that protein aggregation alone is not sufficient to explain the pathology of these disorders. Accumulation of degenerative protein modifications (DPMs) triggered by nonenzymatic spontaneous posttranslational modifications, loss of protein function, protein misfolding, protein aggregation, and their depositions in brain tissues could be key features of multiple neurodegenerative diseases since protein dysfunction is likely to extend beyond these Aβ and *tau* proteins alone. These deleterious protein damages can be caused by dysregulated protein repair and turnover due to hypoxia-ischemia brain injury. Recent epidemiological, clinical, and experimental studies demonstrated that cerebrovascular disease and hypoxic-ischemic brain injury are the primary causes of cognitive impairment and dementia [12–22].

Proteinopathy is the primary cause of dementia, but rarely attempts have been made to determine the complete composition of deposited protein aggregates, to find what promotes the protein aggregation, does proteins other than Aβ are the main culprit, what is the role of DPMs, and how the constituent proteins contribute to plaque formation. The state-of-the-art mass spectrometry-based proteomic technique has the potential to answer these questions. Proteomic techniques can be considered as an integral part of dementia research to identify biomarkers to detect the disorder at the early stage, understand mechanisms that lead to dementia pathogenesis, design new therapeutics, and monitor response of developed treatments. Proteomic discoveries in dementia and current published literature were used as a tool for review. To investigate our question regarding the mechanism of dementia pathogenesis and the role of degenerative protein modifications, we searched PubMed and Scopus for the literature using the following terms: dementia proteomics, amyloidal proteins, dementia proteomic biomarker, neurodegenerative diseases, degenerative protein modification, and posttranslational modification. We then review the returned articles to generate the summary of the mechanism of dementia pathogenesis and the role of degenerative protein modifications in dementia pathogenesis. We provide a review of the most significant findings in the field of dementia with a special focus on DPMs. This chapter aims at providing understanding on dementia pathogenesis through state-of-art proteomics technology and the impact of protein modifications. In the present chapter, we discussed the recent developments and novel proteomic approaches to study the mechanism of dementia pathogenesis, novel insights from neuroproteomic research, mechanism of protein aggregation, and the role of DPMs.

2. Proteomics studies of dementia and AD

Dementia is caused by damage to brain cells, which further interfere with the ability of brain cells to communicate with each other. The broad range of symptoms includes a decline in memory, thinking skills, and decision making. This potentially affects a person's ability to perform everyday activities. According to Alzheimer's association, dementia have several types such as AD, VaD, mixed dementia, Parkinson's Disease (PD), frontotemporal dementia, mild cognitive impairment, posterior cortical atrophy, traumatic brain injury, Down syndrome, Creutzfeldt-Jakob disease, and normal pressure hydrocephalus [23]. These subtypes are associated with damage to specific types of brain cell in particular regions of the brain. For example, hippocampus is the center of learning and memory in the brain, and damage to hippocampus cells results in memory loss, which is one of the earliest symptoms of AD. The presence of aggregated protein plaque is a common clinical manifestation of the diseases, but the specific molecular mechanisms in each type of dementia that trigger neurodegeneration remain a mystery. The main reasons are the lack of well-characterized clinical samples of brain from particular region, suitable technology to isolate plaque and aggregated proteins, the technique that profiles quantitative composition of both soluble and aggregated proteins, and the technique that accurately identifies DPMs. Proteomic technique enables the comprehensive analysis of the protein and its work flow involves the identification of proteins following their separation, digestion by trypsin, determination of the molecular weight of the resulting peptides, and database searching to make the identification and quantification of the proteins as well as the characterization of the DPMs. In addition to label-free proteomic methods, isobaric tags for relative and absolute quantitation (iTRAQ) and tandem mass tag (TMT) protein labeling are widely accepted approaches for quantitative profiling of cell lines and clinical brain tissue samples [24–26]. Proteomics has also been used for the accurate identification of protein modifications [26–31].

2.1. Novel amyloidal protein-enrichment techniques and DPMs

The alteration in protein function and aggregation is the key feature of neurodegenerative diseases. However, what initiates the protein aggregation, and their deposition and formation of insoluble plaque are poorly defined. Due to poor solubility and self-association of these amyloidal plaque proteins, their accurate identification and quantitation in brain tissue extracts are technically challenging. Researchers [32, 33] have attempted to isolate amyloid proteins using detergents or detergent-free buffers. They adopted sequential extraction and quantification by enzyme-linked immunosorbent assay (ELISA), immunoblotting, or immunocytochemistry. But these approaches were unable to determine the aggregation state of the amyloids and complete composition of amyloidal proteins. Recently, Adav et al. [34] successfully developed ultracentrifugation-electrostatic repulsion hydrophilic interaction chromatography (UC-ERLIC)-coupled mass spectrometry-based proteomics technologies to characterize aggregated proteins in human brain tissues affected by dementia. Using a detergent buffer, they extracted soluble proteins, amyloidal proteins, and insoluble aggregated proteins to identify dementia-associated changes in amyloid protein composition, relative abundances, and the extent of DPMs such as deamidation. These authors profiled both soluble and aggregated amyloidal plaque by LC-MS/MS and found significant enrichment of proteins such as S100A9, ferritin, hemoglobin subunits, creatine kinase, and collagen among the aggregated brain proteins. According to their findings, amyloid plaque was enriched in the deamidated variant of protein S100A9. Yet, the following modified protocol (**Figure 1**) could further improve the detection and identification of amyloidal protein profile in clinical samples.

Most DPMs cause small shift in mass and also involve the addition of small chemical motifs to protein side-chain functional group. This causes alterations in charge and hydrophobicity of the peptide/protein. The detection of the DPM-modified peptide/protein is challenging because the DPMs containing peptides in the trypsin-digested protein sample usually exhibit very low stoichiometry; hence, it is very difficult to identify these from high abundant unmodified peptides during LC-MS/MS analysis. However, these DPMs containing peptides with different charges and hydrophilicities can be separated from unmodified peptides by using ion exchange column running in hydrophilic interaction liquid chromatography (HILIC) mode that facilitates the detection and identification by LC-MS/MS [35]. Moreover, the unmodified and modified peptides elute from ion exchange column in a predictable order based on their charge densities in LC-MS/MS mobile phase. Accordingly, the modified and unmodified peptides can be separated by electrostatic-interaction-modified HILIC (emHILIC) methods using weak anion exchange (WAX)/strong anion exchange (SAX) columns in ERLIC mode for online ERLIC-MS/MS analysis, or using weak cation exchange (WCX) columns in electrostatic attraction hydrophilic interaction chromatographic mode (EALIC) for online ERLIC-MS/MS analysis.

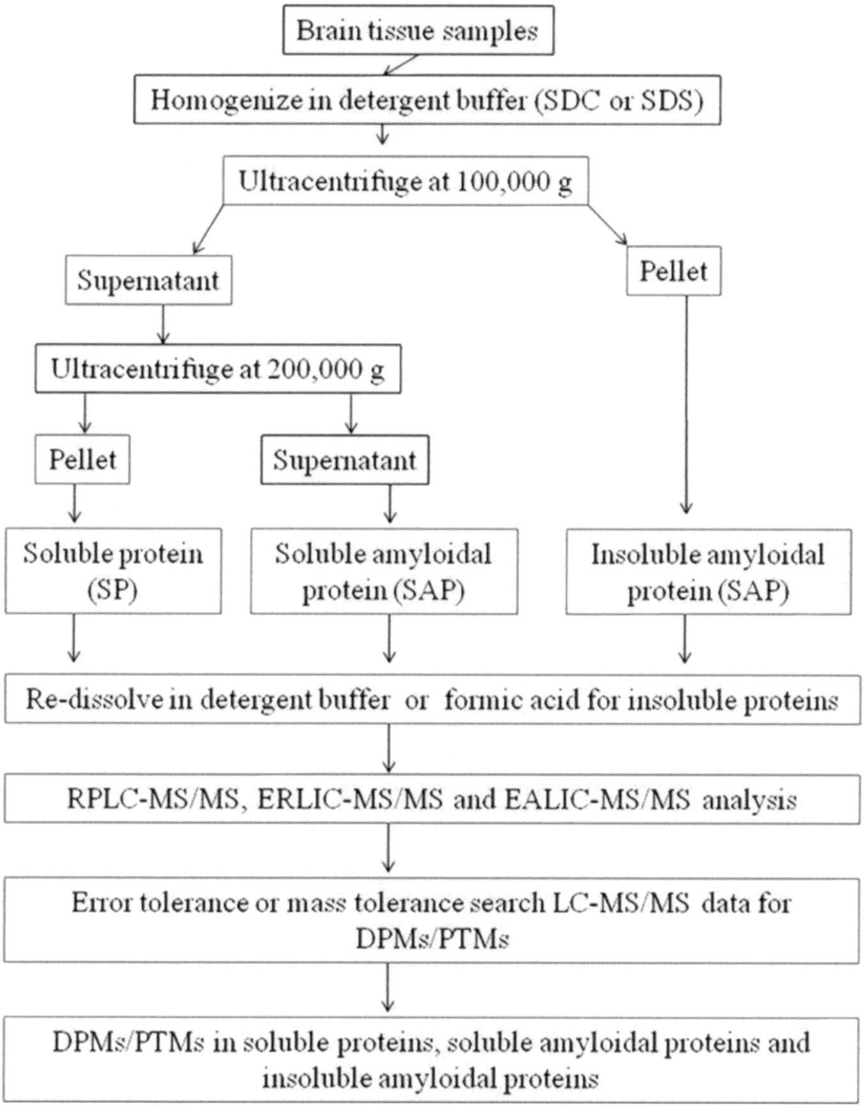

Figure 1. Isolation and identification of both soluble and insoluble amyloid proteins.

2.2. Quantitative clinical proteomics of brain tissue

Protein quantification through the incorporation of stable isotopes has become a vital technology in modern proteomics research. Applying two-dimensional (2D) liquid chromatography coupled with tandem mass spectrometry-based iTRAQ (2D-LC-MS/MS-iTRAQ) technique, Brodmann area 21 of pathologically confirmed cases of VaD and matched non-neurological controls were studied [25]. In the study, 144 differentially expressed proteins including superoxide dismutase, neural cell adhesion molecule, and ATP synthase subunit alpha were characterized to be significantly up-regulated in VaD patients, suggesting a state of hypometabolism and vascular insufficiency along with an inflammatory condition during vascular dementia. iTRAQ quantitative proteomics of brain tissue samples from VaD subjects discovered down-regulation of ion channel proteins including proteins such as V-type proton ATPase subunit D (VATD), ATP synthase, H+ transporting, mitochondrial F0 complex, subunit b-isoform (ATP5F1), Obg-like ATPase 1(OLA1), and V-type proton ATPase subunit F (VATF) [24]. The ion channel protein Na^+–K^+–ATPase exhibits multiple functions including the maintenance of differential membrane potential in neurons, which is an essential feature of the signal transduction. Using proteomics and structural modeling of Na^+–K^+–ATPase, Sze and coworkers [24] showed that the impaired regulation and compromised activity of Na^+–K^+–ATPase contribute to the pathophysiology of VaD. Dysregulated Na^+–K^+–ATPase expression or function have been reported in both animal models and brain tissues in AD, PD, and Huntington's disease (HD) [36].

Synaptic failure is the most common feature observed in both VaD and AD. The loss of synapses and synaptic contacts is also most significant contributor to the cognitive impairment in VaD and other neurodegenerative disease [30, 37]. Similarly, a decline in synapse number in the hippocampal dentate gyrus in AD has been correlated with impairment on a variety of cognitive tests [38]. This suggests that hippocampal degeneration is central to memory loss in AD. Mitochondrial dysfunction is a vital feature of AD, but the fundamental mechanism is still unclear. Mitochondrial dysfunction in neurodegenerative disorders remains a key to the development of oxidative stress. According to Caspersen et al. [39], mitochondrial Aβ-accumulation impairs neuronal function contributing to cellular dysfunction in transgenic (Tg) mice expressing human-mutant amyloid precursor protein (mAPP). During the early stages of AD, a reduced number of mitochondria in neurons [40] and decreased brain glucose metabolism [41] have been reported. As reviewed by Butterfield et al. [42], autopsied AD brain tissue revealed a decreased pyruvate dehydrogenase activity in the parietal, temporal, and frontal cortex. Activities of cytochrome c oxidase and mitochondrial complex IV were significantly low in AD brain.

Dementia risk in women is higher than that in men. Recently, our group [43] applied discovery-based proteomics approach to evaluate gender differences in AD with cerebrovascular disease (CVD) subjects. Quantitative proteomics revealed gender-specific-altered mitochondriome. Proteomic analysis of AD-CVD brain tissues suggested hypercitrullination of arginine and deamidation of glutamine (Gln) in myelin basic protein (MBP) from female patients. It has been revealed that an increased citrullination of MBP is due to the down-regulation of

http://dx.doi.org/10.5772/64693

cathepsin D and other enzymes that degrade the damaged proteins, leading to axonal dysfunction and progressive loss of neuron function [44].

2.3. Insights from hypoxia/ischemia-induced neuropathy

In mild cognitive impairment (MCI) and early phase of AD, a decrease in the cerebral blood flow has been noted and correlated with the symptoms of dementia [45]. At cellular level, a decrease in the blood flow triggers hypoxia. The conditions such as hypoxia/ischemia have been linked to the pathogenesis of AD [46]. Unbiased proteomic analysis of hypoxia-ischemia pathology in numerous disease models and clinical setting including neuronal cell lines [47], a rat model of ischemic middle cerebral artery occlusion [48], a mouse model of cardiovascular disease [49], blood or tissues samples from patients with dementia [24, 26, 30] has provided novel insight into molecular pathology of hypoxia-ischemic injury and confirmed that hypoxia induced mitochondrial dysfunction and oxidative stress, induced epigenetic changes, and dysregulated proteostasis. Thus, oxygen availability is a crucial regulator of cellular metabolism and homeostasis. Proteomic study using ischemic neuronal injury model also identified the dysregulation of proteins such as Park7 and VAP-A implicated in the chronic neurological disorders such as AD and PD [47]. When neuronal cell response to hypoxia and glucose depletion stress was studied by iTRAQ proteomics in hypoxia-ischemic penumbra model, dysregulation of housekeeping proteins, antioxidative defense, chaperone response, and protein metabolism were observed [47]. Proteomic of pathological progression from hypoxia-ischemia brain injury to clinical dementia revealed the dysregulation of energy metabolism, mitochondrial dysfunction, neuro-inflammation, synaptic failure, etc. [24–26, 50]. Further, the activity of α-ketoglutarate dehydrogenase appears to be inhibited in the cerebral cortex of AD patients, and there are substantial evidences indicating that the function of the Krebs cycle is impaired in AD brains [51, 52]. The impact of hypoxia and the γ-aminobutyric acid (GABA) shunt activation in the pathogenesis of AD has been reviewed by Salminen et al. [51]. Restated, neurodegeneration is caused by a progressive cycle of hypoxic-ischemic brain injury that induces DPMs, protein misfolding, and aggregation, leading to cognitive decline and dementia. Hypoxia-inducible transcription factor (HIF) is the key inducer of hypoxia-responsive genes that functions during general development and pathological processes in association with decreased oxygen availability. In hypoxic condition, HIF is accumulated while it is rapidly degraded in normoxic cells. HIF prolyl 4-hydroxylases (HIF-P4Hs, commonly known as PHDs and EglNs) act as oxygen sensing.

Recent studies suggest that neurodegeneration is caused by progressive cycles of hypoxia-ischemic brain injury that induces DPMs, protein misfolding, and aggregation. These processes result in cognitive decline and dementia. The molecular events that drive this proteinopathy preceding dementia symptoms have not yet been well identified. However, unbiased, global, discovery-driven approaches such as proteomics have the potential to uncover the complex molecular pathology of human proteinopathies including dementia. Our groups adopted systematic proteomic studies to investigate hypoxia effects on neuronal cell lines, animal models of ischemic brain injury, human blood plasma samples, and postmortem brain tissues from patients affected by stroke or dementia [47–50, 53–57]. We and other investigators [53–57] have yielded a good progress in understanding how protein DPMs, and protein aggregation induced by hypoxic-ischemic brain injury can promote neurodegeneration in dementia. This "vicious cycle" of brain tissue damage is summarized in **Figure 2**.

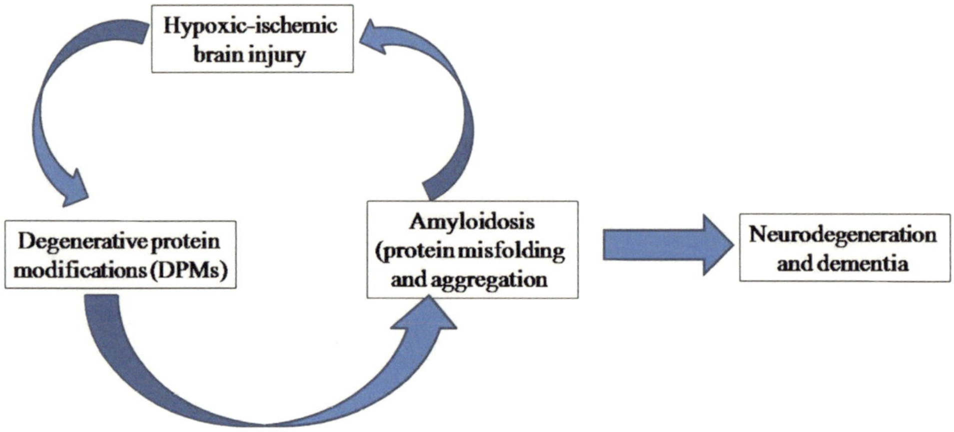

Figure 2. Vicious cycle of hypoxia-ischemic brain injury, degenerative protein modifications, and amyloidosis.

3. DPM studies in brain tissue from dementia patients

DPMs caused by spontaneous chemical reactions can radically alter protein structure and function, promoting pathological progression. Key DPMs including oxidation, deamidation, racemization, glycation, advanced glycation end products, and enzymatic modifications such as citrullination typically alter the charged state and hydrophobicity of the affected protein. This changes charge and hydrophobic nature of protein-promoting protein misfolding and aggregation. Despite the clinical importance of DPMs in neurodegenerative diseases, the mechanism and cause of modifications are poorly understood, largely due to the technical challenges. To define the role of DMPs, accurate identification of protein modification sites is important. However, it is important to avoid the introduction of artificial modification during sample preparation and improve sensitivity and confidence of identifying low-abundant modifications. According to Hao et al. [27, 31], processing proteomic samples at a mild alkaline pH and prolonged incubation at 37°C during trypsin digestion were major causes of nonenzymatic asparagines (Asn)-deamidation. Therefore, these researchers proposed an improved protocol of trypsin digestion in 50 mM ammonium acetate (pH 6) to avoid introduction of artifactual deamidation during sample preparation. Moreover, a sodium deoxycholate (SDC) and ammonium acetate-based buffer (pH 6.5) have been developed to increase protein solubility, to enhance trypsin activity, and to improve the recovery of low-abundant peptides from complex biological samples. This mildly acidic conditions and absence of urea minimized artificial asparagine deamidation and prevented artifactual carbamylation [61].

http://dx.doi.org/10.5772/64693

Under physiological conditions, deamidation of the protein residues asparagines (Asn) and glutamine (Gln) can occur spontaneously and progressively alters protein structure, function, and stability over time. Asn deamidation occurs through the formation of a succinimide ring intermediate, which quickly gets hydrolyzed to D,L-Asp and D,L-isoAsp with isoAsp predominating. Deamidation of Gln occurs much slower since it is thermodynamically less favorable to form a six-membered glutarimide ring. Deamidation causes an increase in the mass of 0.984 Da. The separation of Asp- and isoAsp remains challenging since peptides containing Asp- and isoAsp display the similar mass and hydrophobicity. However, improved ERLIC-LC-MS/MS method allows distinguishing isoAsp-containing peptide from n-Asp-containing peptide prior to their identification. Protein deamidation serves as a versatile molecular clock that can regulates many biological processes. Protein modifications and their biological impacts have been recently reviewed by Hao et al. [27]. Proteins with low turnover rates accumulate nonenzymatic modifications that cannot be repaired, and thus these modifications including deamidation cause age-related changes in biological functions and play major role in aging. Deamidation has been linked with alterations in the structure of human cortical neurons [62]. An accumulation of protein α-synuclein is a pathological characteristic of dementia with Lewy bodies (DLB), PD, AD, and multiple system atrophy (MSA), and can be linked to protein deamidation. The excessive deposition of IsoAsp residues in synapsin 1 and tubulin proteins in VaD [30] suggests that deamidation of synaptic proteins impairs its function and may cause dementia.

3.1. Deamidation of ion channel and other proteins in dementia

The ion channel protein Na^+–K^+–ATPase exhibits multiple functions including the maintenance of differential membrane potential in neurons, which is an essential feature of the signal transduction processes. Dysregulation of Na^+–K^+–ATPase expression or function has been reported in both animal model and human brain tissues affected by AD, PD, and HD. In the study of human brain tissues from patients with VaD, Adav et al. [24] noted deamidation of Na^+–K^+–ATPase subunits in the evolutionary-conserved regions. Using structural model, they located the modification sites and proposed that the disruption of Mg^{2+}– and Cu^{2+}–binding sites impaired electrostatic interactions and function of ion channel proteins in VaD (**Figure 3**). Modification of residues 210 and 220 has been proposed to cause defects in protein phosphorylation and dephosphorylation mechanisms, leading to altered ATP hydrolysis. Deamidation-induced changes in Na^+–K^+–ATPase subunit proteins may lead to defects in membrane excitability and neuronal function. Moreover, the enzyme "protein L-isoaspartate (D-aspartate) O-methyltransferase" (PIMT) functions as a protein repair enzyme and has the potential to recognize these abnormal residues (isoAsp) and convert them to the normal L-Asp form. Thus, deamidation can be repaired. However, according to proteomic analysis of VaD brain tissues, PIMT was also deamidated. Deamidation of PIMT could manipulate its potential to recognize abnormal residues or impair its potential to convert isoaspartyl to the normal L-aspartyl form [24]. In mammalian cells and mouse models lacking repair enzyme PIMT, isoASP accumulation causes hyperactivation of key cell-signaling pathways, weakening animal growth and even fatal seizures [63].

During the characterization of the human brain amyloidal plaque from dementia patients, deamidation of aggregated proteins was noted. The extensively deamidated proteins were S100A9, ferritine, and hemoglobin. In addition to these proteins, proteins such as S100 calcium-binding protein B (S100-B), α2(IV), and α2(I) chains of human collagen, extracellular matrix such as laminin subunit β-2 was found to be deamidated. Further, these authors found deamidated adhesion junction plaque protein dystonin (isoform 3) and many others [34]. Proteins coronin-1A and syntaxin-binding protein 2, which were previously been implicated in the neurodegeneration of the hippocampus, were also found deamidated detected in brain tissue sample of demented patients. Deamidation introduces negative charge at sites of modification. This change in charge promotes protein aggregation and remains as a pathological hallmark of age-related disorders and neurodegenerative diseases. Thus, the multiple deamidated residues of S100A9 (**Figure 3C** and **D**) could introduce a negative charge to form pathological aggregates in the brain. Hence, an accurate identification of DMPs and modification sites is important to understand the role of DPMs in human diseases. A comprehensive investigation including method development for accurate identification of DPMs has been performed for biomedical research [24, 26, 27, 30, 31, 34, 35].

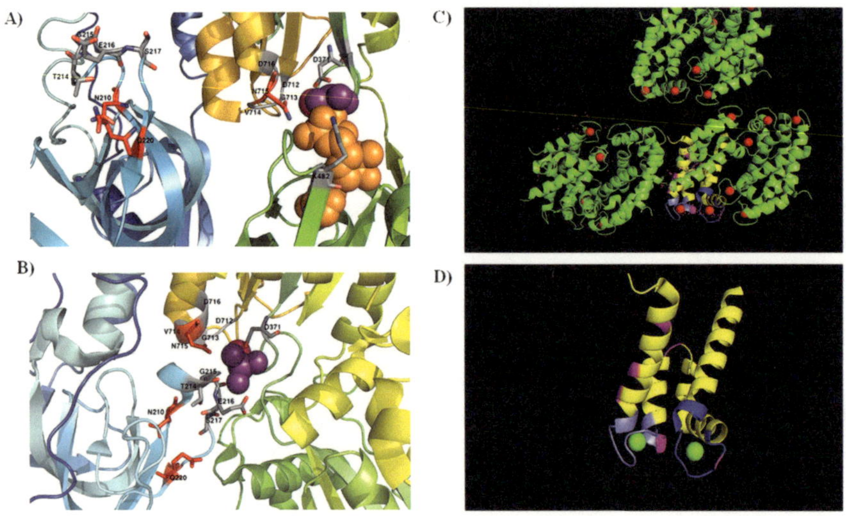

Figure 3. Structural models of Na^+/K^+-ATPase catalytic site in (A) E_1P (PDB ID 4HQJ) and (B) E_2P (2ZXE). Domain A is shown in blue and cyan color, domain P is shown in yellow, while domain N is shown in green. The deamidation sites (N210, D220, and N715) are shown in red color (adapted with permission from Adav et al. [24]). The deamidation sites of protein S100A9 (RCSB Protein Data Bank accession code: 1XK4) are shown in (C). EF hands have been displayed in yellow color and deamidation sites in magenta and blue. EF hands alone are shown in (D).

Loss of synapses is one of the most significant contributors to the cognitive impairment manifest in VaD and other neurodegenerative diseases. Following synapses loss, the remaining synapses alter their shape. According to recent literature [26], synaptic immunoglobulins were perturbed proteins in VaD temporal cortices, while SNAP25 was substantially up-regulated. Further, deamidation studies revealed that the protein synapsin 1 displayed significant accumulation of deamidated asparagine and glutamine residues when compared with age-matched control [30]. The location of the modification site using structural model demonstrated that the deamidation sites in synapsin 1 were likely to induce pathological changes in protein conformation.

4. Proteomic biomarkers of dementia

Mass spectrometry-based proteomics has been widely used for biomarkers of dementia and AD [64]. Proteins such as Aβ40, Aβ42, and their ratio Aβ42:Aβ40 have been linked with AD and dementia [65]. Proteins such as Apolipoprotein E (ApoE) level in serum of AD patients [66], interleukins (IL-1α, IL-6) [67], clusterin [68], and α-1-antichymotrypsin (α-ACT) [69] have been considered as biomarkers of AD. Other than blood, cerebrospinal fluid (CSF), which directly interacts with the space of the brain and reflects biochemical changes that occurs in the brain, has also been used for the biomarker of dementia and AD. Proteins such as phospholipases A2, visinin-like 1, microtubule-associated protein *tau*, neurofilament proteins, and many more that were reviewed by Liu et al. [70] have been considered as CSF biomarkers of AD. The increase in the generation of 2,4-dihydroxybutyrate with the progression of MCI was noted and considered as a promising biomarker of AD [51, 71]. Using human CSF samples and adopting targeted approach, Shi et al [72] proposed a panel consisting of five peptides/proteins such as osteopontin (SPP1), prolow-density lipoprotein receptor-related protein 1 (LRP1), macrophage colony-stimulating factor 1 receptor (CSF1R), ephrin type-A receptor 4 (EPHA4), and metalloproteinase inhibitor 1 (TIMP1) are biomarkers of PD or AD. Alzheimer's Disease Neuroimaging Initiative (ADNI) biomarker core progress has been reviewed by Kang et al. [73].

5. Future outlook and conclusions

Dementia is a global public health challenge that requires urgent action to discover underlying molecular mechanism and to develop cure. Classical biological methods involving analyses of one or several genes have been adopted in the study of the pathogenesis of neurodegenerative disorders. However, it has become clear that neurodegenerative disorders exhibit complex interactions involving wide range of proteins. Proteomics technologies have ushered in a new era in the fields of clinical research by enabling us in identifying and quantifying disease-related protein profiles. Unbiased, global, discovery-driven approaches such as proteomics are well suited to uncover the complex pathology of human proteinopathies such as dementia. Therefore, in this chapter, we exploited state-of-the-art quantitative proteomic profiling of brain proteome, and discussed recent developments in neuroproteomics including DPMs, its impact on protein aggregation that alters protein function and causes deposition, which are key features of dementia and neurodegenerative disorders. To further understand the pathology in depth, along with discovery proteomic approach, targeted proteomics need to be applied to develop cure. In addition, commitments are needed to generate strategies, government policies, programs, and research funding for neurodegenerative diseases. However, obtaining well-characterized clinical samples of specific brain areas remains a major limitation.

Acknowledgements

This work is in part supported by the Singapore Ministry of Education (Tier 2: ARC9/15), NTU-NHG Ageing Research Grant (ARG/14017), and the Singapore National Research Foundation under its CBRG (NMRC/CBRG/0004/2012) administered by the Singapore Ministry of Health's National Medical Research Council.

Author details

Sunil S. Adav and Siu Kwan Sze*

*Address all correspondence to: sksze@ntu.edu.sg

School of Biological Sciences, Nanyang Technological University, Singapore

References

[1] Editorial. Great expectations for dementia research. Lancet Neurol 2016. Available from http://thelancet.com/journals/laneur/article/PIIS1474-4422(15)00394-4/fulltext

[2] Ferri CP, Prince M, Brayne C, Brodaty H, Fratiglioni L, Ganguli M, Hall K, Hasegawa K, Hendrie H, Huang Y, Jorm A, Mathers C, Menezes PR, Rimmer E, Scazufca M. Global prevalence of dementia: A Delphi consensus study. Lancet 2005;366:2112–2117. Doi: 10.1016/s0140-6736(05)67889-0.

[3] WHO. Dementia: A public health priority, dementia report. Available from: http://www.who.int/mental_health/publications/dementia_report_2012/en/

[4] Qiu C, De Ronchi D, Fratiglioni L. The epidemiology of the dementias: An update. Curr Opin Psychiatry 2007;20:380–385. Doi: 10.1097/YCO.0b013e32816ebc7b.

[5] WHO. World Alzheimer's Report 2009. London, Alzheimer's Disease International, 2009.

[6] Corbett A, Williams G, Ballard C. Drug repositioning in Alzheimer's disease. Front Biosci (Schol Ed) 2015;7:184–188.

[7] Corbett A, Pickett J, Burns A, Corcoran J, Dunnett SB, Edison P, Hagan JJ, Holmes C, Jones E, Katona C, Kearns I, Kehoe P, Mudher A, Passmore A, Shepherd N, Walsh F,

Ballard C. Drug repositioning for Alzheimer's disease. Nat Rev Drug Discov 2012;11:833–846. Doi: 10.1038/nrd3869.

[8] Masters CL, Simms G, Weinman NA, Multhaup G, McDonald BL, Beyreuther K. Amyloid plaque core protein in Alzheimer disease and down syndrome. Proc Natl Acad Sci USA 1985;82:4245–4249.

[9] Terry RD, Masliah E, Salmon DP, Butters N, DeTeresa R, Hill R, Hansen LA, Katzman R. Physical basis of cognitive alterations in Alzheimer's disease: Synapse loss is the major correlate of cognitive impairment. Ann Neurol 1991;30:572–580. Doi: 10.1002/ana.410300410.

[10] Arriagada PV, Growdon JH, Hedley-Whyte ET, Hyman BT. Neurofibrillary tangles but not senile plaques parallel duration and severity of Alzheimer's disease. Neurology 1992;42:631–639.

[11] Davis DG, Schmitt FA, Wekstein DR, Markesbery WR. Alzheimer neuropathologic alterations in aged cognitively normal subjects. J Neuropathol Exp Neurol 1999;58:376–388.

[12] Kalaria RN, Ihara M. Dementia: Vascular and neurodegenerative pathways-will they meet? Nat Rev Neurol 2013;9:487–488. Doi: 10.1038/nrneurol.2013.164.

[13] Iadecola C. The pathobiology of vascular dementia. Neuron 2013;80:844–866. Doi: 10.1016/j.neuron.2013.10.008.

[14] Foster V, Oakley AE, Slade JY, Hall R, Polvikoski TM, Burke M, Thomas AJ, Khundakar A, Allan LM, Kalaria RN. Pyramidal neurons of the prefrontal cortex in post-stroke, vascular and other ageing-related dementias. Brain 2014;137:2509–2521. Doi: 10.1093/brain/awu172.

[15] Allan LM, Rowan EN, Firbank MJ, Thomas AJ, Parry SW, Polvikoski TM, O'Brien JT, Kalaria RN. Long term incidence of dementia, predictors of mortality and pathological diagnosis in older stroke survivors. Brain 2011;134:3716–3727. Doi: 10.1093/brain/awr273.

[16] Okamoto Y, Yamamoto T, Kalaria RN, Senzaki H, Maki T, Hase Y, Kitamura A, Washida K, Yamada M, Ito H, Tomimoto H, Takahashi R, Ihara M. Cerebral hypoperfusion accelerates cerebral amyloid angiopathy and promotes cortical microinfarcts. Acta Neuropathol 2012;123:381–394. Doi: 10.1007/s00401-011-0925-9.

[17] Zlokovic BV. Neurovascular pathways to neurodegeneration in Alzheimer's disease and other disorders. Nat Rev Neurosci 2011;12:723–738. Doi: 10.1038/nrn3114.

[18] Quaegebeur A, Segura I, Carmeliet P. Pericytes: Blood-brain barrier safeguards against neurodegeneration? Neuron 2010;68:321–323. Doi: 10.1016/j.neuron.2010.10.024.

[19] Snyder HM, Corriveau RA, Craft S, Faber JE, Greenberg SM, Knopman D, Lamb BT, Montine TJ, Nedergaard M, Schaffer CB, Schneider JA, Wellington C, Wilcock DM, Zipfel GJ, Zlokovic B, Bain LJ, Bosetti F, Galis ZS, Koroshetz W, Carrillo MC. Vascular

contributions to cognitive impairment and dementia including Alzheimer's disease. Alzheimers Dement 2015;11:710–717. Doi: 10.1016/j.jalz.2014.10.008.

[20] Toledo JB, Arnold SE, Raible K, Brettschneider J, Xie SX, Grossman M, Monsell SE, Kukull WA, Trojanowski JQ. Contribution of cerebrovascular disease in autopsy confirmed neurodegenerative disease cases in the national Alzheimer's coordinating centre. Brain 2013;136:2697–2706. Doi: 10.1093/brain/awt188.

[21] Iadecola C. The overlap between neurodegenerative and vascular factors in the pathogenesis of dementia. Acta Neuropathol 2010;120:287–296. Doi: 10.1007/s00401-010-0718-6.

[22] Lo RY, Jagust WJ. Vascular burden and Alzheimer disease pathologic progression. Neurology 2012;79:1349–1355. Doi: 10.1212/WNL.0b013e31826c1b9d.

[23] Alzheimer's Association . Available from: http://www.alz.org/dementia/types-of-dementia.asp

[24] Adav SS, Qian J, Ang YL, Kalaria RN, Lai MKP, Chen CP, Sze SK. ITRAQ quantitative clinical proteomics revealed role of Na+K+-ATPase and its correlation with deamidation in vascular dementia. J Proteome Res 2014;13:4635–4646. Doi: 10.1021/pr500754j.

[25] Datta A, Qian J, Chong R, Kalaria RN, Francis P, Lai MKP, Chen CP, Sze SK. Novel pathophysiological markers are revealed by iTRAQ-based quantitative clinical proteomics approach in vascular dementia. J Proteomics 2014;99:54–67. Doi: 10.1016/j.jprot.2014.01.011.

[26] Gallart-Palau X, Serra A, Sze SK. Uncovering neurodegenerative protein modifications via proteomic profiling. Int Rev Neurobiol 2015;121:87-116. doi: 10.1016/bs.irn.2015.06.002.

[27] Hao P, Adav SS, Gallart-Palau X, Sze SK. Recent advances in mass spectrometric analysis of protein deamidation. Mass Spectrom Rev 2016. (In press) Doi: 10.1002/mas.21491.

[28] Adav SS, Ravindran A, Sze SK. Study of *Phanerochaete chrysosporium* secretome revealed protein glycosylation as a substrate-dependent post-translational modification. J Proteome Res 2014;13:4272–4280. Doi: 10.1021/pr500385y.

[29] Adav SS, Ravindran A, Sze SK. Quantitative proteomic study of *Aspergillus fumigatus* secretome revealed deamidation of secretory enzymes. J Proteomics 2015;119:154–168. Doi: 10.1016/j.jprot.2015.02.007.

[30] Gallart-Palau X, Serra A, Qian J, Chen CP, Kalaria RN, Sze SK. Temporal lobe proteins implicated in synaptic failure exhibit differential expression and deamidation in vascular dementia. Neurochem Int 2015;80:87–98. Doi: 10.1016/j.neuint.2014.12.002.

[31] Hao P, Ren Y, Alpert AJ, Siu KS. Detection, evaluation and minimization of nonenzymatic deamidation in proteomic sample preparation. Mol Cell Proteomics 2011;10(10):O111.009381. Doi:10.1074/mcp.O111.009381.

[32] Izco M, Pesini P, Perez-Grijalba V, Fandos N, Sarasa M. Optimized protocol for amyloid-beta extraction from the brain. J Alzheimers Dis 2013;34:835–839. Doi: 10.3233/jad-121798.

[33] Kuo YM, Emmerling MR, Vigo-Pelfrey C, Kasunic TC, Kirkpatrick JB, Murdoch GH, Ball MJ, Roher AE. Water-soluble abeta (n-40, n-42) oligomers in normal and Alzheimer disease brains. J Biol Chem 1996;271:4077–4081.

[34] Adav SS, Gallart-Palau X, Tan KH, Lim SK, Tam JP, Sze SK. Dementia-linked amyloidosis is associated with brain protein deamidation as revealed by proteomic profiling of human brain tissues. Mol Brain 2016;9:20. Doi: 10.1186/s13041-016-0200-z.

[35] Hao P, Qian J, Dutta B, Cheow ES, Sim KH, Meng W, Adav SS, Alpert A, Sze SK. Enhanced separation and characterization of deamidated peptides with RP-ERLIC-based multidimensional chromatography coupled with tandem mass spectrometry. J Proteome Res 2012;11:1804–1811. Doi: 10.1021/pr201048c.

[36] Mobasheri A, Avila J, Cozar-Castellano I, Brownleader MD, Trevan M, Francis MJ, Lamb JF, Martin-Vasallo P. Na+, K+-ATPase isozyme diversity; comparative biochemistry and physiological implications of novel functional interactions. Biosci Rep 2000;20:51–91.

[37] Scheff SW, Price DA, Schmitt FA, DeKosky ST, Mufson EJ. Synaptic alterations in Ca1 in mild Alzheimer disease and mild cognitive impairment. Neurology 2007;68:1501–1508. Doi: 10.1212/01.wnl.0000260698.46517.8f.

[38] Scheff SW, Price DA, Schmitt FA, Mufson EJ. Hippocampal synaptic loss in early Alzheimer's disease and mild cognitive impairment. Neurobiol Aging 2006;27:1372–1384. Doi: 10.1016/j.neurobiolaging.2005.09.012.

[39] Caspersen C, Wang N, Yao J, Sosunov A, Chen X, Lustbader JW, Xu HW, Stern D, McKhann G, Yan SD. Mitochondrial abeta: A potential focal point for neuronal metabolic dysfunction in Alzheimer's disease. FASEB J 2005;19:2040–2041. Doi: 10.1096/fj.05-3735fje.

[40] Hirai K, Aliev G, Nunomura A, Fujioka H, Russell RL, Atwood CS, Johnson AB, Kress Y, Vinters HV, Tabaton M, Shimohama S, Cash AD, Siedlak SL, Harris PL, Jones PK, Petersen RB, Perry G, Smith MA. Mitochondrial abnormalities in Alzheimer's disease. J Neurosci 2001;21:3017–3023.

[41] Mosconi L. Brain glucose metabolism in the early and specific diagnosis of Alzheimer's disease. FDG-PET studies in MCI and AD. Eur J Nucl Med Mol Imaging 2005;32:486–510. Doi: 10.1007/s00259-005-1762-7.

[42] Butterfield DA, Reed T, Newman SF, Sultana R. Roles of amyloid β-peptide-associated oxidative stress and brain protein modifications in the pathogenesis of Alzheimer's

disease and mild cognitive impairment. Free Rad Biol Med 2007;43:658–677. Doi: 10.1016/j.freeradbiomed.2007.05.037.

[43] Gallart-Palau X, Lee BST, Adav SS, Qian J, Serra A, E. PJ, Lai MKP, Chen CP, Kalaria RN, Sze SK. Gender differences in white matter pathology and mitochondrial dysfunction in Alzheimer's disease with cerebrovascular disease. Mol Brain 2016;17:27. Doi: 10.1186/s13041-016-0205-7.

[44] Bacheva AV, Belogurov AA, Kuzina ES, Serebriakova MV, Ponomarenko NA, Knorre VD, Govorun VM, Gabibov AG. Functional degradation of myelin basic protein. Proteomic approach. Bioorg Khim 2011;37:45–54.

[45] Luckhaus C, Flub MO, Wittsack HJ, Grass-Kapanke B, Janner M, Khalili-Amiri R, Friedrich W, Supprian T, Gaebel W, Modder U, Cohnen M. Detection of changed regional cerebral blood flow in mild cognitive impairment and early Alzheimer's dementia by perfusion-weighted magnetic resonance imaging. Neuroimage 2008;40:495–503. Doi: 10.1016/j.neuroimage.2007.11.053.

[46] Kalaria RN. The role of cerebral ischemia in Alzheimer's disease. Neurobiol Aging 2000;21:321–330.

[47] Datta A, Park JE, Li X, Zhang H, Ho ZS, Heese K, Lim SK, Tam JP, Sze SK. Phenotyping of an in vitro model of ischemic penumbra by iTRAQ-based shotgun quantitative proteomics. J Proteome Res 2010;9:472–484. Doi: 10.1021/pr900829h.

[48] Datta A, Jingru Q, Khor TH, Teo MT, Heese K, Sze SK. Quantitative neuroproteomics of an in vivo rodent model of focal cerebral ischemia/reperfusion injury reveals a temporal regulation of novel pathophysiological molecular markers. J Proteome Res 2011;10:5199–5213. Doi: 10.1021/pr200673y.

[49] Li X, Arslan F, Ren Y, Adav SS, Poh KK, Sorokin V, Lee CN, de Kleijn D, Lim SK, Sze SK. Metabolic adaptation to a disruption in oxygen supply during myocardial ischemia and reperfusion is underpinned by temporal and quantitative changes in the cardiac proteome. J Proteome Res 2012;11:2331–2346. Doi: 10.1021/pr201025m.

[50] Datta A, Akatsu H, Heese K, Sze SK. Quantitative clinical proteomic study of autopsied human infarcted brain specimens to elucidate the deregulated pathways in ischemic stroke pathology. J Proteomics 2013;91:556–568. Doi: 10.1016/j.jprot.2013.08.017.

[51] Salminen A, Jouhten P, Sarajarvi T, Haapasalo A, Hiltunen M. Hypoxia and GABA shunt activation in the pathogenesis of Alzheimer's disease. Neurochem Int 2015;92:13-24. doi: 10.1016/j.neuint.2015.11.005.

[52] Bubber P, Haroutunian V, Fisch G, Blass JP, Gibson GE. Mitochondrial abnormalities in Alzheimer brain: Mechanistic implications. Ann Neurol 2005;57:695–703. Doi: 10.1002/ana.20474.

[53] De Kleijn DPV, Moll FL, Hellings WE, Ozsarlak-Sozer G, De Bruin P, Doevendans PA, Vink A, Catanzariti LM, Schoneveld AH, Algra A, Daemen MJ, Biessen EA, De Jager

W, Zhang H, De Vries JP, Falk E, Lim SK, Van Der Spek PJ, Sze SK, Pasterkamp G. Local atherosclerotic plaques are a source of prognostic biomarkers for adverse cardiovascular events. Arterioscler Thromb Vasc Biol 2010;30:612–619. Doi: 10.1161/ATVBAHA. 109.194944.

[54] Hao P, Ren Y, Pasterkamp G, Moll FL, de Kleijn DPV, Sze SK. Deep proteomic profiling of human carotid atherosclerotic plaques using multidimensional LC-MS/MS. Proteomics Clin Appl 2014;8:631–635. Doi: 10.1002/prca.201400007.

[55] Manavalan A, Mishra M, Sze SK, Heese K. Brain-site-specific proteome changes induced by neuronal p60TRP expression. NeuroSignals 2013;21:129–149. Doi: 10.1159/000343672.

[56] Park JE, Tan HS, Datta A, Lai RC, Zhang H, Meng W, Lim SK, Sze SK. Hypoxic tumor cell modulates its microenvironment to enhance angiogenic and metastatic potential by secretion of proteins and exosomes. Mol Cell Proteomics 2010;9:1085–1099. Doi: 10.1074/mcp.M900381-MCP200.

[57] Ren Y, Hao P, Dutta B, Cheow ESH, Sim KH, Gan CS, Lim SK, Sze SK. Hypoxia modulates a431 cellular pathways association to tumor radioresistance and enhanced migration revealed by comprehensive proteomic and functional studies. Mol Cell Proteomics 2013;12:485–498. Doi: 10.1074/mcp.M112.018325.

[58] Kalaria RN. The role of cerebral ischemia in Alzheimer's disease. Neurobiol Aging 2000;21:321–330. Doi: 10.1016/S0197-4580(00)00125-1.

[59] Kalaria RN, Ihara M. Dementia: Vascular and neurodegenerative pathways—will they meet? Nat Rev Neurol 2013;9:487–488. Doi: 10.1038/nrneurol.2013.164.

[60] Serra A, Zhu H, Gallart-Palau X, Park JE, Ho HH, Tam JP, Sze SK. Plasma proteome coverage is increased by unique peptide recovery from sodium deoxycholate precipitate.Anal Bioanal Chem 2016;408(7):1963-73. doi: 10.1007/s00216-016-9312-7.

[61] Serra A, Zhu H, Cheow E, Gallart-Palau X, Ng JT-Y, Park JE, Kleijn Dd, Ho HH, Tam JP, Sze SK. Increasing proteome coverage through peptide recovery from sodium deoxycholate pellet. J Proteome Res 2015; under review.

[62] Lanthier J, Bouthillier A, Lapointe M, Demeule M, Beliveau R, Desrosiers RR. Downregulation of protein l-isoaspartyl methyltransferase in human epileptic hippocampus contributes to generation of damaged tubulin. J Neurochem 2002;83:581–591.

[63] Kosugi S, Furuchi T, Katane M, Sekine M, Shirasawa T, Homma H. Suppression of protein l-isoaspartyl (d-aspartyl) methyltransferase results in hyperactivation of EGF-stimulated MEK-ERK signaling in cultured mammalian cells. Biochem Biophys Res Commun 2008;371:22–27. Doi: 10.1016/j.bbrc.2008.03.109.

[64] Liu Y, Qing H, Deng Y. Biomarkers in Alzheimer's disease analysis by mass spectrometry-based proteomics. Int J Mol Sci 2014;15:7865–7882. Doi: 10.3390/ijms15057865.

[65] Koyama A, Okereke OI, Yang T, Blacker D, Selkoe DJ, Grodstein F. Plasma amyloid-beta as a predictor of dementia and cognitive decline: A systematic review and meta-analysis. Arch Neurol 2012;69:824–831. Doi: 10.1001/archneurol.2011.1841.

[66] Gupta VB, Laws SM, Villemagne VL, Ames D, Bush AI, Ellis KA, Lui JK, Masters C, Rowe CC, Szoeke C, Taddei K, Martins RN. Plasma apolipoprotein e and Alzheimer disease risk: The AIBL study of aging. Neurology 2011;76:1091–1098. Doi: 10.1212/WNL.0b013e318211c352.

[67] Du Y, Dodel RC, Eastwood BJ, Bales KR, Gao F, Lohmuller F, Muller U, Kurz A, Zimmer R, Evans RM, Hake A, Gasser T, Oertel WH, Griffin WS, Paul SM, Farlow MR. Association of an interleukin 1 alpha polymorphism with Alzheimer's disease. Neurology 2000;55:480–483.

[68] Lambert JC, Heath S, Even G, Campion D, Sleegers K, Hiltunen M, Combarros O, Zelenika D, Bullido MJ, Tavernier B, Letenneur L, Bettens K, Berr C, Pasquier F, Fievet N, Barberger-Gateau P, Engelborghs S, De Deyn P, Mateo I, Franck A, Helisalmi S, Porcellini E, Hanon O, de Pancorbo MM, Lendon C, Dufouil C, Jaillard C, Leveillard T, Alvarez V, Bosco P, Mancuso M, Panza F, Nacmias B, Bossu P, Piccardi P, Annoni G, Seripa D, Galimberti D, Hannequin D, Licastro F, Soininen H, Ritchie K, Blanche H, Dartigues JF, Tzourio C, Gut I, Van Broeckhoven C, Alperovitch A, Lathrop M, Amouyel P. Genome-wide association study identifies variants at CLU and Cr1 associated with Alzheimer's disease. Nat Genet 2009;41:1094–1099. Doi: 10.1038/ng.439.

[69] Guan F, Gu J, Hu F, Zhu Y, Wang W. Association between alpha1-antichymotrypsin signal peptide -15a/t polymorphism and the risk of Alzheimer's disease: A meta-analysis. Mol Biol Rep 2012;39:6661–6669. Doi: 10.1007/s11033-012-1472-8.

[70] Liu Y, Qing H, Deng Y. Biomarkers in Alzheimer's disease analysis by mass spectrometry-based proteomics. Int J Mol Sci 2014;15:7865–7882. Doi: 10.3390/ijms15057865.

[71] Oresic M, Hyotylainen T, Herukka SK, Sysi-Aho M, Mattila I, Seppanan-Laakso T, Julkunen V, Gopalacharyulu PV, Hallikainen M, Koikkalainen J, Kivipelto M, Helisalmi S, Lotjonen J, Soininen H. Metabolome in progression to Alzheimer's disease. Transl Psychiatry 2011;1:e57. Doi: 10.1038/tp.2011.55.

[72] Shi M, Movius J, Dator R, Aro P, Zhao Y, Pan C, Lin X, Bammler TK, Stewart T, Zabetian CP, Peskind ER, Hu SC, Quinn JF, Galasko DR, Zhang J. Cerebrospinal fluid peptides as potential Parkinson disease biomarkers: A staged pipeline for discovery and validation. Mol Cell Proteomics 2015;14:544–555. Doi: 10.1074/mcp.M114.040576.

[73] Kang JH, Korecka M, Figurski MJ, Toledo JB, Blennow K, Zetterberg H, Waligorska T, Brylska M, Fields L, Shah N, Soares H, Dean RA, Vanderstichele H, Petersen RC, Aisen PS, Saykin AJ, Weiner MW, Trojanowski JQ, Shaw LM. The Alzheimer's disease neuroimaging initiative 2 biomarker core: A review of progress and plans. Alzheimers Dement 2015;11:772–791. Doi: 10.1016/j.jalz.2015.05.003.

Chapter 7

Brain Lipids in the Pathophysiology and Treatment of Alzheimer's Disease

Manuel Torres, Xavier Busquets and Pablo V. Escribá

Additional information is available at the end of the chapter

http://dx.doi.org/10.5772/64757

Abstract

Alzheimer's disease (AD) is a neurodegenerative disorder that causes severe and progressive cognitive impairment. The discovery of specific mutations related to AD supported the amyloid cascade hypothesis, which postulates that the accumulation of the amyloid-β (Aβ) peptide triggers neuronal death and dementia. However, most drugs that aim to prevent Aβ accumulation or tau phosphorylation have consistently failed in clinical trials. This would suggest that the amyloid pathology lies downstream of (an)other cellular event(s) that is/are responsible for AD pathogenesis. In this context, several lipid alterations have been described in the brain and in peripheral fluids of patients with AD, suggesting the involvement of lipids in the etiology of this condition. Indeed, the central nervous system (CNS) has the highest lipid content in the body, next to adipose tissue, and it is thought that normalization of brain membrane lipid levels would revert AD-related pathogenic events. In this sense, novel hydroxylated derivatives of docosahexaenoic acid (DHA) such as natural resolvins or synthetic hydroxy-DHA (HDHA, DHALifort) can modulate membrane lipid composition and show remarkable beneficial effects on AD hallmarks, such as prevention of amyloid production and tau phosphorylation, and cognitive restoration in animal models. Therefore, normalization of the neuronal lipid environment by hydroxyl-DHA and/or other lipids may constitute a promising therapy for AD treatment, memory loss and, possibly, other types of dementia.

Keywords: Alzheimer's disease, neurodegeneration, neuroregeneration, hydroxy-DHA, amyloid, tau, neurite dystrophy, inflammation, brain lipids, cholesterol, sphingolipids, lipid rafts, omega-3 PUFAs, HDHA, DHALifort, resolvins, neuroprotectins, lipid biomarkers

1. Introduction

Alzheimer's disease (AD) is the main neurological cause of dementia, and it affects about 46 million people worldwide, mostly elderly adults. The incidence of AD increases exponentially every 5 years from 65 years of age, and it is estimated that 74.7 and 131.5 million people will be living with AD by 2030 and 2050, respectively (World Alzheimer Report, 2015). Patients with AD undergo progressive memory loss, reduced cognitive capacity and eventually, dementia. The debilitating effects of AD, especially at advanced disease stages, impose a substantial financial burden on AD patient's families, primarily due to the cost associated with medical care. However, the etiology of AD still remains largely unclear and although there has been much effort to elucidate the pathophysiological mechanisms underlying this devastating condition over the last 20 years, the principal cause remains unknown, representing an important unmet clinical need. Therefore, AD is undoubtedly one of today's most challenging global public health problems, and there is a pressing need to develop novel therapeutic agents to prevent and treat this disease.

The neuropathological hallmarks of AD include the formation of extracellular senile plaques due to the aggregation of amyloid-β (Aβ; normally associated with local inflammation and dystrophy/swelling of neurites), the formation of intracellular neurofibrillary tangles of hyperphosphorylated tau protein, as well as a loss of synaptic connections and neuronal degeneration [1]. Clinically, AD can be classified into two categories: familial AD (FAD, also known as early-onset AD) and sporadic AD (SAD, also known as late-onset AD). FAD generally accounts for <1% of the total AD cases, and they correspond to a disease variant with onset prior to 65 years of age [2]. This familial form of AD is inherited in an autosomal dominant pattern, and it is caused by mutations in three genes involved in Aβ generation: the amyloid precursor protein (APP), presenilin 1 (PS1) and presenilin 2 (PS2) [3]. In contrast to FAD, no single gene mutation has been found to be directly responsible for the onset and pathogenesis of SAD [4]. For the late-onset cases, the principal risk factors are ageing and the apolipoprotein E (ApoE) allele ε4 (see Section 3.1.).

The identification of clinical mutations in APP and presenilins in association with FAD has contributed to our understanding of AD pathogenesis. APP is a transmembrane protein that undergoes primary enzymatic cleavage by an α- or β-secretase in its extracellular (or intraluminal) domain, as well as secondary cleavage by a γ-secretase within the transmembrane region (**Figure 1**). The metalloproteases ADAM10 and/or ADAM17 appear to be responsible for this α-secretase activity and the aspartyl protease BACE-1 (beta-site APP cleaving enzyme 1) corresponds to the β-secretase activity, whereas γ-secretase is an aspartyl proteolytic complex containing four subunits (PS1 or 2, nicastrin, APH1, and PEN-2) [5]. APP cleavage may be produced by β- and γ-secretases in a pathway known as the amyloidogenic route of APP. First, APP β-cleavage produces soluble APP-β (sAPPβ) and a transmembrane C-terminal fragment known as β-CTF or C99. The latter then undergoes γ-secretase cleavage to generate the APP intracellular domain (AICD) and the Aβ peptide, preferentially the Aβ40 and 42 isoforms. Alternatively, APP may be cleaved by α- and γ-secretases in a pathway known as the non-amyloidogenic route of APP where α-secretase cleaves APP right in the middle of the Aβ sequence (**Figure 1**) to generate soluble APPα (sAPPα) and a transmembrane C-terminal fragment known as α-CTF or C83. The latter undergoes further γ-cleavage to produce AICD and p3 (also known as Aβ17–40/42). In this context, it has been widely reported that FAD mutations induce alterations in APP processing that increased the cellular production of Aβ and augment the Aβ 42/40 ratio. Since mutations in both APP and presenilins are the major causal factors in FAD etiology, altered APP metabolism was assumed to be the principal cause triggering AD, leading to the formulation of the amyloid cascade hypothesis more than 20 years ago. Finally, it is notable that all these participants in APP metabolism, APP and secretases, are membrane-associated proteins influenced by the composition and structure of cell membrane lipids that in turn modulate APP metabolism [6].

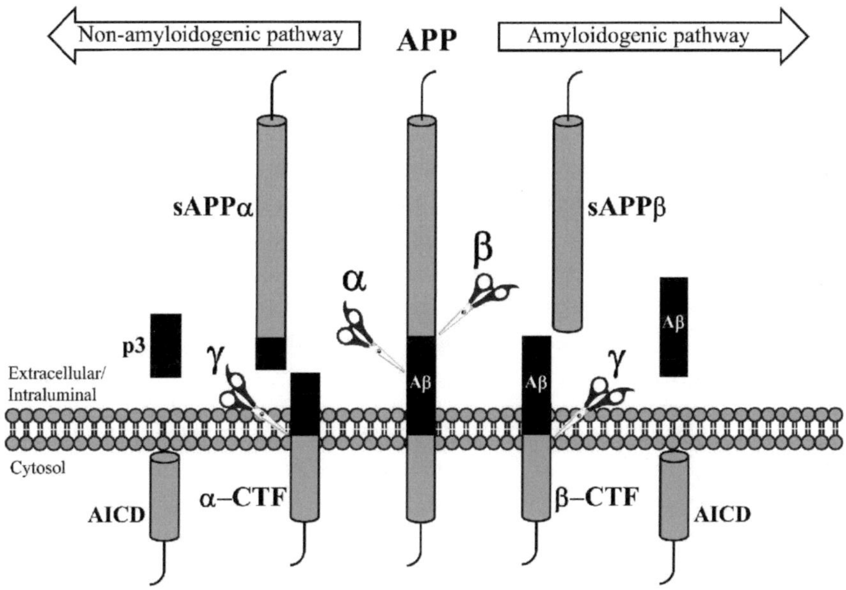

Figure 1. APP processing by secretases. In the non-amyloidogenic pathway, APP is first cleaved by α-secretase at a sequence of amino acids within the Aβ peptide, releasing the sAPPα ectodomain. Further processing of the resulting membrane-associated C-terminal C83 fragment (α-CTF) by γ-secretase leads to the release of the p3 fragment and the APP intracellular domain (AICD). This processing takes place preferentially at the plasma membrane. Conversely, the amyloidogenic pathway is initiated when β-secretase cleaves APP at the amino terminus of the Aβ peptide to release the sAPPβ ectodomain. Further processing of the resulting membrane-associated C-terminal C99 fragment (β-CTF) by γ-secretase releases the Aβ peptide and AICD. This processing normally takes place in acidic cellular compartments like late endosomes. The Aβ peptide produced is normally 40 or 42 amino acids long (Aβ40 or 42) and the Aβ42/40 ratio increases in AD.

2. Historical perspective on the pathophysiology of Alzheimer's disease

For more than 20 years, the accumulation of the Aβ peptide has been considered to be the main cellular/molecular event that triggers AD-related neurodegeneration. Amyloid plaques were first thought to cause AD pathogenesis, and more recently, Aβ-soluble oligomers have gained more attention as key players in AD etiology [7]. Regardless of the form of amyloid, the amyloid cascade hypothesis postulates that Aβ accumulation in the brain is the major upstream event in AD pathophysiology, whereas other neuropathological features are a result of this primary amyloid pathology, including the formation of neurofibrillary tangles, neuroinflammation, synaptic failure, and eventually neural death [8, 9].

According to the amyloid cascade hypothesis, enhanced amyloidogenic activity of secretases and/or reduced clearance of the Aβ peptide may trigger Aβ accumulation. As a result, the secretases involved in Aβ generation have been extensively targeted by the pharmaceutical industry to develop new compounds to treat AD [10]. In particular, the Aβ42/40 ratio may increase due to FAD mutations and this increase enhances oligomer formation, which may in turn impair synaptic function and provoke neuronal degeneration [7]. At the same time, secreted Aβ42 forms primary extracellular Aβ deposits in the brain parenchyma, first as diffuse plaques and later as insoluble fibrillary plaques. A concomitant local inflammatory response develops around these amyloid deposits (involving microglial and astroglial activation), coupled to synaptic spine loss and neurite dystrophy (neuritic pathology) [11, 12]. Over time, these events result in oxidative stress and altered ion homeostasis. Neurofibrillary tangles appear as a consequence of the altered kinase and phosphatase activities that cause tau protein hyperphosphorylation, and likely its subsequent dysfunction in axonal transport, as well as neurite dystrophy [13, 14]. Finally, the cascade ends with extensive synaptic and neuronal dysfunction, which precedes the well-characterized neuronal death associated with the Aβ and tau pathologies [7]. It is this neuronal degeneration that is responsible for memory loss and dementia in patients with AD.

Amyloid burden in the brain parenchyma is closely associated with tau hyperphosphorylation, axonal dystrophy and inflammatory reaction around amyloid plaques (**Figure 2**). Both, inflammation and axonal dystrophy can promote neuronal degeneration [15, 16]. However, it is still largely unknown which of these events (amyloid, inflammation, or neurite dystrophy) appear first during disease development and how these three events are connected. The amyloid cascade hypothesis postulates that amyloid accumulation, first intracellular and then extracellular, leads to the generation of amyloid plaques. Given the close relationship between Aβ plaque number and size with the surrounding dystrophies and gliosis, these two latter events were proposed to progress in conjunction with Aβ plaque formation. However, evidence is now accumulating against the amyloid cascade hypothesis. On the one hand, therapeutic approaches focused on combating amyloid pathology have generally failed to prevent AD progression in clinical trials (see Section 4, [17, 18]), while on the other hand, transgenic AD animal models, mostly created by incorporating human mutated APP and/or PS1 into the animal genome, do not recapitulate all the neuropathological features of AD, and not even the large scale neuronal death that occurs during this pathology [19]. Moreover, the alterations to membrane lipids in neurons of patients with AD suggest that the changes to lipid bilayer could be the first event in the amyloid cascade and related pathways [6]. Indeed, the normalization of membrane lipids is associated with cognitive restoration (see Section 5.2). Accordingly, the amyloid pathology may not actually be the first initial event driving the events that provoke neuronal degeneration.

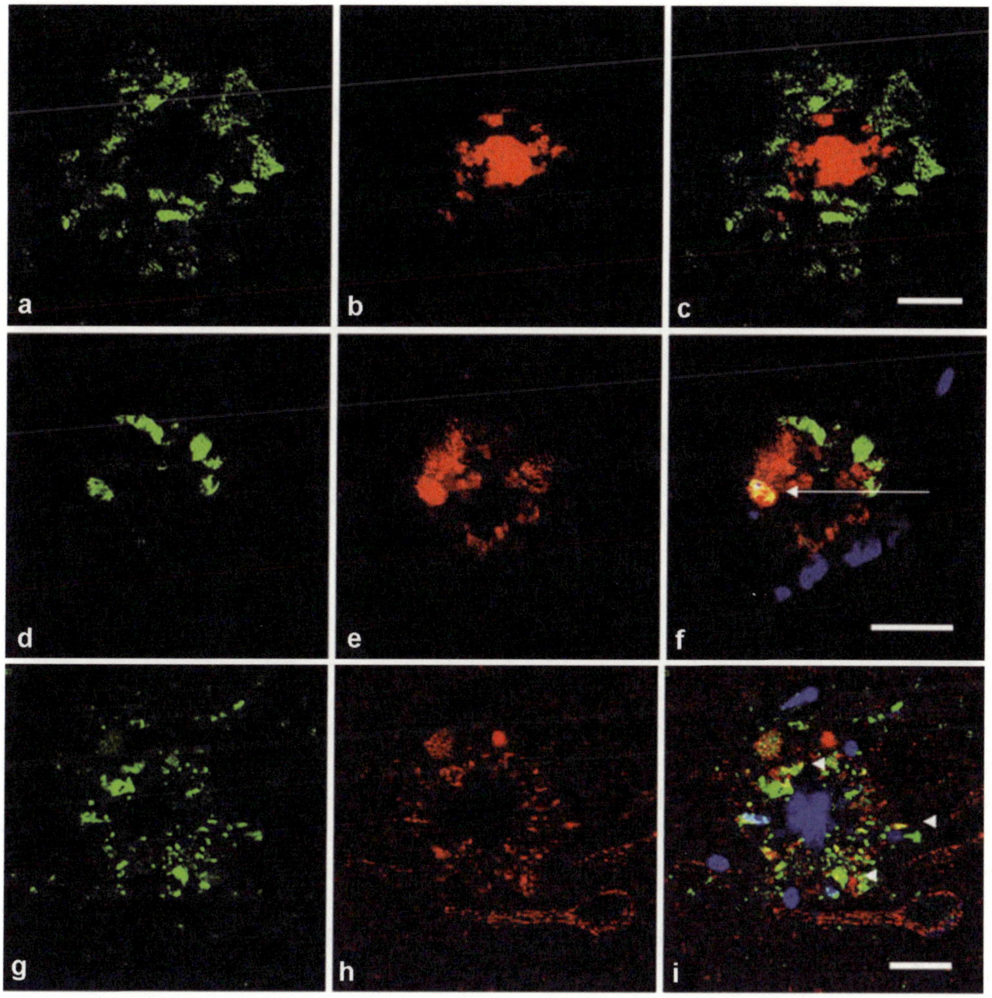

Figure 2. Dystrophic neurites surrounding β-amyloid plaques in AD patient's brain. (a–c) Double-labeling immunofuorescence and confocal microscopy to mitochondrial porin (a; green) and β-amyloid plaques (b; red). Porin immunostaining revealed mitochondrial enrichment in dystrophic neurites surrounding amyloid plaques (c). (d–f) Double-labeling immunofluorescence and confocal microscopy to mitochondrial porin (d; red), and phosphorylated tau (pThr181) (b; green) show co-segregation of porin and hyperphosphorylated tau in dystrophic neurites (long arrow in f). (g–i) Double-labeling immunofuorescence and confocal microscopy to lysosomal associated protein 1 (LAMP-1) (a; green) and mitochondrial porin (b; red). LAMP-1 and porin co-localize in a subset of cellular processes (c; arrowheads) suggesting engulfment of mitochondria into matured autophagic vesicles and participation of lysosomes in its degradation in distrophic neurites. β-Amyloid is stained in blue. Bar 10 μm (a–c and d–f), and 20 μm (g–i). Adapted from [12] with permission of Springer.

It also appears that axon swelling or dystrophy can precede extracellular amyloid deposition in certain animal models, in which autophagic vesicles with all the necessary enzymatic machinery to produce the Aβ peptide are evident [20–23]. In this sense, dystrophic axons have been proposed to be an intracellular source of secreted Aβ that would seed extracellular amyloid plaques. Protein deposits containing APP fragments can be seen in the brain parenchyma of aged wild-type mice, originating from axonal varicosities, further supporting this hypothesis. These data suggest that axonal dystrophy occurs first, leading thereafter to extracellular amyloid deposition in the early stages of the disease. In fact, it has been proposed that neurite dystrophy could reflect a conserved neuroprotective strategy to overcome the age-related accumulation of misfolded proteins, which in turn may represent a molecular mechanism of Aβ plaque deposition that potentially underlies the shift from normal to pathological aging [24, 25]. Nevertheless, Aβ alone may promote axonal atrophy through its interactions with the p75 neurotrophin receptor (p75NTR) in axon membranes [26]. Together, the evidence suggests that dystrophy and extracellular Aβ deposition are involved in a positive feedback loop whereby axon dystrophy is a source of extracellular Aβ, and the latter promotes axonal atrophy.

In terms of neuroinflammation, it is widely accepted that Aβ deposition alone might be sufficient to induce an inflammatory reaction that subsequently contributes to neuronal death and cognitive decline in AD [15]. However, this fact does not necessarily imply that Aβ plaque formation precedes microglial activation in AD. During normal aging, microglial activation aims to clear the misfolded proteins contained in fragmented neurites and aggregated into senile plaques. Interestingly, during AD-related pathological ageing, microglia cells recruited around plaques phagocytose Aβ and this could constitute part of the microglial mechanism to clear misfolded proteins, also during normal ageing [25]. Thus, in a scenario characterized by age-related chronic inflammation, microglia would be highly responsive to further activation which would drive their differentiation toward a classic phenotype characterized by pro-inflammatory cytokine secretion, in turn impairing axon trafficking, promoting Aβ accumulation and cell death [25, 27]. However, this putative role for AD-associated neuroinflammation is not supported by evidence showing that the inflammatory response is not neurotoxic and, indeed, it is even neuroprotective in a transgenic mouse model of AD [28]. In fact, from early in the amyloid pathology, alternative neuroprotective microglia are activated around amyloid plaques supporting neuronal survival, and this alternative phenotype is also present during animal ageing. By contrast, the classic microglial phenotype that is characterized by cytotoxic cytokine secretion only appears at advanced ages, associated with the presence of soluble Aβ oligomers and neuronal loss [27, 28]. Thus, these evidences show that alternative neuroprotective microglia may be present at advanced ages and coexist with classic microglial activation. In summary, although it is widely accepted that neuroinflammation promotes neuronal degeneration, it remains unclear how brain inflammation participates in the shift from normal to pathological ageing.

Hence, determining whether amyloid pathology is the first event in the pathway to AD-associated neuronal degeneration and dementia appears to be a particularly relevant issue, especially after the repeated fiascos in clinical trials of drugs targeting Aβ and related molecular entities. There is a close relationship among Aβ, inflammatory and neurite pathologies in AD because they all appear at early stages of the disease and all three are involved in neuronal death. In the present chapter, we will review how these neuropathological hallmarks are related to AD-associated membrane lipid alterations, as there can now be no shadow of doubt that brain lipids and the pathways they are involved in influence the pathophysiology of AD.

3. Brain lipid alterations in Alzheimer's disease

3.1. Cholesterol and sphingolipid homeostasis in AD

The amyloid cascade hypothesis was postulated because FAD mutations cause Alzheimer's disease, and they induce abnormal APP processing that leads to the well-characterized amyloid pathology [9]. Since the pathological hallmarks are exactly the same for both FAD and SAD, the same cascade of neuropathological events is thought to occur in both these disease variants. However, in addition to the influence of FAD clinical mutations on APP metabolism, these mutations may also have additional effects on other signaling cascades. In fact, presenilins (PSs) are the catalytic center of the γ-secretase complex, which cleaves more than 60 type I membrane proteins (one type of single transmembrane spanning region in integral proteins) [29, 30]. More than 160 clinical mutations have been described for PS1 and most of those that were studied induce loss of function of γ-secretase activity [31, 32]. These mutations may exert additional effects on cellular signaling as a consequence of the altered processing of certain membrane proteins that could influence lipid cellular homeostasis. Interestingly, γ-secretase loss of function induced by the ablation of PSs or by transgenic expression of PS1 mutants provoked a severe imbalance in the cholesterol content of the plasma membrane and intracellular membranes [33, 34]. In this sense, PS ablation increased the overall levels of cholesterol and sphingomyelin (SM) in cells, whereas the local concentration of cholesterol at the plasma membrane was dramatically reduced, resulting in the intracellular accumulation of cholesterol and cholesterol-rich membrane domains, such as lipid rafts [33, 34]. These observations demonstrate the impact of γ-secretase loss of function on the cell membrane lipid composition.

In the human brain, cholesterol is mainly transported in lipoprotein particles that predominantly contain ApoE. Interestingly, ApoE has been identified as a risk factor for SAD suggesting that altered cholesterol transport might also be related to the pathogenesis of late-onset AD [35]. The human ApoE protein is comprised of 299 amino acids and it has three isoforms, namely ApoE2, ApoE3, and ApoE4. The differences between these three isoforms lie in the amino acid residues at positions 112 and 158: ApoE2 (Cys112, Cys158), ApoE3 (Cys112, Arg158), and ApoE4 (Arg112, Arg158). In particular, subjects carrying the ApoE4 allele have a 3- to 4-fold higher risk of developing AD than those who do not carry this allele. Furthermore, ApoE4 was observed to exhibit a gene dose–effect, such that individuals who carry two copies of this allele have an even higher risk of suffering AD and an earlier age of onset. The effects of the ApoE4 isoform on AD risk are maximal between the ages of 60 and 70 years old, ApoE4 allele being present in more than 50% of all AD cases. Conversely, ApoE2 carriers appear to be somewhat protected from AD compared with ApoE3 carriers [36]. In this context, the ApoE4 isoform is less efficient in promoting cholesterol flux in neurons and astrocytes, and it also compromises cell uptake of cholesterol-containing lipoproteins compared with the other ApoE isoforms [37]. Furthermore, individuals carrying the ApoE4 allele accumulate less ApoE lipoprotein in the brain than non-ApoE4 carriers [38]. Hence, the expression of ApoE4 in SAD cases appears to alter cholesterol homeostasis in neurons in a similar way as that induced by γ-secretase loss-of-function in PS1-deficient cells and transgenic models of AD harboring clinical PS1 mutations [33, 34]. In such AD models, the loss of γ-secretase activity leads to impaired uptake of lipoproteins from the extracellular media due to the poor internalization of ApoE receptors like the LDLR (low-density lipoprotein receptor) [34]. In AD patients with the ApoE4 allele, cholesterol uptake would be impaired due to the lower affinity of ApoE4 to bind neuronal lipoprotein receptors, and to the lower concentration of circulating ApoE than in individuals carrying the ApoE2 or ApoE3 alleles [38, 39]. In any case, poorer membrane incorporation of neuronal cholesterol leads to increased *de novo* cholesterol synthesis and an altered neuronal distribution. Thus, altered cholesterol homeostasis is a key aspect of AD pathogenesis and alterations to cholesterol may represent a meeting point in the pathogenesis of FAD and SAD, driving the same neuropathological events in both disease variants, such as increased amyloidogenic APP processing.

The central nervous system (CNS) contains around 25% of the cholesterol in the body and evidence is accumulating that cholesterol homeostasis is indeed associated with AD pathogenesis. High cholesterol and high-density lipoprotein (HDL) in blood plasma are correlated with Aβ load in the brains of patients with AD [40, 41] and that increased cholesterol levels are associated with the incidence of AD [42, 43]. Furthermore, high or low cholesterol levels have often been related to enhanced or diminished Aβ production, respectively, in cell and animal models of AD, although these results are a little controversial [42, 44, 45]. What is more, lipidomic studies have shown that levels of cholesterol, certain cholesterol esters, and certain SM species are upregulated in the brain of patients with AD. This correlation is particularly strong in the case of patients with AD harboring the ApoE4 allele, although some contradictory results have also been reported in this respect [46–49]. Finally, altered cholesterol distribution and transport have been causally linked to neurodegenerative diseases in addition to AD, such as Huntington's and Niemann–Pick Type C diseases [44].

Cholesterol is an essential structural component of cell membranes and one of the major components of the functional membrane microdomains known as lipid rafts, together with sphingolipids such as SM and gangliosides. These microdomains are highly ordered membrane structures that serve as platforms for cell signaling, ligand-receptor binding, protein sorting, and other activities in the cell. Interestingly, amyloidogenic APP processing and Aβ aggregation have been proposed to take place in lipid rafts [50]. In fact, the activities of both BACE-1 and γ-secretase are enhanced in this type of membrane microdomains [51, 52]. In this context, compelling evidence supports the involvement of cholesterol and sphingolipids in the amyloidogenic processing of APP. On the one hand, membrane enrichment of these lipids could alter the biophysical properties of the lipid bilayer, affecting secretase activity in a manner that leads to the production of the longer pathogenic Aβ peptides instead of the shorter p3 peptide [53] (see **Figure 1**). On the other hand, cholesterol and SM storage disorders impair intracellular trafficking of APP, resulting in the accumulation of APP, APP-CTFs, and Aβ in autophagic vesicles of the endolysosomal pathway [54, 55]. Accordingly, impaired distribution of cholesterol and SM is accompanied by the downregulation of proteins involved in endosomal redistribution and fusion to the plasma membrane (SNAREs and RABs) in PS1-deficient cells [33]. These evidences suggest that dysfunctional vesicular trafficking between the plasma membrane and intracellular compartments may be caused by membrane lipid alterations that lead to the neuritic pathology and altered APP processing in FAD transgenic models [33, 56]. Additional studies have also linked shingolipid lysosomal accumulation to autophagic dysfunction and dystrophic neurite formation in AD [55, 57]. Such results indicate that cellular accumulation of sphingolipids could induce key cytopathological changes characteristic of AD, such as alterations to the autophagic/lysosomal system, increased generation of Aβ and accumulation of APP-CTFs in autophagic vesicles at dystrophic neurites, as occurs in an age-dependent manner in transgenic mouse models of AD [58]. Interestingly, a cholesterol-enriched diet in healthy mice also leads to insulin-like growth factor 1 (IGF1) impairment and insulin-mediated pro-survival signaling, which in turn promotes tau hyperphosphorylation in neurons [59]. Together, this evidence suggests that altered cholesterol/sphingolipid homeostasis may promote the neurite pathology, tau hyperphosphorylation, and amyloido-genic APP processing in AD.

Nevertheless, it cannot be ruled out that AD-related membrane lipid alterations can also potentiate the neurotoxicity of the Aβ oligomers in AD patient's brains. In fact, lipid rafts may serve as a platform for the cellular interactions with soluble Aβ oligomers, in turn promoting tau hyperphosphorylation and inhibiting synaptic plasticity by hindering LTP (long-term potentiation) in the brain [60, 61]. Moreover, raft-associated lipids such as cholesterol, SM, and the GM1 ganglioside revert the fibrillar Aβ into soluble oligomers, such that altered cellular lipid homeostasis may actually potentiate the severity of the amyloid pathology in AD [62].

3.2. Polyunsaturated fatty acids in AD

Polyunsaturated fatty acids (PUFAs) are those fatty acids that contain more than one double bond in their backbone. They are abundant in cell membranes, and they are mainly incorpo-rated into membrane phospholipids. The carbon next to the carboxyl group is known as the α carbon, the next one is the β carbon, and so forth, until the final carbon called the ω carbon. Thus, ω-3 fatty acids have the first double bond between the third and fourth C atoms from the ω carbon. For instance, 22:6 ω-3 or 22:6 n-3 (docosahexaenoic acid, DHA) indicates a 22-carbon chain with six double bonds and with the first double bond between the third and fourth carbons from the CH_3 end. The physiological properties of unsaturated fatty acids largely depend on the position of the first unsaturation relative to the end position. The essential fatty acids α-linolenic acid (ALA, 18:3 ω-3) and linoleic acid (LA, 18:2 ω-6) must be incorporated through the diet, and they are the starting point for the synthesis of longer and more unsaturated PUFAs such as arachidonic acid (ARA, 20:4 ω-6), eicosapentaenoic acid (EPA, 20:5 ω-3), and DHA (22:6 ω-3). However, conversion of ALA to longer PUFAs in humans is very inefficient and therefore, these long PUFAs are normally incorporated through the diet, particularly through fish intake [63].

The membranes of the cells in the brain are rich in ω-3 PUFAs such as DHA and EPA. Since AD is a cognitive disorder and DHA is involved in normal cognitive development, the DHA levels in the AD brain have been analyzed extensively. As a result, it is widely accepted that in the human brain AD courses with diminished DHA levels, although a number of discrep-ancies in this respect have also been observed [64]. These discrepancies may reflect the brain region studied as the neurodegeneration associated with AD does not affect all brain areas homogeneously. In the hippocampus, one of the regions primarily affected in AD, decreased DHA levels are associated with reduced levels of PE (phosphatidylethanolamine) or PE plasmalogens [65–69], supporting a relationship between lower DHA levels and cognitive decline in AD. Moreover, there is significant experimental evidence in animal models that hippocampal DHA deficiency or enrichment is associated with reduced or increased learning memory abilities, respectively [70]. At the cellular level, exposure to ω-3 PUFAs enhances synaptic plasticity by increasing LTP and synaptic protein expression, in turn leading to increased dendritic spine density and hippocampal neurogenesis. In addition, ω-3 PUFAs have antioxidant, anti-inflammatory, and anti-apoptotic effects, thereby promoting neuronal survival during normal ageing and in AD. On the other hand, PUFA deficits are related to enhanced amyloidogenic APP processing and cell susceptibility to Aβ neurotoxicity, particularly as ω-3 PUFA deficiency downregulates neuroprotective signaling (e.g., ERK signaling). Therefore, PUFA deficits may enhance neuron degeneration and cognitive impairment in AD [71].

It still remains largely unclear how ω-3 PUFAs exert their cellular functions and consequently, what signaling cascades are impaired in the brain due to their deficiency. Such ω-3 PUFAs maintain the structural functionality of neural cell membranes. Indeed, in consonance with the reduced levels of DHA in the human AD brain, lipid rafts obtained from AD brain cortex also exhibited significantly less DHA than age-matched controls [72]. Interestingly, the biophysical and structural properties of PE and DHA in membranes are opposed to those of cholesterol and SM. Thus, these abnormalities in lipid raft composition may provoke strong modifications to the membrane structure of neurons such as alteration of membrane viscosity, rigidity and thickness, lateral lipid packing, lipid order, and other parameters, which could in turn be relevant to secretase activity and the production of Aβ [73]. Accordingly, decreased PUFA levels in lipid rafts would be coupled to enriched cholesterol and sphingolipids, thereby promoting the detrimental effects on neurons including the neurite dystrophy, tau hyperphosphorylation, and amyloidogenic APP processing that drives neuronal degeneration (see Section 3.1.).

Alternatively, DHA may be released from phospholipids due to the activity of PLA2 (phospholipase A2), acting as a signaling molecule, and DHA can be hydroxylated to produce several secondary bioactive lipids such as resolvins (RVs) and protectins. DHA hydroxylation is mediated through lipoxygenase-15 (LOX-15) or acetylated cyclooxygenase-2 (COX-2) [63]. Compounds derived from DHA are classified as D-series RVs or protectins, while those formed from EPA are designated as E-series RVs. DHA can be hydroxylated on carbon 17 by 15-LOX or acetylated COX-2, leading to stereoselective formation of 17S- or 17R-hydroxy-DHA (17-HDHA), respectively. These derivatives may be further hydroxylated to give rise to trihydroxy derivatives such as the D1, D2, D3, and D4 17-(S/R)-RVs (D-series RVs), and the dihydroxy 17-(R)- and 17(S)-protectin, the latter also known as neuroprotectin D1 (NPD1). EPA can be stereoselectively hydroxylated to 18-(S/R)-hydroxy-EPA (18-HEPA) by cytochrome P450 or acetylated COX-2, which is further processed to form E1, E2 and E3 18-(S/R)-RVs (E-series RVs: **Figure 3**). Both, 17-HDHA and 18-HEPA serve as markers for RVs and protectins, and remarkably, their presence in blood is directly related to the intake of ω-3 PUFAs in animal models [74]. In addition, these PUFA derivatives are thought to exert their biological function by mechanisms that go beyond the simple regulation of lipid membrane composition and structure. In fact, non-esterified DHA, RVs and protectins may bind to different fatty acid (FA) receptors such as the retinoid X receptor (RXR), G protein-coupled receptors (GPCRs), peroxisome proliferator-activated receptors (PPARs), and fatty-acid binding proteins (FABPs). Although the exact signaling cascade mediated by many of these proteins has not been identified, the mechanism of action of DHA or HDHA derivatives like NPD1 has been proposed to involve PPARγ activation. Indeed, NPD1 is known to promote PPARγ activation more intensely than DHA and as such, the neuroprotective effects of DHA may be mediated by NPD1 and/or other DHA-derived hydroxylated bioactive derivatives in the brain [75, 76].

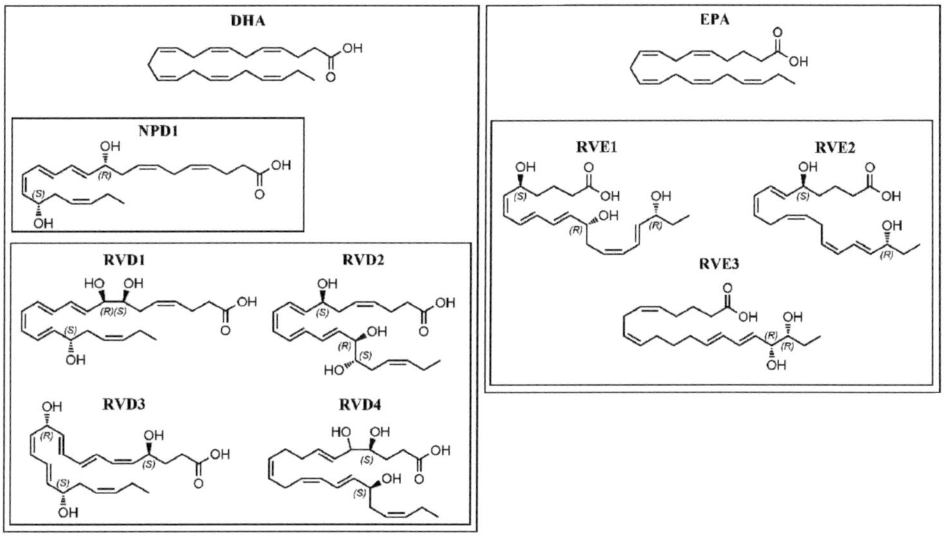

Figure 3. Chemical structure of specialized pro-resolving mediators derived from DHA and EPA ω-3 fatty acids. DHA (docosahexaenoic acid) and EPA (eicosapentaenoic acid) may be released from phospholipids through PLA2 (phospholipase A2) activity and converted into bioactive hydroxylated fatty acids with potent anti-inflammatory properties, known as resolvins and protectins. This conversion may be mediated by several enzymes, including lipoxygenase-15 (LOX-15), acetylated cyclooxigenase-2 (COX-2), and cytochrome P450. Compounds derived from DHA are classified as D-series resolvins (RVs: left panel), while those formed from EPA are designated as E-series resolvins (right panel). Although resolvins normally includes trihydroxy fatty acids, DHA can be also transformed into dihydroxylated compounds denominated as protectins. Within this group, neuroprotectin D1 (NPD1: see left panel) is the best studied DHA-derived hydroxylated compound in terms of AD therapy, and it displays anti-inflammatory, anti-apoptotic, and anti-amyloidogenic properties.

The balance between ω-6 to ω-3 intake has a strong impact on brain health. In Western diets, this ratio is about 10–20:1, while in other cultures and also historically, this ratio has been as low as 1–2:1. Total fat intake as well as the ω-6 to ω-3 ratio in Western diets has increased significantly since the Industrial Revolution, indicating that Western diets are deficient in ω-3 PUFAs [77]. Epidemiological studies, including correlational studies and migration studies, suggest a protective effect against AD of ω-3 PUFAs and fish oil (an important source of ω-3 PUFAs), such that the role of nutrition in preventing AD arouses increasing hope, particularly with reference to ω-3 PUFA dietary intake. One recent meta-analysis reviewed a total of six cohort studies performed in the USA and Europe to address how dietary intake of long-chain ω-3 PUFAs or fish correlates with the incidence of dementia and AD [78]. This meta-analysis found a significant lower risk of AD associated with high fish intake. Such an association was most pronounced when the follow-up period was at least five years and fish intake was 500 g or more per week, such that fish consumption is inversely correlated with AD incidence in a temporal and quantitative manner. A dose–response meta-analysis also showed that for every 100 g per week dietary fish intake the risk of AD falls 11%. This neuroprotective effect of fish intake was mainly attributed to its high long-chain ω-3 PUFA content, particularly DHA [79]. Interestingly, the same meta-analysis also revealed that dietary intake of ω-3 PUFAs alone (not linked to fish consumption) did not lower the risk of dementia or AD. Moreover, an earlier randomized trial reached the same conclusions in patients with mild-to-moderate AD who were administered DHA [80]. Nevertheless, most of the individual studies evaluating the relationships between ω-3 PUFA intake and AD risk suggest there is a potential protective effect of these long ω-3 PUFAs on the incidence of AD, although no significant statistical differences were reached in the pooled analysis.

The discrepancies between fish and ω-3 PUFA consumption in relation to AD incidence may be explained by different factors in terms of the dietary composition or socioeconomic status of the individual. In this context, dietary intake of long-chain ω-3 PUFAs may also be accompanied by the intake of other saturated fats, which would attenuate the neuroprotective effect of ω-3 PUFAs. Alternatively, fish is also a good source of vitamins, essential amino acids and other nutrients, which could in turn be responsible for the beneficial effect attributed to fish in AD prevention. The fact that DHA is converted into bioactive derivatives that mediate its beneficial effects in CNS cannot be overlooked. In this context, the neuroprotective effect of fish intake could be also attributed to PUFA derivatives present in fish, such as hydroxylated forms of PUFAs or PUFA forms easily transformable into bioactive derivatives similar to NPD1 [81]. In fact, fish oil consumption has recently been related to increased levels of total DHA and NPD1-like derivatives in the mouse brain, without any modification of free (unesterified) DHA levels [82]. Hence, fish oil intake promotes elevated levels of NPD1 without affecting basal levels of free DHA in the brain. These data bring to light a central role for ω-3 PUFA hydroxylated bioactive derivatives in the prevention and treatment of AD (see Section 5.2.).

3.3. Specific lipid alterations as potential biomarkers in AD

Modern lipidomic analysis allows a comprehensive atlas to be built up of all the lipid alterations existing in the AD brain. Current laboratory techniques, such as ultra/high pressure liquid chromatography (U/HPLC) and gas chromatography (GC) coupled to mass spectrometry (MS) allow the vast majority of lipids in cells and animal tissues to be studied. Since the brain is the most lipid-enriched organ in the human body, after adipose tissue, alterations in lipid composition might be involved in many neurological disorders, including AD [44]. An in-depth lipidomic analysis performed in the postmortem brain of patients with AD showed heterogeneous changes in lipid metabolism in AD-affected patients [47]. As expected, the cerebellum lipid profile was largely unaffected whereas significant lipid changes were observed in the prefrontal and entorhinal cortex of AD brains when compared with age-matched controls. These changes demonstrate that lipid alterations are restricted to AD-affected brain regions (principally the cortex and hippocampus) and that they are not present in unaffected regions like the cerebellum. Interestingly, the prefrontal cortex displays more severe lipid alterations, with a decrease in PE, LPC (lyso-phosphatidylcholine), and sulfatides, together with elevated levels of ceramides (including glucosyl- and galactosyl-ceramides, Cer) and DAG (diacylglycerol). By contrast, in the entorhinal cortex, significant increases are only evident in LBPA (lysobiphosphatidic acid), SM, ganglioside GM3, and cholesterol esters (ChoE). In addition, polyunsaturated PE 40:6, 38:6, and 38:4 species were markedly downregulated in the prefrontal cortex, whereas there was a general decrease in long-chain fatty acids (≥40C) and a corresponding increase in short-chain fatty acids (≤34C) that is compatible with the lower levels of PE carrying DHA in the brain of patients with AD. Unexpectedly, the entorhinal cortex displays more species of the polyunsaturated lipid pools in PC (phosphatidylcholine) and PE. The different lipid alterations between these two brain regions may reflect different aspects or stages of AD pathophysiology, since the entorhinal cortex is known to be affected earlier and more severely than neocortical areas [83].

AD progresses from a pre-symptomatic stage to mild cognitive impairment (MCI), mild AD and to severe AD with a gradual deterioration in cognitive abilities. Unfortunately, the clinical manifestation of the disease is preceded by a long prodromal phase, during which neuropathological lesions arise, including neuron death. For this reason, clinical diagnosis of AD is unreliable, particularly at early disease stages. Hence, there is a strong need to find peripheral biomarkers to reliably diagnose AD early, thereby enabling early treatment and better therapeutic efficacy. Most approaches to fluid-based biomarker discovery have focused on Aβ42, total tau and phosphorylated tau in cerebrospinal fluid (CSF). Although these are useful to distinguish symptomatic patients from normal controls or other dementias, these CSF biomarkers lack predictive value in preclinical patients, and they are only useful to confirm the clinical diagnosis [84]. Thus, given the brain lipid alterations in AD, lipidomic analysis of lipid derivatives in biological fluids may represent a reliable way to identify non-invasive biomarkers for early AD diagnosis [85].

Of the lipid changes reported in the CSF, plasma, and serum of patients with AD, many do not necessarily correlate with those described previously in the CNS [6]. For instance, free cholesterol and ChoE were reported to be downregulated in the CSF although they are increased in the brain of patients with AD [86] (see Section 3.1.). However, six different long-chain ChoE species in plasma allowed patients with AD to be accurately discriminated from healthy controls (ChoE 32:0, 34:0, 34:6, 32:4, 33:6, and 40:4). These metabolites accumulated more strongly in healthy controls than in MCI, and in MCI than in AD, such that they were proposed as potential biomarkers for early AD diagnosis [87]. Total PC levels and specific PC species have also been proposed as reliable biomarkers, with diminished PC levels in the CSF of patients with AD accompanied by lowered LPC and increased PC hydrolytic products such as glycerophosphocholine and phosphocholine, suggesting that PC breakdown might be enhanced in AD pathogenesis [88]. Notably, a set of 10 PC metabolites was specifically depleted in the plasma of healthy individuals who later suffered phenoconversion towards MCI/AD.

These subjects were diagnosed as AD during a 5-year follow-up even though they displayed no cognitive impairment at entry. The PC species identified were diacyl PC 36:6, 38:0, 38:6, 40:1, 40:2, 40:6, PC acyl-alkyl 40:6, and LPC 18:2, as well as the acylcarnitines (ACs) propionyl AC (C3), and C16:1-OH [89]. It is noteworthy that control subjects (not previously diagnosed with AD) did not display any of these modifications, while already diagnosed patients with AD also showed decreased levels of these PC species. Moreover, downregulation of this panel of lipids predicted phenoconversion from healthy to MCI/AD within a 2–3 year time frame with 90% accuracy [89]. These data were supported by independent studies showing decreased levels of PC 38:4, 38:6, and 40:6 in the plasma or serum of AD subjects [86, 90]. In addition, a variety of peripheral lipid changes were also reported that might potentially be useful for early AD diagnosis, such as lower levels of SM and increased levels of Cers in the plasma or serum of patients with AD. In particular, there were significantly fewer SM species containing long chains (e.g., 22 and 24 carbon atom acyl chains) in AD subjects [86, 91]. In parallel, increased Cer levels were reported in the plasma of patients with AD [91, 92]. SM can be metabolized into Cers, second messengers that regulate cellular differentiation, proliferation and apoptosis. Upregulated levels of Cers were concomitant with significant reductions in SM in the plasma of patients with AD. A correlation between the decrease in SM and the increase in Cers was particularly robust in the ratios of SM and Cer species with identical fatty acyl chains. Cer alterations were particularly evident in mild-to-moderate stages of AD [91]. Moreover, it is noteworthy that upregulated Cer levels were significantly correlated with the onset of memory impairment, supporting the role of Cers as potential AD biomarkers [92].

In conclusion, a wide range of peripheral fluid changes have been described that could be used as biomarkers for early AD diagnosis. However, many of the clinical studies involved are cross-sectional in nature and some of them do not reveal reliable biomarkers to test disease progression. Nevertheless, longitudinal studies with several years of follow-up do identify promising biomarkers for early AD diagnosis that reliably predict cognitive impairment and the onset of AD.

4. Prevention and treatment of Alzheimer's disease

The main risk factors for dementia are age and genetics (see more information about AD risk factors at http://www.alz.org/alzheimers_disease_causes_risk_factors.asp), although other risk factors may also influence the onset of dementia. For instance, since the brain is nourished by a rich network of blood vessels, cardiovascular alterations are considered a risk factor for neurological disorders. In fact, vascular dementia is linked to morphological changes to blood vessels which are in turn present in other types of dementia like AD. Indeed, a healthy cardiovascular system is frequently linked to brain protection [93]. In this context, the control of blood cholesterol levels, blood pressure, and body weight is recommended to maintain good brain health. In fact, high-fat diets and sedentary lifestyles are becoming major concerns in terms of their contribution to the high incidence of dementia in Western society, whereas regular physical exercise and heart-healthy diets are also good habits to lower the risk of dementia [35].

http://dx.doi.org/10.5772/64757

Only two types of drugs are currently available to treat Alzheimer's disease: acetylcholinesterase inhibitors (often shortened to just "cholinesterase inhibitors") and NMDA receptor antagonists. Cholinesterase inhibitors (donepezil, rivastigmine, and galantamine) bind to and reversibly inactivate cholinesterases, inhibiting acetylcholine hydrolysis. Such inhibition results in increased acetylcholine concentrations at cholinergic synapses and indeed, AD involves a substantial loss of cholinergic neurons in the neocortex and hippocampus, which in turn contributes to the AD symptomatology and to memory impairment in particular. Therefore, increased levels of acetylcholine are thought to protect against the death of cholinergic neurons, alleviating AD symptoms [94]. Memantine is a low-affinity voltage-dependent antagonist of glutamatergic NMDA receptors. By binding to the NMDA receptor, memantine inhibits the sustained influx of Ca^{2+} ions from the extracellular milieu, thereby preventing neuronal death by excitotoxicity. Such a pathogenic mechanism can be mediated by the Aβ oligomers that bind to NMDA receptor as agonists, favoring Ca^{2+} influx and neuronal excitotoxicity [95]. Interestingly, memantine preserves physiological receptor activity, such that released glutamate can still mediate receptor activation leading to neuronal depolarization in postsynaptic neurons [96]. However, neither cholinesterase inhibitors nor NMDA antagonists have disease-modifying effects in AD and they are generally viewed as palliative treatments with marginal to minimal clinical efficacy, either alone or in combination. Therefore, only a small percentage of patients with AD respond to these treatments and these responders normally undergo a short period of cognitive stabilization after which they again suffer from the cognitive decline associated to largescale neuronal degeneration [97, 98]. This scenario highlights the unmet clinical need for the treatment of AD and related conditions.

Developing disease-modifying drugs (DMDs) capable of preventing neuron degeneration and thereby counteracting AD progression is one of the most pressing challenges of modern pharmacology. Since the pathological process of AD begins many years before its clinical diagnosis, the optimal time for a disease-modifying therapy may be during the prodromal stage of AD. Therefore, clinical diagnosis of AD must be achieved when patients show no relevant clinical signs. Indeed, the development of DMDs will require the concomitant incorporation of reliable biomarkers to identify early stages of AD (see Section 3.3). Hitherto, no DMDs are available for AD and although several have been tested up to phase 3, none has yet achieved marketing approval. The recurrent failures in clinical trials raise a number of questions about our understanding of AD pathophysiology. In this sense, the amyloid cascade hypothesis has not only influenced the study of AD pathophysiology over the past 2 decades but also, the choice of drug targets (see Section 2). Therefore, most clinical trials have set out to prevent Aβ accumulation, either by inhibiting its production/aggregation or enhancing its clearance, as well as reducing tau phosphorylation [99, 100]. However, it remains unclear if these two hallmarks of AD are a cause or consequence of the disease. In fact, they could lie downstream of previous molecular/cellular alterations, as a result of the disease pathology (damage response proteins) and/or as products of an endogenous protective response to disease-induced damage. Nonetheless, over the past 20 years the main focus of biomedical research and the associated drug discovery programs for AD have targeted brain amyloid or tau hyperphosphorylation, and the associated formation of neurofibrillary tangles [18].

Mutations in the BACE-1 gene have not been related to AD but elevated levels of this enzyme have consistently been found in both the brain and CSF of patients with AD [101–103]. Since β-secretase activity is pathologically elevated in AD, BACE1 inhibition has been addressed as a potential therapeutic approach to combat AD. In fact, both genetic deletion of BACE-1 and administration of a BACE-1 inhibitor rescued cognitive deficits and lowered brain Aβ production in AD mouse models. Interestingly, although BACE-1 has other substrates, its inhibition was apparently free of side effects in AD mice [104, 105]. The latest generation of small molecule BACE-1 inhibitors has achieved satisfactory brain penetration and a robust reduction in cerebral Aβ in preclinical animal models. Furthermore, administration of most of these inhibitors in humans also reduced Aβ and sAPPβ levels, whereas sAPPα (the α-secretase cleavage product) was enhanced in the CSF. This observation is consistent with BACE-1 inhibition since β- and α-secretase compete for APP processing (see **Figure 1**). Many of these BACE-1 inhibitors are still in phase-1 clinical trials where safety and tolerability are tested but some of them are currently in phase 2/3, although no clinical efficacy data are as yet available (**Table 1**). Interestingly, one such drug (LY2886721 from Eli Lilly Company) was discontinued in a phase-2 trial because a number of subjects developed hepatic toxicity, although they were not associated with the mechanism of action of BACE1 [106].

Drug	Synonyms	Company	Mechanism of action	Result of study	Clinical trial ID*	Observations
LY2886721	–	Eli Lilly & Co.	β-Secretase inhibitor	Discontinued in phase 2	NCT01561430	Altered liver biochemistry
AZD3293	LY3314814	Astra Zeneca/ Eli Lilly & Co.	β-Secretase inhibitor	Ongoing in phase 2/3	NCT02245737	–
Verubecestat	MK-8931 MK-8931-009	Merck	β-Secretase inhibitor	Ongoing in phase 2/3	NCT01739348 NCT01953601	–
E2609	–	Eisai/Biogen Idec	β-secretase inhibitor	Ongoing in phase 2	NCT02322021	–
Semagacestat	LY450139	Eli Lilly & Co.	γ-secretase inhibitor	Discontinued in phase 3	NCT01035138 NCT00762411 NCT00594568	Lack of clinical improvement Increased risk of skin cancer and infections.
Avagacestat	BMS-708163	Bristol-Myers Squibb	Notch-sparing γ-secretase inhibitor	Discontinued in phase 3	NCT00890890	Lack of clinical improvement Increased rate of skin cancers
Begacestat	GSI-953	Pfizer	Notch-sparing γ-secretase inhibitor	Phase-1 trial completed	NCT00547560	–

Drug	Synonyms	Company	Mechanism of action	Result of study	Clinical trial ID*	Observations
Tarenflurbil	R-flurbiprofe MPC-7869	Myriad Genetics & Laboratories	γ-Secretase modulator	Discontinued in phase 3	NCT00105547 NCT00380276 NCT00322036	Lack of clinical improvement Low potency and poor brain penetration
Tramiprosate	NC-531 Homotaurine 3APS	Neurochem, Inc	Aβ aggregation inhibitor	Discontinued in phase 3	NCT00314912 NCT00088673 NCT00217763	Lack of clinical improvement
Scyllo-inositol	AZD-103 ELND005	Elan Corporation, Speranza Therapeutics, Transition Therapeutics, Inc.	Aβ aggregation inhibitor	Discontinued in phase 2	NCT00568776 NCT00934050	Lack of clinical improvement
Rosiglitazone	Avandia	GlaxoSmithKline	Anti-diabetic drug Aβ clearance enhancer	Discontinued in phase 3	NCT00428090 NCT00550420	Lack of clinical improvement
AN-1792	AIP 001	Janssen Pfizer	Aβ-targeted active immunotherapy	Discontinued in phase 2	NCT00021723	Brain inflammation Aseptic meningoencephalitis
Bapineuzumab	AAB-001	Janssen Pfizer	Aβ-targeted passive immunotherapy	Discontinued in phase 3	NCT00676143 NCT00667810 NCT00998764 NCT00996918	Lack of clinical improvement
Solanezumab	LY2062430	Eli Lilly & Co.	Aβ-targeted passive immunotherapy	Ongoing in phase 3	NCT00905372 NCT00904683 NCT01127633 NCT01900665	–
Gantenerumab	RO4909832 RG1450	Chugai Pharmaceutical Co. Ltd. Hoffmann-La Roche	Aβ-targeted passive immunotherapy	Ongoing in phase 3	NCT01224106 NCT02051608	–
Aducanumab	BIIB037	Biogen	Aβ-targeted passive immunotherapy	Ongoing in phase 3	NCT02477800 NCT02484547	–
Ponezumab	PF-04360365	Pfizer	Aβ-targeted passive immunotherapy	Discontinued in phase 2	NCT00722046 NCT00945672	Lack of clinical improvement

Drug	Synonyms	Company	Mechanism of action	Result of study	Clinical trial ID*	Observations
Valproate	Depakote, Depakene	Abbott Laboratories	Tau phosphorylation inhibitor	Discontinued in phase 3	NCT00071721	Lack of clinical improvement Brain volume loss
Lithium **	Lithium carbonate	Public institutions	Tau phosphorylation inhibitor	Ongoing in phase 2	ISRCTN72046462 (see at isrctn.com) NCT01055392 NCT02129348 NCT00088387	Discrepant results reported Apparently effective in early AD (amnestic MCI) but not in mild-to-moderate AD
Epothilone D	BMS-241027	Bristol-Myers Squibb	Microtubule stabilizer	Discontinued in phase 1	NCT01492374	No reasons reported regarding discontinuation in phase 1
TPI 287	–	Cortice Biosciences	Microtubule stabilizer	Ongoing in phase 1	NCT01966666	
Methylthioninium (MT)	Methylene Blue Rember TM TRx-0014	TauRx Therapeutics Ltd	Tau aggregation inhibitor	Discontinued in phase 2	NCT00684944 NCT00515333	Discrepant results reported Blinding of phase-2 trial has been questioned
LMT-X	Methylene Blue TRx-0237	TauRx Therapeutics Ltd	Tau aggregation inhibitor	Phase 3 completed	NCT01689233 NCT01689246 NCT01626378	No results available as yet
ACI-35	–	AC Immune SA Janssen	Tau-targeted active immunotherapy	Phase 1 completed	ISRCTN13033912 (see at isrctn.com)	–
AADvac1	Axon peptide 108 conjugated to KLH	Axon Neuroscience SE	Tau-targeted active immunotherapy	Ongoing phase 1	NCT02031198	–
RG7345	RO6926496	Roche	Tau-targeted passive immunotherapy	Discontinued in phase 1	NCT02281786	No reasons reported regarding discontinuation in phase 1

Some data in this table are available at http://www.alzforum.org/therapeutics/.
*Clinical trial IDs were obtained from Clinicaltrials.gov unless specified.
**Information regarding the clinical use of lithium was obtained from [121, 122] and Clinicaltrials.gov.

Table 1. Developed disease-modifying drugs for AD treatment in clinical trials.

Clinical mutations in PS1 are supposed to induce a loss of γ-secretase function that in turn prevents Aβ generation and increases the Aβ 42/40 ratio (an increase in the longer vs. shorter Aβ isoforms) [31]. Such loss of function is then translated into increased neuronal Aβ production, which is further potentiated with the ageing in AD mice harboring FAD mutations [23, 58]. This pathological mechanism is associated with accumulation of autophagic vesicles in axonal dystrophies surrounding amyloid plaques, which are principally formed by long hydrophobic isoforms of Aβ like Aβ42. Therefore, γ-secretase inhibition or modulation has also been studied as a plausible therapeutic approach against AD, although non-specific effects hinder the development of γ-secretase inhibitors (GSI) as DMDs given that γ-secretase also cleaves several type-I transmembrane proteins such as the Notch receptor, N-cadherin, ErbB4, and p75NTR (see Section 2).

Semagacestat was the first GSI to undergo clinical trials, and it reduced Aβ concentrations in the mouse CNS and human plasma [107, 108]. Two large phase-3 trials with semagacestat were prematurely interrupted due to serious adverse events, including hematological alterations, and an increased risk of skin cancer and infections that were attributed to inhibition of the Notch signaling pathway. Furthermore, a worsening of cognition was observed in AD-treated patients [109]. Notch-sparing GSIs (second generation inhibitors) and modulators (agents that shift γ-secretase cleavage from longer to shorter Aβ species without affecting Notch cleavage) were then designed for clinical development. Avagacestat and begacestat were first conceived as notch-sparing GSIs that supposedly display greater selectivity for APP than for Notch cleavage [10], although this was recently reported not to be the case [31]. Therefore, these drugs are also likely to fail and indeed, the poor clinical efficacy of Avagacestat was coupled to an increased rate of skin cancers, again suggesting side effects attributable to Notch signaling inhibition (see **Table 1**). Finally, some non-steroidal anti-inflammatory drugs (NSAIDs) modulate γ-secretase (GSMs), decreasing the abundance of Aβ42 while increasing that of Aβ38. Tarenflurbil (the R-enantiomer of flurbiprofen) was tested in a phase-3 trial but it did not slow cognitive decline in patients, while it did increase the frequency of dizziness, anemia, and infection. This failure of tarenflurbil was attributed to its low potency and poor brain penetration [10, 99].

Aggregation of Aβ monomers into higher molecular weight oligomers is thought to be a key neurotoxic event leading to neurodegeneration in the amyloid pathology [7]. For this reason, some DMDs also target this conversion to fight AD. Tramiprosate and scyllo-inositol are two compounds that prevent the transition from Aβ monomers to oligomers, thus favoring Aβ clearance from the brain by insulin-degrading enzyme (IDE) and neprilysin [110]. In addition, scyllo-inositol can also directly bind to Aβ oligomers, promoting their dissociation. Both these drugs have been involved in phase-2 clinical trials and both reduced Aβ42 levels in the CSF of treated patients. In a larger phase-3 study, tramiprosate failed to induce clinical improvement, and thus, further clinical evaluation is still necessary. Scyllo-inositol, also failed to produce significant clinical improvement in a phase-2 trial. Rosiglitazone is an anti-diabetic drug that improves spatial learning and memory abilities, and it mildly decreases Aβ42 brain levels by activating PPARγ and upregulating IDE in AD mice [111]. This drug was involved in phase-2 and phase-3 clinical trials, although the inconclusive results in phase 2 were followed by a lack of clinical efficacy in a larger phase-3 study [99, 112].

Another therapeutic approach to promote Aβ clearance was based on immunization toward Aβ. Active immunization by vaccination stimulates the immune response to promote antibody formation against pathogenic forms of Aβ, such as Aβ42. Active Aβ immunotherapy has been studied since 1999 when the generation of Aβ antibodies was shown to produce clearance of cerebral Aβ by phagocytic microglia in animal models [113]. Unfortunately, this revolutionary approach soon suffered its first setback in a phase-2 trial to test active immunization using full length human Aβ42 peptide, with some patients developing brain inflammation with aseptic meningoencephalitis and provoking the termination of the clinical study [99]. Passive immunotherapy is an alternative strategy and recent approaches were based on shorter Aβ immunogens, such as the humanized monoclonal antibody to Aβ1–5, bapineuzumab, which binds to both soluble and fibrillar forms of Aβ. Despite the evidence of adverse effects in phase-1 trials, bapineuzumab advanced to phases 2 and 3 where it failed to demonstrate clinical efficacy in patients with AD. Another antibody against Aβ is Solanezumab, a humanized monoclonal antibody against Aβ16–24 that preferentially binds to soluble Aβ. In phase-2 trials, solanezumab was found to be safe while increasing plasma and CSF levels of Aβ40 and Aβ42, an indication of decreased plaque load in the brain. However, solanezumab had no effect on behavioral outcomes. Despite the lack of efficacy in phase 2, the antibody advanced to phase-3 trials in patients with mild-to-moderate AD where the primary endpoints, both cognitive and functional, were not achieved [18]. Many other humanized antibodies have been developed, directed at different regions of the Aβ peptide, some entering phase-3 trials (Gantenerumab and Aducanumab) and others having been discontinued (Ponezumab; **Table 1**).

According to the amyloid cascade hypothesis, Aβ accumulation precedes and drives tau hyperphosphorylation via the activation of different kinases, including cyclin dependent kinase 5 (CDK5) and glycogen synthase kinase 3β (GSK3β) [14, 114]. Tau hyperphosphorylation is thought to destabilizes neuronal microtubules, impairing axonal transport and leading to neurite pathology, finally resulting in deficient synaptic function and neuronal death [115, 116] (see Section 2). In this context, DMDs were developed to inhibit tau phosphorylation, as well as compounds that prevent tau aggregation. GSK3β is the main enzyme involved in tau hyperphosphorylation, and lithium and valproate are both drugs that inhibit GSK3β and reduce tau phosphorylation in animal models [117]. Unexpectedly, valproate impaired the cognitive and functional status, and it was also associated with a reduced brain volume in patients with AD receiving the drug in clinical trials [118]. Lithium is neuroprotective in animal models of AD, not only via the inhibition of GSK-3β but also through the remodeling of Aβ plaques, leading to a decrease in the number of dystrophic axons, reduced neuronal degeneration and improved cognitive scores in AD mice [119, 120]. However, no conclusions have been reached regarding the clinical efficacy of lithium for AD treatment. Some clinical trials failed to demonstrate a protective effect of lithium on cognitive performance, although a more recent clinical study showed that lithium reduced cognitive decline patients with early AD (amnesic MCI) [121, 122]. Tau hyperphosphorylation compromises its ability to bind to microtubules in AD, provoking microtubule instability. In this sense, epothilone D and TPI

287, synthetic paclitaxel-derived microtubule-stabilizing drugs with good BBB permeability, were assessed in phase-1 trials of safety and tolerability. Unfortunately, epothilone D was recently discontinued (see **Table 1**). Tau hyperphosphorylation also provokes tau aggregation which is also considered a key neurotoxic event in AD [123]. LMT-X is a new version of methylene blue, a compound that was tested and discontinued in a phase-2 trial to treat AD. LMT-X is an inhibitor of tau aggregation that specifically disrupts tau-tau interactions in the microtubule binding region. In a phase-2 trial, this new drug slowed down the cognitive decline in a subgroup of patients, and it is now being tested in phase-3 trials, although information about clinical efficacy is not yet available [124, 125]. Finally, two tau-derived peptide vaccines that stimulate active immunization entered phase I studies: AADvac1 and ACI-35. AADvac1 is a synthetic peptide corresponding to a naturally occurring, truncated and misfolded form of tau. ACI-35 is a liposomal vaccine containing a synthetic peptide corresponding to human protein tau sequence 393–408 (numbering according to the tau 2N4R isoform), with phosphorylated S396 and S404 residues. Vaccination with these peptides improves neurobehavioral deficits in AD rodents while ACI-35 is characterized by a rapid and robust polyclonal antibody response specific to phosphorylated tau in WT and AD mice [125]. In addition, passive immunization has also been investigated using a humanized monoclonal antibody targeting pS422 phospho-tau. In AD mice, chronic administration of this antibody reduced hyperphosphorylated tau accumulation [126], although clinical studies with this antibody were recently discontinued in phase 1 (see **Table 1**).

The aforementioned therapeutic approaches summarize the attempts to develop DMDs based on the amyloid cascade hypothesis, principally focused on Aβ and hyperphosphorylated tau protein. With several anti-amyloid drugs now having failed in late stage clinical trials, many critical voices in the scientific community have questioned the validity of the amyloid hypothesis to explain the pathophysiology of AD and as platform on which to develop DMDs for AD therapy. Moreover, the incidence of serious side effects observed in human trials is another drawback to the clinical development of these types of drugs, particularly when many of these adverse effects are associated with the mechanism of action of the compounds tested. However, the amyloid hypothesis cannot be disregarded due the lack of reliable biomarkers to detect efficacy at early stages, and because many of the compounds in clinical trials cross the BBB poorly or cause side effects that forced trials to be discontinued before efficacy could be evaluated [18, 127].

5. The role of brain lipids in preventing and treating Alzheimer's disease

5.1. Therapeutic approaches based on inhibitors of cholesterol biosynthesis

Over the last 2 decades, the relationship between cholesterol levels and the risk of developing AD has become more evident, in turn encouraging the use of statins to treat or prevent AD (see Section 3.1.). Statins are a group of drugs used to treat hypercholesterolemia as they inhibit HMG-CoA reductase, the principal enzyme involved in cholesterol synthesis. In animal models of AD, simvastatin administration to guinea pigs decreased brain and CSF Aβ levels, an effect that is reversed by discontinuing the treatment [128]. By contrast, simvastatin failed to modify brain levels of Aβ in other studies but it improved the cognitive capacity of transgenic AD mice [129]. Thus, it appears that simvastatin can possibly prevent cognitive decline in AD mice without affecting amyloidogenic APP processing, in turn suggesting that the amyloid pathology may be a consequence more than the primary causal agent of AD, possibly due to changes in membrane lipids. In another study, lovastatin and pravastatin reduced the amount of Aβ in the brains of AD mice, while simultaneously increasing the levels of sAPPα [130]. Therefore, the results of preclinical research into these drugs are encouraging, although the outcome of human studies has been inconsistent, in part due to the differences in study design and data analysis [131].

While several observational studies in human subjects support the hypothesis that statins may prevent AD development, other studies argue against such effects [132]. Nevertheless, some clinical trials are investigating the use of statins in AD, such as simvastatin or atorvastatin. The first trial to analyze the effect of simvastatin on cognitive scores and APP processing was completed in 2003. This clinical study was performed over 12 weeks on patients with AD, and it reported changes in APP metabolites in the CSF: sAPPα and sAPPβ levels were significantly reduced but not those of Aβ or tau. Remarkably, a significant cognitive improvement in response to simvastatin treatment was found in patients with AD [133]. Unexpectedly, subsequent results based on a 12 month treatment failed to show such cognitive improvements in the same patients, even though cholesterol metabolism was altered in the brain [134]. Unfortunately, a later larger trial performed on 406 mild-to-moderate AD patients also failed to identify clinical benefits of simvastatin (the multicenter CLASP trial). This CLASP trial (clinicaltrials.gov ID: #NCT00053599) evaluated the safety and efficacy of an 18 month treatment with simvastatin to prevent AD progression. Once again, simvastatin treatment lowered lipid levels but it did not slow the progressive AD-related decline in cognitive performance [135]. Despite the apparent lack of clinical improvement on cognition in patients with AD, the University of Wisconsin (Madison, USA) evaluated simvastatin in cognitively normal people at risk of developing FAD. This study (ESPRIT study: clinicaltrials.gov ID: #NCT00486044), compared the changes in CSF Aβ and cognitive scores following simvastatin or placebo administration, as well as markers of cholesterol metabolism and inflammation. Again, no specific effect of simvastatin was observed on CSF Aβ or tau levels but a improvement in terms of cognitive performance was reported [136]. As a result, a follow-up study attempted to evaluate similar outcome measures after a longer course of simvastatin (the SHARP study; clinicaltrials.gov ID: #NCT00939822). Additional clinical trials with a more precise methodological design are also being developed to define the clinical efficacy of simvastatin. For instance, the SIMaMCI study (clinicaltrials.gov ID: #NCT00842920) on 445 subjects assesses the time until participants suffer phenoconversion to dementia, with conversion being defined as an increase in the Clinical Dementia Rating (CDR) score above 0.5. The trial also focuses on the change in cognitive scores from a healthy state to MCI and dementia.

Other clinical studies have assessed atorvastatin, lovastatin, and pravastatin in AD. The only clinical trial showing cognitive improvement associated with atorvastatin administration was a phase-2 pilot study comparing a 1-year course of atorvastatin to a placebo in patients with mild-to-moderate-AD who were also taking a cholinesterase inhibitor and vitamin E (clinicaltrials.gov: #NCT00024531). This study reported trends towards benefits on cognition and function [137, 138], leading to a larger phase-3 randomized trial involving 640 patients to confirm the potential clinical benefits of atorvastatin in patients with mild-to-moderate AD also treated with donepezil (the LEADe study; clinicaltrial.gov ID: #NCT00151502). Unfortunately, no clinical benefit was observed after 18 months of treatment [139, 140], and this was considered the definitive trial on atorvastatin regarding symptomatic AD treatment. It is worth noting that APP metabolites were not assessed in these studies and that decreased circulating cholesterol, as well as improved neurovascular response and cerebral blood flow were found in atorvastatin-treated patients with AD (clinicaltrials.gov: #NCT00751907) [141]. Lovastatin has been less frequently studied in randomized AD trials, and it was shown to be efficient in reducing serum Aβ levels in patients AD, although no cognitive evaluations were performed (clinicaltrial.gov: #NCT00046358) [142]. In the case of pravastatin, APP processing was not analyzed and the cognitive evaluation of treated patients revealed no significant improvement relative to the placebo group (clinicaltrial.gov: # NCT00303277) [143].

The substantial variability in outcome from these human studies makes it difficult to ascertain whether statins might have a beneficial role in preventing or treating AD. One possible reason to explain such inconsistency relates to the ability of statins to cross the BBB and enter the brain. In this respect, the chemical structure of statins can vary greatly, which justifies why some of them cross the BBB better than others. Accordingly, simvastatin and lovastatin appear to cross the BBB via passive diffusion, whereas pravastatin depends on an active transport system. Although this could justify the lack of clinical effect of pravastatin in clinical trials, it is also true that pravastatin reduced Aβ load in AD mice, suggesting that pravastatin does reach the brain and exert its pharmacological effects [130, 144]. In this sense, clinical studies have investigated different statins with substantial variation in BBB permeability, making it difficult to reconcile the conflicting findings in the literature.

Another confounding factor would be the AD patient's ApoE genotype which may affect the effectiveness of statins in AD prevention and treatment. In fact, individuals with the ApoE4 allele may experience less benefit from statin treatment in terms of cholesterol levels than others with the E2 or E3 alleles [145]. Therefore, although some trials in humans have taken the ApoE genotype into account, not all do. In addition, statins have a number of pleitropic effects on physiology and metabolism besides lowering cholesterol levels. For instance, statins can alter the expression of genes related to cell growth, signaling, trafficking, and apoptosis, which in turn can potentially affect the results of trials. In this sense, inhibition of HMG-CoA reductase activity can lead to decreased isoprenylation of proteins which in turn may cause a variety of downstream effects [146]. Thus, low isoprenoid levels may inhibit the secretory APP pathway leading to intracellular accumulation of APP metabolites that bias their analysis in the CSF or plasma [147].

In summary, cholesterol-lowering drugs such as statins have potential therapeutic effects for the treatment of AD. Based on preclinical studies in animal models and clinical trials in humans, statins represent a valuable group of compounds with promising therapeutic effects in AD. However, individual statins show different outcomes in terms of APP metabolism and cognitive improvement. In part, these disparities may be explained by the variability in BBB permeability and the different biochemical effects of these drugs observed to date.

5.2. Therapeutic approaches based on PUFAs

Neuroprotective effects of long-chain ω-3 PUFAs (see Section 3.2.) encouraged a number of clinical trials to assess the effects of ω-3 fatty acid administration to patients with AD over a defined time period, particularly focusing on the cognitive benefits of DHA and EPA. Interestingly, decreases in plasma DHA are associated with cognitive decline in healthy elderly adults and DHA administration to these patients improved the physiological memory loss and cognitive decline that frequently appears in the elderly [148] (clinicaltrials.gov ID: #NCT0027813). However, DHA administration to patients with AD did not significantly improve cognitive scores [80] (clinicaltrials.gov ID: #NCT00440050). Another randomized study involving administration of a commercially available fish oil as source of DHA and EPA only improved cognition in a small subgroup of patients with very mild cognitive dysfunction, with no clear beneficial effects in most patients [149] (clinicaltrials.gov ID: #NCT00211159). Finally, the most recent trial was carried out on a small group of patients with mild-to-moderate AD who were administered fish oil containing DHA and EPA. In this pilot study, significant recovery of cognitive capacity was evident in the patients treated with fish oil (with or without lipoic acid supplementation) [150] (clinicaltrials.gov ID: #NCT00090402). Together, these studies indicate that DHA supplementation may represent a plausible therapeutic approach for the treatment of the physiological age-related cognitive decline, although it is unclear what type of ω-3 PUFAs could be used to treat AD. Some of these discrepancies in the different randomized studies may reflect the source of the ω-3 PUFAs administered to the patients. As yet there is no consensus with regards the defined sources of ω-3 PUFAs or a standard ratio or dose of DHA and EPA: Quinn et al. [80] evaluated 2 g/day DHA, Freund-Levi et al. [149] evaluated the effect of fish oil administration with a DHA and EPA content of 1.7 and 0.6 g/day, respectively (EPAX 1500 TG; Pronova Biocare, Norway), and Shinto et al. [150] evaluated a fish oil daily dose containing 675 mg DHA and 975 mg EPA, the latter trial being the only efficacious treatment against AD in humans and having a different DHA:EPA ratio with respect to the former.

It is likely that differences in the source of ω-3 PUFAs together with variable DHA:EPA ratios might explain the variation in the results observed when treating AD patients with long-chain ω-3 PUFAs. Moreover, the presence of mercury in some fish oil supplements may provoke some neurological problems that could counteract the beneficial effects of DHA and related compounds. In this context, ω-3 PUFAs also exert their physiological function through the production of hydroxylated bioactive derivatives, such as NPD1 (see Section 3.2.). In fact, it has been demonstrated that NPD1 levels are dramatically reduced in the AD brain, even more so than DHA [68]. These data suggest that abnormally low levels of DHA in AD would be accompanied by impaired conversion of this fatty acid into NPD1 and other RVs. In fact, reduced levels of 15-LOX, the key enzyme involved in the generation of the D-series RVs and protectins, were observed in the brain of patients with AD, in turn demonstrating that lipid second messenger generation from DHA is impaired in AD [68]. Assuming that the conversion of DHA into hydroxylated derivatives is needed to mediate DHA-related physiological activity, such 15-LOX modifications could at least partially explain why DHA administration did not improve cognition in patients with AD. In this context, it is noteworthy that some cognitive improvement was observed when fish oil alone was used as the source of ω-3 PUFAs, suggesting that these oils might contain other PUFAs that impart neuroprotection independently of DHA and EPA (hydroxylated PUFAs such as RVs or other PUFA derivatives) [81]. This hypothesis is supported by the high efficacy of HDHA(see below DHALifort) on cognitive score and by the aforementioned epidemiological meta-analysis showing an inverse correlation between AD incidence and fish oil intake but not with DHA/EPA (ω-3 PUFA) intake (see Section 3.2) [78].

DHA-derived NPD1 produces many beneficial effects in animal and cell models of AD [75]. On the one hand, NPD1 suppresses Aβ42 peptide shedding by downregulating BACE-1 activity while enhancing α-secretase activity, thereby upregulating sAPPα levels and shifting the cleavage of APP from the amyloidogenic to the non-amyloidogenic pathway. Thus, NPD1 stimulated secretion of sAPPα strengthens neurotrophic signaling and prevents Aβ oligomer neurotoxicity, which may in turn be accompanied by a number of beneficial effects, such as the prevention of neuronal and axonal injury, improved neuronal plasticity, and enhanced learning memory [151–153]. In addition, like other RVs, NPD1 also displays anti-inflammatory properties. Indeed, NPD1 administration decreases Aβ42-triggered expression of the pro-inflammatory COX-2 and of B-94 (a TNF-α-inducible pro-inflammatory factor), and it prevents apoptosis in cultured cells by upregulating the expression of anti-apoptotic members of the Bcl-2 protein family.

The neuroprotective properties of NPD1 have encouraged the development of new pharmacological approaches based on hydroxylated derivatives of ω-3 PUFAs to treat AD. Regardless of the use of natural RVs and protectins to treat inflammatory and neurodegenerative diseases [154], synthetic ω-3-PUFA bioactive hydroxyl derivatives have also been used to treat such disorders. This kind of therapeutic approach, aimed at modulating brain lipids to treat neurological diseases, is framed within so-called membrane lipid therapy (MLT) [155–157]. In this context, a novel hydroxylated derivative named HDHA (2-hydroxy-docosahexanoic acid) has been proposed as a promising therapeutic approach to treat AD. HDHA (DHALifort; PharmaConcept, Hungary) administration influences the brain lipid composition, increasing the PE species carrying long-chain PUFAs, which are significantly reduced in patients with AD (see Section 3.3.). Upon normalization of the membrane lipid composition by HDHA treatment, the membrane structure recovers the presence of liquid-disordered prone membrane structures [158] (**Figure 4**). These lipid changes are paralleled with a reduction in Aβ accumulation and tau hyperphosphorylation, and recovery of cognitive scores in a transgenic mouse model of AD (5xFAD mice) [159, 160] (see **Figure 4**).

HDHA also enhances the survival of neuron-like cells exposed to different insults, such as oligomeric Aβ and NMDA-mediated neurotoxicity (*in vitro*), and it promotes hippocampal neuronal cell proliferation in 5XFAD mice *in vivo* [159, 160], suggesting that HDHA induced neuroregeneration both *in vivo* and *in vitro*, which in part may explain its efficacy against neurodegeneration and memory loss. As part of its mechanism of action, HDHA dampens the binding affinity of oligomeric and fibrillar Aβ to lipid-raft membrane domains. Moreover, it enhances the unfolded protein response (UPR) and autophagy in neuron-like cells, which in turn may promote neuronal survival [160, 161]. In this sense, although the molecular role of autophagy in AD is complex and still largely unknown, it is thought that activation of salvage autophagy would avoid the intracellular accumulation of Aβ and its precursors by reducing the neuritic pathology (see **Figure 2**) [162, 163]. Therefore, the pleitropic effects of HDHA have proven beneficial to treat AD, suggesting that its molecular target is an upstream entity such as the membrane lipid bilayer. Thus, the normalization of the PE, DHA, cholesterol, and SM content mediated by HDHA would restore membrane lipid structure, which in turn would regulate amyloidogenic secretase activity tau phosphorylation and neuronal degeneration.

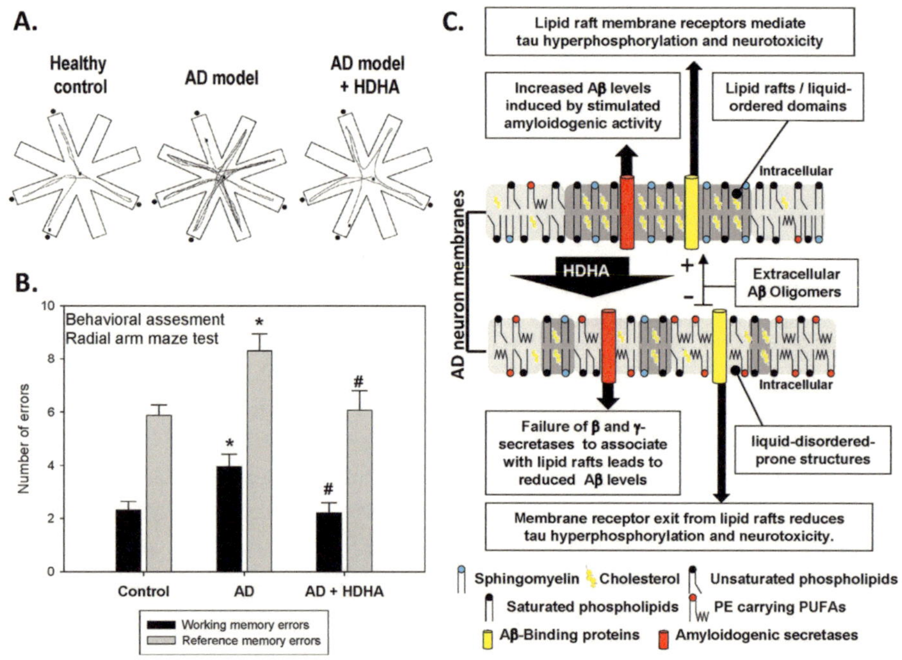

Figure 4. Proof of concept for the use of HDHA in AD mice and the proposed molecular mechanism of action. (A) Diagrams showing representative outlines of control and AD mice (5xFAD mice) that received HDHA or the vehicle alone, in the Radial Arm Maze test (RAM). A black point at the end of one arm represents where the mice find a food pellet. (B) Quantitative analysis of test performance is addressed by quantifying working (reentry of an arm already visited) and reference (entry into an unbaited arm) memory errors. Both parameters increased significantly in AD mice while HDHA treatment prevented such behavioral impairment until cognitive scores were almost totally reverted to those of the controls. Bars represent the mean ± SEM. One-way ANOVA followed by Bonferroni's post hoc test: *$p < 0.05$, difference relative to healthy controls; #: $p < 0.05$ difference relative to the untreated AD group. C) Postulated mechanism of action for HDHA. HDHA enriches brain membranes in PE carrying DHA and other long PUFAs. These lipid changes may influence the structure of the cell membrane by promoting the appearance of liquid-disordered prone structures and potentially preventing AD-related cell signaling by: (i) downregulating APP amyloidogenic processing and Aβ-induced tau protein hyperphosphorylation; and (ii) decreasing neuron vulnerability to extracellular toxic agents such as oligomeric Aβ. Together, this evidence supports a neuroprotective role of HDHA that may be associated with the improved cognitive capabilities observed in AD mice. Adapted from [159, 160].

Interestingly, the cellular heat shock response (HSP) depends on the plasma membrane composition, such that increased membrane fluidity is related to enhanced expression of heat-shock proteins (HSP) [164]. In this context, these proteins (particularly Hsp70, Hsp60, and Hsp27) are involved in the mechanism of action of lithium in compacting Aβ plaques, lowering the density of dystrophic neurites and preventing neuronal degeneration in a mouse model of AD [119]. Therefore, lipid derivatives like HDHA that enhance membrane fluidity might also reduce the neurite pathology and prevent neuronal loss in AD via a mechanism involving Hsp expression. Regardless of amyloid production and the neuritic pathology, inflammation is also a key player in AD. In this sense, another synthetic hydroxyl derivative of ARA, 2-HARA (2-hydroxy-arachidonic acid) is a COX-1 and COX-2 inhibitor [165]. The inhibitory effect over COX-1 has been related to alternative microglia activation, as well as reduced Aβ production and tau hyperphosphorylation in a transgenic model of AD [166]. Thus, 2-HARA may be a promising therapeutic approach to mitigate the inflammatory component of AD, driving microglia activation towards an alternative neuroprotective phenotype, and reducing AD-related amyloid and tau pathologies. To summarize, MLT is a therapeutic concept targeting membrane lipids that could be used to treat neurological disorders such as AD. In this context, recent findings about ω-3 PUFA RV-like mediators, such as HDHA and 2-HARA, offer a wide range of possibilities to design new bioactive compounds to treat neurodegenerative diseases.

6. Concluding remarks

After adipose tissue, the human brain is the organ with the largest amount of lipids in the body. There is compelling evidence that lipid homeostasis is altered in AD, suggesting that the plasma membrane lipid composition and structure plays a critical role in the pathophysiology of AD and hence in its therapy. Therefore, lipid alterations might be responsible for other downstream neuropathological hallmarks of AD, including amyloid and neurite pathologies, as well as inflammation and neuron loss, which eventually causes the cognitive deterioration evident in patients with AD. Accordingly, a number of clinical trials have been set up to investigate how the regulation of cholesterol and PUFA hydroxyl derivatives such as HDHA may constitute promising therapeutic approaches to treat this devastating condition.

7. Review criteria

The PubMed database (NCBI, National Library of Medicine, USA) was searched for relevant, both original and review, articles using the keywords mentioned at the beginning of the present chapter either by separate or with multiple combinations. The papers were selected accordingly to their adhesion to the main subject of the present review and the expert authors' knowledge of the field. In addition, interesting and useful information has been achieved from http://www.alzforum.org/ and http://clinicaltrials.gov/, as well as from books at the Library of the University of the Balearic Islands (Palma de Mallorca, Spain).

Acknowledgements

Springer is the original publisher of images shown in **Figure 2**. These pictures were reproduced with permission from Springer and were adapted from [12] (please see full credits in the reference list). The authors wish to thank the original publisher as well as the original authors (Dr. Isidre Ferrer and co-workers) for allowing reproduction of these images in the present work. Information concerning clinical trials of several drugs has been obtained from the website http://www.alzforum.org/therapeutics. This work was supported in part by grants from the Spanish Ministerio de Economía y Competitividad (BIO2010-21132, IPT-010000-2010-16, BIO2013-49006-C2-1-R, RTC-2015-3542, RTC-2015-4094 to PVE and XB), with co-financing from EU FEDER funds, by grants to Research Groups of Excellence from the Govern de les Illes Balears, Spain (PVE), and by the Marathon Foundation (Spain). MT was a recipient of a Torres-Quevedo contract from the Spanish Ministerio de Economía y Competitividad.

Conflict of interest

MT was supported by a Torres-Quevedo Research Contract granted to Lipopharma Therapeutics, S.L., from the Ministerio de Economía y Competitividad (Spanish Government). Lipopharma Therapeutics, S.L., is a spin-off company from the University of the Balearic Islands.

Author details

Manuel Torres[1,2*], Xavier Busquets[1] and Pablo V. Escribá[1*]

*Address all correspondence to: manuel.torres.phd@gmail.com and Pablo.escriba@uib.es

1 Laboratory of Molecular Cell Biomedicine, University of the Balearic Islands, Palma de Mallorca, Spain

2 Lipopharma Therapeutics S.L., Palma de Mallorca, Spain

References

[1] Castellani RJ, Rolston RK, Smith MA. Alzheimer disease. Dis Mon. 2010;56(9):484–546.

[2] Annaert W, Cupers P, Saftig P, De Strooper B. Presenilin function in APP processing. Ann N Y Acad Sci. 2000;920:158–64.

[3] Price DL, Sisodia SS. Mutant genes in familial Alzheimer's disease and transgenic models. Annu Rev Neurosci. 1998;21:479–505.

[4] Harman D. Alzheimer's disease pathogenesis: role of aging. Ann N Y Acad Sci. 2006;1067:454–60.

[5] De Strooper B. Proteases and proteolysis in Alzheimer disease: a multifactorial view on the disease process. Physiol Rev. 2010;90(2):465–94.

[6] Xiang Y, Lam SM, Shui G. What can lipidomics tell us about the pathogenesis of Alzheimer disease? Biol Chem. 2015;396(12):1281–91.

[7] Haass C, Selkoe DJ. Soluble protein oligomers in neurodegeneration: lessons from the Alzheimer's amyloid beta-peptide. Nat Rev Mol Cell Biol. 2007;8(2):101–12.

[8] Hardy JA, Higgins GA. Alzheimer's disease: the amyloid cascade hypothesis. Science. 1992;256(5054):184–5.

[9] Hardy J, Selkoe DJ. The amyloid hypothesis of Alzheimer's disease: progress and problems on the road to therapeutics. Science. 2002;297(5580):353–6.

[10] De Strooper B, Vassar R, Golde T. The secretases: enzymes with therapeutic potential in Alzheimer disease. Nat Rev Neurol. 2010;6(2):99–107.

[11] Duyckaerts C, Delatour B, Potier M-C. Classification and basic pathology of Alzheimer disease. Acta Neuropathol. 2009;118(1):5–36.

[12] Pérez-Gracia E, Torrejón-Escribano B, Ferrer I. Dystrophic neurites of senile plaques in Alzheimer's disease are deficient in cytochrome c oxidase. Acta Neuropathol. 2008;116(3):261–8.

[13] Jin M, Shepardson N, Yang T, Chen G, Walsh D, Selkoe DJ. Soluble amyloid beta-protein dimers isolated from Alzheimer cortex directly induce Tau hyperphosphorylation and neuritic degeneration. Proc Natl Acad Sci U S A. 2011;108(14):5819–24.

[14] Spires-Jones TL, Stoothoff WH, de Calignon A, Jones PB, Hyman BT. Tau pathophysiology in neurodegeneration: a tangled issue. Trends Neurosci. 2009;32(3):150–9.

[15] Heneka MT, O'Banion MK. Inflammatory processes in Alzheimer's disease. J Neuroimmunol. 2007;184(1–2):69–91.

[16] Nixon RA. Autophagy, amyloidogenesis and Alzheimer disease. J Cell Sci. 2007;120(Pt 23):4081–91.

[17] Krstic D, Knuesel I. The airbag problem-a potential culprit for bench-to-bedside translational efforts: relevance for Alzheimer's disease. Acta Neuropathol Commun. 2013;1:62.

[18] Mullane K, Williams M. Alzheimer's therapeutics: continued clinical failures question the validity of the amyloid hypothesis-but what lies beyond? Biochem Pharmacol. 2013;85(3):289–305.

[19] Wong PC, Cai H, Borchelt DR, Price DL. Genetically engineered mouse models of neurodegenerative diseases. Nat Neurosci. 2002;5(7):633–9.

[20] Yu WH, Cuervo AM, Kumar A, Peterhoff CM, Schmidt SD, Lee J-H, et al. Macroautophagy – a novel Beta-amyloid peptide-generating pathway activated in Alzheimer's disease. J Cell Biol. 2005;171(1):87–98.

[21] Zhang X-M, Cai Y, Xiong K, Cai H, Luo X-G, Feng J-C, et al. Beta-secretase-1 elevation in transgenic mouse models of Alzheimer's disease is associated with synaptic/axonal pathology and amyloidogenesis: implications for neuritic plaque development. Eur J Neurosci. 2009;30(12):2271–83.

[22] Doehner J, Genoud C, Imhof C, Krstic D, Knuesel I. Extrusion of misfolded and aggregated proteins--a protective strategy of aging neurons? Eur J Neurosci. 2012;35(12):1938–50.

[23] Sanchez-Varo R, Trujillo-Estrada L, Sanchez-Mejias E, Torres M, Baglietto-Vargas D, Moreno-Gonzalez I, et al. Abnormal accumulation of autophagic vesicles correlates with axonal and synaptic pathology in young Alzheimer's mice hippocampus. Acta Neuropathol. 2012;123(1):53–70.

[24] Mattson MP, Magnus T. Ageing and neuronal vulnerability. Nat Rev Neurosci. 2006;7(4):278–94.

[25] Krstic D, Knuesel I. Deciphering the mechanism underlying late-onset Alzheimer disease. Nat Rev Neurol. 2013;9(1):25–34.

[26] Knowles JK, Rajadas J, Nguyen T-VV, Yang T, LeMieux MC, Vander Griend L, et al. The p75 neurotrophin receptor promotes amyloid-beta(1–42)-induced neuritic dystrophy *in vitro* and *in vivo*. J Neurosci. 2009;29(34):10627–37.

[27] Heneka MT, Carson MJ, El Khoury J, Landreth GE, Brosseron F, Feinstein DL, et al. Neuroinflammation in Alzheimer's disease. Lancet Neurol. 2015;14(4):388–405.

[28] Jimenez S, Baglietto-Vargas D, Caballero C, Moreno-Gonzalez I, Torres M, Sanchez-Varo R, et al. Inflammatory response in the hippocampus of PS1M146L/APP751SL mouse model of Alzheimer's disease: age-dependent switch in the microglial phenotype from alternative to classic. J Neurosci. 2008;28(45):11650–61.

[29] Wakabayashi T, De Strooper B. Presenilins: members of the gamma-secretase quartets, but part-time soloists too. Physiology (Bethesda). 2008;23:194–204.

[30] De Strooper B, Annaert W. Novel research horizons for presenilins and γ-secretases in cell biology and disease. Annu Rev Cell Dev Biol. 2010;26:235–60.

[31] Chávez-Gutiérrez L, Bammens L, Benilova I, Vandersteen A, Benurwar M, Borgers M, et al. The mechanism of γ-Secretase dysfunction in familial Alzheimer disease. EMBO J. 2012;31(10):2261–74.

[32] Bentahir M, Nyabi O, Verhamme J, Tolia A, Horré K, Wiltfang J, et al. Presenilin clinical mutations can affect gamma-secretase activity by different mechanisms. J Neurochem. 2006;96(3):732–42.

[33] Thimiri Govinda Raj DB, Ghesquière B, Tharkeshwar AK, Coen K, Derua R, Vanderschaeghe D, et al. A novel strategy for the comprehensive analysis of the biomolecular composition of isolated plasma membranes. Mol Syst Biol. 2011;7:541.

[34] Tamboli IY, Prager K, Thal DR, Thelen KM, Dewachter I, Pietrzik CU, et al. Loss of gamma-secretase function impairs endocytosis of lipoprotein particles and membrane cholesterol homeostasis. J Neurosci. 2008;28(46):12097–106.

[35] Martins IJ, Hone E, Foster JK, Sünram-Lea SI, Gnjec A, Fuller SJ, et al. Apolipoprotein E, cholesterol metabolism, diabetes, and the convergence of risk factors for Alzheimer's disease and cardiovascular disease. Mol Psychiatry. 2006;11(8):721–36.

[36] Bu G. Apolipoprotein E and its receptors in Alzheimer's disease: pathways, pathogenesis and therapy. Nat Rev Neurosci. 2009;10(5):333–44.

[37] Martins IJ, Berger T, Sharman MJ, Verdile G, Fuller SJ, Martins RN. Cholesterol metabolism and transport in the pathogenesis of Alzheimer's disease. J Neurochem. 2009;111(6):1275–308.

[38] Poirier J. Apolipoprotein E, cholesterol transport and synthesis in sporadic Alzheimer's disease. Neurobiol Aging. 2005;26(3):355–61.

[39] Rapp A, Gmeiner B, Hüttinger M. Implication of apoE isoforms in cholesterol metabolism by primary rat hippocampal neurons and astrocytes. Biochimie. 2006;88(5):473–83.

[40] Launer LJ, White LR, Petrovitch H, Ross GW, Curb JD. Cholesterol and neuropathologic markers of AD: a population-based autopsy study. Neurology. 2001;57(8):1447–52.

[41] Pappolla MA, Bryant-Thomas TK, Herbert D, Pacheco J, Fabra Garcia M, Manjon M, et al. Mild hypercholesterolemia is an early risk factor for the development of Alzheimer amyloid pathology. Neurology. 2003;61(2):199–205.

[42] Puglielli L, Tanzi RE, Kovacs DM. Alzheimer's disease: the cholesterol connection. Nat Neurosci. 2003;6(4):345–51.

[43] Whitmer RA, Sidney S, Selby J, Johnston SC, Yaffe K. Midlife cardiovascular risk factors and risk of dementia in late life. Neurology. 2005;64(2):277–81.

[44] Vetrivel KS, Thinakaran G. Membrane rafts in Alzheimer's disease beta-amyloid production. Biochim Biophys Acta. 2010;1801(8):860–7.

[45] Ledesma MD, Dotti CG. Amyloid excess in Alzheimer's disease: what is cholesterol to be blamed for? FEBS Lett. 2006;580(23):5525–32.

[46] Bandaru VVR, Troncoso J, Wheeler D, Pletnikova O, Wang J, Conant K, et al. ApoE4 disrupts sterol and sphingolipid metabolism in Alzheimer's but not normal brain. Neurobiol Aging. 2009;30(4):591–9.

[47] Chan RB, Oliveira TG, Cortes EP, Honig LS, Duff KE, Small SA, et al. Comparative lipidomic analysis of mouse and human brain with Alzheimer disease. J Biol Chem. 2012;287(4):2678–88.

[48] Cutler RG, Kelly J, Storie K, Pedersen WA, Tammara A, Hatanpaa K, et al. Involvement of oxidative stress-induced abnormalities in ceramide and cholesterol metabolism in brain aging and Alzheimer's disease. Proc Natl Acad Sci U S A. 2004;101(7):2070–5.

[49] Ledesma MD, Abad-Rodriguez J, Galvan C, Biondi E, Navarro P, Delacourte A, et al. Raft disorganization leads to reduced plasmin activity in Alzheimer's disease brains. EMBO Rep. 2003;4(12):1190–6.

[50] Lai AY, McLaurin J. Mechanisms of amyloid-Beta peptide uptake by neurons: the role of lipid rafts and lipid raft-associated proteins. Int J Alzheimers Dis. 2010;2011:548380.

[51] Kalvodova L, Kahya N, Schwille P, Ehehalt R, Verkade P, Drechsel D, et al. Lipids as modulators of proteolytic activity of BACE: involvement of cholesterol, glycosphingolipids, and anionic phospholipids *in vitro*. J Biol Chem. 2005;280(44):36815–23.

[52] Holmes O, Paturi S, Ye W, Wolfe MS, Selkoe DJ. Effects of membrane lipids on the activity and processivity of purified γ-secretase. Biochemistry. 2012;51(17):3565–75.

[53] Askarova S, Yang X, Lee JCM. Impacts of membrane biophysics in Alzheimer's disease: from amyloid precursor protein processing to Aβ peptide-induced membrane changes. Int J Alzheimer's Dis. 2011;2011:134971.

[54] Runz H, Rietdorf J, Tomic I, de Bernard M, Beyreuther K, Pepperkok R, et al. Inhibition of intracellular cholesterol transport alters presenilin localization and amyloid precursor protein processing in neuronal cells. J Neurosci. 2002;22(5):1679–89.

[55] Tamboli IY, Hampel H, Tien NT, Tolksdorf K, Breiden B, Mathews PM, et al. Sphingolipid storage affects autophagic metabolism of the amyloid precursor protein and promotes Abeta generation. J Neurosci. 2011;31(5):1837–49.

[56] Lazarov O, Morfini GA, Pigino G, Gadadhar A, Chen X, Robinson J, et al. Impairments in fast axonal transport and motor neuron deficits in transgenic mice expressing familial Alzheimer's disease-linked mutant presenilin 1. J Neurosci. 2007;27(26):7011–20.

[57] Boland B, Kumar A, Lee S, Platt FM, Wegiel J, Yu WH, et al. Autophagy induction and autophagosome clearance in neurons: relationship to autophagic pathology in Alzheimer's disease. J Neurosci. 2008;28(27):6926–37.

[58] Torres M, Jiménez S, Sánchez-Varo R, Navarro V, Trujillo-Estrada L, Sánchez-Mejias E, et al. Defective lysosomal proteolysis and axonal transport are early pathogenic events that worsen with age leading to increased APP metabolism and synaptic Abeta in transgenic APP/PS1 hippocampus. Mol Neurodegener. 2012;7:59. Epub 2012/11/24.

[59] Bhat NR, Thirumangalakudi L. Increased tau phosphorylation and impaired brain insulin/IGF signaling in mice fed a high fat/high cholesterol diet. J Alzheimers Dis. 2013;36(4):781–9.

[60] Rushworth JV, Griffiths HH, Watt NT, Hooper NM. Prion protein-mediated toxicity of amyloid-β oligomers requires lipid rafts and the transmembrane LRP1. J Biol Chem. 2013;288(13):8935–51.

[61] Kuperstein I, Broersen K, Benilova I, Rozenski J, Jonckheere W, Debulpaep M, et al. Neurotoxicity of Alzheimer's disease Aβ peptides is induced by small changes in the Aβ42 to Aβ40 ratio. EMBO J. 2010;29(19):3408–20.

[62] Martins IC, Kuperstein I, Wilkinson H, Maes E, Vanbrabant M, Jonckheere W, et al. Lipids revert inert Abeta amyloid fibrils to neurotoxic protofibrils that affect learning in mice. EMBO J. 2008;27(1):224–33.

[63] Ibarguren M, López DJ, Escribá PV. The effect of natural and synthetic fatty acids on membrane structure, microdomain organization, cellular functions and human health. Biochim Biophys Acta. 2014;1838(6):1518–28.

[64] Plourde M, Fortier M, Vandal M, Tremblay-Mercier J, Freemantle E, Bégin M, et al. Unresolved issues in the link between docosahexaenoic acid and Alzheimer's disease. Prostaglandins Leukot Essent Fatty Acids. 2007;77(5–6):301–8.

[65] Söderberg M, Edlund C, Kristensson K, Dallner G. Fatty acid composition of brain phospholipids in aging and in Alzheimer's disease. Lipids. 1991;26(6):421–5.

[66] Prasad MR, Lovell MA, Yatin M, Dhillon H, Markesbery WR. Regional membrane phospholipid alterations in Alzheimer's disease. Neurochem Res. 1998;23(1):81–8.

[67] Han X, Holtzman DM, McKeel DW. Plasmalogen deficiency in early Alzheimer's disease subjects and in animal models: molecular characterization using electrospray ionization mass spectrometry. J Neurochem. 2001;77(4):1168–80.

[68] Lukiw WJ, Cui J-G, Marcheselli VL, Bodker M, Botkjaer A, Gotlinger K, et al. A role for docosahexaenoic acid-derived neuroprotectin D1 in neural cell survival and Alzheimer disease. J Clin Invest. 2005;115(10):2774–83.

[69] Astarita G, Jung K-M, Berchtold NC, Nguyen VQ, Gillen DL, Head E, et al. Deficient liver biosynthesis of docosahexaenoic acid correlates with cognitive impairment in Alzheimer's disease. PLoS One. 2010;5(9):e12538.

[70] Belkouch M, Hachem M, Elgot A, Van AL, Picq M, Guichardant M, et al. The pleiotropic effects of omega-3 docosahexaenoic acid on the hallmarks of Alzheimer's disease. J Nutr Biochem. 2016;38:1–11.

[71] Su H-M. Mechanisms of n-3 fatty acid-mediated development and maintenance of learning memory performance. J Nutr Biochem. 2010;21(5):364–73.

[72] Martín V, Fabelo N, Santpere G, Puig B, Marín R, Ferrer I, et al. Lipid alterations in lipid rafts from Alzheimer's disease human brain cortex. J Alzheimers Dis. 2010;19(2):489–502.

[73] Shaikh SR. Biophysical and biochemical mechanisms by which dietary N-3 polyunsaturated fatty acids from fish oil disrupt membrane lipid rafts. J Nutr Biochem. 2012;23(2):101–5.

[74] Serhan CN. Pro-resolving lipid mediators are leads for resolution physiology. Nature. 2014;510(7503):92–101.

[75] Stark DT, Bazan NG. Neuroprotectin D1 induces neuronal survival and downregulation of amyloidogenic processing in Alzheimer's disease cellular models. Mol Neurobiol. 2011;43(2):131–8.

[76] Zhao Y, Calon F, Julien C, Winkler JW, Petasis NA, Lukiw WJ, et al. Docosahexaenoic acid-derived neuroprotectin D1 induces neuronal survival via secretase- and PPARγ-mediated mechanisms in Alzheimer's disease models. PLoS One. 2011;6(1):e15816.

[77] Simopoulos AP. Evolutionary aspects of diet, the omega-6/omega-3 ratio and genetic variation: nutritional implications for chronic diseases. Biomed Pharmacother. 2006;60(9):502–7.

[78] Wu S, Ding Y, Wu F, Li R, Hou J, Mao P. Omega-3 fatty acids intake and risks of dementia and Alzheimer's disease: a meta-analysis. Neurosci Biobehav Rev. 2015;48:1–9.

[79] Barberger-Gateau P, Raffaitin C, Letenneur L, Berr C, Tzourio C, Dartigues JF, et al. Dietary patterns and risk of dementia: the Three-City cohort study. Neurology. 2007;69(20):1921–30.

[80] Quinn JF, Raman R, Thomas RG, Yurko-Mauro K, Nelson EB, Van Dyck C, et al. Docosahexaenoic acid supplementation and cognitive decline in Alzheimer disease: a randomized trial. JAMA. 2010;304(17):1903–11.

[81] Hong S, Tjonahen E, Morgan EL, Lu Y, Serhan CN, Rowley AF. Rainbow trout (Oncorhynchus mykiss) brain cells biosynthesize novel docosahexaenoic acid-derived resolvins and protectins—mediator lipidomic analysis. Prostaglandins Other Lipid Mediat. 2005;78(1–4):107–16.

[82] Afshordel S, Hagl S, Werner D, Röhner N, Kögel D, Bazan NG, et al. Omega-3 polyunsaturated fatty acids improve mitochondrial dysfunction in brain aging—impact of Bcl-2 and NPD-1 like metabolites. Prostaglandins Leukot Essent Fatty Acids. 2015;92:23–31.

[83] Gómez-Isla T, Price JL, McKeel DW, Morris JC, Growdon JH, Hyman BT. Profound loss of layer II entorhinal cortex neurons occurs in very mild Alzheimer's disease. J Neurosci. 1996;16(14):4491–500.

[84] Ritter A, Cummings J. Fluid biomarkers in clinical trials of Alzheimer's disease therapeutics. Front Neurol. 2015;6:186.

[85] Khan TK, Alkon DL. Peripheral biomarkers of Alzheimer's disease. J Alzheimers Dis. 2015;44(3):729–44.

[86] Orešič M, Hyötyläinen T, Herukka S-K, Sysi-Aho M, Mattila I, Seppänan-Laakso T, et al. Metabolome in progression to Alzheimer's disease. Transl Psychiatry. 2011;1:e57.

[87] Proitsi P, Kim M, Whiley L, Pritchard M, Leung R, Soininen H, et al. Plasma lipidomics analysis finds long chain cholesteryl esters to be associated with Alzheimer's disease. Transl Psychiatry. 2015;5:e494.

[88] Walter A, Korth U, Hilgert M, Hartmann J, Weichel O, Hilgert M, et al. Glycerophosphocholine is elevated in cerebrospinal fluid of Alzheimer patients. Neurobiol Aging. 2004;25(10):1299–303.

[89] Mapstone M, Cheema AK, Fiandaca MS, Zhong X, Mhyre TR, MacArthur LH, et al. Plasma phospholipids identify antecedent memory impairment in older adults. Nat Med. 2014;20(4):415–8.

[90] Olazarán J, Gil-de-Gómez L, Rodríguez-Martín A, Valentí-Soler M, Frades-Payo B, Marín-Muñoz J, et al. A blood-based, 7-metabolite signature for the early diagnosis of Alzheimer's disease. J Alzheimers Dis. 2015;45(4):1157–73.

[91] Han X, Rozen S, Boyle SH, Hellegers C, Cheng H, Burke JR, et al. Metabolomics in early Alzheimer's disease: identification of altered plasma sphingolipidome using shotgun lipidomics. PLoS One. 2011;6(7):e21643.

[92] Mielke MM, Bandaru VVR, Haughey NJ, Rabins PV, Lyketsos CG, Carlson MC. Serum sphingomyelins and ceramides are early predictors of memory impairment. Neurobiol Aging. 2010;31(1):17–24.

[93] Zambón D, Quintana M, Mata P, Alonso R, Benavent J, Cruz-Sánchez F, et al. Higher incidence of mild cognitive impairment in familial hypercholesterolemia. Am J Med. 2010;123(3):267–74.

[94] Kása P, Rakonczay Z, Gulya K. The cholinergic system in Alzheimer's disease. Prog Neurobiol. 1997;52(6):511–35.

[95] Texidó L, Martín-Satué M, Alberdi E, Solsona C, Matute C. Amyloid β peptide oligomers directly activate NMDA receptors. Cell Calcium. 2011;49(3):184–90.

[96] Rogawski MA, Wenk GL. The neuropharmacological basis for the use of memantine in the treatment of Alzheimer's disease. CNS Drug Rev. 2003;9(3):275–308.

[97] Raina P, Santaguida P, Ismaila A, Patterson C, Cowan D, Levine M, et al. Effectiveness of cholinesterase inhibitors and memantine for treating dementia: evidence review for a clinical practice guideline. Ann Intern Med. 2008;148(5):379–97.

[98] Kaduszkiewicz H, Zimmermann T, Beck-Bornholdt H-P, van den Bussche H. Cholinesterase inhibitors for patients with Alzheimer's disease: systematic review of randomised clinical trials. BMJ. 2005;331(7512):321–7.

[99] Salomone S, Caraci F, Leggio GM, Fedotova J, Drago F. New pharmacological strategies for treatment of Alzheimer's disease: focus on disease modifying drugs. Br J Clin Pharmacol. 2012;73(4):504–17.

[100] Caraci F, Bosco P, Leggio GM, Malaguarnera M, Drago F, Bucolo C, et al. Clinical pharmacology of novel anti-Alzheimer disease modifying medications. Curr Top Med Chem. 2013;13(15):1853–63.

[101] Zetterberg H, Andreasson U, Hansson O, Wu G, Sankaranarayanan S, Andersson ME, et al. Elevated cerebrospinal fluid BACE1 activity in incipient Alzheimer disease. Arch Neurol. 2008;65(8):1102–7.

[102] Hébert SS, Horré K, Nicolaï L, Papadopoulou AS, Mandemakers W, Silahtaroglu AN, et al. Loss of microRNA cluster miR-29a/b-1 in sporadic Alzheimer's disease correlates with increased BACE1/beta-secretase expression. Proc Natl Acad Sci U S A. 2008;105(17):6415–20.

[103] O'Connor T, Sadleir KR, Maus E, Velliquette RA, Zhao J, Cole SL, et al. Phosphorylation of the translation initiation factor eIF2alpha increases BACE1 levels and promotes amyloidogenesis. Neuron. 2008;60(6):988–1009.

[104] Chang W-P, Huang X, Downs D, Cirrito JR, Koelsch G, Holtzman DM, et al. Beta-secretase inhibitor GRL-8234 rescues age-related cognitive decline in APP transgenic mice. FASEB J. 2011;25(2):775–84.

[105] Ohno M, Sametsky EA, Younkin LH, Oakley H, Younkin SG, Citron M, et al. BACE1 deficiency rescues memory deficits and cholinergic dysfunction in a mouse model of Alzheimer's disease. Neuron. 2004;41(1):27–33.

[106] Vassar R. BACE1 inhibitor drugs in clinical trials for Alzheimer's disease. Alzheimers Res Ther. 2014;6(9):89.

[107] Henley DB, May PC, Dean RA, Siemers ER. Development of semagacestat (LY450139), a functional gamma-secretase inhibitor, for the treatment of Alzheimer's disease. Expert Opin Pharmacother. 2009;10(10):1657–64.

[108] Bateman RJ, Siemers ER, Mawuenyega KG, Wen G, Browning KR, Sigurdson WC, et al. A gamma-secretase inhibitor decreases amyloid-beta production in the central nervous system. Ann Neurol. 2009;66(1):48–54.

[109] Doody RS, Raman R, Farlow M, Iwatsubo T, Vellas B, Joffe S, et al. A phase 3 trial of semagacestat for treatment of Alzheimer's disease. N Engl J Med. 2013;369(4):341–50.

[110] Numata K, Kaplan DL. Mechanisms of enzymatic degradation of amyloid Beta microfibrils generating nanofilaments and nanospheres related to cytotoxicity. Biochemistry. 2010;49(15):3254–60.

[111] Pedersen WA, McMillan PJ, Kulstad JJ, Leverenz JB, Craft S, Haynatzki GR. Rosiglitazone attenuates learning and memory deficits in Tg2576 Alzheimer mice. Exp Neurol. 2006;199(2):265–73.

[112] Gold M, Alderton C, Zvartau-Hind M, Egginton S, Saunders AM, Irizarry M, et al. Rosiglitazone monotherapy in mild-to-moderate Alzheimer's disease: results from a randomized, double-blind, placebo-controlled phase III study. Dement Geriatr Cogn Disord. 2010;30(2):131–46.

[113] Schenk D, Barbour R, Dunn W, Gordon G, Grajeda H, Guido T, et al. Immunization with amyloid-beta attenuates Alzheimer-disease-like pathology in the PDAPP mouse. Nature. 1999;400(6740):173–7.

[114] Hanger DP, Anderton BH, Noble W. Tau phosphorylation: the therapeutic challenge for neurodegenerative disease. Trends Mol Med. 2009;15(3):112–9.

[115] Kanaan NM, Pigino GF, Brady ST, Lazarov O, Binder LI, Morfini GA. Axonal degeneration in Alzheimer's disease: when signaling abnormalities meet the axonal transport system. Exp Neurol. 2013;246:44–53.

[116] Nixon RA, Wegiel J, Kumar A, Yu WH, Peterhoff C, Cataldo A, et al. Extensive involvement of autophagy in Alzheimer disease: an immuno-electron microscopy study. J Neuropathol Exp Neurol. 2005;64(2):113–22.

[117] Tariot PN, Aisen PS. Can lithium or valproate untie tangles in Alzheimer's disease? J Clin Psychiatry. 2009;70(6):919–21.

[118] Fleisher AS, Truran D, Mai JT, Langbaum JBS, Aisen PS, Cummings JL, et al. Chronic divalproex sodium use and brain atrophy in Alzheimer disease. Neurology. 2011;77(13):1263–71.

[119] Trujillo-Estrada L, Jimenez S, De Castro V, Torres M, Baglietto-Vargas D, Moreno-Gonzalez I, et al. *In vivo* modification of Abeta plaque toxicity as a novel neuroprotective lithium-mediated therapy for Alzheimer's disease pathology. Acta Neuropathol Commun. 2013;1(1):73.

[120] Mudher A, Shepherd D, Newman TA, Mildren P, Jukes JP, Squire A, et al. GSK-3beta inhibition reverses axonal transport defects and behavioural phenotypes in Drosophila. Mol Psychiatry. 2004;9(5):522–30.

[121] Forlenza OV, Diniz BS, Radanovic M, Santos FS, Talib LL, Gattaz WF. Disease-modifying properties of long-term lithium treatment for amnestic mild cognitive impairment: randomised controlled trial. Br J Psychiatry. 2011;198(5):351–6.

[122] Hampel H, Ewers M, Bürger K, Annas P, Mörtberg A, Bogstedt A, et al. Lithium trial in Alzheimer's disease: a randomized, single-blind, placebo-controlled, multicenter 10-week study. J Clin Psychiatry. 2009;70(6):922–31.

[123] Lasagna-Reeves CA, Castillo-Carranza DL, Sengupta U, Sarmiento J, Troncoso J, Jackson GR, et al. Identification of oligomers at early stages of tau aggregation in Alzheimer's disease. FASEB J. 2012;26(5):1946–59.

[124] Pritchard SM, Dolan PJ, Vitkus A, Johnson GVW. The toxicity of tau in Alzheimer disease: turnover, targets and potential therapeutics. J Cell Mol Med. 2011;15(8):1621–35.

[125] Grüninger F. Invited review: drug development for tauopathies. Neuropathol Appl Neurobiol. 2015;41(1):81–96.

[126] Collin L, Bohrmann B, Göpfert U, Oroszlan-Szovik K, Ozmen L, Grüninger F. Neuronal uptake of tau/pS422 antibody and reduced progression of tau pathology in a mouse model of Alzheimer's disease. Brain. 2014;137(Pt 10):2834–46.

[127] De Strooper B, Chávez Gutiérrez L. Learning by failing: ideas and concepts to tackle γ-secretases in Alzheimer's disease and beyond. Annu Rev Pharmacol Toxicol. 2015;55:419–37.

[128] Fassbender K, Simons M, Bergmann C, Stroick M, Lutjohann D, Keller P, et al. Simvastatin strongly reduces levels of Alzheimer's disease beta -amyloid peptides Abeta 42 and Abeta 40 *in vitro* and *in vivo*. Proc Natl Acad Sci U S A. 2001;98(10):5856–61.

[129] Li L, Cao D, Kim H, Lester R, Fukuchi K-I. Simvastatin enhances learning and memory independent of amyloid load in mice. Ann Neurol. 2006;60(6):729–39.

[130] Chauhan NB, Siegel GJ, Feinstein DL. Effects of lovastatin and pravastatin on amyloid processing and inflammatory response in TgCRND8 brain. Neurochem Res. 2004;29(10):1897–911.

[131] Shepardson NE, Shankar GM, Selkoe DJ. Cholesterol level and statin use in Alzheimer disease: I. Review of epidemiological and preclinical studies. Arch Neurol. 2011;68(10): 1239–44.

[132] Shepardson NE, Shankar GM, Selkoe DJ. Cholesterol level and statin use in Alzheimer disease: II. Review of human trials and recommendations. Arch Neurol. 2011;68(11): 1385–92.

[133] Sjögren M, Gustafsson K, Syversen S, Olsson A, Edman A, Davidsson P, et al. Treatment with simvastatin in patients with Alzheimer's disease lowers both alpha- and beta-cleaved amyloid precursor protein. Dement Geriatr Cogn Disord. 2003;16(1):25–30.

[134] Hoglund K, Thelen KM, Syversen S, Sjogren M, von Bergmann K, Wallin A, et al. The effect of simvastatin treatment on the amyloid precursor protein and brain cholesterol

metabolism in patients with Alzheimer's disease. Dement Geriatr Cogn Disord. 2005;19(5–6):256–65.

[135] Sano M, Bell KL, Galasko D, Galvin JE, Thomas RG, van Dyck CH, et al. A randomized, double-blind, placebo-controlled trial of simvastatin to treat Alzheimer disease. Neurology. 2011;77(6):556–63.

[136] Carlsson CM, Gleason CE, Hess TM, Moreland KA, Blazel HM, Koscik RL, et al. Effects of simvastatin on cerebrospinal fluid biomarkers and cognition in middle-aged adults at risk for Alzheimer's disease. J Alzheimers Dis. 2008;13(2):187–97.

[137] Sparks DL, Sabbagh MN, Connor DJ, Lopez J, Launer LJ, Browne P, et al. Atorvastatin for the treatment of mild to moderate Alzheimer disease: preliminary results. Arch Neurol. 2005;62(5):753–7.

[138] Sparks DL, Sabbagh MN, Connor DJ, Lopez J, Launer LJ, Petanceska S, et al. Atorvastatin therapy lowers circulating cholesterol but not free radical activity in advance of identifiable clinical benefit in the treatment of mild-to-moderate AD. Curr Alzheimer Res. 2005;2(3):343–53.

[139] Feldman HH, Doody RS, Kivipelto M, Sparks DL, Waters DD, Jones RW, et al. Randomized controlled trial of atorvastatin in mild to moderate Alzheimer disease: LEADe. Neurology. 2010;74(12):956–64.

[140] Jones RW, Kivipelto M, Feldman H, Sparks L, Doody R, Waters DD, et al. The Atorvastatin/Donepezil in Alzheimer's Disease Study (LEADe): design and baseline characteristics. Alzheimers Dement. 2008;4(2):145–53.

[141] Carlsson CM, Xu G, Wen Z, Barnet JH, Blazel HM, Chappell RJ, et al. Effects of atorvastatin on cerebral blood flow in middle-aged adults at risk for Alzheimer's disease: a pilot study. Curr Alzheimer Res. 2012;9(8):990–7.

[142] Friedhoff LT, Cullen EI, Geoghagen NS, Buxbaum JD. Treatment with controlled-release lovastatin decreases serum concentrations of human beta-amyloid (A beta) peptide. Int J Neuropsychopharmacol. 2001;4(2):127–30.

[143] Shepherd J, Blauw GJ, Murphy MB, Bollen ELEM, Buckley BM, Cobbe SM, et al. Pravastatin in elderly individuals at risk of vascular disease (PROSPER): a randomised controlled trial. Lancet. 2002;360(9346):1623–30.

[144] Tsuji A, Saheki A, Tamai I, Terasaki T. Transport mechanism of 3-hydroxy-3-methylglutaryl coenzyme A reductase inhibitors at the blood-brain barrier. J Pharmacol Exp Ther. 1993;267(3):1085–90.

[145] Carmena R, Roederer G, Mailloux H, Lussier-Cacan S, Davignon J. The response to lovastatin treatment in patients with heterozygous familial hypercholesterolemia is modulated by apolipoprotein E polymorphism. Metabolism. 1993;42(7):895–901.

[146] Johnson-Anuna LN, Eckert GP, Keller JH, Igbavboa U, Franke C, Fechner T, et al. Chronic administration of statins alters multiple gene expression patterns in mouse cerebral cortex. J Pharmacol Exp Ther. 2005;312(2):786–93.

[147] Cole SL, Grudzien A, Manhart IO, Kelly BL, Oakley H, Vassar R. Statins cause intracellular accumulation of amyloid precursor protein, beta-secretase-cleaved fragments, and amyloid beta-peptide via an isoprenoid-dependent mechanism. J Biol Chem. 2005;280(19):18755–70.

[148] Yurko-Mauro K, McCarthy D, Rom D, Nelson EB, Ryan AS, Blackwell A, et al. Beneficial effects of docosahexaenoic acid on cognition in age-related cognitive decline. Alzheimers Dement. 2010;6(6):456–64.

[149] Freund-Levi Y, Eriksdotter-Jönhagen M, Cederholm T, Basun H, Faxén-Irving G, Garlind A, et al. Omega-3 fatty acid treatment in 174 patients with mild to moderate Alzheimer disease: OmegAD study: a randomized double-blind trial. Arch Neurol. 2006;63(10):1402–8.

[150] Shinto L, Quinn J, Montine T, Dodge HH, Woodward W, Baldauf-Wagner S, et al. A randomized placebo-controlled pilot trial of omega-3 fatty acids and alpha lipoic acid in Alzheimer's disease. J Alzheimers Dis. 2014;38(1):111–20.

[151] Jimenez S, Torres M, Vizuete M, Sanchez-Varo R, Sanchez-Mejias E, Trujillo-Estrada L, et al. Age-dependent accumulation of soluble amyloid beta (Abeta) oligomers reverses the neuroprotective effect of soluble amyloid precursor protein-alpha (sAPP(alpha)) by modulating phosphatidylinositol 3-kinase (PI3K)/Akt-GSK-3beta pathway in Alzheimer mouse model. J Biol Chem. 2011;286(21):18414–25.

[152] Fragkouli A, Papatheodoropoulos C, Georgopoulos S, Stamatakis A, Stylianopoulou F, Tsilibary EC, et al. Enhanced neuronal plasticity and elevated endogenous sAPPα levels in mice over-expressing MMP9. J Neurochem. 2012;121(2):239–51.

[153] Thornton E, Vink R, Blumbergs PC, Van Den Heuvel C. Soluble amyloid precursor protein alpha reduces neuronal injury and improves functional outcome following diffuse traumatic brain injury in rats. Brain Res. 2006;1094(1):38–46.

[154] Lorente-Cebrián S, Costa AGV, Navas-Carretero S, Zabala M, Laiglesia LM, Martínez JA, et al. An update on the role of omega-3 fatty acids on inflammatory and degenerative diseases. J Physiol Biochem. 2015;71(2):341–9.

[155] Escribá PV. Membrane-lipid therapy: a new approach in molecular medicine. Trends Mol Med. 2006;12(1):34–43.

[156] Escribá PV, Busquets X, Inokuchi J-I, Balogh G, Török Z, Horváth I, et al. Membrane lipid therapy: modulation of the cell membrane composition and structure as a molecular base for drug discovery and new disease treatment. Prog Lipid Res. 2015;59:38–53.

[157] Nicolson GL, Ash ME. Lipid replacement therapy: a natural medicine approach to replacing damaged lipids in cellular membranes and organelles and restoring function. Biochim Biophys Acta. 2014;1838(6):1657–79.

[158] Ibarguren M, López DJ, Encinar JA, González-Ros JM, Busquets X, Escribá PV. Partitioning of liquid-ordered/liquid-disordered membrane microdomains induced by the fluidifying effect of 2-hydroxylated fatty acid derivatives. Biochim Biophys Acta. 2013;1828(11):2553–63.

[159] Fiol-Deroque MA, Gutierrez-Lanza R, Terés S, Torres M, Barceló P, Rial RV, et al. Cognitive recovery and restoration of cell proliferation in the dentate gyrus in the 5XFAD transgenic mice model of Alzheimer's disease following 2-hydroxy-DHA treatment. Biogerontology. 2013;14(6):763–75.

[160] Torres M, Price SL, Fiol-Deroque MA, Marcilla-Etxenike A, Ahyayauch H, Barceló-Coblijn G, et al. Membrane lipid modifications and therapeutic effects mediated by hydroxydocosahexaenoic acid on Alzheimer's disease. Biochim Biophys Acta. 2014;1838(6):1680–92.

[161] Torres M, Marcilla-Etxenike A, Fiol-deRoque MA, Escribá PV, Busquets X. The unfolded protein response in the therapeutic effect of hydroxy-DHA against Alzheimer's disease. Apoptosis. 2015;20(5):712–24.

[162] Yang D-S, Stavrides P, Mohan PS, Kaushik S, Kumar A, Ohno M, et al. Reversal of autophagy dysfunction in the TgCRND8 mouse model of Alzheimer's disease ameliorates amyloid pathologies and memory deficits. Brain. 2011;134(Pt 1):258–77.

[163] Schaeffer V, Lavenir I, Ozcelik S, Tolnay M, Winkler DT, Goedert M. Stimulation of autophagy reduces neurodegeneration in a mouse model of human tauopathy. Brain. 2012;135(Pt 7):2169–77.

[164] Török Z, Crul T, Maresca B, Schütz GJ, Viana F, Dindia L, et al. Plasma membranes as heat stress sensors: from lipid-controlled molecular switches to therapeutic applications. Biochim Biophys Acta. 2014;1838(6):1594–618.

[165] Lopez DH, Fiol-Deroque MA, Noguera-Salvà MA, Terés S, Campana F, Piotto S, et al. 2-hydroxy arachidonic Acid: a new non-steroidal anti-inflammatory drug. PLoS One. 2013;8(8):e72052.

[166] Choi S-H, Aid S, Caracciolo L, Minami SS, Niikura T, Matsuoka Y, et al. Cyclooxygenase-1 inhibition reduces amyloid pathology and improves memory deficits in a mouse model of Alzheimer's disease. J Neurochem. 2013;124(1):59–68.

Chapter 8

Beta Amyloid Peptides: Extracellular and Intracellular Mechanisms of Clearance in Alzheimer's Disease

Luis F. Hernández-Zimbrón, Elisa Gorostieta-Salas, Mei-Li Díaz-Hung, Roxanna Pérez-Garmendia, Gohar Gevorkian and Hugo Quiroz-Mercado

Additional information is available at the end of the chapter

http://dx.doi.org/10.5772/64744

Abstract

Alzheimer's disease (AD) is a neurodegenerative disease and the most common form of dementia, characterized by the overproduction and accumulation of different amyloid-β peptide peptides (Aβ) within different areas in the brain conducting to memory loss and dementia. The Aβ cascade hypothesis of AD was originally proposed by Selkoe in 1991 by the theory that accumulation of Aβ42 is the initial trigger for neurodegeneration. The Aβ cascade hypothesis assumes that changes in the production or accumulation of Aβ are responsible for AD pathology. Different Aβ clearance mechanisms are also affected by AD pathology. Studies from the past years have revealed that the blocking of Aβ production is not effective for reducing the brain Aβ levels. However, the relevance of Aβ clearance in AD, especially in late-onset sporadic AD (LOAD), has been heightened, and the study of the Aβ clearance mechanisms has elucidated new possible therapeutic targets. This chapter summarizes recent data underlying the idea of the reduced Aβ clearance and subsequent Aβ spread in AD. We discuss the Aβ clearance mechanisms altered in AD, and the Aβ clearance through autophagy in more detail, a more recent mechanism proposed, and the new strategies to eliminate Aβ42 inducing autophagy.

Keywords: β-amyloid peptide, alzheimer's disease, clearance, autophagy, neurodegeneration

1. Introduction

The removal of accumulated amyloid peptide in the brain is carried out by several mechanisms. The clearance of Aβ by nonenzymatic pathway is performed as follows: the total flux of the interstitial fluid (ISF) into the cerebrospinal fluid (CSF) accompanied by the ISF drainage pathway, phagocytosis by microglial or astrocytic cells, and a mechanism named peripheral sink (transport through the blood vessel walls into the circulation); the last one could be regulated by different receptors.

The enzymatic pathway uses the proteolytic machinery in the brain in order to clean the Aβ excess and includes the participation of multiple Aβ-degrading enzymes (ADE) implicated in the clearance of the different Aβ peptides, which include neprilysin, insulin-degrading enzyme, matrix metalloproteinase-9, glutamate carboxypeptidase II, the mitochondrial human preprotease, and others.

Finally, the last Aβ clearance mechanism involved in the Aβ degradation is related with the proteasome and Aβ degradation by autophagy. The proteasome is important for the degradation of worn out and misfolded proteins. Decreased proteasome activity has been implicated in Alzheimer's disease (AD) and proteasome inhibition induces autophagy. Autophagy is a catabolic process involved in the degradation of aberrant organelles and macromolecules, into double membrane vesicles, and delivers it to lysosomes for degradation and the eventual recycling of the resulting macromolecules, and more recently, autophagy has been related with Aβ clearance, but it is still unknown whether autophagy is beneficial or deleterious to AD neurons as the autophagosome has been suggested as a site of amyloid-β (Aβ) generation. In addition, there is little information about the autophagic processes on neurons or microglia involved in the degradation of amyloid peptides.

A series of studies on the Aβ clearance mechanism provide new insight into the pathogenesis of AD at the molecular level and suggest a new target for the development of novel therapeutics. There are a lot of publications dealing with signaling pathways of Aβ synthesis and related enzymes but the identification of molecules responsible for Aβ clearance pathways and their mechanistic links to AD is still a matter of debate. The recent results have shown that Aβ-degrading enzymes have played an important role in reducing AD pathology in both cell and animal models. However, the induction of intracellular clearance of Aβ42 by autophagy is becoming an important proposed mechanism to improve the degradation of Aβ peptides.

2. Methods

2.1. Literature review

This chapter reviews the current available information about beta amyloid clearance mechanisms. We performed a systematic review and exploratory analysis of articles in order to identify, select, and synthesize all high-quality research evidence and arguments relevant to the mechanisms of clearance of beta amyloid peptides form CNS in Alzheimer´s disease. By high-quality evidence we mean the whole of peer-reviewed articles in indexed journals to guarantee the quality and reliability of data in this chapter. Specifically, a manual literature search was carried out using the Medline, NCBI, and Embase databases. The following text words and MeSH headings were used in this search: "beta amyloid 1-42", "beta amyloid 3-42", and "beta amyloid 11-42", "clearance", "degradation", "enzymatic clearance", "microglial activation", "autophagy", and combinations of these terms, and the search was extended for papers referenced by other papers, papers and authors known by reputation, and papers from personal databases.

3. Alzheimer´s disease: a brief description and pathological markers (Aβ1-42, 3-42, 11-42)

Alzheimer's disease (AD) is the most common cause of dementia in the elderly population. It is characterized by a progressive atrophy in several brain areas such as the entorhinal cortex, hippocampus, corpus callosum, and also areas outside the limbic system [1]. This process is irreversible and results in memory loss, inability to learn, performing calculation, unbalanced perception of space, and depression. AD is classified in three stages: mild, moderate, and severe.

AD commences with signs of mild cognitive impairment characterized by memory loss, poor judgment, mood swings, repetitive questions, and difficulty in doing mathematical calculations. The symptoms of moderate AD include the inability to learn new things, difficulty to recognized people, hallucinations, delusions, paranoia, and impulsive behavior. Finally, severe AD patients are dependent and bedridden [2].

Pathological hallmarks of AD include the presence of neurofibrillary tangles, senile plaques, neuronal death, synapsis loss, astrogliosis in the enthorinal cortex, hippocampus, amygdala, and frontal, temporal, parietal, and occipital cortex [3].

Neurofibrillary tangles are intracellular deposits of paired helical filaments formed by hyperphosphorylated tau protein. On the other hand, senil plaques are present as diffuse plaques composed of amorphous extracellular deposits of amyloid β (Aβ) that lacks neurites and neuritic plaques composed of extracellular deposits of insoluble Aβ surrounded by dystrophic neurites, reactive astrocytes, and activated microglia [3, 4].

The etiology of AD is not yet fully understood, but genetic and environmental factors are involved in the disease pathogenesis and progression. Early-onset, so-called familial AD occurs in 1% of cases that are linked to autosomal dominant mutation in amyloid β precursor protein (APP), presenillin (PSEN) 1, and PSEN2. The rest of AD cases are sporadic, the late-onset form (so-called "sporadic AD"). There are also genetic risk factors associated with late-onset AD, for example, the presence of the ε4 allele of the gene for apo-lipoprotein E, which has been shown to increase the probability of the development of AD, whereas the presence of an ε2 allele appears to protect against the disease [5, 6]. Nongenetic risk factors include cerebrovascular changes (hemorrhagic or ischemic), hypertension, type 2 diabetes, and metabolic syndrome [4].

Aβ is generated from the amyloid precursor protein, an ~105 kDa single-pass transmembrane glycoprotein found at presynaptic and postsynaptic terminals in the brain. APP gene in human is located on chromosome 21 and alternative splicing of APP transcript generates 8 isoform, of which the 695, 751, and 770 amino acids forms are the most common [7]. APP695 is predominantly expressed in neurons, especially during neuronal differentiation whereas APP751 and APP770 are more ubiquitous, although during brain injury their expression increases in astrocytes and microglia [8]. APP plays an important role in neuronal functions such as synapse formation, neuronal migration, neurite outgrowth, synaptic plasticity, synaptic transmission and learning, and memory [9]. APP is synthetized in endoplasmic reticulum and is modified in the Golgi apparatus. The ectodomain contains part of the Aβ sequence, which extends into the transmembrane domain.

Proteolytic processing of APP includes two different pathways (**Figure 1**): (1) nonamyloidogenic processing and (2) amyloidogenic processing. The first is the cleavage by α-secretase within the Aβ domain releasing a soluble α-secretase-released N-terminal of APP (sAPPα) and generating a truncated APP CTF (αCTF or C83). The latter is subsequently intramembrane cut by γ-secretase, which liberates a truncated Aβ peptide called p3 and generates the APP intracellular domain (AICD). This process stops the production of β-amyloid peptide and prevents its deposition in plaques. On the other hand, APP can be cleaved by β-secretase at the beginning of Aβ sequence liberating a soluble sAPPβ and generating a membrane-associated C-terminal fragment (βCTF or C99) whose subsequent cleavage by γ-secretase activity results in the generation of Aβ peptides ranging in length from 38 to 42 residues, where Aβ1-42 is the most neurotoxic form [10–13]. The resulting peptides are liberated into extracellular fluids such as cerebrospinal fluid (CSF), plasma, or interstitial fluid [14].

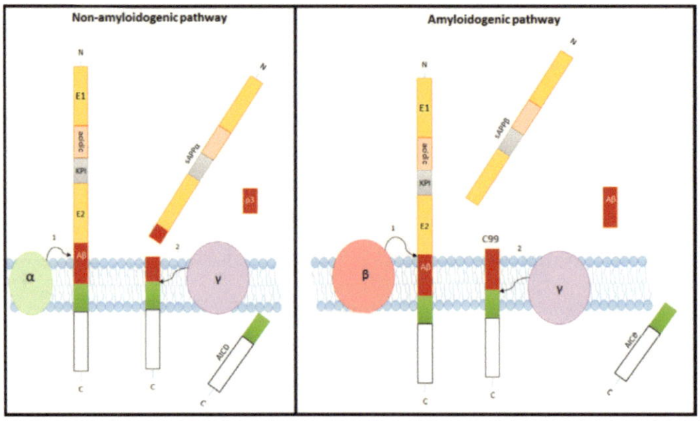

Figure 1. APP schematic structure and processing by secretases.

Mutation in APP molecule has differential effect depending on the location of the mutated residue. Amino acid substitution flanking the Aβ region close to β-secretase cleavage site like

http://dx.doi.org/10.5772/64744

Swedish mutation modulates the rate of enzymatic processing of APP maintaining the ratio Aβ-42/Aβ-40. In contrast, mutation occurring in close proximity to γ-secretase cleavage site (such as the so-called Austrian, Iranian, French, German, London, and Florida mutations) is associated with increasing production of Aβ-42 and lower levels of Aβ-40 [15]. Mutations in the mid region of Aβ domain affect the primary sequence of Aβ peptide resulting in enhanced aggregation propensity. Some of these intraAβ mutations can lead to mixed amyloid pathologies: marked cerebral angiopathy and marked amyloid plaque formation [11]. The α-secretase activity is mediated by a series of membrane-bound proteases, which are member of the ADAM (a disintegrin and metalloprotease) family. In neuron, the principal constitutive α-secretase activity is exerted by ADAM10. The processing of APP by α-secretase is postulated to be protective in the context of AD because the enzymes cleave within the Aβ sequence, thereby preventing the production of Aβ [16].

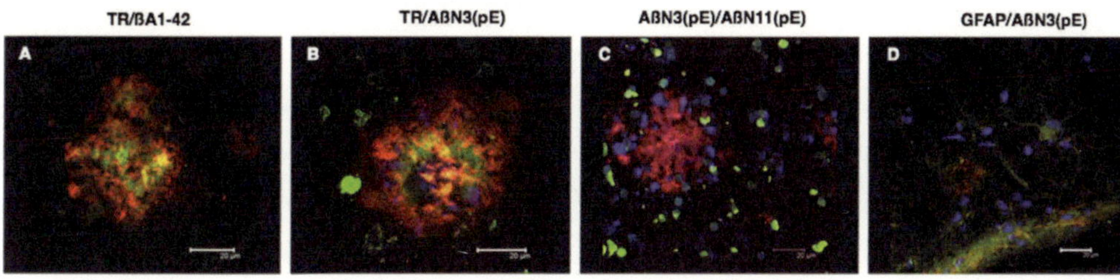

Figure 2. Amyloid plaques of 1-42, AβN3(pE), and AβN11(pE) present in human brain. (A) Merge (yellow) between βA1-42 plaque (green) and the fibrillar βA1-42 marker TR (red). (B) Merge (yellow) between AβN3(pE) plaque (green) and TR (red). (C) Merge between AβN3(pE) (green), AβN11(pE) (red), and the nuclear marker DAPI (blue). (D) Merge between AβN3(pE) (red) and the glial cell marker GFAP (green) showing a glial cell surrounding AβN3(pE) aggregates. These amyloid aggregates were observed in 50 mm thick brain tissue sections of temporal cortex from AD patients. Scale bar represents 20 μm; A–D.

The major neuronal β-secretase, termed BACE-1, is a transmembrane 501 amino acid aspartyl protease. After synthesis, BACE-1 is transported to the cell surface via the endoplasmic reticulum and Golgi. APP and BACE-1 are both endocytosed where the APP cleavage occurs as the optimum pH of BACE is 3.5–4.4. Mutations of BACE-1 have not been identified in familial AD cases, but the activity of BACE is increased in both familial and sporadic AD [17]. The γ-secretase activity is executed by a high molecular weight, membrane-embedded protein complex consisting of PSEN, nicastrin, anterior pharynx defective (APH1), and presenilin enhancer (PEN2), although PSEN seems to provide the active core γ-secretase complex functioning as an aspartyl protease [18]. In mammals, two homologous, PSEN1 and PSEN2, are found whose mutation alters the biochemical character of the γ-secretase complex and its interaction with APP substrate to skew the transmembrane cleavage toward longer more aggregation-prone forms of Aβ, increasing the ratio Aβ-42/Aβ-40, which is associated to early onset of AD [19]. The proteolytic APP processing preferentially generates Aβ1-40/1-42; however, there is a great diversity of Aβ peptides depending on γ-secretase and shorter peptides resulting from γ-secretase activity upon C99. In addition, a significant proportion of Aβ consist of N-terminal truncated/modified species, which increase the Aβ propensity to form aggregates [14, 20] with the most prominent forms identified starting at position 3 or 11 and possessing N-terminal pyroglutamic acid (pyroE), generated by glutamic acid [21]. The N-terminal truncated Aβ3-42/Aβ3 is generated by the zinc-metalloprotease neutral endopeptidase or neprilysin (NeP)-40 cleaving Aβ between Arg-2 and Glu-3. On the other hand, BACE-1 is also capable of cleaving between Tyr-10 and Glu-11, leading to the release of Aβ11-42/Aβ11-40 peptides [22]. Then, the GluN-terminal undergoes N-terminal pyroglutamate (pGlu) modification catalyzed by glutaminylcyclase (**Figure 2**) [23].

4. Aβ structure

The native conformation of Aβ is an unfolded protein. Aβ forms amyloid fibrils by folding from the native random-coil-rich state to α-helical-rich intermediate, and finally to a β-sheet-rich amyloid monomer that self-assembles into the fibrils [24].

Another protein closely related to AD pathology is the tau protein. This is encoded in mapt gene, located on chromosome 17q21. Several tau isoforms are generated by alternative splicing, creating high and low isoforms. The human central nervous system expresses six low molecular weight isoform ranging from 352 to 441 amino acids [25].

Tau is a neuronal cytosolic protein whose function is to promote microtubules polymerization and stabilization. In addition, Tau has importance in maintaining an appropriate morphology of neurons and it appear to modulate axonal transport [26, 27].

Domains of Tau are defined on the basis of their microtubule interaction and their amino acid character. The C-terminal domain (assembly domain) binds microtubules while the N-terminal domain projects away from microtubule (projection domain). The overall amino acid tau composition is hydrophilic, consistent with its unfolded character; however, the N-terminal is predominantly acidic and the C-terminal roughly neutral, which is important for microtubule interaction. The middle region is a proline-rich domain which is targets of many proline-directed kinases and binding sites for proteins with SH3 domains [28]. Tau is highly regulated and is subject to multiple post-translational modifications. Phosphorylation is the most common tau post-translational modification described resulted from the equilibrium between the amount and activity of protein kinases and phosphatases.

Hyperphosphorylation of tau is not only associated with the disease, but is also employed by the neuron to downregulate its activity transiently and reversibly where required, for example during development, anesthesia, and hypothermia. It is the nonreversible nature of the abnormal hyperphosphorylation of tau in AD and other tauopathies that results in an involuntary slowing down of neuronal activity and a consequent chronic progressive neurodegeneration [29]. Increased tau phosphorylation decreased its affinity for microtubules resulting in an abnormal increase in the levels of the free (unbound) Tau fraction; next small nonfibrillary tau deposits (normally referred to as "pretangles") are formed followed by structural rearrangement involving the formation of the characteristic pleated β-sheet structures, which finally form the neurofibrillary tangles by self-assemble [26].

5. Clearance mechanisms

5.1. Alzheimer's disease clearance: is microglia involved?

Since Alois Alzheimer described the disease in 1907 several therapeutic options have been developed. The therapeutic treatments available today treat the symptoms without targeting the cause of the disease [30] and as a consequence the disease follows it's natural course [31]. Cholinesterase inhibitors and memantine are FDA-approved therapies against the cognitive symptoms for AD [32]. These drugs favor short-term cognitive benefits, so even though patients are receiving the ideal treatment, they will return to their baseline cognitive decline [33].

Since the amyloid cascade was described research for a disease modifying therapy is being aimed toward the study of Aβ. β-Secretase inhibitors have been tested in an attempt to reduce the production of Aβ. It was demonstrated that β-secretase inhibitors reduced plasma and CSF levels of Aβ but concerns have emerged about potential side effects with chronic administration [34].

One of the most recent strategies, known for its ability to reduce the accumulation of Aβ and promote a cognitive benefit in preclinical trials, is the immunotherapy. The immunotherapeutic approach can be classified as either active or passive. Passive immunotherapy refers to the administration of anti-Aβ antibodies, bypassing the patient need to mount an immunological response toward Aβ. Active immunotherapy involves the administration of full length Aβ or peptide fragments conjugated to a carrier protein, with a T-cell epitope and with an adjuvant in order to stimulate the patient own immune response. The basis of both immunotherapeutic approaches relies on the recognition of Aβ aggregates by specific anti-Aβ antibodies [35].

Extensive studies of active and passive immunization with Aβ showed promising benefits. Schenk et al. were the first to report the beneficial effects of Aβ immunotherapy in a preclinical study with active immunization in PDAPP mouse. The immunization with Aβ reduced levels of cerebral amyloid and produced high serum antibody titers. A year later Morgan et al. reported that Aβ immunization improved behavioral performance in learning and memory tasks [36]. Passive immunization studies showed that antibodies were able to enter the central nervous system, 0.01% of the peripherally administered antibodies, bind plaques, and induce clearance of preexisting amyloid lesions. Passive immunization of PDAPP mice led to reduce plaque burden, increase blood circulating Aβ, and improve cognitive performance [37]. Immunotherapy via active or passive immunization against Aβ peptides has shown to be very successful in reducing Aβ aggregates in AD animal models [38–41]. The immunotherapeutic approach was translated to clinical trials by ELAN/Wyeth in 2000. After a few immunized subjects, the trial was stopped due to the development of meningoencephalitis in 6% of immunized AD patients [42]. The postmortem analysis of participants, who died from causes not related to the immunization, showed patchy clearance of amyloid plaques in the brain [43]. These areas of clearance were accompanied by Aβ immunoreactive microglia cells, supporting the hypothesis that Aβ-specific antibodies may lead to the phagocytosis of Aβ by microglia cells [39].

The involvement of microglia in clearance of Aβ aggregates after immunotherapy has been demonstrated through several studies. After a single injection of anti-Aβ antibody to APP mice, the antibodies were found associated not only with amyloid deposits but also with microglia surrounding the plaques [44]. Wilcock et al. reported that 24 and 72 hours after the injection of anti-Aβ antibodies to Tg2576 APP mice there was a reduction in fibrillar amyloid deposits and showed an increase in microglial activation, evaluated by CD45, a protein tyrosine phosphatase commonly used as a marker for microglia activation, and MHC-II staining. Intracraneal injections of anti-Aβ antibodies to APP mice demonstrated that the increase in CD45 expression of microglia is evident after the clearance of diffuse deposits and is parallel with the clearance of fibrillar deposits [36]. The temporal association of fibrillar amyloid loss with microglia activation suggests some causal role for microglial activation in the process [45]. In 2004 Wilcock reported that 1 month after the administration of anti-Aβ antibodies to APP transgenic mice an increase in CD45 expression on microglia surrounding amyloid deposits in both the hippocampus and frontal cortex. After 2 months of treatment there was an additional increase in CD45 not only in microglia surrounding amyloid plaques but also in microglia associated with soluble aggregate [46, 47]. This microglial activation also takes form of an increased transcript level of proinflammatorycyctokines and iNOS [47].

The role of microglia in the clearance of amyloid deposits after the administration of anti-Aβ antibodies was analyzed *in vivo* through the generation of the CX3CR1-GFP protein. CX3XR1 is a gene specifically expressed in microglia in the CNS [48]. After administration of an anti-Aβ antibody that recognizes both aggregated and soluble Aβ, PDAPP mice contained more levels of CX3CR1-GFP positive cells and these cells had twice as many protruding processes from their cell bodies. These changes were detected surrounding amyloid plaques and amyloid deposits associated with blood vessels. These changes were also seen with the microglia marker Iba-1 and with CD45 staining [49]. When Fab fragments of the antibody were injected there was no effect on the number of microglia CX3CR1-GFP positive cells or on microglia morphology, suggesting that the Fc is required to elicit the microglial changes observed in the mouse treated with the full-length antibody [49].

One of the mechanisms for plaques clearance is by anti-Aβ immunotherapy through FcγR-mediated phagocytosis of plaques by microglia [50]. After administration of anti-Aβ antibodies to APP mice there was an increase in FcRII and FcRIII on microglia. The microglia expressing the FcR were associated with amyloid plaques and with diffuse aggregates [46]. When examined in *an ex vivo* assay with sections of PDAPP or AD brain tissue, antibodies against Aβ-activated microglia cells clear amyloid plaques through FcR-mediated phagocytosis and subsequent peptide degradation [39]. Anti-Aβ antibodies with binding affinity for FcγR increased the Aβ oligomer induced p38MAPK activity in microglia [51]. The p38MAPK pathway is responsible for the upregulation of proinflamatory cytokines in microglia, such as TNF-α and IL-1β [52].

After the role of microglia in anti-Aβ antibodies amyloid clearance was proposed, and the effect of microglia inhibition was assessed. The anti-Mac-1-saporin immunotoxin was used to kill activated microglia in APP mice. The elimination of activated microglia reduced Aβ clearance by anti-Aβ antibodies, although appreciable clearance was still present [53]. This suggests that microglia, dependent and independent mechanisms, are likely involved in the clearance of amyloid aggregates following immunotherapy [54]. Additional mechanisms for clearance of amyloid peptides are possible *in vivo*. If Fab2 fragments, which fail to activate microglia, are injected in transgenic mice, the clearance of Aβ deposits is blocked, but the clearance of diffuse aggregates is unaffected [46]. These data suggest that the clearance of diffuse aggregates may proceed by the catalytic dissolution mechanism proposed by Solomon [50], who postulated that direct interaction of antibodies with Aβ may lead to the disruption of aggregates [55]. This process does not depend on FcR activation. Even though there are several non-Fc-dependent mechanisms for the removal of Aβ aggregates, previous studies demonstrate, through the analysis of microglial cells and frozen tissue sections, that the Fc-mediated mechanism is dominant in the removal of amyloid deposits [39].

Even though the involvement of microglia is important for the removal of amyloid deposits, the activation of microglia by anti Aβ antibodies is accompanied with microhemorrhages and edema. It has been proposed that microglia activation by antibodies induces damage to the vasculature and to the neurons [50]. The prevention of microhemorrhages is achieved when antibodies with reduced affinity for FcγR are used. This was shown by using Crenezumab, a humanized antibody with lower affinity for all FcγR; this antibody promotes a reduction in microglial activation, limiting the release of inflammatory cytokines to avoid side effects, such as vasogenic edema. In the phase I of the safety trial, no vasogenic edema or microhemorrhage were found (Clinicaltrials.gov). The current immunotherapeutic approaches for AD are directed to the design of an optimized antibody that could separate the phagocytic and inflammatory response, promoting an efficient clearance of Aβ aggregates the induction of the detrimental proinflammatory citokyne release [56].

6. Intracellular mechanisms

6.1. βA peptides degradation by autophagy

Cellular homeostasis largely depends on the proteostasis network. Under normal conditions, this network senses and rectifies disturbances in the proteome to restore homeostasis in cells. The main players in proteostasis maintenance are chaperones and two proteolitic systems: the ubiquitin-proteasome and the autophagy system.

Although there are some differences in this proteolitic systems, substrates of the ubiquitin-proteasomes pathway are predominantly short-live proteins and misfolded or damaged proteins. Meanwhile, the autophagy substrates are long-live proteins and multiple proteins organized into oligomeric complex or aggregates that cannot be degraded by others systems [53].

In this sense, macroautophagy (hereafter referred to as autophagy) has been characterized as a catabolic process that engulfs aberrant organelles, misfolded proteins, and protein aggregates into double membrane vesicles (named autophagosomes) and delivers it to lysosomas [54]. The correct function of this catabolic process is very important because it is the only known mechanism that eukaryotic cells possess to degrade protein aggregates and the only one by which entire organelles such as mitochondria and peroxisomes are recycled. Several studies proposed that autophagy helps to relieve the proteotoxic stress of misfolded proteins by degrading toxic oligomers in the cytosol [55].

Posmitotic cells like neurons are highly dependent on autophagy. Mainly because once neurons mature and become postmitotic, they lose their ability to dilute insults by cell division. Thus, neuronal survival heavily depends on housekeeping processes to maintain cellular quality control [56]. In this regard, the loss of autophagy particularly in neurons causes the accumulation of ubiquitin-positive inclusion bodies and triggers a process of neurodegeneration [57]. Evidence points that dysfunction in the autophagy processes is part of Alzheimer's disease pathogenesis [58] and the clearance of autophagic vacuoles and lysosomal degradation of Aβ could prevent the intracellular accumulation.

6.2. Autophagy

Nowadays it is recognized that autophagy has a fundamental role in homeostasis through the degradation of components that would be toxics for the cell.

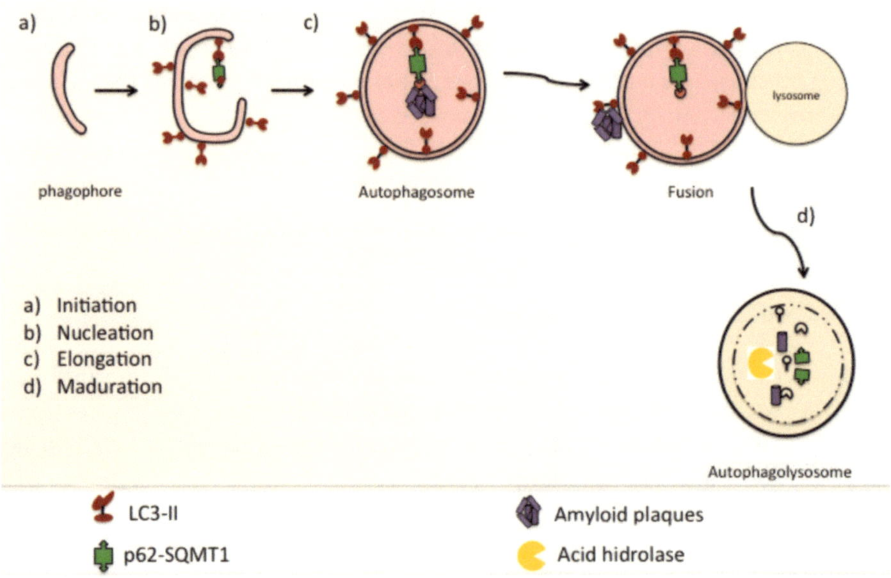

Figure 3. Autophagy elimination of Aβ plaques. Autophagy is the only known mechanisms that eukaryotic cells possess to degrade Aβ aggregates.

Autophagy is a complex process that requires a series of coordinated steps. In the first place, the formation of a vesicle isolation called phagophore is described. After the phagophore formation, it elongates around the cytoplasmatic components selected for degradation. The recognition of the components that will be degraded and the closing of the vesicle are dependent on the lipidated form of LC3 protein (microtubule-associated protein light chain 3). The lipidated form of LC3 is associated with the outer and inner membranes of the autophagosome and has become a reliable method for monitoring autophagy and autophagy-related processes [59].

Finally, the late stage of autophagy or maturation depends on the successful fusion of autophagosome with lysosome. This fusion allows contact of autophagosome cargo with lysosomal hydrolases and consequently the degradation of the components that in some cases are recycled.

These steps are fundamentaly important for the autophagic flux (defined as the continuous series of events since the cargo is engulf until it is degraded). Any event that alters the autophagic flux also alters the degradation process and consequently leads to the accumulation of autophagosomes (**Figure 3**).

6.3. Autophagy and Alzheimer's disease

Autophagic vacuoles are uncommon in neurons of the healthy brain because this process is constitutive active in neurons and the efficient clearance of autophagosomes keeps their presence low [60]. Moreover, in AD there is an accumulation of autophagic vesicles preferentially in dystrophic neuritis [61]. This evidence suggests that some of the later steps in the autophagic process is altered; this idea is supported by the observation that the lysosomal hidrolases are increased and abnormally distributed in AD brain indicating the defective maturation of autophagosomes [62]. Additionally, it was observed that acidification of lysosomes causes an autophagosome accumulation without altering the induction [62].

6.4. Why autophagy is altered in AD?

It is not clear, but it has been demonstrated, that a large number of autophagic vacuoles are observed in dystrophic neuritis before extracellular Aβ deposition in neurons of AD patients and transgenic mouse models [63, 64]. This suggests that autophagy dysfunction leads to the accumulation of Aβ, avoiding proper degradation.

Inductors of autophagy as trehalosa (a natural disaccharide that block glucose transporters) could rescue the AD-like phenotype in APP/PS1 transgenic mice. In this sense, trehalosa treatment significantly improves the performance of memory and learning tasks. In accordance with behavioral test, Aβ deposits were significantly reduced in hippocampus [65].

In addition, the induction of autophagy by rapamicyn (an mTORC1 complex inhibitor) in PD/APP transgenic mice improves the cognitive performance through the degradation of extracellular Aβ depositions.

In this model, autophagy induction was higher in the hippocampus of transgenic mice compared with nontransgenic mice [66]. This suggests that autophagy dysfunctions could be reversed through the pharmacological stimulation and these inductions have beneficial effects by promoting Aβ degradation. Different studies have been performed finding that rapamycin reduces the accumulation of Aβ levels and fibrillar aggregates approximately 40–50% in 3XAD-Tg mice and APP transgenic mice [67].

Morphological evidence shows that APP and Aβ peptide are colocalized with LC3-positive autophagosomes and autophagy induction shows a greater colocalization of Aβ in autophagic vacuoles, suggesting a more active degradation [68]. However, the mechanism by which autophagy can degrade extracellular amyloid plaque content is unknown. But autophagic process of microglia (the resident macrophages in the brain) seems to play an important role.

The degradation of extracellular amyloid content through microglia involves at the first step phagocytosis; once Aβ peptide is in the cytosol it is exposed to be recognized by LC3-II via optineurin (an adaptor protein). LC3-II/OPTN recognition allows Aβ degradation via the autophagic–lysosomal system [69].

The exact pathology of AD is still unknown, but it is widely believed that the deposition of Aβ is one of the main causes leading to the degeneration and death of neurons. So, finding alternatives that avoid Aβ accumulation or enhance its degradation could be a strong therapeutic target. In this sense, autophagy seems to be the first line of defense to face accumulation but it is not clear how autophagy dysfunctions are related to Aβ aggregation or if Aβ overproduction directly induces autophagy defects.

6.5. Differential autophagy activation by monomers and oligomers

Some observations have demonstrated that a large number of autophagic vacuoles are observed in dystrophic neuritis before extracellular Aβ depositions in the neurons of AD patients and murine models of AD [70], but recently it has been demonstrated that Aβ monomers and oligomers differentially modulate autophagy in neurons. In a different way, monomers stimulate autophagy increasing autophagosome rates and the elevation of LC3-II protein levels, but at the same time monomers impaired lysosomal pathway affecting the autophagy flux. These events resulted in autophagosome accumulation. On the other hand, Aβ oligomers cause a less pronounced increase in LC3-II protein levels and does not affect the autophagy flux [58], suggesting that defects in autophagy could be the result of an increase in amyloid monomers.

Enhancing autophagic clearance of toxic protein aggregates through rapamycin or trehalosa ameliorates protein aggregation, neuron survival, and this is reflected in the improvement of cognitive skills. However, converging evidence suggests that improvement in autophagic flux through stimulation is a promising therapeutic intervention, and this field is still developing.

In other words, there are barely some studies showing the degradation by autophagy of the N-truncated beta amyloid peptide [71–74]. Recently, it has been determined that pE3-Aβ is strongly reduced in the TgCRND8 mice fed with a normal diet supplemented with the antioxidant Oleurupein (OLE) and that such a decrease likely reflects the parallel reduction of QC expression. In addition, their model of (Aβ) peptide deposition displayed strongly improved performance in behavioral and cognitive tests, reduced inflammatory response, and recovered dysfunctions of transgene-induced long-term potentiation (LTP) in the CA1 hippocampal area. These effects were induced, at least in part, by a strong activation of autophagy. All these results suggest new perspectives for AD not only at the prevention but also at the therapeutic level [75–77].

7. β-Amyloid peptides altered clearance in loss vision in AD

Until now, we have been discussing the altered clearance mechanisms of beta amyloid peptides in AD. However, these peptides are involved in other pathological mechanisms during the development and progression of AD. Recently, the βA42 peptide has been involved in vision loss and its presence in the retina has been proposed as an early diagnostic marker for AD [78–80]. The presence of multiple βA42 reservoirs in the eye, especially in the retina environment, also induces different pathologies that lead to deficient vision as blindness [81, 82]. Pathologies such as age-related macular degeneration (AMD) and cataracts may contribute to the local inflammatory events involved in the formation of local deposits of lipids and beta amyloid peptide called drusens, atrophy of retinal pigment epithelium, lens degeneration, and photoreceptor cell death [82, 83]. In this section of the chapter, we will discuss the most recent findings emerging from the altered mechanisms of beta amyloid clearance in the eye.

As mentioned above, one of the principal degradation mechanism of amyloid beta peptides is the enzymatic pathway. In the brain, the principal βA-degrading enzymes are neprilysin, endothelin-converting enzyme (ECE), insulin-degrading enzyme (IDE), angiotensin-converting enzyme (ACE), and in mitochondria the enzyme is called hPreP [84]. However, in the eye the presence of the Neprilysin specifically in the lens [82] has been described. In other words, it has been reported that autophagy could be involved in the degradation of beta amyloid peptides through the internalization in clathrin-positive endosomes. However, these mechanisms have not been totally elucidated and current research is being performed in order to probe it in the eye [85, 86]. Finally, as mentioned above, antibeta amyloid antibody therapy is a currently applicable treatment. In the eye, this therapy was designed to target the C-terminal fragment of βA42 in a mouse model of AMD resulting in a protective effect. All this mechanisms of Alzheimer pathophysiology can contribute to vision degeneration, suggesting further that therapeutics targeting Aβ proteases or induced autophagy may be applicable to avoid vision loss.

8. Conclusions

As discussed in this chapter, there are some βA clearance mechanisms that are altered in Alzheimer´s disease. A large number of evidence exists about the βA1-42 clearance mechanism. However, despite of this, there is a lack of evidence related to the βA3-42 and βA11-42 degradation mechanisms. The principal βA variants detected in the human brain are A1-40 and A1-42; however, a significant proportion of AD brain A also consists of N-terminal-truncated species and the latest hypothesis pointing that they are seeding species. For this reason, N-terminal peptides represent highly desirable and abundant therapeutic targets.

We have an urgent need to perform immunotherapy strategies directed against N-truncated/pyroglutamate-modified βA peptides and consider them for vaccine development for AD. These kinds of analysis may provide promising diagnostic and therapeutic tools, targeting all pathological amyloid species involved in AD in the future.

In other words, autophagy is a hot topic in the recent years, enhancing autophagic clearance of toxic protein aggregates through rapamycin or trehalosa ameliorates protein aggregation and neuron survival, and this is reflected in the improvement of cognitive skills. However, converging evidence suggests that the improvement in the autophagic flux through stimulation is a promising therapeutic intervention that is still developing. Importantly, the combination of different strategies targeting simultaneously different pathological pathways, "systems therapeutics", might be more appropriate for a multifactorial disease like AD. For example, we should try to design an anti-βA, anti-tau, anti-inflammatory, anti-oxidative stress, and autophagy enhancing strategy in preclinical trials with a hope to translate them to human research.

Interestingly, there is no information about the presence of the N-truncated species of beta amyloid peptides in the eye. The big question is: Why? Is not there relevance? Or only has not been studied? More research in this topic is urgently needed in order to improve the quality of life of patients with AD.

Author details

Luis F. Hernández-Zimbrón[1*], Elisa Gorostieta-Salas[2], Mei-Li Díaz-Hung[3], Roxanna Pérez-Garmendia[4], Gohar Gevorkian[5] and Hugo Quiroz-Mercado[1]

*Address all correspondence to: lfhernandez@unam.mx

1 Research Department, Association to Prevent Blindness in Mexico "Luis Sanchez Bulnes Hospital" Mexico City, Mexico

2 Neuroscience Division, Institute of Cellular Physiology, National Autonomous University of Mexico, Mexico City, Mexico

3 Neuroimmunochemistry Department, International Center of Neurological Restoration, La Havana, Cuba

4 Surgery Department, Faculty of Medicine, National Autonomous University of Mexico, Mexico City, Mexico

5 Immunology Department, Biomedical Research Institute, National Autonomous University of Mexico, Mexico City, Mexico

References

[1] Du AT, Schuff N, Kramer JH et al.Higher atrophy rate of entorhinal cortex than hippocampus in AD. Neurology.2004;62:422–427. DOI: 10. 1212/01.WNL.0000106462. 72282. 90

[2] Bhat Shreya RAU, Dadmehr N,Adeli H. Clinical neurophysiological and automated EEG-based diagnosis of the Alzheimer's disease. European Neuro. 2015;74:202–210. DOI: 10.1159/000441447

[3] Lovell MA, Markesbery WR. Oxidative DNA damage in mild cognitive impairment and late-stage Alzheimer's disease. Nucleic Acids Res. 2007;35(22):7497–7504. DOI: 10.1093/nar/gkm821

[4] Reitz C, Mayeux R. Alzheimer disease: epidemiology, diagnostic criteria, risk factors and biomarkers. Biochem Pharmacol. 2014;88(4):640–651. DOI:10.1016/j.bcp. 2013.12.024

[5] Revett TJ, Baker GB, Jhamandas J, Kar S. Glutamate system, amyloid ss peptides and tau protein: functional interrelationships and relevance to Alzheimer disease pathology. J Psychiatry Neurosci. 2013;38(1):6–23. DOI: 10.1503/jpn.110190

[6] Shinohara M, Fujioka S, Murray ME, Wojtas A, Baker M, Rovelet-Lecrux A, et al. Regional distribution of synaptic markers and APP correlate with distinct clinicopathological features in sporadic and familial Alzheimer's disease. Brain. 2014;137(Pt 5): 1533–1549. DOI: http://dx.doi.org/10.1093/brain/awu046

[7] O'Brien RJ, Wong PC. Amyloid precursor protein processing and Alzheimer's disease. Annu Rev Neurosci. 2011;34:185–204. DOI:10.1146/annurev-neuro-061010-113613

[8] Kummer MP, Heneka MT. Truncated and modified amyloid-beta species. Alzheimer's Resand Ther. 2014;6(28):1581–1591. DOI:10.1046/j.1471-4159.2003.01818.x

[9] Gautam V, D'Avanzo C, Berezovska O, Tanzi RE, Kovacs DM. Synaptotagmins interact with APP and promote Abeta generation. Mol Neurodegener. 2015;10:31. DOI: 10.1186/ s13024-015-0028-5

[10] Bayer TA, Wirths O. Intracellular accumulation of amyloid-Beta-a predictor for synaptic dysfunction and neuron loss in Alzheimer's disease. Front Aging Neurosci. 2010;2:8. DOI:10.3389/fnagi.2010.00008

[11] Haass C, Kaether C, Thinakaran G, Sisodia S. Trafficking and proteolytic processing of APP. Cold Spring Harb Perspect Med. 2012;2(5):a006270. DOI: 10.1101/cshperspect.a006270

[12] Pluta R, Furmaga-Jablonska W, Maciejewski R, Ulamek-Koziol M, Jablonski M. Brain ischemia activates beta-and gamma-secretase cleavage of amyloid precursor protein:

significance in sporadic Alzheimer's disease. Mol Neurobiol. 2013;47(1):425–434. DOI: 10.1007/s12035-012-8360-z

[13] Tabaton M, Tamagno E. The molecular link between beta-and gamma-secretase activity on the amyloid beta precursor protein. Cell Mol Life Sci. 2007;64(17):2211–2218. DOI: 10.1007/s00018-007-7219-3

[14] Heneka MPKaMT. Truncated and modified amyloid-beta species. Alzheimer's Research and Therapy. 2014;6(3):28. DOI: 10.1186/alzrt258

[15] Rostagno A, Holton JL, Lashley T, Revesz T, Ghiso J. Cerebral amyloidosis: amyloid subunits, mutants and phenotypes. Cell Mol Life Sci. 2010;67(4):581–600. DOI: 10.1007/s00018-009-0182-4

[16] De Strooper B, Vassar R, Golde T. The secretases: enzymes with therapeutic potential in Alzheimer disease. Nat Rev Neurol. 2010;6(2):99–107. DOI:10.1038/nrneurol.2009.218

[17] Venugopal C, Demos CM, Rao KJ, Pappolla MA and Sambamurti K. Beta-secretase: structure, function and evolution. CNS and neuro disorders drug targets. 2008;7(3):278. DOI: http://dx.doi.org/10.2174/187152708784936626

[18] Lipinski MM, Zheng B, Lu T, Yan Z, Py BF, Ng A, … and Yuan J. Genome-wide analysis reveals mechanisms modulating autophagy in normal brain aging and in Alzheimer's disease. PNAS. 2010;107(32).14164–14169. DOI:10.1073/pnas.1009485107/-/DCSupplemental

[19] De Strooper B, Iwatsubo T, Wolfe MS. Presenilins and gamma-secretase: structure, function and role in Alzheimer Disease. Cold Spring Harb Perspect Med. 2012;2(1):a006304. DOI: 10.1101/cshperspect.a006304

[20] Wirths O, Bethge T, Marcello A, Harmeier A, Jawhar S, Lucassen PJ, et al. Pyroglutamate Abeta pathology in APP/PS1KI mice, sporadic and familial Alzheimer's disease cases. J Neural Transm (Vienna). 2010;117(1):85–96. DOI: 10.1007/s00702-009-0314-x

[21] Jonson M, Pokrzywa M, Starkenberg A, Hammarstrom P, Thor S. Systematic Abeta analysis in drosophila reveals high toxicity for the 1–42, 3–42 and 11–42 Peptides and Emphasizes N-and C-Terminal Residues. PLoS One. 2015;10(7):e0133272. DOI: 10.1371/journal.pone.0133272

[22] Bayer TA, Wirths O. Focusing the amyloid cascade hypothesis on N-truncated Abeta peptides as drug targets against Alzheimer's disease. Acta Neuropathol. 2014;127(6):787–801. DOI: 10.1007/s00401-014-1287-x

[23] Hook V, Schechter I, Demuth HU, Hook G. Alternative pathways for production of beta-amyloid peptides of Alzheimer's disease. Biol Chem. 2008;389(8):993–1006. DOI: 10.1515/BC.2008.124,

[24] Ow SY, Dunstan DE. A brief overview of amyloids and Alzheimer's disease. Protein Sci. 2014;23(10):1315–1331. DOI: 10.1002/pro.2524

[25] Lee G, Leugers CJ. Tau and tauopathies. Prog Mol Biol Transl Sci. 2012;107:263–293. DOI: 10.1016/B978-0-12-385883-2.00004-7

[26] Ballatore C, Lee VM, Trojanowski JQ. Tau-mediated neurodegeneration in Alzheimer's disease and related disorders. Nat Rev Neurosci. 2007;8(9):663–672. DOI:10.1038/nrn2194

[27] Wang Y, Martinez-Vicente M, Kruger U, Kaushik S, Wong E, Mandelkow EM, et al. Tau fragmentation, aggregation and clearance: the dual role of lysosomal processing. Hum Mol Genet. 2009;18(21):4153–4170. DOI: 10.1093/hmg/ddp367

[28] Mandelkow EM, Mandelkow E. Biochemistry and cell biology of tau protein in neurofibrillary degeneration. Cold Spring Harb Perspect Med. 2012;2(7):a006247. DOI: 10.1101/cshperspect.a006247

[29] Iqbal K, Liu F, Gong CX, Alonso Adel C, Grundke-Iqbal I. Mechanisms of tau-induced neurodegeneration. Acta Neuropathol. 2009;118(1):53–69. DOI: 10.1007/s00401-009-0486-3

[30] Lobello K, Ryan JM, Liu E, Rippon G, Black R. Targeting beta amyloid: a clinical review of immunotherapeutic approaches in Alzheimer's disease. Int J Alzheimers Dis. 2012;20(12):628070.http://dx.doi.org/10.1155/2012/628070

[31] Masliah BSaE. Immunotherapy for Alzheimer's disease: past, present and future. Frontiers in Aging Neurosci. 2014;6(114):1–7. DOI: 10.3389/fnagi.2014.00114

[32] Aisen PS, Cummings Jand Schneider LS. Symptomatic and nonamyloid/tau based pharmacologic treatment for Alzheimer disease. Cold Spring Harbor Perspectin Med. 2012;2(3). DOI: 10.1101/cshperspect.a006395

[33] Lang AE. Clinical trials of disease-modifying therapies for neurodegenerative diseases: the challenges and the future. Nature medicine. 2010;16(11):1223–1226. DOI: 10.1038/nm.2220

[34] Vassar R. BACE1 inhibitor drugs in clinical trials for Alzheimer's disease. Alzheimer's Resand **Ther. 2014;6(89). DOI: 10.1186/s13195-014-0089-7

[35] Masliah CALaE. Can Alzheimer disease be prevented by amyloid-β immunotherapy? Nat Rev Neurol. 2010;6(6):108–119. DOI:10.1038/nrneurol.2009.219

[36] Dave Morgan DMD, Paul E Gottschall, Kenneth E Ugen CD, John H, Karen D, Paul J, Giovanni DC, Donna W, Karen C, Jaime Hatcher CH, Marcia Gand Gary W Arendash. Ab peptide vaccination prevents memory loss in an animal model of Alzheimer's disease. Lett Nat. 2000;408:982–985. DOI:10.1038/35050116

[37] Richard E, Hartman YI, Kelly R Bales, Steven M. Paul, David F Wozniak and David M. Holtzman. Treatment with an amyloid- antibody ameliorates plaque

load, learning deficits and hippocampal long-term potentiation in a mouse model of Alzheimer's disease. Neurobiol Dis. 2005;25(26):6213–6220. DOI: 10.1523/JNEUROSCI.0664-05.2005

[38] Dale Schenk RB, Whitney D, Grace G, Henry Grajeda TG, Kang Hu, Jiping H, Kelly Johnson-Wood KK, Dora K, Mike Lee ZL, Ivan L, Ruth M, Linda Mutter FS, George S, Nicki V, Christopher Vandevert SW, Mark W, et al. Immunization withamyloid-b attenuates Alzheimer′s disease-like pathology in the PDAPP mouse. Nature. 1999;400(6740):173–177. DOI:10.1038/22124

[39] Bard F, Cannon C, Barbour R, Burke R L, Games D, Grajeda H, and Khan K. Peripherally administered antibodies against amyloid β-peptide enter the central nervous system and reduce pathology in a mouse model of Alzheimer disease. Nature Medicine. 2000;6(8):916–919. DOI:10.1038/78682

[40] Manuel Buttini EM, Robin B, Henry G, Ruth M, Kelly JW, Karen K, Peter S, Stephen F, Dale S and Dora G. Β-amyloid immunotherapy prevents synaptic degeneration in a mouse model of Alzheimer's disease. Neurobiol Dis. 2005;25(40):9096–9101. 10.1523/JNEUROSCI.1697-05.2005

[41] Ronald B, DeMattos KRB, David J Cummins, Jean-Cosme D, Steven M Paul, Holtzman aDM. Peripheral anti-Ab antibody alters CNS and plasma Ab clearance and decreases brain Ab burden in a mouse model of Alzheimer's disease. PNAS 2001 98(15):8850–8855. DOI: 10.1073/pnas.151261398

[42] Orgogozo JM, Gilman S, Dartigues JF, Laurent B, Puel M, Kirby LC, and Michel BF. Subacute meningoencephalitis in a subset of patients with AD after A42 immunization. Neurology. 2003;61:46–54. DOI: 10.1212/01.WNL.0000073623. 84147. A8

[43] Masliah E, Hansen L, Adame A, Crews L, Bard F, Lee C, and Schenk D. A vaccination effects on plaque pathology in the absence of encephalitis in Alzheimer disease. Neurology. 2005;64(1):129–131. DOI: http://dx. doi. org/10. 1212/01.WNL.0000148590. 39911. DF

[44] Wang A, Das P, Switzer RC, Golde TEand Jankowsky JL. Robust amyloid clearance in a mouse model of Alzheimer's disease provides novel insights into the mechanism of amyloid- immunotherapy. The J Neurosci. 2011;31(11):4124–4136. DOI: 10.1523/JNEUROSCI.5077-10.2011

[45] Wilcock DM, Gordon MN, Ugen KE, Gottschall PF, DiCarlo G, Dickey Cand Hardy J. Number of A β inoculations in APP+ PS1 transgenic mice influences antibody titers, microglial activation and congophilic plaque levels. DNA and cell biol. 2001;20(11):731–736. DOI:10.1089/10445490152717596.

[46] Wilcock DM, Munireddy SK, Rosenthal A, Ugen KE, Gordon MN and Morgan D. Microglial activation facilitates Aβ plaque removal following intracranial anti-Aβ antibody administration. Neurobiol dise. 2004;15(1):11–20. DOI:10.1016/j.nbd.2003.09.015

[47] Wilcock DM, Zhao Q, Morgan D, Gordon MN, Everhart A, Wilson JGand Colton CA. Diverse inflammatory responses in transgenic mouse models of Alzheimer's disease and the effect of immunotherapy on these responses. ASN neuro. 2011;3(5). DOI: 10.1042/AN20110018

[48] Nimmerjahn A, Kirchhoff Fand Helmchen F. Resting microglial cells are highly dynamic surveillants of brain parenchyma in vivo. Science 2005;308(5726):1314–1318. DOI: 10.1126/science.1110647

[49] Koenigsknecht-Talboo Jand Landreth G. E. Microglial phagocytosis induced by fibrillar β-amyloid and IgGs are differentially regulated by proinflammatory cytokines. The J neurosci. 2005;25(36):8240–8249. DOI: 10.1523/JNEUROSCI.1808-05.2005

[50] Morgan D, Gordon MN, Tan J, Wilcock Dand Rojiani AM. Dynamic complexity of the microglial activation response in transgenic models of amyloid deposition: implications for Alzheimer therapeutics. J Neuropatholand Exper Neurol. 2005;64(9):743–753. DOI: http://dx.doi.org/10.1097/01.jnen.0000178444.33972.e0

[51] Adolfsson O, Pihlgren M, Toni N, Varisco Y, Buccarello AL, Antoniello K, et al. An effector-reduced anti-beta-amyloid (Abeta) antibody with unique abeta binding properties promotes neuroprotection and glial engulfment of Abeta. J Neurosci. 2012;32(28):9677–9689. DOI: 10.1523/JNEUROSCI.4742-11.2012

[52] Bachstetter AD, Xing B, de Almeida L, Dimayuga ER, Watterson DM and Van Eldik LJ. Microglial p38a MAPK is a key regulator of proinflammatory cytokine up-regulation induced by toll-like receptor (TLR) ligands or beta-amyloid (Ab). J Neuroinflammation. 2011;8:79. DOI: 10.1186/1742-2094-8-79

[53] Garcia-Alloza M, Robbins EM, Zhang-Nunes SX, Purcell SM, Betensky RA, Raju S, Prada C, Greenberg SM, Bacskai BJ, Frosch MP. Characterization of amyloid deposition in the APPswe/PS1dE9 mouse model of Alzheimer disease.Neurobiol Dis. 2006;24:516–524. [PubMed: 17029828]. DOI:10.1016/j.nbd.2006.08.017

[54] Boche D andNicoll JA. (2008). SYMPOSIUM: Clearance of Aβ from the Brain in Alzheimer' Disease: the role of the immune system in clearance of Aβ from the Brain. Brain Patholo. 2008; 18(2):267–278. DOI:10.1111/j.1750-3639.2008.00134.x

[55] Solomon B, Koppel R, Hanan E, et al. Monoclonal antibodies inhibit in vitro fibrillar aggregation of the Alzheimer beta-amyloid peptide. Proc Natl Acad Sci U S A. 1996;93:452–455. http://www.ncbi.nlm.nih.gov/pmc/articles/PMC40256/

[56] Fuller JP, Stavenhagen JB, Christensen S, Kartberg F, Glennie MJ andTeeling JL. Comparing the efficacy and neuroinflammatory potential of three anti-abeta antibodies. Actaneuropathologica.2015;130(5): 699–711. DOI: 10.1007/s00401-015-1484-257

[57] Kaushik Sand Cuervo AM. Proteostasis and aging. Nat Med. 2015;21(12):1406–1415. DOI:10.1038/nm.4001

[58] Menzies FM, Fleming A. Compromised autophagy and neurodegenerative diseases. Nat Rev Neurosci. 2015;16(6):345–357. DOI:10.1038/nrn3961

[59] Milisav I, Suput D, Ribaric S. Unfolded protein response and macroautophagy in Alzheimer's, Parkinson's and Prion diseases. Molecules. 2015;20(12):22718–22756. DOI: 10.3390/molecules201219865

[60] Larsen KE, & Sulzer, D. Autophagy in neurons a review. Histo Histopatho.2002;17:897–908. http://hdl.handle.net/10201/20821

[61] Komatsu M, Waguri S, Chiba T, Murata S, Iwata JI, Tanida I and Tanaka K. Loss of autophagy in the central nervous system causes neurodegeneration in mice. Nature. 2006;441(7095):880–884. DOI:10.1038/nature04723

[62] Correia SC, Resende R, Moreira PI, Pereira CM. Alzheimer's disease-related misfolded proteins and dysfunctional organelles on autophagy menu. DNA Cell Biol. 2015;34(4): 261–273. DOI:10.1089/dna.2014.2757

[63] Mehrpour M, Esclatine A, Beau I and Codogno P. Overview of macroautophagy regulation in mammalian cells. Cell Res. 2010;20(7):748–762. DOI: 10.1038/cr.2010.82

[64] Nixon RA, Yang DS. Autophagy failure in Alzheimer's diseaselocating the primary defect. Neurobiol Dis. 2011;43(1):38–45. DOI:10.1016/j.nbd.2011.01.021

[65] Rami A. Review: autophagy in neurodegeneration: firefighter and/or incendiarist? Neuropathol Appl Neurobiol. 2009;35(5):449–461. DOI:10.1111/j.1365-2990.2009.01034.x

[66] Nilsson P, Saido TC. Dual roles for autophagy: degradation and secretion of Alzheimer's disease Aβ peptide. Bioessays. 2014;36(6):570–578. DOI:10.1002/bies.201400002

[67] Yu WH, Cuervo AM, Kumar A, Peterhoff CM, Schmidt SD, Lee JH, et al. Macroautophagya novel Beta-amyloid peptide-generating pathway activated in Alzheimer's disease. J Cell Biol. 2005;171(1):87–98. DOI: 10.1083/jcb.200505082

[68] Yu WH, Kumar A, Peterhoff C, Shapiro Kulnane L, Uchiyama Y, Lamb BT, et al. Autophagic vacuoles are enriched in amyloid precursor protein-secretase activities: implications for β-amyloid peptide over-production and localization in Alzheimer's disease. The Int J Biochemand Cell Biol. 2004;36(12):2531–2540. DOI:10.1016/j.biocel.2004.05.010

[69] Du J, Liang Y, Xu F, Sun B, Wang Z. Trehalose rescues Alzheimer's disease phenotypes in APP/PS1 transgenic mice. J Pharm Pharmacol. 2013;65(12):1753–1756. DOI:10.1111/jphp.12108

[70] Spilman P, Podlutskaya N, Hart MJ, Debnath J, Gorostiza O, Bredesen D, et al. Inhibition of mTOR by rapamycin abolishes cognitive deficits and reduces amyloid-beta levels in a mouse model of Alzheimer's disease. PLoS One. 2010;5(4):e9979. http://dx.doi.org/10.1371/journal.pone.0009979

[71] Majumder S, Richardson A, Strong R and Oddo S. Inducing autophagy by rapamicina before but not after the formation of plaques and tangles ameliorates congitive deficits. PLoS One. 2011;6(9):25416. http://dx.doi.org/10.1371/journal.pone.0025416

[72] Caccamo A, Majumder S, Richardson A, Strong R, Oddo S. Molecular interplay between mammalian target of rapamycin (mTOR), amyloid-betaand Tau: effects on cognitive impairments. J Biol Chem. 2010;285(17):13107–13120. DOI: 10.1074/jbc.M110.100420

[73] Cho MH, Cho K, Kang HJ, Jeon EY, Kim HS, Kwon HJ, et al. Autophagy in microglia degrades extracellular beta-amyloid fibrils and regulates the NLRP3 inflammasome. Autophagy. 2014;10(10):1761–1775.http://dx.doi.org/10.4161/auto.29647

[74] Guglielmotto M, Monteleone D, Piras A, Valsecchi V, Tropiano M, Ariano S, et al. Aβ1-42 monomers or oligomers have different effects on autophagy and apoptosis. Autophagy. 2014;10(10):1827–1843. DOI:10.4161/auto.30001

[75] Ewald CY, Li C. Understanding the molecular basis of Alzheimer's disease using a Caenorhabditis elegans model system. Brain Struct Funct. 2010;214(2–3):263–283.DOI 10.1007/s00429-009-0235-3

[76] Luccarini I, Grossi C, Rigacci S, Coppi E, Pugliese AM, Pantano D, et al. Oleuropein aglycone protects against pyroglutamylated-3 amyloid-ss toxicity: biochemical, epigenetic and functional correlates. Neurobiol Aging. 2015;36(2):648–663. DOI: 10.1016/j.neurobiolaging.2014.08.029

[77] Rigacci S, Miceli C, Nediani C, Berti A, Cascella R, Pantano Dand Stefani M. Oleuropein aglycone induces autophagy via the AMPK/mTOR signalling pathway: a mechanistic insight. Oncotarget. 2015;6(34):35344–35357. DOI:10.18632/oncotarget.6119

[78] Koronyo-Hamaoui M, Koronyo Y, Ljubimov AV, Miller CA, Ko MK, Black KL, Schwartz M, Farkas DL. Identification of amyloid plaques in retinas from Alzheimer's patients and noninvasive in vivo optical imaging of retinal plaques in a mouse model. Neuroimage. 2011 Jan;54Suppl(1):S204–S217. PubMed.

[79] Alexandrov PN, Pogue A, Bhattacharjee S, Lukiw WJ. Retinal amyloid peptides and complement factor H in transgenic models of Alzheimer's disease. Neuroreport. 2011 Aug 24;22(12):623–627. PubMed.

[80] Tian T, Zhang B, Jia Y, Li Z. Can the lens model provide a biomarker for Alzheimer's disease? Brain Pathol. 2013 Nov;23(6):696. PubMed.

[81] Goldstein LE, Muffat JA, Cherny RA, Moir RD, Ericsson MH, Huang X, Mavros C, Coccia JA, Faget KY, Fitch KA, Masters CL, Tanzi RE, Chylack LT, Bush AI. Cytosolic beta-amyloid deposition and supranuclear cataracts in lenses from people with Alzheimer's disease. Lancet. 2003 Apr 12;361(9365):1258–1265. PubMed.

[82] Li G, Percontino L, Sun Q, Qazi AS, Frederikse PH. Beta-amyloid secretases and beta-amloid degrading enzyme expression in lens. Mol Vis. 2003 May 1;9:179–183. PubMed.

[83] Anderson DH, Talaga KC, Rivest AJ, Barron E, Hageman GS and Johnson LV. Characterization of β amyloid assemblies in drusen: the deposits associated with aging and age-related macular degeneration. Exp Eye Res. 2004;78(2):243–256.

[84] Wang DS, Dickson DW andMalter JS. β-Amyloid degradation and Alzheimer's disease. BioMed Res Int., 2006, 1–12.

[85] Soura V, Stewart-Parker M, Williams TL, Ratnayaka A,Atherton J, Gorringe K et al. Visualization of co localizationin Abeta42-administered neuroblastoma cells reveal-slysosome damage and autophagosome accumulationrelated to cell death. Biochem J. 2012;441(2):579–590.

[86] Wu F, Yao PJ. Clathrin-mediated endocytosis andAlzheimer's disease: an update. Ageing Res Rev. 2009;8(3):147–149.

Chapter 9

Alzheimer's Disease: From Animal Models to the Human Syndrome

Erika Orta-Salazar, Isaac Vargas-Rodríguez,
Susana A Castro-Chavira,
Alfredo I. Feria-Velasco and Sofía Díaz-Cintra

Additional information is available at the end of the chapter

http://dx.doi.org/10.5772/64619

Abstract

Some animal models, genetically modified (such as murine) and sporadic (as others species), enable the study of the origin of specific lesions observed in human neurodegenerative diseases. In particular, Alzheimer's disease (AD) models have been designed to test the hypothesis that certain lesions are associated with functional and morphological changes beginning with memory loss and impairment in activities of daily life. This review compares and evaluates the phenotypes of different AD animal models, on the basis of the specific objectives of each study, with the purpose of encompassing their contributions to the comprehension of the AD signs and symptoms in humans. All these models contribute to the comprehension of the human AD mechanisms regarding the heterogeneity of AD phenotypes: the overlap between AD and age-related changes, the variability of AD onset (early or late), the probable reactiveness of amyloid-β and tau proteins, the scarcity of senile plaques and/or neurofibrillary tangles in some AD cases, the spatial correlation of the pathology and cerebral blood vessels, and the immunological responses (microglial aging) and synaptopathy. Altogether, these considerations may contribute to find therapies to treat and prevent this disease.

Keywords: Alzheimer's disease, nutritional risk, murine, human, genetic Alzheimer's disease, sporadic Alzheimer's disease

1. Introduction

Alzheimer's disease (AD) is one of the major progressive and irreversible neurodegenerative diseases associated with aging [1]. The first case was identified by Dr. Alois Alzheimer in 1901 who presented the clinical and neuropathological characteristics of this disease on November 3, 1906 at the 37th meeting of the Society of Southwest German Psychiatrists in Tübingen, Germany [2]. AD is a progressively degenerative disease that destroys the patient's functional capacity and is the primary cause for loss of functional capacity among the elderly in developed countries [3]. AD accounts for 60–80% of all dementia cases, as described in the Organisation for Economic Cooperation and Development (OECD) report. The number of people worldwide living with AD was estimated at between 27 million and 36 million in 2016 [4, 5]. AD symptoms worsen over time at a variable rate; on average; AD patients live between 4 and 8 years after diagnosis, but they could live until 20 years, depending on various factors. Once installed, three main stages of pathological progression of AD have been defined, namely early, middle and late.

In the early stage, a person may have memory lapses, such as forgetting familiar words or names, losing or misplacing a valuable object, or being unable to plan or organize. The middle stage is the longest and can last many years. The person with middle stage AD may confuse words, become easily frustrated or angry, and has increased difficulty expressing thoughts and performing routine tasks. In late stage or severe dementia, the person loses the ability to respond to the environment, to carry on a conversation and, eventually, to control movement; memory and cognitive skills continue to worsen, personality changes may occur and individuals need extensive help with daily activities [5]. According to the age of onset, AD can be classified as: early-onset or familial AD accounting for only 5–10 % of AD cases, or late-onset or sporadic AD accounting for the rest of the AD cases. Familial AD is associated with mutations in the genes for presenilin (PS) 1 and 2 and/or amyloid precursor protein (APP); its symptoms appear at 30–50 years of age, whereas the majority of sporadic cases develop after age 65 [6].

AD is a multifactorial disease that is a pathologically and etiologically complex. There are a few causative genes which have been linked to the relatively small proportion of patients with early-onset familial AD [7]. The molecular analysis of families with early-onset AD has made it possible to identify mutations in genes associated with the disease: APP, PS 1 and PS 2, and the mean onset age is 45. Mutations in Apolipoprotein E $\varepsilon 4$ (Apo E $\varepsilon 4$) genes are present in 15–20% of AD cases appearing after 65 years of age. Three additional genes.

There are numerous hypotheses to explain the appearance of sporadic AD, such as head trauma, neuroinflammation, poor dietary habits and the lack of exercise, but the cause is still unknown [8, 9]. A possible explanation is that the abundant knowledge of AD biochemistry has not yet been well integrated into the cellular context of brain [10].

In order to elucidate the AD etiology, animal models that have genetic mutations linked to familial AD and show the same disease progression pattern have been developed. These models are either based on: (1) the overexpression of APP and secretases [11, 12]; (2) mutated APP [13, 14]; or (3) the overexpression of human APP (hAPP) together with mutated forms of

http://dx.doi.org/10.5772/64619

PS [15]. Notwithstanding these mutations, such mouse models rarely develop neurofibrillary tangles (NFTs). To simulate tau pathology, a microtubule-associated protein tau (MAPT) mutation associated with frontotemporal dementia is included in the 3xTg-AD mouse, in which the expression of hAPP and mutated forms of PS and tau are combined [16, 17]. Currently, at least 11 rodent models that exhibit AD characteristics, such as Aβ accumulation, tau pathology, neuronal loss and pathophysiology of glial cells, are being studied [6, 18].

2. Methods

For the AD definition, relevant representative book chapters, journal articles and a web page were selected aiming to first summarize the basics of well-established knowledge on Alzheimer's disease that included its biochemical, neuropathological and physiological features. Then, a literature search with the computerized PubMed data base was conducted in February, 2016 with no limit of date. We used the following search terms: (Malnutrition AND Senescence), (Malnutrition AND Alzheimer), and (Senescence). Then, relevant references cited in papers found via this search were reviewed. Studies were selected if they either provided updated information on the AD basics or regarding the biological mechanisms underlying Alzheimer's disease. Case studies were excluded. A total of 170 journal articles, four book chapters and a web page were selected.

3. Histopathological brain changes in AD

Autopsy studies examining the incidence of neuropathological lesions and clinical symptoms reveal that AD often occurs in conjunction with other pathologies, specifically, vascular and Lewy body dementias. The overlap of pathologies suggests the existence of common pathophysiological mechanisms [19].

In AD brains, many cellular and molecular changes coincide with changes in the proteins and genes implicated. The two primary lesions associated with AD are NFTs and the senile plaques first described by Alois Alzheimer. Graeber and co-workers explained in 1998 that the tissue sections of cerebral cortex from Auguste D had numerous NFTs and many amyloid plaques, especially in the upper cortical layer of the brain [20]. In this tissue, NFTs can be seen as accumulations of abnormally phosphorylated tau protein within the perikaryal cytoplasm of cortical neurons, and senile plaques consist of a central core of amyloid-β (Aβ), a 4-kD peptide, surrounded by abnormally configured neuronal processes or neurites; the neurites are localized similarly in animal models such as the PDAPP first model, which develops plaques and cognitive deficits similar to those in humans [13].

These histopathological features start in the temporal lobe and extend to the Meynert nucleus that projects to the hippocampus and to the frontal, parietal and occipital cortices, all of which have important roles in the control of cognitive functions; gradually, these lesions destroy a person's memory and ability to learn, to reason, to communicate and to carry out daily activities

[21, 22]. The first histopathological lesion is the intracellular NFT, which consists largely of twisted, hyperphosphorylated filaments of the microtubule-associated protein tau. The second lesion type is the extracellular plaque of differently sized, small amyloid peptides called Aβ that are derived via sequential proteolytic cleavages of APP [23]. The two types of lesions seem to form independently, with tangles appearing first [24]. Affected regions typically exhibit synaptic and neuronal loss, with cholinergic and glutamatergic neurons being the most affected [25], as well as inflammation, gliosis, oxidative stress and neuronal dystrophy [8].

3.1. Brain atrophy and traumatic brain injury

New technologies based on structural and functional neuroimaging and on the biochemical analysis of cerebrospinal fluid have established interesting correlates of intracerebral amyloidosis in individuals with mild, pre-dementia symptoms.

Whole brain volume changes are used as surrogate markers for AD neuropathology in clinical studies; the extent to which these changes can be attributed to pathological features of AD in the aging brain may be established using other signs of brain atrophy in patients showing cognitive impairment [26]. The relationship between pathology and brain atrophy is not simple and linear; neither is the distinction between normal aging and the disease, which is a complicated issue. Aging, dementia diagnosis and AD pathologies closely correlate with enlargement of the brain ventricles but not with reduced total brain volume. Ventricle enlargement may be a response to various conditions and reflect changes in both white and gray matter of the brain, and may be related to cerebrovascular disease and AD. Clinically, brain atrophy in AD patients precedes symptoms. Researchers have proposed using brain atrophy as a surrogate marker for pathology in clinical trials and longitudinal studies. For example, decreased hippocampal volume is considered an acceptable marker in people with mild cognitive impairment (MCI) and at early stages of AD.

It is well established that AD leads to nerve cell death and tissue loss throughout the brain. As more neurons die, more brain regions are affected and over time, the brain shrinks dramatically leading to functional impairment. The atrophy pattern involves white matter and largely spares the isocortex and hippocampus, which is different from that reported in AD patients [27]. The atrophy of the medial temporal lobe, including the entorhinal cortex, amygdala and hippocampus, is closely related to impairment for forming new memories. The hippocampus in AD patients may lose 3–4% of its volume in a year, whereas average loss in a normal brain is less than 1%. Thus, these hippocampal alterations are one of the best-established signs of AD. Furthermore, the hippocampus is more susceptible to reduced blood flow, which occurs in cortical amyloid angiopathy.

Some studies evaluating brain atrophy in the transgenic PDAPP mouse model found a reduction in hippocampal volume and severe atrophy or agenesis of fiber tracts, fornix and corpus callosum [28–30]. ApoE ε4 is associated with increased risk of sporadic AD and of conversion from mild cognitive impairment to AD. ApoE ε4 also plays an important role in brain atrophy and memory impairment by modulating amyloid production and deposition [31].

http://dx.doi.org/10.5772/64619

Microglia is the innate immune cell in the brain that, as a result of brain injury like infection or traumatic injury, produces cytokines and may remain primed in a state where a second stimulus produces an exaggerated activation (hyper-reactivity). This response may be triggered by traumatic brain injury, infection or aging [32, 33], which are risk factors for developing AD. Hyper-activated microglia is importantly involved in this process [33–35].

3.2. Neuronal and synaptic loss

Extracellular accumulation of Aβ protein and intracellular accumulation of tau in brain tissues have been described in animal models of AD, as well as in some mechanical stress-based diseases with different mechanisms, such as traumatic brain injury, arterial hypertension and normal pressure hydrocephalus.

Numerous studies dealing with AD have shown evidence for synaptic dysfunction, which correlates with cognitive decline along with an abundance of plaques or tangles [36]. Synapse abnormalities in AD brain tissue were first described by Gonatas and colleagues [37]. Quantitative ultrastructural and immunohistochemical *postmortem* studies of brain samples from patients with MCI to early-mild AD confirmed previous results that synapse loss was an early structural finding that correlated with AD severity. These studies showed a marked loss of synaptic proteins, such as synaptophysin, SV2 and p65, in the brains of AD patients [38–41]. Numerous factors have been associated with increased risk of AD: diabetes, hypertension, smoking, obesity and dyslipidemia [3].

Dysfunction of synaptic communication in cortical and hippocampal networks has been suggested as one of the neuropathological hallmarks of the early stages of AD and has been increasingly referred to as a "synaptopathy", in which the soluble oligomeric Aβ peptide plays a pivotal role in disrupting synaptic function and, thus, in neuronal network activity [42, 43]. In addition, high levels of soluble Aβ oligomers show a strong correlation with synaptic dysfunction, which contributes to neurodegeneration. This reflects the loss or damage to synapses that occurs as the disease progresses, which in turn produces functional degeneration of specific neuronal circuits and consequent aberrant activity in neural networks; however, the exact mechanisms are still unknown. One possibility is the immediate-early gene Arc/Arg3.1 (early-expression activity-regulated cytoskeletal gene, here referred to as Arc), one of the genes known to be vital for memory consolidation and synaptic plasticity. Also, the mapping of Arc expression patterns in brain networks has been extensively used as a marker of memory-relevant neuronal activity history. A recent study by Morin et al. proposes that in 3xTg-AD mice, intraneuronal Aβ expression in the hippocampus could increase unspecific neuronal activation and subsequent Arc protein expression, which might impair further memory-stabilizing processes [44]. Understanding the link between intracellular Aβ and Arc/Arg3.1 protein function should help disentangle the molecular and cellular mechanisms underlying episodic memory deficits during the early phases of AD and could clarify the role of disrupted hippocampal excitability in memory retrieval deficits occurring in early-stage AD-like pathology.

3.3. Synaptopathy

Activated Arc/Arg3.1 is targeted to the post-synaptic density of synaptically active dendritic spines where it associates with polysomes. Arc interacts with endophilin 2/3 and dynamin, contributing to α-amino-3-hydroxyl-5-methyl-4-isoxazole-propionate (AMPA) type glutamate receptor (AMPAR) modulation by enhancing receptor endocytosis. The Arc-endosome also traffics APP and physically associates with PS 1, thereby increasing the amount of activity-dependent Aβ [45]. This may be a positive feedback mechanism in which removal of the AMPAR from the synapse will produce a significant loss of dendritic spines and synaptic activity, resulting in synaptic failure similar to that observed in AD. Activity of the *N*-methyl-D-aspartate receptor (NMDAR) in the hippocampus is also known to be crucial for long-term spatial memory formation and to play a role in AD pathogenesis. The NMDAR is localized at synaptic and extra-synaptic sites where it has diverse functions, from modulating memory strength to neurotoxicity and neuroprotection, and one of the components of the NMDAR-associated signaling complex is Arc/Arg3.1. Other postsynaptic elements are the lipid rafts (subdomains of the plasma membrane that contain high concentrations of cholesterol and glycosphingolipids), which are involved in cell signaling and with the NMDAR complex. Thus, physiological and pathological events such as ischemia and spatial learning can induce movements of NMDAR signaling complexes between the postsynaptic density and lipid raft subdomains. Synaptopathy and lipid raft disruption may be related to the onset of episodic memory deficits during the early stages of AD [46–48]. In order to analyze this possibility, studies have been initiated to determine the content of NMDA and AMPA receptors as well as Arc/Arg3.1 levels in the lipid raft microdomains of the 3xTg-AD murine model of AD at the pre-plaque stage and to understand perturbations in neurons, which may help to explain the synaptic plasticity deficits and long-term memory impairments observed in AD models.

4. Proteins in the pathophysiology of AD

4.1. The amyloid precursor protein (APP)

The APP is a type 1 transmembrane glycoprotein of 110–130 kDa, one of the most abundant proteins in the central nervous system (CNS), and is cut by α-secretase within the sequence of amino acids that comprise the Aβ peptide, precluding formation of amyloid peptides [49]. In the amyloidogenic pathway, APP is cleaved instead by β-secretase, releasing a smaller N-terminal fragment (sAPPβ) and a longer C-terminal fragment (C99) that contains the full amyloidogenic sequence of amino acids. A further cleavage of APP by γ-secretase yields the Aβ peptide. In brain, there is an equilibrium between Aβ peptide production and its clearance [50]. How Aβ is removed from the brain is not entirely clear, but is mediated by two proteins: apolipoprotein E (APOE) and the insulin-degrading enzyme (IDE) that may inhibit its aggregation [51]. Disadvantageous genetic polymorphisms (such as the ε4 allele of APOE) and pathological conditions related to abnormal IDE homeostasis (e.g., diabetes mellitus) that may favor the amyloidogenic cleavage of APP and/or decrease Aβ clearance from the brain will therefore facilitate Aβ accumulation in neural tissues and the downstream effects of the amyloid cascade [52].

4.2. Deposition of Aβ

Aβ is produced by endoproteolysis, post-translational processing of the amyloid precursor protein (APP), which is achieved by the sequential cleavage of APP by groups of enzymes or enzyme complexes termed α-, β- and γ-secretases [53]. The first transgenic mouse (PDAPP) model that developed amyloid plaque pathology was generated by Games and colleagues to express human APP containing mutations associated with early-onset AD; results obtained in these mice support a primary role for APP/Aβ in the genesis of AD and show they could provide a preclinical model for testing therapeutic drugs [13]. Since then, other mouse models have been created that recapitulate all aspects of AD including processing of the APP. However, not all APP transgenic mice have cognitive impairment, cellular loss and other AD characteristics, and they fail to replicate the full human disease. Some models actually confirm that the reduction of Aβ is insufficient to rescue memory function once downstream processes are underway. Conversely, other studies in mice predict that immunization against Abfix might prevent cognitive decline if administered early enough [54]. Also, Schenk et al. [55] studied transgenic mouse models and reported that their active immunization alleviated the burden of amyloid plaque, suggesting a potential therapeutic strategy [56].

Brain injury is reported to accelerate Aβ deposition and exacerbate Alzheimer's disease associated with impairment of cognition prior to the emergence of Aβ plaques. However, the relationships between Aβ levels (Aβ 40, A β42, or the ratio of Aβ 42 to Aβ 40), gender, age and cognitive function were measured in five mouse models (Tg2576, APP, PS 1, APP(OSK)-Tg, 3xTg-AD), see reference [57]. They used behavior tests such as escape latency times in the Morris water maze or exploratory preference percentage in the novel object recognition test. Tg2576 mice, overexpressing human APP_{695} concentration six times greater than that of normal mouse APP levels, show higher levels of Aβ40 and Aβ42 and Aβ deposits that begin at 9 months of age [58]. The APP models express hAPPSw and APP751 isoforms under the control of the murine Thy1 promoter. As a result, this mouse exhibits levels of human APP seven times greater than that of wild-type mice, and its Aβ plaques begin at 6 months of age. The APP(OSK)-Tg mouse expresses APP harboring the Osaka (E693) mutation, and it exhibits intraneuronal Aβ oligomers and memory impairment from 8 months of age. The PS 1 model expresses human PS with the mutation M146L or M146V via the PDGF-β promoter and higher levels of endogenous mouse Aβ1-42/43 [59]. The 3xTg-AD, triple-transgenic model exhibits both Aβ and tau pathologies and mimics human AD [60]. Thus, the possible role of Aβ in AD cognitive decline needs to be further investigated, fueled by other possible hypotheses and explanations [57].

4.3. Apolipoprotein E

Genetic association studies reveal that several genes such as ApoE are associated with multiple age-related disorders, indicating that these genes could play a crucial role in their causation. The e4 allele of the apolipoprotein E (ApoE) gene is the best-known genetic risk factor for AD, because it has been suggested to affect both Aβ and NFT pathology in AD. ApoE is a 34-kDa lipid-binding protein that functions in the transport of triglycerides and cholesterol in multiple tissues by interacting with lipoprotein receptors on target cells; these functions are particularly critical for the central nervous system where ApoE transport of cholesterol is important for the maintenance of myelin and neuronal membranes [60]. Polymorphism of the ApoE gene has been implicated in many chronic cardiovascular (myocardial infarction, hypertension, coronary heart) and neuronal diseases. The ApoE ε4 genotype not only is a risk factor for cardiovascular disease but also it combines synergistically with age, atherosclerosis, peripheral vascular disease or type-2 diabetes to increase the risk of AD [62–66].

The ApoE gene is expressed most highly in the liver and brain; genome-wide association studies have confirmed the ε4 allele of ApoE as the strongest genetic risk factor for AD [67, 68], because over 60% of persons with AD harbor at least one ApoE-ε4 allele, and recent data indicate complex interactions between age, ApoE genotype and gender [61]. In reference [69], Dowell et al. used NMR to study two age groups: a young group (average age, 21 years) and a mid-age group (average age, 50 years); they reported that there are regional white matter brain volume and cortical thickness differences between genotype groups at each age. They raised the possibility that an over-engagement with these regions by e4+ individuals in youth may have a neurogenic effect that is observable later in life. According to a genome-wide association study of cerebrospinal fluid (CSF) from AD subjects, several single nucleotide polymorphisms (SNPs) in the ApoE gene region of the brain were also associated with phosphorylated tau (p tau) elevated levels in the CSF. When cerebrospinal fluid levels of Aβ 1–42 were analyzed together with tau/p tau, a significant correlation was found with SNPs of the ApoE gene. ApoE is also a crucial regulator of the innate immune system, which promotes pro-inflammatory responses that could exacerbate AD pathogenesis [70].

In 2002, Colton et al. demonstrated that ApoE regulates the production of nitric oxide (NO), a critical cytoactive factor released by active macrophages. Thus, due to greater NO production, ApoE4 carriers characteristically have high levels of oxidative/nitrosative stress and a higher incidence of AD, a mechanism that explains the genetic association between ApoE4 and human diseases [71].

4.4. Tau accumulation

Besides the accumulation of soluble and toxic Aβ-aggregates, tau accumulation causes oxidative stress and mitochondrial dysfunction, and it is linked to the initiation of the tau cascade. The tauopathies are a group of degenerative diseases with histopathology characterized by filamentary inclusions composed of tau protein in neurons (NFT pathology). These are abundant in many neurodegenerative diseases, including AD, Pick's disease, argyrophilic grain disease and frontotemporal dementia with parkinsonism linked to chromosome 17 (FTDP-17) [72]. In AD, the presence of neurofibrillary tangles (NFT) composed of tau is prominent, and their density correlates with neuronal loss and clinical severity [72, 74]. Dystrophic neurites are all sites of accumulation of pathological paired helical filaments (PHFs) that appear to be central to neurofibrillary degeneration of neuropathology and that contain

http://dx.doi.org/10.5772/64619

(the microtubule-associated protein) tau as an integral structural component [75–78]. Also, tau processing in AD, leading to the formation of paired helical filaments, is driven by aggregation and polymerization, and appears to be associated with abnormal phosphorylation and truncation processes [79]. Mouse models expressing the P301L mutation causing neurofibrillary degeneration have been generated to study neurofibrillary pathologies [80]; and this mutation facilitates the development in transgenic mice of tauopathies [81–83] that recapitulate human tauopathies [83]; these mice provided the opportunity to test experimentally whether the distribution or timing of neurofibrillary pathology is influenced by the pathogenic mutations that cause AD. However, the physiology of tau protein is different in adult mice and humans; because mouse brain contains only isoforms like 4R, while in normal adult human there is a balance between 3R and 4R isoforms [85].

There is a clear link between type 2 diabetes mellitus and AD, and the use of antidiabetic drugs such as metformin has been proposed as a potential therapy for AD. There is also experimental evidence that metformin may have beneficial effects on cognition [86]. However, it remains unknown whether, in the absence of insulin resistance or diabetes, chronic treatment with metformin ameliorates tau pathology and behavioral performance in a transgenic model of neurodegenerative tauopathy *in vivo.* A recent study by Barini et al. shows how metformin modulates tau pathology in vivo. In P301S mice, they found similar levels of tau and ptau in the cortex and hippocampus with or without metformin, but metformin enhanced hyperactive behavior in the open field test. Due to dual actions on tau phosphorylation and aggregation, metformin may unpredictably impact the development of tauopathy in elderly diabetic patients at risk for AD [87].

In order to elucidate the molecular mechanisms underlying the post-translational modifications of Aβ and tau, several transgenic mouse models have been developed. One of these models is the 3xTg-AD transgenic mouse, carrying three transgenes encoding the APPSWE, S1M146V and TauP301L proteins. Ontiveros-Torres et al. reported the hippocampal accumulation of fibrillar Aβ as a function of age and hyperphosphorylation patterns of TauP301L at both its N- and C-termini: the expression of activated protein kinases and mediators of inflammation was monitored from 3 to 28 months as well. These authors reported that the accumulation of Aβ oligomers results in an inflammatory environment that upregulates kinases involved in hyperphosphorylation of the TauP301L polypeptide. The 3xTg-AD mouse is an excellent model for further studying pathological modifications of key factors in AD [88].

5. Hypotheses explaining AD

5.1. Developmental origins of health and adult disease in dementia

Today, an increasing number of epidemiological, clinical and experimental studies suggest an association between toxicant and drug exposure during the perinatal period and the development of metabolic-related diseases and neurotoxicity later in life. A study called 'The developmental origins of health and adult disease' (DOHaD) addressed fundamental issues in the emerging areas of lifetime neurotoxicity testing, differential vulnerable periods of exposure, non-monotonic dose-response effects and neurotoxic risk assessment. Neurotoxicity during central nervous system development results in permanent changes.

The DOHaD hypothesis proposes an association of early fetal environment with adult size, later ischemic heart disease, hypertension, metabolism, diabetes and insulin resistance, which are risk factors for dementia, obesity and deficits in behavior and learning [89–91]. Aβ-derived diffusible ligands (ADDL) also contribute to insulin deficits and insulin resistance in the brain of AD patients, and ADDL levels can be used to diagnose AD [92].

The brain of patients with AD has deficits in cerebral glucose utilization due to insulin/IGF resistance associated with increased oxidative stress, DNA damage, reactive oxygen species and mitochondrial dysfunction. The consequences of insulin and IGF resistance in the brain compromise neuronal survival, energy production, gene expression, and cerebral plasticity [93]. Thus, inhibition of insulin/IGF signaling mediates AD neurodegeneration by an increase in activity of kinases which phosphorylate tau; accumulation of AβPP – Aβ; mitochondrial dysfunction; generation of reactive oxygen and nitrogen species, oxidative and endoplasmic reticulum stress, and signaling through pro-inflammatory and pro-apoptotic cascades [93, 94].

Since Hoyer [95] proposed that the deficits in cerebral glucose utilization and energy metabolism worsen with progression in cognitive impairment. In addition, Steen et al. proposed that chronic deficits in insulin signaling mediate the pathogenesis of AD [96]. Additionally, AD could be regarded as a brain disorder that has composite features of type 1 (insulin deficiency) and type 2 (insulin resistance) diabetes. Thus, AD could be referred to as "type 3 diabetes", because both molecular and biochemical consequence overlap with type 1 and type 2 diabetes [94, 97]. Recently, experimental studies consider that glucose hypometabolism is an early and persistent sign of AD because brains present features of impaired insulin signaling, a model using intracerebroventricular streptozotocin injections (icv STZ model) to generate sporadic AD that emulates the AD characteristics of Aβ deposits on the wall of meningeal and cortical blood vessels, mitochondrial abnormalities and oxidative stress [98].

5.2. Mitochondria, aging and AD

A major risk factor in patients who progress to dementia is aging, which is characterized by defects in energy metabolism and mitochondrial function. Mitochondrial dysfunction is a hallmark of aging, and it plays a central role not only in Alzheimer's but also in Parkinson's disease [99]; it causes the accumulation of soluble and toxic Aβ-aggregates and oxidative stress, and it is linked to the initiation of the tau cascade. In addition, signaling from the nucleus to mitochondria may be crucial for the regulation of mitochondrial function and aging, possibly contributing to the development of age-associated diseases such as AD. Mitochondria not only play a central role in metabolic pathways, they also regulate cell fate through crosstalk between autophagy and apoptosis. Macroautophagy (autophagy) and apoptosis are intimately interconnected and determine whether cells survive or die [100].

On the other hand, genes define a baseline mitochondrial function, where maternal mtDNA contributes more, and environmental factors determine the rate of mitochondrial function, with less durability producing faster brain aging. Mitochondrial function influences AD, APP expression and processing and Aß accumulation [101, 102]. Also in familiar AD (FAD), the impaired mitochondrial function is caused by PS (either PS 1 or PS 2) mutations, but about 10% are inherited, most of the cases are sporadic AD (SAD). Both FAD and SAD share the features of accumulated extra and intracellular Aβ plaques, as well as intracellular NFTs and cell atrophy and cell death, suggesting a common pathogenic origin on the basis of the intracellular Ca^{2+}-homeostasis disruption tested in a mutant PS with a mitochondrial dysfunction with potential cell death [103]. Xie et al. used APP/PS1 transgenic mice to study the temporal relationship among Aβ plaque deposition, oxidative stress, and cell death, identified Aβ as the mediator of oxidative stress and subsequent neurodegeneration. Oxidative stress began in neurites and was followed by the appearance of Aβ plaques in the surrounding tissue ultimately leading to oxidation in neuronal soma, but the oxidized neurites survived for several weeks. The oxidation in neuronal soma was associated with caspase-dependent apoptosis [104]. In addition, intermediate cellular players, including astrocytes or microglia, responded to amyloid deposits with chemokine or cytokine signaling which, in turn, led to oxidation in neurites.

The Glutamate (Glu) and mitochondria have a relationship in oxidative stress that underlies AD; Glu is an important neurotransmitter in neurons and glial cells, and is strongly dependent on calcium homeostasis and mitochondrial function [105]. Mitochondrial deficits occur early in AD, even before plaque formation [106]. Decreased expression of cytochrome c oxidase (COX) and pyruvate dehydrogenase (PDH) has also been detected in postmortem brain tissue of patients with AD, as well as in animal models. Substances used to maintain brain metabolism in the 3xTg-AD mouse model, such as icariin active component of the traditional Chinese herbal medicine *Epimedium*, could modulate neuronal cell activity, preserve mitochondria and functional synaptic proteins, inhibit Abfix expression and improve cognitive functions in AD mice [107].

5.3. Nutrition and AD

Genetic and environmental factors are particularly important for the sporadic form of AD. Diets rich in saturated fatty acids and alcohol but deficient in antioxidants and vitamins appear to promote the onset of the disease. In contrast, diets rich in antioxidants, vitamins B6, B12 and folate, unsaturated fatty acids, and fish suppress its onset [108]. During the last decade, many investigations have shown metabolic disturbances (obesity and metabolic syndrome) to be risk factors for the development of dementias and even AD [109]. Obesity is related to vascular diseases, and there is increasing evidence linking vascular risk factors to dementia and AD [109]. Instead of exploring the effect of its subcomponents, several studies have assessed the relationship between metabolic syndrome as a whole and the risk of AD or cognitive decline [111–113]. The cellular mechanisms involved in the AD associated with metabolic alterations are now becoming more understandable. It is well known that an optimal supply of nutrients is necessary to maintain normal functioning of the brain. Thus, the impact of poor nutrition (overweight, obesity) on the development of AD and the importance of good nutrition as a preventive strategy to reduce the incidence of dementias and AD are clear.

Malnutrition is associated with increased morbidity and mortality in patients with AD, with sleep disturbances, psychological problems, immobility, falls and increased hospitalization risk [114]. Normal human aging is also associated with vitamin deficiencies. One study in an Alzheimer transgenic mouse (VCT2+/-APP/PSEN1) found decreased ascorbic acid and increased oxidative stress in the brain as well as for Alzheimer's disease [115].

Antioxidant nutrients may help to protect these affected brain regions. Plasma vitamin C levels are lower in subjects with dementia compared to controls, supporting the free radical theory of oxidative neuronal damage [116]. Despite years of scientific, medical and clinical advances in this area, much work remains to discover specific nutritional interventions for the prevention of AD. Promising agents such as vitamins, energy substrates, flavonoids, lipids and modified diets functioning as antioxidants, metabolic enhancers, immune modulators and direct disease-modifying agents await further investigation [117].

5.4. Malnutrition and senescence hypothesis of AD progression

It is well known that adequate nutrition is an important factor in order to maintain cognitive function, particularly during aging. Malnutrition is among the risk factors for developing mild cognitive impairment and AD in which a cognitive decline is correlated with synaptic loss. The synapses are part of the neuronal membrane and are continuously being remodeled; therefore, ensuring the availability of sufficient levels of nutritional precursors (i.e., uridine monophosphate, choline and omega-3 fatty acids) to make the phospholipids required to build neuronal membranes may reduce synaptic degeneration in AD. Also, B-vitamins, phospholipids and other micronutrients act as cofactors to enhance the supply of precursors required to make neuronal membranes and synapses. Vitamin D has a role in brain physiology as well, for instance, by promoting neurotransmission, neurogenesis, synaptogenesis, amyloid clearance and preventing neuronal death [118].

Undernutrition during early life results in deficits in the spatial learning capacity of the animals [118], as shown by a wide variety of behavioral tests, and it is known to cause changes in the developing brain that affect the morphology, particularly in the granule cells of the dentate gyrus [120–122]. Prenatal malnutrition and chronic malnutrition in the aged rats cause abnormal mitochondrial, swollen Golgi membrane system, increase in multivesicular bodies and lypofuscine density in neurons of the hippocampus [123]. Since the mitochondrion is responsible for the production of ATP, its dysfunction induces a senescence response [124]. Furthermore, mitochondrial autophagocytosis is believed to be a major contributor to lipofuscin formation [125]. Autophagocytosis of mitochondria is also prominent in AD, because the accumulated autophagic vacuoles in dystrophic neurites contribute to the local production of Aβ within plaques, and the generalized increase in autophagy in the neuropil could be a significant source of Aβ overproduction in the AD brain. Thus, a link between mitochondrial dysfunction/oxidative stress and autophagy has been reported to occur in AD [126]. In addition, lipofuscin can be used as a biomarker to detect senescence [127], since it is one of the "age pigments", autofluorescent cell products from lysosomes that diverge in number and size among brain regions.

The increase in lipid components is possibly due to modifications in neuronal metabolism with age [128]. In Ref. [129], Giacone et al. proposed the "lipofuscin hypothesis of AD", in which the first step in the genesis of senile plaques is the release of lipofuscin free into the neuropil, where it cannot be rapidly degraded due to its biochemical characteristics. Therefore, the lipofuscin may persist in the extracellular milieu, giving rise to a focal impairment that can initiate the senile plaque and serving as a source of Aβ oligomers for a prolonged period of time. This idea is supported by the hydrophobic and insoluble characteristics of lipofuscin, which mimic those of substances that are the most effective in inducing an innate immune response [130]; the rate of lipofuscin formation is also closely related to oxidative stress [131].

5.5. Senescence hypothesis and microglial aging

Cellular senescence is a terminal phase of mitotic cells characterized by permanent cell-cycle arrest; it can be induced by a variety of stressors, including reactive oxygen species. One hypothesis is that senescent cells contribute to aging by altering cells and its secretory phenotype, as well as to the development of age-associated diseases such as AD [132].

It has been suggested that neuroinflammation, mediated by the brain's innate immune system, contributes to AD neuropathology and exacerbates the course of the disease. Some studies found that a systemic immune challenge during late gestation predisposes mice to develop AD-like neuropathology during aging when there are elevated levels of inflammatory cytokines and hippocampal amyloid precursor protein (APP), altered tau phosphorylation and missorting to somatodendritic compartments. All these effects produced significant impairments in working memory in old age [34]. Also, AD and brain aging share common molecular changes, and AD could be a form of accelerated brain aging. In addition, in AD senescent mechanisms are present in all cells, including glia and neurons. Evidence indicates that vascular impairment is a fundamental contributor to AD pathology, and platelets are generally considered a key element because they represent the link between Aβ deposition, peripheral inflammation and endothelial senescence. AD is superimposed onto the normal process of aging and one important facet of aging is the accumulation of senescent cells that lose the ability to proliferate, and also release cytokines and proteases, collectively known as the senescence-associated secretory phenotype, which contribute to the chronic inflammatory environment seen in the old age [133]. In brain, astrocytes clearly play a role in modulating neuronal function and survival in health but in disease are senescent [134]. Also, human astrocyte lines expressing the toxic form of Aβ rapidly reached a senescent state in vitro [135].

In the other hand, observations suggest that chronic systemic inflammation induces in middle-aged rats intense neuroinflammation evoked by senescent-type microglia and may contribute to the initiation and progression of AD, resulting in cognitive impairment. Also, with chronic inflammatory bone disorders, pro-inflammatory blood cells and bacterial components including lipopolysaccharides (LPS), activate the receptors localized on the surface of leptomeningeal cells, which in turn activate brain-resident microglia to evoke neuroinflammation [136]. Furthermore, the maternal immune response predisposes the offspring to develop neuropsychiatric disorders and can prime microglia cells to produce high levels of cytokines with a second stimulus [137]. Prenatal immune activation of offspring changes the integrity of the gastrointestinal barrier [138], which probably increases exposure to antigens with pathogen-associated molecular patterns, such as LPS. Exposure to Poly (I:C) on the late gestational day can alter cognitive performance in the adult or aged animals [34, 139]. High-fat diets can also cause metabolic endotoxemia (an increased LPS concentration in plasma from microbiota in the gut) with a pro-inflammatory response [140]. This gut microbiota LPS accelerates aging, with an increase in the concentration of pro-inflammatory cytokines and of protein 16 (p16), which is a senescence biomarker in the colon [141]. The senescent cells produce chemokines, cytokines, growth and differentiation factors and matrix-remodeling enzymes, collectively known as the senescence-associated secretory phenotype [142, 143], which can contribute to tissue dysfunction [142] as Alzheimer's diseases [144]. The possible mechanism is that chronic systemic inflammatory challenges induce differential age-dependent microglial responses. Microglia are the resident immune cells in the brain, providing its first line of defense and initiating the release of pro-inflammatory mediators to trigger neuroinflammation in response to autoimmune injury, infection, ischemia, toxic insults and trauma. They recognize a broad spectrum of molecular targets, such as glycolipids, lipoproteins, nucleotides, abnormally processed peptides, modified or aggregated proteins (i.e., Aβ), inflammatory cytokines, and damaged neurons, which are the strongest inducers of microglia activation [145]. In Ref. [99], Wu et al. propose a strong relationship between nutrients, microglia, aging and brain based on the concept of "microglia ageing." This concept considers microglia as the key contributor to the acceleration of cognitive decline, which is the major sign of brain aging. Senescent microglia display morphological changes: fewer and shorter processes, increased soma volume, and formation of spheroid swellings, collectively referred to as "dystrophic microglia." Furthermore, inflammation induces oxidative stress and DNA damage, leading to the overproduction of reactive oxygen species, including macrophages and microglia and promoting aging. Therefore, providing early treatment of inflammatory disorders and controlling microglia aging, may delay the onset and limit the severity and/or progression of AD [136].

Animal models are used to test changes in microglia. For example, in adult APP/PS1 mice, exercise enhances memory test performance and is associated with increased numbers of cholinergic and serotoninergic neurons, and reduced Aβ levels and microglia activation [146]. Dietary restriction also appears to attenuate age-related activation of microglia, resulting in beneficial effects on neurodegeneration and cognitive decline [147]. Dietary restriction suppresses LPS-induced secretion of inflammatory cytokines, and shifts hypothalamic signaling pathways to an anti-inflammatory bias [148].

5.6. β-Amyloidopathy and neuroinflammation in the pathogenesis of age-related AD

The study of the aging organism allowed selection of a group of neurodegenerative diseases which have a similar mechanism of pathogenesis, including the pathological processes of protein aggregation and deposition in nerve tissue. The AD pathogenesis in β-amyloidopathy is a manifestation of proteinopathy leading to cytotoxicity, neurodegeneration and the development of pathological apoptosis activated by the formation of intracellular Aβ [166].

Proteinopathy-induced cell senescence is caused by the accumulation of misfolded proteins and activation of the innate immune system, with the production of pro-inflammatory cytokines, chemokines and oxidative stress that trigger chronic inflammation and ultimately, senescence. Components of SASP and proteinopathy can induces more senescent cells. These cells are resistant to apoptosis, but can die by autophagy. Senescent cells can be the link between Aß and secondary proteinopathies such as tau, α-synuclein and TDP-43 [149]. Indirect evidence that infection could be a cause of AD has been reported, and it was suggested that invasion by a virus could cause activation of microglia and pericytes and ultimately, amyloid deposition [150].

Systemic infections and persistent neuroinflammation are risk factors for developing AD [151]. Mice injected on gestational day 17 with poly I:C (a mimic of virus exposure) show, at 15 months, an increase in APP and its proteolytic fragments, hyperphosphorylation of tau without NFTs and the absence of significant Aβ accumulation, but these parameters have not yet been determined in aged mice [34]. Indirect evidence that infection could be a cause of AD has been reported by Wisniewski et al., who suggested that invasion by a virus could cause activation of microglia and pericytes and ultimately, amyloid deposition [152].

The infectious hypothesis is suggested by the altered blood-brain barrier and the activation of neuroinflammation in the brain, which could decrease Aß peptide clearance. For example, infection by *Helicobacter pylori* is acquired during childhood and often persists for life, inducing a chronic gastric inflammation that remains asymptomatic but can induce systemic inflammation and increase homocysteine levels, contributing to the risk of AD. In animal models of AD (5xFAD), in which glutamate excitotoxicity through NMDA receptors involves neuroinflammation, however, apart from Aβ reductions, improvements were no longer observed in the 5xFAD model during advanced stages of the disease, which may reflect the limited efficacy of memantine in clinical settings [153].

5.7. Amyloid cascade hypothesis

The amyloid cascade hypothesis postulates that memory deficits are caused by increased brain levels of Aβ peptide, which are derived from the larger amyloid precursor protein (APP) by sequential proteolytic processing [154]. This hypothesis is a neuron-centric, linear and quantitative model postulating direct cause and consequences in a cascade initiated by Abfix deposition and leading progressively to Tau pathology, synaptic dysfunction, inflammation, neuronal loss and ultimately, to dementia. Earlier AD mouse models have generated a wealth of information that has significantly improved our knowledge about AD; however, the amyloid cascade hypothesis remains controversial, because the majority of these models are based on transgenic overexpression of APP in combinations with different familial AD-associated mutations in APP or PS 1. Overexpression of APP generates elevated Aβ levels to mimic the Aβ amyloidosis of AD brains, but concomitant with this it produces non-physiological effects and a number of undesirable side effects. One strategy is to introduce mutations into the mouse APP gene and new models (APP^{NL-F} and APP^{NLG-F}) that develop robust Aβ amyloidosis, which induces synaptic degeneration and memory impairments [155].

The quantitative aspects of the hypothesis imply that reducing the number of Aβ-plaques or the concentration of Aβ-oligomers should be sufficient to halt progression of AD. Thus, a minor increase in the $A\beta_{42}$:$A\beta_{40}$ ratio stabilizes toxic oligomeric species with intermediate conformations. The toxic impact of these Abfix species on the synapse but can spread into cells, producing neuronal death; Kuperstein et al. [156], suggest that there is a dynamic equilibrium between toxic and non-toxic intermediates.

In addition, it is well known that diffusible Aβ oligomers are the major toxic agents in AD, and both monomers and oligomers are important for the early diagnosis of dementia because they are potential predictors for the progression of AD and are useful to evaluate new drugs against AD [157, 158].

A quarter to a third of older people has amyloid burdens without symptoms of dementia [159]. Various APP transgenic mice do not have all the characteristics of AD: they exhibit little or no neuron loss and not all of them develop cognitive impairments, even if for three-quarters of their lives they have deposits of amyloid, suggesting that Aβ alone is not sufficient. Thus, they are a model of asymptomatic AD [159, 160].

6. Animal models for AD study

AD investigations have been conducted traditionally by studying human brains (autopsy) or by producing specific brain lesions in mice. The generation of animal models is particularly relevant, because they have been designed to test neurodegeneration with characteristics similar to those in the human brain, allowing us to design new therapeutic approaches. These models are key tools for in-depth studies of neurodegenerative diseases like AD.

Many studies of AD are based on experimental models in mice since their genome is nearly 99% homologous with human [161]. Transgenic mouse models recapitulate the major hallmarks of AD and have been utilized since the early 1990s to explore in detail mechanisms underlying the disease pathology; they have provided excellent opportunities to analyze the bases for the temporal evolution of AD brains and to delineate the basic mechanisms that cause cellular dysfunction.

At present, there are many transgenic mouse and knockout models to analyze certain aspects of AD pathology, allowing the exploration of uncharted territories; they have revealed new pathogenic possibilities, many of which have not yet been demonstrated in humans. On the other hand, some discrepancies between the data obtained in the mice and in man remain unexplained [162]. Mice lack certain important aspects of AD; for example, age is an important factor in AD, but these animals have a short life, between 2 and 4 years. Also, the amyloid protein in mice, derived from proteolysis of the APP precursor, is different from that in human [163]. In spite of that, diverse studies in this mouse model showed the presence of soluble Aβ oligomers at prefibrillar stages that can act as toxic ligands at postsynaptic compartments, driving the synaptic in neuronal populations localized in similar areas to those affected in the human pathology with memory alterations. They have also been instrumental in validating dug targets in special cerebral areas to control memory.

The triple transgenic (3xTg-AD) mouse, which develops pathologies associated with AD, was created in 2003 (**Figure 1**). To produce this model, Oddo's team simultaneously microinjected two genes (APP and tau) into single-cell PS1M146V mouse embryos (transgenic mice that overexpress human or wild-type APP, and are hybrids from the 129/C57BL6 strain). These mice develop both amyloid plaques and NFT-like pathology in a progressive and age-dependent manner associated with anatomical and temporal analogously to that observed in the human AD brain [16]. In this 3xTg-AD, Aβ deposits initiate in the cortex and progress to the hippocampus with aging (**Figure 2**). Amyloid accumulation is localized in the basal neocortex as well as in entorhinal areas, but this accumulation can also expand into the hippocampus. The conformational or hyperphosphorylation changes characteristic of tau pathology occur particularly in pyramidal neurons of the hippocampal CA1 subfield and in cortical structures (**Figure 3**) and evolve in the AD brain [164].

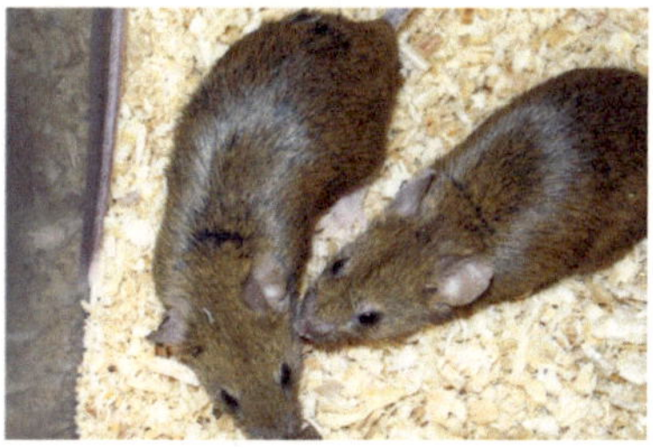

Figure 1. Triple transgenic mouse (3xTg-AD).

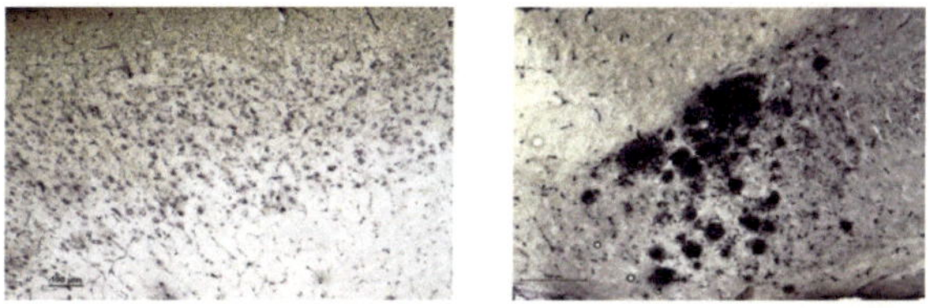

Figure 2. Photomicrographs of the amyloid beta in triple transgenic mouse in the cerebral cortex of 11-month-old female showing the staining for amyloid beta aggregates mice stained by immunohistochemistry using a BAM-10 antibody.

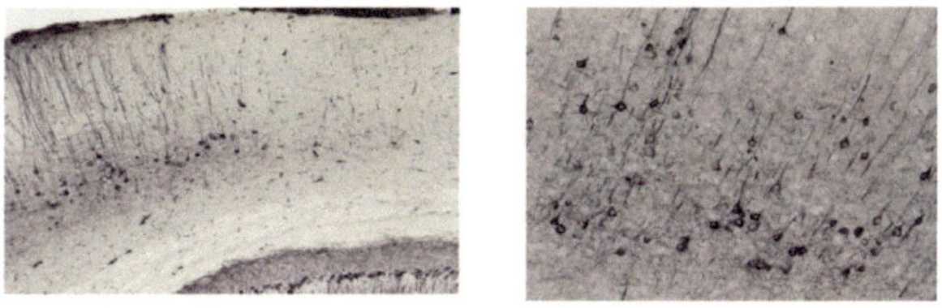

Figure 3. Photomicrographs of the cerebral cortex of an 11-month-old female mouse stained by immunohistochemistry using 499 tau antibody, showing the presence of human tau protein in two magnifications.

Another characteristic of the 3xTg-AD mouse is that the brain regions severely affected, including the hippocampus, entorhinal cortex, amygdala, neocortex, and some subcortical areas such as basal forebrain where the acetylcholine (Ach) neurotransmitter is altered in the brains of individuals with mild AD due to low choline acetyltransferase (ChAT) activity [165–167].

The 3xTg-AD mouse has fewer ChAT-immunopositive neurons in the Meynert nucleus (primary source of cholinergic neurons), as well as a reduced density of ChAT-positive cholinergic fibers projecting to the primary motor cortex and the CA1 area of the hippocampus [168]. These cognitive dysfunctions are caused by massive loss of cholinergic neurons in the anterior basal brain, the area most vulnerable to the development of the pathological characteristics associated with AD. Alterations in cholinergic neurotransmission in the patients' neocortex and hippocampus are associated with the early stages of memory loss [168]. We also found a 50% reduction in nest-building quality (a task controlled by the hippocampus), associated with a significant increase in damaged neurons in the CA1 hippocampal area (26%) compared to wild-type mice [170]. The decreased ability to carry out activities of daily living (humans) or to perform nest building correctly (3xTg-AD mice) are behavioral symptoms that can be studied and related to anatomical and morphological signs in the complex Alzheimer's disease syndrome.

6.1. Sporadic models for Alzheimer's study

A variety of animals can serve as experimental models of AD, which are valuable tools for the design of new therapeutic strategies and to explore some other aspects of the disease, as some specimens develop amyloid plaques in their brain and cognitive dysfunctions similar to those of AD. Like humans, dogs develop amyloid plaques in their brains with advancing age, and some specimens suffer sporadic cases of Alzheimer's disease, age-related cognitive impairment with loss of short-term memory or working memory, changes in behavior, irritability, incontinence, and orientation problems [171]. Sarasa cloned and sequenced the canine APP, finding it virtually identical to human APP, including the peptide sequence corresponding to β-amyloid peptide. They analyzed the presence and distribution of amyloid plaques in the brains of healthy young and old dogs with severe cognitive dysfunction. With specific antibodies against AB40 and AB42, they found that the old demented animals had many amyloid and more mature plaques than older control dogs [163].

A nontransgenic rodent *Octodon degus*, which develops hallmarks of AD, could be a natural model to understand how sporadic AD, between 12 and 36 months of age, develop the accumulation of Aβ oligomers and phosphorylated tau proteins. Moreover, age-related changes in Aβ oligomers and tau phosphorylation levels are correlated with decreases in spatial and object recognition memory, postsynaptic function, and synaptic plasticity [172].

Sparks and Schreurs proposed studying AD in rabbits fed a diet rich in cholesterol and copper. These animals develop amyloid plaques in their brains and deficiencies in learning complex tasks. They exhibit increased immunoreactivity to amyloid β in neurons, the presence of extracellular plaques in the meninges, microgliosis, apoptosis, vascular activation of SOD, rupture of the blood-brain barrier and elevated brain levels of cholesterol; these data provide strong support for the suggestion that copper is implicated in the accumulation of Abfix [173].

Alzheimer's disease is of special interest to neuroscientists, not only because it is the most common of the brain degenerations but also because it is a multifactorial disorder of unknown etiology. In addition, recent evidence supports the hypothesis that persistent chronic infections produce increased Aβ (amyloidosis) in brain, and may be mediated by a response of the innate immune system. This hypothesis may give an explanation of the common pathogenic mechanisms and inflammatory gene polymorphisms involved in both AD and type 2 diabetes. In both diseases amyloidosis, that is, the accumulation of insoluble aggregates of fibrillar proteins, occurs in various organs and is often associated with bacterial infections [174]. Thus, the accumulation of intraneuronal amyloid-β peptide (Aβ) appears to be an early event in AD, suggesting its important role in the neurodegenerative process of AD, because Aβ aggregates, particularly oligomers, may lead to synaptic dysfunction and neuronal loss, which are associated with memory and neural plasticity loss. Transgenic animal models are established to study the pathological role of intracellular Aβ and to screen for drugs against Aβ aggregation and associated toxicity, and they suggest that soluble, nonfibrillar Aβ oligomers may induce synaptic failure early in AD. Despite their undoubted value, the transgenic models rely on genetic manipulations that represent the inherited and familial but not the most abundant, sporadic form of AD [175].

7. Conclusions

This review poses a historical overview of the pathology of Alzheimer's disease and provides an up to date of its features. Then, a molecular and histological follow-up of the proteins most strongly associated with this pathology is delivered. Finally, the diverse molecular and cellular current hypotheses seeking to disentangle the mechanisms of Alzheimer's disease and supported by research in animal models are analyzed. These models have been extremely useful in elucidating the mechanisms of Alzheimer's disease, including the numerous factors and conditions that contribute to the pathogenesis, which may have important implications providing new insight for current and future strategies to treat Alzheimer's disease and to reduce or delay its onset by preventing infection, inflammation and amyloidosis.

Acknowledgements

The authors would like to thank Azucena Aguilar for technical assistance, genotyping and colony management; special thanks to INB Units (Proteogenomics, Vivarium, Microscopy and Behavior). They also thank Dr. Dorothy Pless for proofreading of this manuscript. This work was supported in part by CONACYT: CB2012/178841, CB-2015-01/255399 and DGAPA-UNAM IN203616 and IN203616 to SDC.

Author details

Erika Orta-Salazar[1], Isaac Vargas-Rodríguez[1], Susana A Castro-Chavira[1], Alfredo I. Feria-Velasco[2] and Sofía Díaz-Cintra[1*]

*Address all correspondence to: yodi@unam.mx

1 Institute of Neurobiology (INB), Developmental Neurobiology and Neurophysiology UNAM-JuriquillaQuerétaro, México

2 Laboratory of Cellular Neurobiology, Department of Cellular and Molecular Biology, CUCBA, University of Guadalajara Zapopan Jalisco, México

References

[1] Wolkow CA, Zou SM, Mattson P. Aging of the Nervous System, In: Wolf N S, editor. The Comparative Biology of Aging, Springer, 2010: p. 319–352. DOI:10.1007/978-90-481-3465-6.

[2] Goedert M, Spillantini MG. A century of Alzheimer's disease, Science. 2006;314:777–781. DOI:10.1126/science.1132814.

[3] Mayeux R, Stern Y. Epidemiology of Alzheimer disease. Cold Spring Harb Perspect Med. 2012;2(8). DOI: 10.1101/cshperspect.a006239.

[4] Suzman J, Beard RE. 2011. Global Health and Aging. National Institute on Aging, National Institutes of Health, U.S. Department of Health and Human Services, and World Health Organization.

[5] World Health Organization, Dementia: a public health priority, Dementia. 2012; 112. DOI:978 92 4 156445 8.

[6] Dzamba D, Harantova L, Butenko O, Anderova M. Glial cells—the key elements of Alzheimer's disease, Curr Alzheimer Res. 2016; 13 (8): 894–911. [Epub ahead of print]

[7] Choonara YE. Pillay V, du Toit L C, Modi G, Naidoo D, Ndesendo VM, Sibambo SR. Trends in the molecular pathogenesis and clinical therapeutics of common neurodegenerative disorders. Int J Mol Sci. 2009; 2510–2557. DOI:10.3390/ijms10062510.

[8] Amtul Z. Why therapies for Alzheimer's disease do not work: do we have consensus over the path to follow? Ageing Res Rev. 2016; 25: 70–84.

[9] Zetterberg H, Mattsson N. Understanding the cause of sporadic Alzheimer's disease Exp Rev Neurother. 2014;14: 621–630.

[10] De Strooper B, Karran E. Review. The cellular phase of Alzheimer's disease, Cell. 2016;164:603–615. DOI:10.1016/j.cell.2015.12.056.

[11] Quon D, Wang Y, Catalano R, Scardina JM, Murakami K. Formation of beta-amyloid protein deposits in brains of transgenic mice, Nature. 1991;352:239–241.

[12] Xu ZQ, Huang H, Chen YL, Gao YY, Xu J, Marshall C, Cai ZY. Different expression patterns of amyloid-β protein precursor secretases in human and mouse hippocampal neurons: a potential contribution to species differences in neuronal susceptibility to amyloid-β pathogenesis. J Alzheimers Dis. 2016;51:179–195. DOI:10.3233/JAD-150634.

[13] Games D, Adams D, Alessandrini R, Barbour R, Borthelette P, Blackwell C, Carr T, Clemens J, Donaldson T, Gillespie F et al. Alzheimer-type neuropathology in transgenic mice overexpressing V717F β-amyloid precursor protein. Nature. 1995;373(6514):523-537.

[14] Zhao L, Liu S, Wang Y, Zhang Q, Zhao W, Wang Z. Effects of curculigoside on memory impairment and bone loss via anti-oxidative character in APP / PS1 mutated transgenic Mice. PLoS One. 2015;10(7): e0133289. DOI:10.1371/journal.pone.0133289.

[15] Borchelt R C, Thinakaran G, Eckman CB, Lee MK, Davenport F, Ratovitsky T, et al., Familial Alzheimer's disease-linked presenilin 1 variants elevate A 1 – 42 / 1 – 40 ratio in vitro and in vivo. Neuron 1996;17: 1005–1013.

[16] Oddo S, Caccamo A, Shepherd JD, Murphy MP, Golde TE, Kayed R, et al., Triple-transgenic model of Alzheimer's disease with plaques and tangles: intracellular A and synaptic dysfunction. Neuron 2003;39: 409–421.

[17] Oddo S. Amyloid deposition precedes tangle formation in a triple transgenic model of Alzheimer's disease, Neurobiol Aging. 2003;24:1063–1070. DOI:10.1016/j.neurobiolaging.2003.08.012.

[18] Alzforum, http://www.alzforum.org/research-models. 2014.

[19] Lucke-Wold BP, Turner RC, Logsdon AF, Simpkins JW, Alkon DL, Smith KE, Chen YW, Tan Z, Huber JD, Rosen CL. Common mechanisms of Alzheimer's disease and ischemic stroke: the role of protein kinase C in the progression of age-related neurodegeneration. J Alzheimers Dis. 2015;43(3):711-724. DOI: 10.3233/JAD-141422.

[20] Graeber MP, Kösel S, Grasbon-Frodl E, Möller HJ. Histopathology and APOE genotype of the first Alzheimer disease patient, Auguste D. Neurogenética. 1998;1:223–228.

[21] Whitehouse PJ, Price DL, Clark AW, Coyle JT. Alzheimer disease: evidence for selective loss of cholinergic neurons in the nucleus basalis. Ann Neurol. 1981;10:122–126.

[22] Mufson, S.E. Counts, S.E. Perez, S.D. Ginsberg, Cholinergic system during the progression of Alzheimer's disease: therapeutic implications, Exp Rev Neurother. 2008; 8:1703–1718. DOI:10.1586/14737175.8.11.1703.

[23] Selkoe DG. Alzheimer's disease: genes, proteins, and therapy. Physiol Rev. 2001;81:741–766.

[24] Price JC, Morris JC. Tangles and plaques in nondemented aging and "preclinical" Alzheimer's Disease. Ann Neurol. 1999;45: 358–368. DOI:10.1002/1531-8249(199903)45.

[25] Mattson MP. Pathways towards and away from Alzheimer's disease. Nature. 2004;430: 631–639. DOI:10.1038/nature02621.

[26] Erten-Lyons D, Dodge HH, Woltjer R, Silbert LC, Howieson DB; Kramer P, Kaye JA., Neuropathological basis of age-associated brain atrophy, JAMA Neurol. 2013;70:616–622. DOI:10.1001/jamaneurol.2013.1957.

[27] Delatour M, Guégan M, Volk A, Dhenain M. In vivo MRI and histological evaluation of brain atrophy in APP/PS1 transgenic mice. Neurobiol Aging. 2006;27:835–847.

[28] Gonzalez-Lima F, Berndt JD, Valla JE, Games D, Reiman EM. Reduced corpus callosum, fornix and hippocampus in PDAPP transgenic mouse model of Alzheimer's disease. Neuroreport. 2001;12(11):2375–2379.

[29] Redwine JM, Kosofsky B, Jacobs RE, Games D, Reilly JF, Morrison JH, Young WG, Bloom FE. Dentate gyrus volume is reduced before onset of plaque formation in PDAPP mice: a magnetic resonance microscopy and stereologic analysis. Proc Natl Acad Sci USA. 2002;100(3): 1381-1386.

[30] Valla J, Schneider LE, Gonzalez-Lima M, Reiman EM. Nonprogressive transgene-related callosal and hippocampal changes in PDAPP mice. Neuroreport. 2006;17:29–32.

[31] Yin J, Turner GH, Coons SW, Maalouf M, Reiman EM, Association of amyloid burden, brain atrophy and memory deficits in aged apolipoprotein ε4 mice. Curr Alzheimer Res. 2014;11:283–290. DOI:PMID: 24694076.

[32] Norden DM, Muccigrosso MM, Godbout JP. Neuropharmacology microglial priming and enhanced reactivity to secondary insult in aging, and traumatic CNS injury, and neurodegenerative disease. Neuropharmacology. 2015;96:29–41. DOI:10.1016/j.neuropharm.2014.10.028.

[33] Witcher KG, Eiferman DS, Godbout JP. Priming the inflammatory pump of the CNS after traumatic brain injury. Trends Neurosci. 2015;38:609–620. DOI:10.1016/j.tins.2015.08.002.

[34] Krstic D, Madhusudan A, Doehner J, Vogel P, Notter T, Imhof C, Manalastas A, Hilfiker M, Pfister S, Schwerdel C, Riether C, Meyer U, Knuesel I. Systemic immune challenges trigger and drive Alzheimer-like neuropathology in mice. J Neuroinflammation. 2012;9:1-23. DOI: 10.1186/1742-2094-9-151.

[35] Mhatre SD, Tsai CA, Rubin AJ, James ML, Andreasson KI. Microglial malfunction: the third rail in the development of Alzheimer's disease. Trends Neurosci. 2015;38:621–636.

[36] Lazarov O, Robinson J, Tang YP, Hairston IS, Korade-Mirnics Z, Lee VM, Hersh LB, Sapolsky RM, Mirnics K, Sisodia SS. Environmental enrichment reduces Abeta levels and amyloid deposition in transgenic mice. Cell 2005;120:701–713. DOI:10.1016/j.cell.2005.01.015.

[37] Gonatas NK. Axonic and synaptic lesions in neuropsychiatric disorders. Nature. 1967;214(5086):352-5. PubMed PMID: 6032829.

[38] Masliah E, Terry R. The role of synaptic proteins in the pathogenesis of disorders of the central nervous system. Brain Pathol. 1993;3(1):77-85. Review. DOI:PMID: 8269086.

[39] Masliah E, Terry RD, DeTeresa RM, Hansen LA. Immunohistochemical quantification of the synapse-related protein synaptophysin in Alzheimer disease. Neurosci Lett. 1989;103(2):234–239.

[40] Scheff SW, Price DA. Synapse loss in the temporal lobe in Alzheimer's disease. Ann Neurol. 1993;33(2):109-199.

[41] Scheff SW, Price DA. Sparks DL. Quantitative assessment of possible age-related change in synaptic numbers in the human frontal cortex. Neurobiol Aging. 2001;22:355–365. DOI:10.1016/S0197-4580(01)00222-6.

[42] Walsh DM, Selkoe DJ. Deciphering the molecular basis of memory failure in Alzheimer's disease. Neuron 2004;44: 181–193.

[43] Walsh DM, Selkoe DJ. Oligomers? A decade of discovery. J. Neurochem. 2007;101:1172–1184. DOI:10.1111/j.1471-4159.2006.04426.x.

[44] Morin JP, Cerón-Solano G, Velázquez-Campos G, Pacheco-López G, Bermúdez-Rattoni F. Spatial memory impairment is associated with intraneural amyloid-β immunoreactivity and dysfunctional Arc expression in the hippocampal-CA3 region of a transgenic mouse model of Alzheimer's disease. J Alzheimer Dis. 2016;51: 69–79. DOI:PMID: 26836189.

[45] Wu J, Petralia RS, Kurushima H, Patel H, Jung MY, Volk L, Chowdhury S, Shepherd JD, Dehoff M, Li Y, Kuhl D, Huganir RL, Price DL, Scannevin R, Troncoso JC, Wong PC, Worley PF. Arc/Arg3.1 regulates an endosomal pathway essential for activity-dependent β-amyloid generation. Cell. 2011;147:615–628. DOI:10.1016/j.cell.2011.09.036.

[46] Kerrigan, A.D. Randall, H.L. A new player in the "synaptopathy" of Alzheimer's disease– Arc/Arg 3.1. Front Neurol 2013;4:1–7. DOI:10.3389/fneur.2013.00009.

[47] Marin R, Rojo JA, Fabelo N, Fernandez CE, Diaz M. Lipid raft disarrangement as a result of neuropathological progresses: a novel strategy for early diagnosis? Neuroscience. 2013;245:26–39. DOI:10.1016/j.neuroscience.2013.04.025.

[48] Delint-Ramirez I, Fernández E, Bayés A, Kicsi E, Komiyama NH, Grant SG. In vivo composition of NMDA receptor signaling complexes differs between membrane

subdomains and is modulated by PSD-95 and PSD-93. J Neurosci. 2010;30:8162–8170. DOI:10.1523/JNEUROSCI.1792-10.2010.

[49] Braak H, Braak E. Evolution of neuronal changes in the course of Alzheimer's disease. J Neural Transm Suppl. 1998;53:127-40. Review. PubMed PMID: 9700651.

[50] Roberts GW, Gentleman SM, Lynch A, Murray L, Landon M, Graham DI. Beta amyloid protein deposition in the brain after severe head injury: implications for the pathogenesis of Alzheimer's disease. J Neurol Neurosurg Psychiatry. 1994;57: 419–425.

[51] Recuero M, Serrano E, Bullido MJ, Valdivieso F. Abeta production as consequence of cellular death of a human neuroblastoma overexpressing APP. FEBS Lett. 2004;570:114–118. DOI:10.1016/j.febslet.2004.06.025.

[52] Schmitt, HP. epsilon-Glycation, APP and Abeta in ageing and Alzheimer disease: a hypothesis. Med Hypotheses. 2006;66:898–906. DOI:10.1016/j.mehy.2005.11.016.

[53] Rosenkranz SC, Geissen M, Härter K, Szalay B, Ferrer I, Vogel J, Smith S, Glatzel M. Amyloid-precursor-protein-lowering small molecules for disease modifying therapy of Alzheimer's disease. PLoS One. 2013;18:8(12):e82255. DOI:10.1371/journal.pone.0082255.

[54] Zahs KH. Ashe KH, "Too much good news" – are Alzheimer mouse models trying to tell us how to prevent, not cure, Alzheimer's disease? Trends Neurosci. 2010;33:381–389. DOI:10.1016/j.tins.2010.05.004.

[55] Schenk D, Barbour R, Dunn W, Gordon G, Grajeda H, Guido T, Hu K, Huang J, Johnson-Wood K, Khan K, Kholodenko D, Lee M, Liao Z, Lieberburg I, Motter R, Mutter L, Soriano F, Shopp G, Vasquez N, Vandevert C, Walker S, Wogulis M, Yednock T, Games D, Seubert P. Immunization with amyloid- b attenuates Alzheimer- disease-like pathology in the PDAPP mouse. Nature. 1999;400:173–177.

[56] Awasthi M, Singh S, Pandey VP, Dwivedi UN. Alzheimer's disease: an overview of amyloid beta dependent pathogenesis and its therapeutic implications along with in silico approaches emphasizing the role of natural products. J Neurol Sci. 2016;361:256–271. DOI:10.1016/j.jns.2016.01.008.

[57] Foley JA, Cocchini G, Logie RH, Della Sala S. No dual-task practice effect in Alzheimer's disease. Memory 2015;23(4): 518–528.

[58] Westerman MA, Cooper-Blacketer D, Mariash A, Kotilinek L, Kawarabayashi T, Younkin LH, Carlson GA, Younkin SG, Ashe KH. The relationship between Abeta and memory in the Tg2576 mouse model of Alzheimer's disease. J Neurosci. 2002;22(5): 1858-1867.

[59] Lok K, Zhao H, Zhang C, He N, Shen H, Wang Z, Zhao W, Yin M. Effects of accelerated senescence on learning and memory, locomotion and anxiety-like behavior in APP/PS1 mouse model of Alzheimer's disease. J Neurol Sci. 2013;335:145–154. DOI:10.1016/j.jns.2013.09.018.

[60] Sterniczuk R, Antle MC, Laferla FM, Dyck RH. Characterization of the 3xTg-AD mouse model of Alzheimer's disease: part 2. Behavioral and cognitive changes. Brain Res. 2010; 1348:149–55. DOI: 10.1016/j.brainres.2010.06.011.

[61] Haan J, Roos RA, Bakker E. No protective effect of apolipoprotein E epsilon 2 allele in Dutch hereditary cerebral amyloid angiopathy. Ann Neurol. 1995; 37(2):282. DOI: 10.1002/ana.410370223.

[62] Peila R, Rodriguez BL, Launer LJ; Honolulu-Asia Aging Study. Type 2 diabetes, APOE gene, and the risk for dementia and related pathologies: the Honolulu-Asia Aging Study. Diabetes. 2002;51(4):1256-1262

[63] Irie F, Fitzpatrick AL, Lopez OL, Kuller LH, Peila R, Newman AB, Launer LJ. Enhanced risk for Alzheimer disease in persons with type 2 diabetes and APOE epsilon4: the Cardiovascular Health Study Cognition Study. Arch Neurol. 2008;65(1):89-93. DOI: 10.1001/archneurol.2007.29.

[64] Matsuzaki T, Sasaki K, Tanizaki Y, Hata J, Fujimi K, Matsui Y, Sekita A, Suzuki SO, Kanba S, Kiyohara Y, Iwaki T. Insulin resistance is associated with the pathology of Alzheimer disease: the Hisayama study. Neurology. 2010;75:764–770. DOI: 10.1212/WNL.0b013e3181eee25f.

[65] Siegel G, Mockenhaupt FH, Behnke AL, Ermilov E, Winkler K, PriesAR, Malmsten M, Hetzer R, Saunders R, Lindman B. Lipoprotein binding to anionic biopolyelectrolytes and the effect of glucose on nanoplaque formation in arteriosclerosis and Alzheimer's disease. Adv Colloid Interface Sci. DOI:10.1016/j.cis.2016.02.001.

[66] Harold D, Abraham R, Hollingworth P, Sims R, Gerrish A, Hamshere ML, Pahwa JS, Moskvina V, Dowzell K, Williams A, et al. Genome-wide association study identifies variants at CLU and PICALM associated with Alzheimer's disease. Nat Genet. 2010;41:1088–1093. DOI:10.1038/ng.440.Genome-wide.

[67] Lambert JC, Heath S, Even G, Campion D, Sleegers K, Hiltunen M, Combarros O, Zelenika D, Bullido MJ, Tavernier B, Letenneur L, et al. Genome-wide association study identifies variants at CLU and CR1 associated with Alzheimer's disease. Nat Genet. 2009;41(10):1094-1099. DOI:ng.439 [pii]\r10.1038/ng.439.

[68] Dowell NG, Evans SL, Tofts PS, King SL, Tabet N, Rusted JM. Jennifer. Structural and resting-state MRI detects regional brain differences in young and mid-age healthy APOE-e4 carriers compared with non-APOE-e4 carriers. 2016 NMR Biomed. 2016;29:1–18. DOI: 10.1002/nbm.3502.

[69] Liu CC, Kanekiyo T, Xu H, Bu G. Apolipoprotein E and Alzheimer disease: risk, mechanisms and therapy. Nat Rev Neurol. 2013;9(2):106-18. DOI: 10.1038/nrneurol.2012.263.

[70] Colton CA, Brown CM, Cook D, Needham LK, Xu Q, Czapiga M, Saunders AM, Schmechel DE, Rasheed K, Vitek MP. APOE and the regulation of microglial nitric

oxide production: a link between genetic risk and oxidative stress. Neurobiol Aging. 2002;23:777–785. DOI:10.1016/S0197-4580(02)00016-7.

[71] Goedert M, Jakes R. Mutations causing neurodegenerative tauopathies. Biochim Biophys Acta. 2005;1739(2-3):240-250. Review DOI:10.1016/j.bbadis.2004.08.007.

[72] Gómez-Isla T, Hollister R, West H, Mui S, Growdon JH, Petersen RC, Parisi JE, Hyman BT. Neuronal loss correlates with but exceeds neurofibrillary tangles in Alzheimer's disease. Ann Neurol. 1997;41:17–24. PMID: 9005861.

[73] Kril JJ, Patel S, Harding AJ, Halliday GM. Neuron loss from the hippocampus of Alzheimer's disease exceeds extracellular neurofibrillary tangle formation. Acta Neuropathol. 2002; 103(4):370–376. DOI:10.1007/s00401-001-0477-5.

[74] Kondo J, Honda T, Mori H, Hamada Y, Miura R, Ogawara M, Ihara Y. The carboxyl third of tau is tightly bound to paired helical filaments. Neuron. 1988; 1(9):827–834. DOI:10.1016/0896-6273(88)90130-4.

[75] Braak H, Braak E. Neuropathological stageing of Alzheimer-related changes. Acta Neuropathol. 1991;82(4): 239–259.

[76] Braak H, Braak E. Frequency of stages of Alzheimer-related lesions in different age categories. Neurobiol Aging. 1997;18(4):351-357. PubMed PMID:9330961.

[77] Mena R, Edwards PC, Harrington CR, Mukaetova-Ladinska EB, Wischik CM. Staging the pathological assembly of truncated tau protein into paired helical filaments in Alzheimer's disease. Acta Neuropathol. 1996;91: 633–641. DOI:10.1007/s004010050477.

[78] Mena R and Luna-Muñoz J. Stages of pathological tau-protein processing in Alzheimer's disease: from soluble aggregations to polymerization into insoluble tau-PHFs, in: R.B. Maccioni, G. Perry (Eds.), Current Hypotheses and Research Milestones in Alzheimer's Disease. 2005: p. 247. DOI: 10.1007/978-0-387-87995-6.

[79] Terwel D, Lasrado R, Snauwaert J, Vandeweert E, Van Haesendonck C, Borghgraef P, Van Leuven F. Changed conformation of mutant Tau-P301L underlies the moribund tauopathy, absent in progressive, nonlethal axonopathy of Tau-4R/2N transgenic mice. J Biol Chem. 2005;280:3963–3973. DOI:10.1074/jbc.M409876200.

[80] Lewis J, Dickson DW, Lin WL, Chisholm L, Corral A, Jones G, Yen SH, Sahara N, Skipper L, Yager D, Eckman C, Hardy J, Hutton M, McGowan E. Enhanced neurofibrillary degeneration in transgenic mice expressing mutant tau and APP. Science. 2002;293(5534):1487-1491. DOI:10.1126/science.1062097.

[81] Higuchi M, Ishihara T, Zhang B, Hong M, Andreadis A, Trojanowski J, Lee VM. Transgenic mouse model of tauopathies with glial pathology and nervous system degeneration. Neuron. 2002;35:433–446.

[82] Lewis J, McGowan E, Rockwood J, Melrose H, Nacharaju P, Van Slegtenhorst M, Gwinn-Hardy K, Paul Murphy M, Baker M, Yu X, Duff K, Hardy J, Corral A, Lin WL, Yen SH, Dickson DW, Davies P, Hutton M. Neurofibrillary tangles, amyotrophy and

progressive motor disturbance in mice expressing mutant (P301L) tau protein. Nat Genet. 2000;25(4):402-405. Erratum in: Nat Genet. 2000;26(1):127.

[83] Götz J, Chen F, van Dorpe J, Nitsch RM. Formation of neurofibrillary tangles in P3011 tau transgenic mice induced by Abeta 42 fibrils. Science. 2007;293(5534) 91–103. DOI: 10.1111/j.1750-3639.2007.00051.x.

[84] Lewis J, Dickson DW, Lin WL, Chisholm L, Corral A, Jones G, Yen SH, Sahara N, Skipper L, Yager D, Eckman C, Hardy J, Hutton M, McGowan E. Enhanced neurofibrillary degeneration in transgenic mice expressing mutant tau and APP. Science. 200;29;(5534):1487-1491.

[85] Pintana H, Apaijai N, Pratchayasakul W, Chattipakorn N, Chattipakorn SC. Effects of metformin on learning and memory behaviors and brain mitochondrial functions in high fat diet induced insulin resistant rats. Life Sci. 2012;91:409–414. DOI:10.1016/j.lfs.2012.08.017.

[86] Barini E, Antico O, Zhao Y, Asta F, Tucci V, Catelani T, Marotta R, Xu H, Gasparini L. Metformin promotes tau aggregation and exacerbates abnormal behavior in a mouse model of tauopathy. Mol Neurodegener. 2016;11(1)16. DOI:10.1186/s13024-016-0082-7.

[87] Ontiveros-Torres MA, Labra-Barrios M L, Díaz-Cintra S, Vázquez-Aguilar A, Moreno-Campuzano S, Flores-Rodríguez P, Luna-Herrera C, Mena R, Perry, G, Florán-Garduño B, Luna-Muñoz JL. Fibrillar amyloid-β accumulation triggers an inflammatory mechanism leading to hyperphosphorylation of the carboxyl-terminal end of tau polypeptide in the hippocampal formation of the 3×Tg-AD transgenic mouse. J Alzheimer's Dis. DOI: 10.3233/JAD-150837.

[88] Cottrell EC, Ozanne SE. Early life programming of obesity and metabolic disease. Physiol Behav. 2007; 94: 17–28. DOI:10.1016/j.physbeh.2007.11.017.

[89] Miller DB, O'Callaghan JP. Do early-life insults contribute to the late-life development of Parkinson and Alzheimer diseases? Metabolism 2008;57:44–49. DOI:10.1016/j.metabol.2008.07.011.

[90] Whalley LJ, Dick FD, McNeill G. A life-course approach to the aetiology of late-onset dementias. Lancet Neurol. 2006;5:87–96.

[91] Mittal K, Katare DP. Shared links between type 2 diabetes mellitus and Alzheimer's disease: a review. Diabetes Metab. Syndr. DOI:10.1016/j.dsx.2016.01.021.

[92] De La Monte SM, Metabolic derangements mediate cognitive impairment and Alzheimer's disease: role of peripheral insulin-resistance diseases. Panminerva Med. 2012;54(3):171-178.

[93] de la Monte SM. Type 3 Diabetes is sporadic Alzheimer's disease: mini-review. Eur Neuropsychopharmacol. 2014;24:1954–1960. DOI:10.1016/j.euroneuro.2014.06.008.

[94] Hoyer S, Nitsch R, Oesterreich K. Predominant abnormality in cerebral glucose utilization in late-onset dementia of the Alzheimer type: a cross-sectional comparison

against advanced late-onset and incipient early-onset cases. J Neural Transm Park Dis Dement Sect. 1991;3:1–14.

[95] Steen E, Terry BM, Rivera EJ, Cannon JL, Neely TR, Tavares R, Xu XJ, Wands JR, de la Monte SM. Impaired insulin and insulin-like growth factor expression and signaling mechanisms in Alzheimer's disease—is this type 3 diabetes? J Alzheimers Dis. 2005; 7:63–80.

[96] Rivera EJ, Goldin A, Fulmer N, Tavares R, Wands JR, de la Monte SM. Insulin and insulin-like growth factor expression and function deteriorate with progression of Alzheimer's disease: link to brain reductions in acetylcholine, J Alzheimers Dis. 2005;8:247–68.

[97] Grieb P, Intracerebroventricular streptozotocin injections as a model of Alzheimer's disease: in search of a relevant mechanism. Mol. Neurobiol. 2016;53(3)1–12. DOI: 10.1007/s12035-015-9132-3

[98] Wu Z, Yu J, Zhu A, Nakanishi H. Nutrients, microglia aging, and brain aging. Oxid Med Cell Longev. 2016:7498528. DOI:10.1155/2016/7498528.

[99] Fang EF, Scheibye-Knudsen M, Chua KF, Mattson MP, Croteau DL, Bohr VA. Nuclear DNA damage signalling to mitochondria in ageing. Nat Rev Mol Cell Biol. 2016;17(5): 308-321. DOI:10.1038/nrm.2016.14.

[100] Grimm A, Friedland K, Eckert A. Mitochondrial dysfunction: the missing link between aging and sporadic Alzheimer's disease, Biogerontology. 2016;17(2):1–16.

[101] Swerdlow RH, Burns JM, Khan SM. The Alzheimer's disease mitochondrial cascade hypothesis: progress and perspectives. Biochim Biophys Acta - Mol. Basis Dis. 2014;1842:1219–1231. DOI:10.1016/j.bbadis.2013.09.010.

[102] Toglia P, Cheung KH, Mak DD, Ullah G. Impaired mitochondrial function due to familial Alzheimer's disease-causing presenilins mutants via Ca(2+) disruptions. Cell Calcium. DOI:10.1016/j.ceca.2016.02.013.

[103] Xie H, Hou S, Jiang J, Sekutowicz M, Kelly J, Bacskai BJ. Rapid cell death is preceded by amyloid plaque-mediated oxidative stress. Proc Natl Acad Sci USA. 2013;110(19): 7904-7909. DOI:10.1073/pnas.1217938110.

[104] Cassano T, Pace L, Bedse G, Lavecchia AM, De Marco F, Gaetani S, Serviddio G. Glutamate and Mitochondria: two prominent players in the oxidative stress-induced neurodegeneration. Curr Alzheimer Res. 2016;13:185–197.

[105] Du H, Guo L, Yan S, Sosunov AA, McKhann GM, Yan SS. Early deficits in synaptic mitochondria in an Alzheimer's disease mouse model. Proc Natl Acad Sci USA. 2010;107:18670–18675. DOI:10.1073/pnas.1006586107.

[106] Chen YJ, Zheng HY, Huang XX, Han SX, Zhang DS, Ni JZ, He XY. Neuroprotective effects of icariin on brain metabolism, mitochondrial functions, and cognition in triple-

transgenic Alzheimer's disease mice. CNS Neurosci Ther. 2016;22(1): 63–73. DOI: 10.1111/cns.12473.

[107] Luchsinger JA, Noble JM, Scarmeas N. Diet and Alzheimer's disease. Curr Neurol Neurosci Rep. 2007;7(5):366-372.

[108] Emmerzaal TL, Kiliaan AJ, Gustafson DR. 2003–2013: a decade of body mass index, Alzheimer's disease, and dementia. J Alzheimers Dis. 2015;43:739–755. DOI: 10.3233/JAD-141086.

[109] Kivipelto M, Ngandu T, Fratiglioni L, Viitanen M, Kåreholt I, Winblad B, Helkala EL, Tuomilehto J, Soininen H, Nissinen A. Obesity and vascular risk factors at midlife and the risk of dementia and Alzheimer disease. Arch Neurol. 2005; 62(10):1556-1560. PubMed PMID: 16216938.

[110] Yaffe K, Weston AL, Blackwell T, Krueger KA. The metabolic syndrome and development of cognitive impairment among older women. Arch Neurol. 2009;66:324–328. DOI: 10.1001/archneurol.2008.566.

[111] Raffaitin C, Gin H, Empana JP, Helmer C, Berr C, Tzourio C, Portet F, Dartigues JF, Alpérovitch A, Barberger-Gateau P., Metabolic syndrome and risk for incident Alzheimer's disease or vascular dementia: the Three-City Study. Diabetes Care. 2009;32(1):169-174. DOI: 10.2337/dc08-0272.

[112] Solfrizzi V(1), Scafato E, Capurso C, D'Introno A, Colacicco AM, Frisardi V, Vendemiale G, Baldereschi M, Crepaldi G, Di Carlo A, Galluzzo L, Gandin C, Inzitari D, Maggi S, Capurso A, Panza F. Metabolic syndrome and the risk of vascular dementia: the Italian Longitudinal Study on Ageing. J Neurol Neurosurg Psychiatry. 2010;8: 433–440. DOI: 10.1136/jnnp.2009.181743

[113] Yildiz D, Büyükkoyuncu Pekel N, Kiliç AK, Tolgay EN, Tufan F. Malnutrition is associated with dementia severity and geriatric syndromes in patients with Alzheimer disease. Turk J Med Sci. 2015;45(5):1078–1081. DOI:10.3906/sag-1406-76.

[114] Warner TA, Kang JQ, Kennard JA, Harrison FE. Low brain ascorbic acid increases susceptibility to seizures in mouse models of decreased brain ascorbic acid transport and Alzheimer's disease. Epilepsy Res. 2015;110:20-25. DOI: 10.1016/j.eplepsyres.2014.11.017.

[115] Charlton KE, Rabinowitz TL, Geffen LN, Dhansay MA. Lowered plasma vitamin C, but not vitamin E, concentrations in dementia patients. J Nutr Health Aging. 2004;8(2): 99-107.

[116] Swaminathan A. Jicha GA. Nutrition and prevention of Alzheimer's dementia. Front Aging Neurosci. 2014;6: 1–13. DOI:10.3389/fnagi.2014.00282.

[117] Brouwer-Brolsma EM, de Groot LC. Vitamin D and cognition in older adults: an update of recent findings, Curr Opin Clin Nutr Metab Care. 2015;18:11–6. DOI: 10.1097/MCO.0000000000000114.

[118] Bedi KS. Spatial learning ability of rats undernourished during early postnatal life. Physiol. Behav. 1992;51: 1001–1007.

[119] Cintra L, Díaz-Cintra S, Galván A, Kemper T, Effects of protein undernutrition on the dentate gyrus in rats of three age groups. Brain Res. 1990;532:271–277. PMID: 2282520.

[120] Levitsky DA, Strupp BJ. Malnutrition and the brain: changing concepts, changing concerns. J Nutr. 1995;125: 2212S–2220S.

[121] Almeida SS, Tonkiss J, Galler JR. Prenatal protein malnutrition affects avoidance but not escape behavior in the elevated T-maze test. Physiol Behav. 1996;60: 191–195. DOI: 10.1016/0031-9384(95)02209-0.

[122] Castro-Chavira AS, Aguilar-Vázquez AR, Martínez-Chávez Y, Palma L, Padilla-Gómez E, Diaz-Cintra S. Effects of chronic malnourishment and aging on the ultrastructure of pyramidal cells of the dorsal hippocampus. Nutr Neurosci. 2015;1–8. DOI: 10.1179/1476830515Y.0000000009.

[123] Wiley CD, Velarde MC, Lecot, Liu S, Sarnoski EA, Freund A, Shirakawa K, Lim HW, Davis SS, Ramanathan A, Gerencser AA, Verdin E, Campisi J. Mitochondrial dysfunction induces senescence with a distinct secretory phenotype. Cell Metab. 2015;23(2): 303-314. DOI: 10.1016/j.cmet.2015.11.011

[124] Gray DA, Woulfe J. Lipofuscin and aging: a matter of toxic waste. Sci Aging Knowl Environ. 2005;5: re1. DOI:10.1126/sageke.2005.5.re1.

[125] Moreira PI, Carvalho C, Zhu X, Smith MA, Perry G. Mitochondrial dysfunction is a trigger of Alzheimer's disease pathophysiology. Biochim Biophys Acta. 2010;1802: 2–10. DOI:10.1016/j.bbadis.2009.10.006.

[126] Georgakopoulou EA(1), Tsimaratou K, Evangelou K, Fernandez Marcos PJ, Zoumpourlis V, Trougakos IP, Kletsas D, Bartek J, Serrano M, Gorgoulis VG. Specific lipofuscin staining as a novel biomarker to detect replicative and stress-induced senescence. A method applicable in cryo-preserved and archival tissues. Aging (Albany NY). 2013;5: 37–50.

[127] Merlo S, Nakayama AB, Brusco J, Rossi MA, Carlotti CG Jr, Moreira JE. Lipofuscin granules in the epileptic human temporal neocortex with age. Ultrastruct Pathol. 2015;39:378–384. DOI:10.3109/01913123.2015.1043416.

[128] Giaccone G, Orsi L, Cupidi C, Tagliavini F. Lipofuscin hypothesis of Alzheimer's disease. Dement Geriatr Cogn Dis Extra. 2012;1: 292–296. DOI:10.1159/000329544.

[129] Seong SY, Matzinger P. Hydrophobicity: an ancient damage-associated molecular pattern that initiates innate immune responses. Nat Rev Immunol. 2004; 4: 469–478. DOI:10.1038/nri1372.

[130] Brunk UT, Terman A. Lipofuscin: mechanisms of age-related accumulation and influence on cell function, Free Radic Biol Med. 2002;33: 611–619. DOI:10.1016/S0891-5849(02)00959-0.

[131] Naylor RM, Baker DJ, van Deursen JM. Senescent cells: a novel therapeutic target for aging and age-related diseases. Clin Pharmacol Ther. 2013;93:105–116. DOI:10.1038/clpt.2012.193.

[132] Campisi J, d'Adda di Fagagna F. Cellular senescence: when bad things happen to good cells. Nat. Rev. Mol. Cell Biol. 2007;8:729–740. DOI:10.1038/nrm2233.

[133] Chinta SJ, Lieu CA, Demaria M, Laberge RM, Campisi J, Andersen JK. Environmental stress, ageing and glial cell senescence: a novel mechanistic link to Parkinson's disease? J. Intern. Med. 2013;273:429–436. DOI:10.1111/joim.12029.

[134] Bhat R, Crowe EP, Bitto A, Moh M, Katsetos CD, Garcia FU, Johnson FB, Trojanowski JQ, Sell C, Torres C. Astrocyte senescence as a component of Alzheimer's disease. PLoS One. 2012;7:1–10. DOI:10.1371/journal.pone.0045069.

[135] Wu Z, Nakanishi H. Lessons from microglia aging for the link between inflammatory bone disorders and Alzheimer's disease. J Immunol Res. 2015; 471342. DOI: 10.1155/2015/471342.

[136] Bilbo SD, Schwarz JM. Early-life programming of later-life brain and behavior: a critical role for the immune system. Front Behav Neurosci. 2009; 3:14. DOI:10.3389/neuro.08.014.2009.

[137] Hsiao EY, McBride SW, Hsien S, Sharon G, Hyde ER, McCue T, Codelli JA, Chow J, Reisman SE, Petrosino JF, Patterson PH, Mazmanian SK. Microbiota modulate behavioral and physiological abnormalities associated with neurodevelopmental disorders. Cell. 2013;155:1451–1463. DOI:10.1016/j.cell.2013.11.024.

[138] Meyer U, Nyffeler M, Engler A, Urwyler A, Schedlowski M, Knuesel I, Yee BK, Feldon J. The time of prenatal immune challenge determines the specificity of inflammation-mediated brain and behavioral pathology. J Neurosci. 20056;26: 4752–4762.

[139] Cani PD, Amar J, Iglesias MA, Poggi M, Knauf C, Bastelica D, Neyrinck AM, Fava F, Tuohy KM, Chabo C, Waget A, Delmée E, Cousin B, Sulpice T, Chamontin B, Ferrières J, Tanti JF, Gibson GR, Casteilla L, Delzenne NM, Alessi MC, Burcelin R. Metabolic endotoxemia initiates obesity and insulin resistance. Diabetes. 2007;56: 1761–1772. DOI: 10.2337/db06-1491.P.D.C.

[140] Kim K, Jeong JJ, Yoo SY, Kim DH. Gut microbiota lipopolysaccharide accelerates inflamm-aging in mice. BMC Microbiol. 2016;16:16-19. DOI: 10.1186/s12866-016-0625-7.

[141] van Deursen JM. The role of senescent cells in ageing. Nature. 2014;509:439–446. DOI: 10.1038/nature13193.

[142] Vicente R, Mausset-Bonnefont AL, Jorgensen C, Louis-Plence P, Brondello JM. Cellular senescence impact on immune cell fate and function. Aging Cell. DOI: 10.1111/acel.12455.

[143] Streit WJ, Xue QS. Alzheimer's disease, neuroprotection, and CNS immunosenescence. Front Pharmacol. 2012;3 138. DOI:10.3389/fphar.2012.00138.

[144] von Bernhardi R, Eugenín-von Bernhardi, Eugenín J. Microglial cell dysregulation in brain aging and neurodegeneration, Front Aging Neurosci. 2015;7:124. DOI:10.3389/fnagi.2015.00124.

[145] Ke HC, Huang HJ, Liang KC, Hsieh-Li HM. Selective improvement of cognitive function in adult and aged APP/PS1 transgenic mice by continuous non-shock treadmill exercise. Brain Res. 2011;1403:1–11. DOI: 10.1016/j.brainres.2011.05.056

[146] Morgan T. Wong A. Finch C. Anti-inflammatory mechanisms of dietary restriction in slowing aging processes, in: N.Y. Mobbs C.V. (New York (Ed.), Mech. Diet. Restrict. Aging Dis. 2007: pp. 83–97. DOI:10.1159/000096557.

[147] Ke HC, Huang HJ, Liang KC, Hsieh-Li HM. Selective improvement of cognitive function in adult and aged APP/PS1 transgenic mice by continuous non-shock treadmill exercise. Brain Res. 2011;1403:1-11. DOI: 10.1016/j.brainres.2011.05.056.

[148] Golde TE, Miller VM. Proteinopathy-induced neuronal senescence: a hypothesis for brain failure in Alzheimer's and other neurodegenerative diseases. Alzheimers Res Ther. 2009;1(2): 5. DOI:10.1186/alzrt5.

[149] Wisniewski HM, Moretz RC, Lossinsky AS. Evidence for induction of localized amyloid deposits and neuritic plaques by an infectious agent. Ann Neurol. 1981;10:517–522. DOI:10.1002/ana.410100605.

[150] Honma T, Hatta K, Hitomi Y, Kambayashi Y, Hibino Y, Konoshita T, Nakamura H. Increased systemic inflammatory interleukin-1 and interleukin-6 during agitation as predictors of Alzheimer's disease. Int J Geriatr Psychiatry. 2013;28:233–241. DOI: 10.1002/gps.3816.

[151] Wisniewski T, Ghiso J, Frangione B. Alzheimer's disease and soluble A beta. Neurobiol Aging. 1994;15:143–52. DOI:10.1016/0197-4580(94)90105-8.

[152] Devi L, Ohno M. Cognitive benefits of memantine in Alzheimer's 5XFAD model mice decline during advanced disease stages. Pharmacol Biochem Behav. 2016;144: 60–66. DOI:10.1016/j.pbb.2016.03.002.

[153] Hardy J, Selkoe DJ. The amyloid hypothesis of Alzheimer's disease: progress and problems on the road to therapeutics. Science. 2002;297: 353–356. DOI:10.1126/science.1072994.

[154] Nilsson P, Saito T, Saido TC. New mouse model of Alzheimer's. ACS Chem Neurosci. 2014;5: 499–502. DOI:10.1021/cn500105p.

[155] Kuperstein I, Broersen K, Benilova I, Rozenski J, Jonckheere W, Debulpaep M, Vandersteen A, Segers-Nolten I, Van Der Werf K, Subramaniam V, Braeken D, Callewaert G, Bartic C, D'Hooge R, Martins IC, Rousseau F, Schymkowitz J, De Strooper B. Neurotoxicity of Alzheimer's disease Aβ peptides is induced by small changes in the Aβ42 to Aβ40 ratio. EMBO J. 2010. 29: 3408–3420. DOI:10.1038/emboj.2010.211.

[156] Zhou Y, Liu L, Hao Y. Detection of Aβ monomers and oligomers: early diagnosis of Alzheimer's disease. Chem Asian J. 2016;11:805–817. DOI: 10.1002/asia.201501355.

[157] Szaruga M, Veugelen S, Benurwar M, Lismont S, Sepulveda-Falla D, Lleo A, Ryan NS, Lashley T, Fox NC, Murayama S, Gijsen H, De Strooper B, Chávez-Gutiérrez L. Qualitative changes in human γ-secretase underlie familial Alzheimer's disease. J Exp Med. 2015. 212(12):2003-2013. DOI:10.1084/jem.20150892.

[158] Herrup K. The case for rejecting the amyloid cascade hypothesis. Nat Neurosci. 2015. 18(6):794–799. DOI: 10.1038/nn.4017.

[159] Ashe KH, Zahs KR. Review probing the biology of Alzheimer 's disease in mice. Neuron. 2010. 66:631–645. DOI:10.1016/j.neuron.2010.04.031.

[160] Manzano S, González J, Marcos A, Payno M, Villanueva C, Matías-Guiu J. Experimental models in Alzheimer's disease. Neurologia. 2009;24:255–252.

[161] Duyckaerts C, Potier MC, Delatour B. Alzheimer disease models and human neuropathology: similarities and differences. Acta Neuropathol. 2007;115:5-38. DOI:10.1007/s00401-007-0312-8.

[162] Sarasa M. Experimental models for Alzheimer's disease research. Rev Neurol. 2006;42:297–301.

[163] Janelsins MC, Mastrangelo MA, Park KM, Sudol KL, Narrow WC, Oddo S, LaFerla FM, Callahan LM, Federoff HJ, Bowers WJ. Chronic neuron-specific tumor necrosis factor-alpha expression enhances the local inflammatory environment ultimately leading to neuronal death in 3xTg-AD mice. Am. J. Pathol. 2008;173:1768–1782. DOI:10.2353/ajpath.2008.080528.

[164] Mufson EJ, Ginsberg SD, Ikonomovic MD, DeKosky ST. Human cholinergic basal forebrain: chemoanatomy and neurologic dysfunction. J Chem Neuroanat. 2003;26:233–242. DOI:10.1016/S0891-0618(03)00068-1.

[165] Geula C, Nagykery N, Nicholas A, Wu CK. Cholinergic neuronal and axonal abnormalities are present early in aging and in Alzheimer disease. J Neuropathol Exp Neurol. 2008;67:309–318. DOI:10.1097/NEN.0b013e31816a1df3.

[166] Ikonomovic MD, Klunk WE, Abrahamson EE, Wuu J, Mathis CA, Scheff SW, Mufson EJ, DeKosky ST. Precuneus amyloid burden is associated with reduced cholinergic activity in Alzheimer disease. Neurology. 2011;77:39–47. DOI:10.1212/WNL.0b013e3182231419.

[167] Orta-Salazar E, Aguilar-Vázquez A, Martínez-Coria H, Luquín-De Anda S, Rivera-Cervantes S, Beas-Zarate C, Feria-Velasco A, Diaz Cintra S. REST/NRSF-induced changes of ChAT protein expression in the neocortex and hippocampus of the 3xTg-AD mouse model for Alzheimer's disease. Life Sci. 2014;116:83–89. DOI: 10.1016 / j.lfs.2014.09.013

[168] Boissie F, Faucheux B, Agid Y, Hirsch EC. Choline acetyltransferase mRNA expression in the striatal neurons of patients with Alzheimer 's disease. Neurosci Lett. 1997;225:169–172.

[169] Orta-Salazar E, Feria-Velasco A, Medina-Aguirre G, Morphological analysis of the hippocampal region associated with an innate behaviour task in the transgenic mouse model (3xTg-AD) for Alzheimer disease. Neurologia. 2013;28:497–502. DOI: 10.1016/j.nrl.2013.01.014.

[170] Ruehl WW, Bruyette DS, DePaoli A, Cotman CW, Head E, Milgram NW, Cummings BJ. Canine cognitive dysfunction as a model for human age-related cognitive decline, dementia and Alzheimer's disease: clinical presentation, cognitive testing, pathology and response to 1-deprenyl therapy. Prog Brain Res. 1995;106:217–225.

[171] Ardiles AO, Tapia-Rojas CC, Mandal M, Alexandre F, Kirkwood A, Inestrosa NC, Palacios AG. Postsynaptic dysfunction is associated with spatial and object recognition memory loss in a natural model of Alzheimer's disease. Proc Natl Acad Sci USA. 2012;109:13835–13840. DOI:10.1073/pnas.1201209109.

[172] Sparks DL, Schreurs BG. Trace amounts of copper in water induce beta-amyloid plaques and learning deficits in a rabbit model of Alzheimers's disease. Proc Natl Acad Sci USA. 2003;100:11065-11069.

[173] Miklossy J, McGeer PL. Common mechanisms involved in Alzheimer's disease and type 2 diabetes: a key role of chronic bacterial infection and inflammation. Aging (Albany NY) 2016; 8:575-88. DOI: 10.18632/aging.100921..

[174] Duff, F. Suleman F. Transgenic mouse models of Alzheimer's disease: how useful have they been for therapeutic development? Brief Funct Genomic Proteomic. 2004;3: 47–59. http://www.ncbi.nlm.nih.gov/entrez/query.fcgi?cmd=Retrieve&db=PubMed&dopt=Citation&list_uids=15163359.

Chapter 10

Risk Factors for Alzheimer's Disease

Dongming Cai and Farida El Gaamouch

Additional information is available at the end of the chapter

http://dx.doi.org/10.5772/64270

Abstract

Alzheimer's disease (AD) is the most common form of dementia in the elderly. Currently there is no effective treatment available. Senile plaques and neurofibrillary tangles are hallmarks of AD pathology, and patients demonstrate cognitive complaints with deficits in various neuropsychological domains. Familial AD (FAD) accounts for 0.5% of all AD cases and usually presents before the age of 65 years. Approximately 50% of the FAD patients carry mutations in one of the following genes: APP, PSEN1, and PSEN2. Inheriting any of these genetic mutations increases $A\beta_{42}$ production, which has been linked to AD pathogenesis. Late-onset AD represents the majority of AD cases, with evidence suggesting impaired Aβ clearance. However, the etiology of late-onset AD is more complex. Several findings suggest that multiple risk genes and factors may contribute to the pathogenesis of LOAD. In this chapter, we elaborate some of these factors and their involvements in the development of AD.

Keywords: Alzheimer's disease, risk genes, risk factors

1. Introduction

Alzheimer's disease (AD) is the most commonly diagnosed dementia in aging individuals older than 65 years [1]. The typical clinical symptoms include progressive cognitive decline and memory impairments. The hallmarks of the disease include aggregation of insoluble Aβ peptides and hyper-phosphorylated tau, resulting in the formation of amyloid plaques and neurofibrillary tangles (NFT), respectively, in the brain. Several studies including sequencing, meta-analysis, and genome-wide association studies have highlighted more than 20 AD-associated loci, as well as several molecular pathways altered in AD pathology.

2. Complexity of the disease

Alzheimer's disease is a complex multifactorial disorder, in which genetic predisposition and environmental factors interact with disease processes. The genetic polymorphism of amyloid precursor protein (APP) or genetic mutations of presenilin 1 (PSEN1) [2] or presenilin 2 (PSEN2) are well known to be the major genetic causes of familial early-onset AD (EOAD) [3–6]. These mutations have been shown to induce a preferential generation of $A\beta_{42}$ with a high propensity for aggregation [7]. On the other hand, the most common genetic risk factor for sporadic AD is the apolipoprotein E (APOE) gene (located on chromosome 19) [8]. Subsequent genome-wide association studies identified several new risk genes [9–11]: the gene for clusterin (CLU) also known as apolipoprotein J (localized on chromosome 8), the gene encoding the complement component (3b/4b) receptor 1 (CR1) (located on chromosome 1), the gene encoding PI-binding clathrin assembly protein (PICALM) (located on chromosome 11), the gene encoding the bridging integrator 1 (BIN1) (located on chromosome 2), and the disabled homolog 1 (DAB1) (located on chromosome 1). Later studies identified additional novel risk loci associated with late-onset AD such as SORL1, TREM2, MS4A, ABCA1 and 7, and CD33 [12]. The implication of these newly identified genes in the disease mechanism(s) are yet to be elucidated, with some evidence suggesting possible involvements in clearance dysfunction, lipid metabolism [13] (El gaamouch et al., 2016 in press), immune response and APP metabolism [14].

Studies conducted on cohorts composed of normal and AD twins not only showed the impact of genetic factors in AD [15], but also revealed a considerable importance of environmental factors in disease onset and development [16]. Environmental factors include socio-demographic factors such as age, level of study, life style, physical activity, eating habits, and tobacco or alcohol consumption. Other comorbidities related to life style such as hypertension, dyslipidemia, and diabetes have also been associated with AD pathogenesis.

In this chapter, we elaborate some of these AD risk genes and environmental factors, as well as their involvements in the pathogenesis of AD based on the state of our current knowledge.

3. Aβ and tau

Aβ isoforms are 39–43 amino acid peptides present as soluble $A\beta_{40}$ or insoluble $A\beta_{42}$. In physiological condition, $A\beta_{40}$ represents more than 90% of Aβ while $A\beta_{42}$ levels are less than 5%. A possible function of Aβ under physiological conditions may be inhibiting γ-secretase activity to generate more Aβ in a negative feedback control mechanism [17]. However, under pathological conditions, $A\beta_{42}$ which is found in high concentrations in AD patients is prone to aggregate lacking the ability to inhibit γ-secretase [18–20].

Aggregated Aβ peptides, either soluble oligomers or fibrils, could induce a cascade of cellular events such as apoptosis [21–24], oxidative injury [24–26], alterations in kinase or phosphatase activities [26–29], microglial activation [30–32], and mitochondrial dysfunction [33–35], which trigger neuronal death [36, 37].

The role of Aβ in AD pathogenesis has been extensively investigated by a large number of studies. However, only Aβ accumulation is not sufficient to induce AD pathology. AD pathogenesis requires tau protein accumulation and deposits [38, 39]. Some evidence supports the notion that Aβ deposition induces tau pathology by promoting the intra-neuronal formation of NFT which consist of hyper-phosphorylated tau proteins. However, whether Aβ directly interacts with tau aggregates is still under debate [40].

Tau has been identified 40 years ago as a microtubule-associated protein by Weingarten et al [41]. Tau is a highly soluble neuronal protein [42] mainly located in the axons, which promotes microtubule polymerization and stabilization [43]. There are six isoforms expressed in the central nervous system [44]. Under physiological conditions, tau plays an important role in the regulation of axonal transport, neuronal signaling pathways, DNA protection, and synaptic function [45–47]. During early stages of development, tau isoforms are highly phosphorylated [44], and it is hypothesized that fibrillary deposits of hyper-phosphorylated tau contribute to synaptic dysfunction in AD [48].

4. APP, PS, and other genes involved in Aβ biogenesis

As stated above, accumulation and aggregation of Aβ peptide are part of the starting steps of AD. The accumulation can result from Aβ overproduction or an alteration of its clearance. Aβ peptide is derived from APP as a result of sequential cleavage by β- and γ-secretases [49]. Its elimination is mediated through proteolysis and/or lysosome degradation system.

Forty well-known APP gene missense mutations within Aβ coding regions or close to the processing sequence, are shown to result in an increase of Aβ fibril deposition [50, 51] accounting for an autosomal form of the disease: EOAD [52]. Among these mutations, A673V and E693D mutations have been associated to the autosomal recessive EOAD [37, 53], while 30 other dominant mutations were involved in autosomal dominant EOAD [53].

Interestingly, a recent study conducted on the Icelander population highlighted a mutation on APP gene that has a neuroprotective role in AD. It was reported that the A673T mutation of APP, which is close to BACE1 proteolytic site, protects against cognitive loss and AD development in old individuals. They also showed that this mutation reduced levels of $A\beta_{40}$ and $A\beta_{42}$ by approximately 40%. These results were later confirmed by another separate study [54].

APP is subjected to two independent proteolysis [55] known as non-amyloidogenic and amyloidogenic pathways. In non-amyloidogenic pathway, APP is cleaved by α-secretase ADAM within the Aβ amino acid sequence, thus preventing the formation of amyloid peptide fragment [5, 56–58]. ADAM belongs to the disintegrin and metalloproteinase domain protein family [59–61], and ADAM10 is the most represented α-secretase isoform in the brain. A few rare ADAM10 mutations have been associated with LOAD with evidence suggesting that these mutations disrupt α-secretase and increase Aβ deposition [62]. The amyloidogenic pathway is mediated by both β- and γ-secretases to generate Aβ. The γ-secretase, which catalyzes APP cleavage into toxic Aβ fragments, is formed by a complex formation of four components: PSEN1, PSEN2, nicastrin, APH-1, and PEN2 [53].

While APP mutations account for a small part of EOAD, mutations on PSEN1/PSEN2 have been identified as critical genes in EOAD [63], which are shown to increase $A\beta_{42}/A\beta_{40}$ ratios and promote $A\beta_{42}$ accumulation [64, 65]. After proteolytic cleavage of full-length presenilin to generate N-terminal and C-terminal fragments and assembly into γ-secretase complex, γ-secretase is transported to cell surface where it acts on APP processing and cleavage. Both PSEN1 and 2 mutations increase formation of Aβ species and deposition of amyloid plaques [63, 66, 67]. PSEN1 mutations by altering APP γ-secretase cleavage site promote $A\beta_{42}$ generation [68]. PSEN2 mutations lead to AD with a slower progression than PSEN1 mutations [67].

Besides their role in APP processing, presenilins are involved in many other cellular functions such as Notch signaling and differentiation [69], calcium homeostasis [70], gene expression via interaction with transcriptional coactivators like CREB-binding protein [71]. It was reported that PSEN1 exhibited neuroprotective functions through ephrin-B [72], and that defects in these functions with genetic modifications are implicated in AD pathogenesis. In AD transgenic animal models, APP mutations or in combination with presenilin 1 mutations induced Aβ plaque formation similarly to what were seen in AD human brains [73]. Interestingly, comparatively to sporadic AD cases, patients with PSEN1 mutations had more senile plaques and NFTs developed in their brains, suggesting that PSEN1 may enhance tau deposition as well [74].

5. Genetic risk factors in sporadic AD

Among all identified genetic factors involved in the disease, APOE gene has been extensively studied over the past decade or so. APOE is a major risk gene associated with AD, is located on chromosome 19 [75], and encodes for apolipoprotein E, a 34-kDa lipid binding protein involved in triglycerides and cholesterol transport [76–81]. Three ApoE isoforms which differ by single amino acid substitutions have been found in humans: ApoE2, ApoE3, and ApoE4. ApoE4 carriers present with high levels of cholesterol and LDL in the plasma, which predispose the carriers to cardiovascular disease and AD [82]. ApoE4 carriers contribute to about 50% of AD cases. While ApoE2 decreases the risk and delays the onset of AD [53], ApoE4 multiplies the risk of EOAD and late-onset AD (LOAD) by approximately 3-fold for heterozygous and 10-fold for homozygous carriers [62]. ApoE4 is shown to increase amyloid plaque formation by altering Aβ clearance [83] and promoting fibrillary aggregations [84].

New methods of genetic mapping of single-nucleotide polymorphisms (SNP) provided new information regarding genes involved in increasing or decreasing the risk of AD. Besides well-established AD risk genes described above, nine additional AD-related genes including complement receptor 1 (CR1), bridging integrator 1 (BIN1), clusterin (CLU), phosphatidylinositol-binding clathrin assembly protein (PICALM), MS4A4/MS4A6E, CD2AP, CD33, EPHA1, and ATP-binding cassette transporter (ABCA7) have been unveiled by genome-wide association and sequencing studies [85, 86].

The CR1 gene polymorphism rs6656401 was the first found to be associated with AD in European population [85]. A study conducted on two Canadian cohorts further showed that polymorphisms in CR1 (rs6656401 and rs3818361), BIN1 (rs7561528), and CD33 (rs3865444) are highly associated with LOAD [87]. The CD33 polymorphism seems to provide neuroprotection against AD through inhibition of CD33 expression with a subsequent decrease in brain $A\beta_{42}$ levels [88].

Recent studies have also identified a risk gene: the triggering receptor expressed on myeloid cells 2 (TREM2) encodes an immune receptor preferentially expressed in microglia, which are involved in inflammation and phagocytosis [89–91]. TREM2 is localized in cerebral regions where AD pathologies exhibit [90, 92, 93]. Some evidence suggests that activated TREM2 is involved in Aβ clearance during AD [94, 95]. A study reported that TREM2 mutations prevent its physiological function in Aβ clearance [90]. Autosomal recessive loss-of-function mutations of TREM2 are associated with increased risks of AD leading to development of early-onset dementia [96].

TREM2 receptor is found to be cleaved in the ectodomain to release a soluble fragment (sTREM2) that is detectable in cerebrospinal fluid (CSF) [96, 97]. A cross-sectional study reported that sTREM2 levels in the CSF of AD patients were higher than in controls while TREM2 variant (R136Q, D87N, Q33X, or T66M) carriers exhibited lower levels of CSF sTREM2. Interestingly, R47H variant carriers displayed significantly higher levels of CSF sTREM2 than non-carriers, suggesting that this variant different from other variants, increases AD risk through a mechanism not necessarily involving TREM2 protein expression. This study also showed that elevated sTREM2 levels in the CSF were strongly correlated with levels of tau and hyper-phosphorylated tau but not with $A\beta_{42}$ levels [96, 98]. These observations have been reproduced by another study [97], implicating that elevated CSF sTREM2 levels could be used as a potential biomarker for early symptomatic phase of AD.

ATP-binding cassette subfamily B member (ABCB) gene has been reported to play a role in AD pathogenesis as well. ABCB encodes P-glycoprotein (P-gp) which is essential for Aβ clearance, and its inhibition as a consequence of genetic polymorphisms prevented Aβ clearance in an AD mouse model [99]. Decrease in P-gp expression levels was found to correlate with increased Aβ deposition [100].

Finally, a recent meta-analysis in combination with sequencing study identified five novel genes associated with AD: HLA-DRB5–HLA-DRB1, PTK2B, SORL1, SLC24A4-RIN3, and DSG2 [101]. Their functional roles in disease mechanisms are yet to be characterized.

6. Epigenetic alterations in AD

Epigenetic variabilities such as histone modifications, DNA methylation/demethylation, and microRNA regulation have been reported not only in the aging processes of different tissues but also in neurodegenerative diseases such as AD. These epigenetic changes might play a pathogenic role in disease mechanism [102–108].

6.1. Histone modifications

A few recent studies reported histone modifications in AD [105, 109, 110]. For example, histone acetylation such as H4 acetylation was decreased in APP/PS1 transgenic mice, which might be involved in cognitive deficits [109, 111, 112]. Another study reported increased H3 and H4 acetylation in the 3xTg-AD mouse model compared to wild-type mice [113]. Levels of phosphorylated histone proteins such as HDAC6 and H3S10 were found to be increased in AD brain regions and neurons [114, 115]. Finally, levels of methylation, acetylation, and phosphorylation of histone H3 were showed to be elevated in AD individual cortex [116].

6.2. DNA methylation/demethylation

Genes containing CpG islands are methylated in their promoter regions. Differences in methylation have been reported in APP, BACE, PS1, and APOE genes [105, 107]. For example, one study showed that methylation in APP promoter region was decreased in the brains of old AD patients compared to young [117]. Evidence suggests that hypo-methylated promoter region of APP gene was correlated with an increased Aβ production [118], which resulted in an increase of the genome-wide hypo-methylation, leading to upregulation of neuro-inflammation and apoptosis genes, subsequently applying a positive feedback control on Aβ production [105].

The changes in DNA methylation at PSEN1 and APOE promoter regions are variable based on results from different studies. PSEN1 promoter may be up- or downregulated by DNA methylation in AD [119, 120]. PSEN1 promoter hypo-methylation increased PSEN1 expression which resulted in an elevated Aβ production [121]. The APOE gene presents a duality in its structure; while its 5′-promoter CpG site is hypo-methylated, the 3′-CpG island is hyper-methylated. Wang et al. suggested that aberrant epigenetic modifications in these CpG sites may contribute to LOAD [105, 118]. High levels of CLU (APOJ) gene, due to high methylation of CpG regions in the promoter of CLU, were observed in AD and might be associated with disease severity and clinical progression [122].

Tau promoter region was also found to be affected by methylation changes during AD [117]. For example, $A\beta_{25-35}$ induced demethylation and increased tau phosphorylation and NFTs formation [123], which may be resulted from hypo-methylation of protein phosphatase 2A (PP2A) [102, 103, 124].

Recently, Sánchez-Mut et al. studied CpG 5′-region gene methylation patterns in different brain regions of AD mouse models and found hyper-methylation of three new target genes which could be involved in AD: thromboxane A2 receptor (TBXA2R), sorbin and SH3 domain containing 3 (SORBS3), and spectrin β4 (SPTBN4) [125]. Finally, genes involved in cell cycle and apoptosis were found to be modulated by DNA methylation and upregulated in AD neurons and aging AD brains [105].

6.3. miRNAs regulation in AD

MicroRNAs (miRNAs) are noncoding regulatory RNAs that are known to modulate ~60% of genome via post-transcriptional gene silencing. The alterations in epigenetic modulations by miRNAs may promote abnormal expression of genes involved in AD [126, 127]. For example, Kumar et al. discovered a unique signature of seven circulating miRNAs in the plasma that could differentiate AD from non-AD individuals with >95% accuracy [128]. Similarly, another miRNA-based signature from blood samples has been reported, which allowed disease detection with 93% accuracy and 95% specificity [129]. It was also reported that four miRNAs (miRNA-9, miRNA-125b, miRNA-146a, miRNA-155) were involved in pathogenic signaling in AD brains and increased levels of these miRNAs were found in the CSF and brain samples of AD patients [130].

Within an exhausted list of miRNAs in AD pathogenesis, some directly regulate APP mRNA [105]. For example, miR-101 subexpression decreased APP levels and Aβ plaque formation in neurons [131]. Conversely, miR-16 over-expression may trigger an impaired APP expression [132]. miR-124 was reported to alter splicing of APP exons 7 and 8 in neurons [133], and to regulate BACE1 expression [112]. Over-expression of miR-29c, miR-298, miR-328, and miR-195 reduced BACE1 expression and thereby decreased Aβ generation [134–136].

Several miRNAs were found to regulate tau expression. For example, miR-132 was downregulated in some tauopathies [133]. miR-9, miR-124, and miR-15a were reported to be downregulated in AD, affecting tau levels [78, 133]. The miR-15/ERK1 pathway that modulates tau hyper-phosphorylation was found to be downregulated in AD brains [78]. Altered levels of miR-26a in AD inhibited GSK-3β expression and thus affected production of NFT and Aβ in AD [137–139]. In a mouse model with impaired miRNA production, tau was highly phosphorylated leading to NFT formation in mouse brains [140]. Finally, downregulation of miR-212 was involved in NFT density in AD [139, 141].

7. Gender differences

Sex difference has a strong impact on AD risk. More than 60% of AD individuals are composed of postmenopausal women [76, 77]. Two decades ago, a study showed that APOE4 risk for AD was higher in women. Women expressing just one allele of APOE4 presented the same risk to develop AD as men with two APOE4 alleles [142]. This observation has been confirmed by other studies [142–145]. APOE4 women with a single allele had a fourfold increase in risks of having AD, similarly as men with two copies of APOE4 allele [143]. APOE4 homozygous women exhibited the greatest risk of developing AD and the shortest age of onset when compared to APOE2 or 3 carriers [142, 143, 145]. The gender effects on rate of cognitive decline were also reported in APOE4 female carriers compared to men. For example, APOE4 heterozygous women displayed a faster decline in cognitive deterioration than elderly heterozygous men [142]. Compared to men, APOE4 female carriers presented with a reduced neuronal network connectivity in the anterior cingulate cortex which is structurally connected to medial temporal lobe, showing reduced glucose metabolism [146]. Payami et al. showed that APOE4 female mild cognitive impairment (MCI) patients displayed higher levels of CSF tau/Aβ ratios and tau than male MCI carriers [143]. APOE4 female carriers suffering from mild AD were more prone to have high burden of Aβ plaques and NFT than AD male carriers [147].

Finally, estrogen receptor (ER) has been shown to regulate the risk of AD [80, 148]. Two ERs are involved in this regulation: ERα and β. While ERβ was found to downregulate APOE gene and protein expression, ERα acted on upregulation of APOE expression. Genetic polymorphisms in both ER (rs4986938) and (rs2234693) have been associated with high risks of AD [148].

8. Environmental factors

Cohort studies have shown that educational levels play a critical role in neurodegenerative diseases. A lower education level was found to be associated with a higher risk of developing dementia [149–151]. Based on the hypothesis of cerebral cognitive reserve, intellectual training as indicated by educational levels could contribute to the development of neural networks through densification of synapses and increase of brain vascularization [152]. Intellectual solicitation could then maintain dense networks in working conditions according to "Use it or Lose it" principle. Besides levels of knowledge acquired during youth, intellectual stimulation as frequent practice of intellectual activities in adulthood [153] and older ages [154] appears to be associated with a lower risk of dementia.

Lifestyle has an impact on the risk to develop AD as well. Longitudinal studies conducted in Europe and USA demonstrated positive effects of wealth activities such as social, physical, and intellectual activities on decreased risks of AD [155]. Recent longitudinal studies conducted in general population reported an association of regular practice and/or sustained physical activities with lower risks of cognitive decline and dementia [156–160].

Vascular diseases are precipitating factors for AD. The relationship between blood pressure and dementia is complex [161]. Some epidemiological studies suggest that depending on the period of life hypertension appeared (before or after age of 65), high blood pressure did not exhibit homogeneous effects on the risk of dementia. For example, untreated hypertension around age of 50 increased the risk of developing dementia by four-fold compared to individuals with normal blood pressure [162].

Cholesterol, as an essential component of the brain, plays a critical role in regulation of amyloid plaque formation. However, results from numerous studies of the relationship between cholesterol levels and AD were rather contradictory [163]. Some studies showed that high levels of cholesterol were found to increase risks of dementia by two-fold. This hypothesis led to clinical trials testing the use of statins which lower cholesterol production as treatment of AD. Besides cholesterol, hyperglycemia affects the risks of developing vascular dementia and AD. The risk of dementia was increased by up to three-fold among individuals with diabetes [164].

Finally, the effect of nutrition on AD becomes a growing interest in recent years [164, 165]. Food intake plays a decisive role in the onset of systemic diseases such as hypertension, hyperlipidemia, diabetes, and cardiovascular disease which are closely associated to the risk of AD. Several cohort studies showed a relationship between antioxidant intake and lower risks of dementia and cognitive decline. Aging studies conducted in Europe demonstrated protective roles of fish consumption, which is rich in omega 3 polyunsaturated fatty acids (PUFA). The risk of cognitive decline was decreased in individuals displaying high omega 3 PUFA levels [166–168]. Interactions between fat dietary intake and genetic characteristics (including genes involved in lipid metabolism and transport) are implicated in this phenomenon. For example, similar dietary intakes did not exhibit the same effects on cognitive function in individuals with different genetic heritage. Moreover, conflicted observations were reported from longitudinal studies of the association between nutrient involved in the cycle of homocysteine (including vitamins B6, B12, and folate) and the risk of dementia and/or cognitive deficit.

9. Conclusion

It is clear that Alzheimer's disease (AD) that affects a growing number of individuals is a complex disease endowed with different facets. In this chapter, we summarize the state of knowledge in matters of research on AD based on studies that have contributed to major discoveries in the field. We provide a global overview about current understanding of the disease.

As we enunciated it above, there is a strong genetic predisposition to AD. Mutations and polymorphism in key genes such as APP, PSEN, and APOE affect different aspects of disease pathogenesis such as accumulation of aggregating proteins, defective clearance mechanism, lipid dyshomeostasis, neuronal dysfunction, and synaptic dysfunction. Environmental factors, which most of the time during evolution are responsible for genetic mutations, interact with genetic risk factors and contribute to AD development. Gender difference also has a considerable impact on the apparition of AD.

The complexity and multiplicity of these risk factors make AD an extremely difficult disease to treat. In fact, as of today, even if we have a better knowledge regarding some of these factors, researchers continue to discover new players. These findings raise the question of whether these factors are linked together, which ones are causes or consequences of the disease, how do they act: independently, or in an event cascade starting from a unique triggering factor. Many therapeutic approaches aimed at reducing clinical symptoms or preventing the disease have been developed and tested in clinical trials over the years. However, we have to acknowledge the fact that before we establish the cause and effect link between all these risk factors, and possibly provide a case-by-case treatment of the disease to individuals, it may be difficult to establish an effective treatment based on the heterogeneity of AD individuals.

10. Methods

Article research was performed using Pubmed database and key words such as Alzheimer's disease, environmental factors, and genes were used for database search of articles published from 1975 to 2016. Articles relevant for the review were selected based on different criteria such as topics of interests, scientific rigor, and reproducibility of results.

Acknowledgements

This work was supported in whole or in part by funding from Alzheimer Association (NIRP14-304720), Department of Veteran Affairs RR&D SPiRE (1I21RX001558-01A1), and NIH R01 (1R01AG048923-01) for DC.

Author details

Dongming Cai[1,2,3*] and Farida El Gaamouch[1,2]

*Address all correspondence to: dongming.cai@mssm.edu

1 Research & Development, James J Peters VA Medical Center, Bronx, NY, USA

2 Department of Neurology, Icahn School of Medicine at Mount Sinai, Alzheimer Disease Research Center, New York, NY, USA

3 The Central Hospital of Wuhan, Wuhan, China

References

[1] Gatz M, Reynolds CA, Fratiglioni L, Johansson B, Mortimer JA, Berg S, et al. Role of genes and environments for explaining Alzheimer disease. Arch Gen Psychiatry. 2006;63(2):168–74.

[2] Sobhanifar S, Schneider B, Lohr F, Gottstein D, Ikeya T, Mlynarczyk K, et al. Structural investigation of the C-terminal catalytic fragment of presenilin 1. Proc Natl Acad Sci U S A. 2010;107(21):9644–9.

[3] Chartier-Harlin MC, Crawford F, Houlden H, Warren A, Hughes D, Fidani L, et al. Early-onset Alzheimer's disease caused by mutations at codon 717 of the beta-amyloid precursor protein gene. Nature. 1991;353(6347):844–6.

[4] Goate A, Chartier-Harlin MC, Mullan M, Brown J, Crawford F, Fidani L, et al. Segregation of a missense mutation in the amyloid precursor protein gene with familial Alzheimer's disease. Nature. 1991;349(6311):704–6.

[5] Gandy S, Caporaso G, Buxbaum J, Frangione B, Greengard P. APP processing, A beta-amyloidogenesis, and the pathogenesis of Alzheimer's disease. Neurobiol Aging. 1994;15(2):253–6.

[6] Sahlin C, Lord A, Magnusson K, Englund H, Almeida CG, Greengard P, et al. The Arctic Alzheimer mutation favors intracellular amyloid-beta production by making amyloid precursor protein less available to alpha-secretase. J Neurochem. 2007;101(3):854–62.

[7] Bekris LM, Yu CE, Bird TD, Tsuang DW. Genetics of Alzheimer disease. J Geriatr Psychiatry Neurol. 2010;23(4):213–27.

[8] Lambert JC, Amouyel P. Genetic heterogeneity of Alzheimer's disease: complexity and advances. Psychoneuroendocrinology. 2007;32(Suppl 1):S62–70.

[9] Lambert JC, Heath S, Even G, Campion D, Sleegers K, Hiltunen M, et al. Genome-wide association study identifies variants at CLU and CR1 associated with Alzheimer's disease. Nat Genet. 2009;41(10):1094–9.

[10] Harold D, Abraham R, Hollingworth P, Sims R, Gerrish A, Hamshere ML, et al. Genome-wide association study identifies variants at CLU and PICALM associated with Alzheimer's disease. Nat Genet. 2009;41(10):1088–93.

[11] Hu X, Pickering E, Liu YC, Hall S, Fournier H, Katz E, et al. Meta-analysis for genome-wide association study identifies multiple variants at the BIN1 locus associated with late-onset Alzheimer's disease. PLoS One. 2011;6(2):e16616.

[12] Allen M, Zou F, Chai HS, Younkin CS, Crook J, Pankratz VS, et al. Novel late-onset Alzheimer disease loci variants associate with brain gene expression. Neurology. 2012;79(3):221–8.

[13] Zhu L, Zhong M, Elder GA, Sano M, Holtzman DM, Gandy S, et al. Phospholipid dysregulation contributes to ApoE4-associated cognitive deficits in Alzheimer's disease pathogenesis. Proc Natl Acad Sci U S A. 2015;112(38):11965–70.

[14] De Strooper B, Karran E. The cellular phase of Alzheimer's disease. Cell. 2016;164(4): 603–15.

[15] Gatz M, Mortimer JA, Fratiglioni L, Johansson B, Berg S, Reynolds CA, et al. Potentially modifiable risk factors for dementia in identical twins. Alzheimers Dement. 2006;2(2): 110–7.

[16] Bird TD. Genetic factors in Alzheimer's disease. N Engl J Med. 2005;352(9):862–4.

[17] Kamenetz F, Tomita T, Hsieh H, Seabrook G, Borchelt D, Iwatsubo T, et al. APP processing and synaptic function. Neuron. 2003;37(6):925–37.

[18] Burdick D, Soreghan B, Kwon M, Kosmoski J, Knauer M, Henschen A, et al. Assembly and aggregation properties of synthetic Alzheimer's A4/beta amyloid peptide analogs. J Biol Chem. 1992;267(1):546–54.

[19] Gravina SA, Ho L, Eckman CB, Long KE, Otvos L, Jr., Younkin LH, et al. Amyloid beta protein (A beta) in Alzheimer's disease brain. Biochemical and immunocytochemical analysis with antibodies specific for forms ending at A beta 40 or A beta 42(43). J Biol Chem. 1995;270(13):7013–6.

[20] Kim J, Kleizen B, Choy R, Thinakaran G, Sisodia SS, Schekman RW. Biogenesis of gamma-secretase early in the secretory pathway. J Cell Biol. 2007;179(5):951–63.

[21] Small DH, Mok SS, Bornstein JC. Alzheimer's disease and Abeta toxicity: from top to bottom. Nat Rev Neurosci. 2001;2(8):595–8.

[22] Morishima Y, Gotoh Y, Zieg J, Barrett T, Takano H, Flavell R, et al. Beta-amyloid induces neuronal apoptosis via a mechanism that involves the c-Jun N-terminal kinase pathway and the induction of Fas ligand. J Neurosci. 2001;21(19):7551–60.

[23] Roth KA. Caspases, apoptosis, and Alzheimer disease: causation, correlation, and confusion. J Neuropathol Exp Neurol. 2001;60(9):829–38.

[24] Zhu N, Lin J, Wang K, Wei M, Chen Q, Wang Y. Huperzine A protects neural stem cells against Abeta-induced apoptosis in a neural stem cells and microglia co-culture system. Int J Clin Exp Pathol. 2015;8(6):6425–33.

[25] Yatin SM, Varadarajan S, Link CD, Butterfield DA. In vitro and in vivo oxidative stress associated with Alzheimer's amyloid beta-peptide (1–42). Neurobiol Aging. 1999;20(3): 325–30; discussion 39–42.

[26] Varadarajan S, Yatin S, Aksenova M, Butterfield DA. Review: Alzheimer's amyloid beta-peptide-associated free radical oxidative stress and neurotoxicity. J Struct Biol. 2000;130(2–3):184–208.

[27] Mark RJ, Hensley K, Butterfield DA, Mattson MP. Amyloid beta-peptide impairs ion-motive ATPase activities: evidence for a role in loss of neuronal Ca2+ homeostasis and cell death. J Neurosci. 1995;15(9):6239–49.

[28] Ezeani M, Omabe M. A new perspective of lysosomal cation channel-dependent homeostasis in Alzheimer's disease. Mol Neurobiol. 2016;53(3):1672–8.

[29] Heneka MT, Carson MJ, El Khoury J, Landreth GE, Brosseron F, Feinstein DL, et al. Neuroinflammation in Alzheimer's disease. Lancet Neurol. 2015;14(4):388–405.

[30] Weggen S, Eriksen JL, Das P, Sagi SA, Wang R, Pietrzik CU, et al. A subset of NSAIDs lower amyloidogenic Abeta42 independently of cyclooxygenase activity. Nature. 2001;414(6860):212–6.

[31] Neniskyte U, Neher JJ, Brown GC. Neuronal death induced by nanomolar amyloid beta is mediated by primary phagocytosis of neurons by microglia. J Biol Chem. 2011;286(46):39904–13.

[32] Liu S, Liu Y, Hao W, Wolf L, Kiliaan AJ, Penke B, et al. TLR2 is a primary receptor for Alzheimer's amyloid beta peptide to trigger neuroinflammatory activation. J Immunol. 2012;188(3):1098–107.

[33] Anandatheerthavarada HK, Biswas G, Robin MA, Avadhani NG. Mitochondrial targeting and a novel transmembrane arrest of Alzheimer's amyloid precursor protein impairs mitochondrial function in neuronal cells. J Cell Biol. 2003;161(1):41–54.

[34] Devi L, Prabhu BM, Galati DF, Avadhani NG, Anandatheerthavarada HK. Accumulation of amyloid precursor protein in the mitochondrial import channels of human Alzheimer's disease brain is associated with mitochondrial dysfunction. J Neurosci. 2006;26(35):9057–68.

[35] Barsoum MJ, Yuan H, Gerencser AA, Liot G, Kushnareva Y, Graber S, et al. Nitric oxide-induced mitochondrial fission is regulated by dynamin-related GTPases in neurons. EMBO J. 2006;25(16):3900–11.

[36] Hardy J, Selkoe DJ. The amyloid hypothesis of Alzheimer's disease: progress and problems on the road to therapeutics. Science. 2002;297(5580):353–6.

[37] Walsh DM, Klyubin I, Fadeeva JV, Cullen WK, Anwyl R, Wolfe MS, et al. Naturally secreted oligomers of amyloid beta protein potently inhibit hippocampal long-term potentiation in vivo. Nature. 2002;416(6880):535–9.

[38] Le MN, Kim W, Lee S, McKee AC, Hall GF. Multiple mechanisms of extracellular tau spreading in a non-transgenic tauopathy model. Am J Neurodegener Dis. 2012;1(3): 316–33.

[39] Avila J, Lucas JJ, Perez M, Hernandez F. Role of tau protein in both physiological and pathological conditions. Physiol Rev. 2004;84(2):361–84.

[40] Musiek ES, Holtzman DM. Three dimensions of the amyloid hypothesis: time, space and 'wingmen'. Nat Neurosci. 2015;18(6):800–6.

[41] Weingarten MD, Lockwood AH, Hwo SY, Kirschner MW. A protein factor essential for microtubule assembly. Proc Natl Acad Sci U S A. 1975;72(5):1858–62.

[42] Trojanowski JQ, Schuck T, Schmidt ML, Lee VM. Distribution of tau proteins in the normal human central and peripheral nervous system. J Histochem Cytochem. 1989;37(2):209–15.

[43] Gotz J, Xia D, Leinenga G, Chew YL, Nicholas H. What renders TAU toxic. Front Neurol. 2013;4:72.

[44] Goedert M, Spillantini MG, Jakes R, Rutherford D, Crowther RA. Multiple isoforms of human microtubule-associated protein tau: sequences and localization in neurofibrillary tangles of Alzheimer's disease. Neuron. 1989;3(4):519–26.

[45] Sultan A, Nesslany F, Violet M, Begard S, Loyens A, Talahari S, et al. Nuclear tau, a key player in neuronal DNA protection. J Biol Chem. 2011;286(6):4566–75.

[46] Pooler AM, Usardi A, Evans CJ, Philpott KL, Noble W, Hanger DP. Dynamic association of tau with neuronal membranes is regulated by phosphorylation. Neurobiol Aging. 2012;33(2):431 e27–38.

[47] Mondragon-Rodriguez S, Trillaud-Doppia E, Dudilot A, Bourgeois C, Lauzon M, Leclerc N, et al. Interaction of endogenous tau protein with synaptic proteins is regulated by N-methyl-D-aspartate receptor-dependent tau phosphorylation. J Biol Chem. 2012;287(38):32040–53.

[48] Frandemiche ML, De Seranno S, Rush T, Borel E, Elie A, Arnal I, et al. Activity-dependent tau protein translocation to excitatory synapse is disrupted by exposure to amyloid-beta oligomers. J Neurosci. 2014;34(17):6084–97.

[49] Bettens K, Sleegers K, Van Broeckhoven C. Current status on Alzheimer disease molecular genetics: from past, to present, to future. Hum Mol Genet. 2010;19(R1):R4–R11.

[50] Citron M, Oltersdorf T, Haass C, McConlogue L, Hung AY, Seubert P, et al. Mutation of the beta-amyloid precursor protein in familial Alzheimer's disease increases beta-protein production. Nature. 1992;360(6405):672–4.

[51] Di Fede G, Catania M, Morbin M, Rossi G, Suardi S, Mazzoleni G, et al. A recessive mutation in the APP gene with dominant-negative effect on amyloidogenesis. Science. 2009;323(5920):1473–7.

[52] Kutoku Y, Ohsawa Y, Kuwano R, Ikeuchi T, Inoue H, Ataka S, et al. A second pedigree with amyloid-less familial Alzheimer's disease harboring an identical mutation in the amyloid precursor protein gene (E693delta). Intern Med. 2015;54(2):205–8.

[53] Guerreiro RJ, Gustafson DR, Hardy J. The genetic architecture of Alzheimer's disease: beyond APP, PSENs and APOE. Neurobiol Aging. 2012;33(3):437–56.

[54] Kokawa A, Ishihara S, Fujiwara H, Nobuhara M, Iwata M, Ihara Y, et al. The A673T mutation in the amyloid precursor protein reduces the production of beta-amyloid protein from its beta-carboxyl terminal fragment in cells. Acta Neuropathol Commun. 2015;3:66.

[55] Bohm C, Chen F, Sevalle J, Qamar S, Dodd R, Li Y, et al. Current and future implications of basic and translational research on amyloid-beta peptide production and removal pathways. Mol Cell Neurosci. 2015;66(Pt A):3–11.

[56] Ray B, Long JM, Sokol DK, Lahiri DK. Increased secreted amyloid precursor protein-alpha (sAPPalpha) in severe autism: proposal of a specific, anabolic pathway and putative biomarker. PLoS One. 2011;6(6):e20405.

[57] Sahlin C, Pettersson FE, Nilsson LN, Lannfelt L, Johansson AS. Docosahexaenoic acid stimulates non-amyloidogenic APP processing resulting in reduced Abeta levels in cellular models of Alzheimer's disease. Eur J Neurosci. 2007;26(4):882–9.

[58] Thinakaran G, Koo EH. Amyloid precursor protein trafficking, processing, and function. J Biol Chem. 2008;283(44):29615–9.

[59] Asai M, Hattori C, Szabo B, Sasagawa N, Maruyama K, Tanuma S, et al. Putative function of ADAM9, ADAM10, and ADAM17 as APP alpha-secretase. Biochem Biophys Res Commun. 2003;301(1):231–5.

[60] Fahrenholz F, Gilbert S, Kojro E, Lammich S, Postina R. Alpha-secretase activity of the disintegrin metalloprotease ADAM 10. Influences of domain structure. Ann N Y Acad Sci. 2000;920:215–22.

[61] Fuwa H, Takahashi Y, Konno Y, Watanabe N, Miyashita H, Sasaki M, et al. Divergent synthesis of multifunctional molecular probes to elucidate the enzyme specificity of dipeptidic gamma-secretase inhibitors. ACS Chem Biol. 2007;2(6):408–18.

[62] Suh J, Choi SH, Romano DM, Gannon MA, Lesinski AN, Kim DY, et al. ADAM10 missense mutations potentiate beta-amyloid accumulation by impairing prodomain chaperone function. Neuron. 2013;80(2):385–401.

[63] Sherrington R, Rogaev EI, Liang Y, Rogaeva EA, Levesque G, Ikeda M, et al. Cloning of a gene bearing missense mutations in early-onset familial Alzheimer's disease. Nature. 1995;375(6534):754–60.

[64] Bergmans BA, De Strooper B. gamma-secretases: from cell biology to therapeutic strategies. Lancet Neurol. 2010;9(2):215–26.

[65] Chavez-Gutierrez L, Bammens L, Benilova I, Vandersteen A, Benurwar M, Borgers M, et al. The mechanism of gamma-secretase dysfunction in familial Alzheimer disease. EMBO J. 2012;31(10):2261–74.

[66] Sudoh S, Kawamura Y, Sato S, Wang R, Saido TC, Oyama F, et al. Presenilin 1 mutations linked to familial Alzheimer's disease increase the intracellular levels of amyloid beta-protein 1-42 and its N-terminally truncated variant(s) which are generated at distinct sites. J Neurochem. 1998;71(4):1535–43.

[67] Levy-Lahad E, Wasco W, Poorkaj P, Romano DM, Oshima J, Pettingell WH, et al. Candidate gene for the chromosome 1 familial Alzheimer's disease locus. Science. 1995;269(5226):973–7.

[68] Scheuner D, Eckman C, Jensen M, Song X, Citron M, Suzuki N, et al. Secreted amyloid beta-protein similar to that in the senile plaques of Alzheimer's disease is increased in vivo by the presenilin 1 and 2 and APP mutations linked to familial Alzheimer's disease. Nat Med. 1996;2(8):864–70.

[69] Steiner H, Capell A, Leimer U, Haass C. Genes and mechanisms involved in beta-amyloid generation and Alzheimer's disease. Eur Arch Psychiatry Clin Neurosci. 1999;249(6):266–70.

[70] Zatti G, Burgo A, Giacomello M, Barbiero L, Ghidoni R, Sinigaglia G, et al. Presenilin mutations linked to familial Alzheimer's disease reduce endoplasmic reticulum and Golgi apparatus calcium levels. Cell Calcium. 2006;39(6):539–50.

[71] Francis YI, Stephanou A, Latchman DS. CREB-binding protein activation by presenilin 1 but not by its M146L mutant. Neuroreport. 2006;17(9):917–21.

[72] Barthet G, Dunys J, Shao Z, Xuan Z, Ren Y, Xu J, et al. Presenilin mediates neuroprotective functions of ephrinB and brain-derived neurotrophic factor and regulates ligand-induced internalization and metabolism of EphB2 and TrkB receptors. Neurobiol Aging. 2013;34(2):499–510.

[73] Armstrong RA. Plaques and tangles and the pathogenesis of Alzheimer's disease. Folia Neuropathol. 2006;44(1):1–11.

[74] Shepherd CE, Gregory GC, Vickers JC, Brooks WS, Kwok JB, Schofield PR, et al. Positional effects of presenilin-1 mutations on tau phosphorylation in cortical plaques. Neurobiol Dis. 2004;15(1):115–9.

[75] Lyall DM, Harris SE, Bastin ME, Munoz Maniega S, Murray C, Lutz MW, et al. Alzheimer's disease susceptibility genes APOE and TOMM40, and brain white matter integrity in the Lothian Birth Cohort 1936. Neurobiol Aging. 2014;35(6):1513 e25–33.

[76] Brookmeyer R, Gray S, Kawas C. Projections of Alzheimer's disease in the United States and the public health impact of delaying disease onset. Am J Public Health. 1998;88(9): 1337–42.

[77] Brookmeyer R, Johnson E, Ziegler-Graham K, Arrighi HM. Forecasting the global burden of Alzheimer's disease. Alzheimers Dement. 2007;3(3):186–91.

[78] Hebert LE, Weuve J, Scherr PA, Evans DA. Alzheimer disease in the United States (2010–2050) estimated using the 2010 census. Neurology. 2013;80(19):1778–83.

[79] Mayeux R, Stern Y, Ottman R, Tatemichi TK, Tang MX, Maestre G, et al. The apolipoprotein epsilon 4 allele in patients with Alzheimer's disease. Ann Neurol. 1993;34(5): 752–4.

[80] Wang JM, Irwin RW, Brinton RD. Activation of estrogen receptor alpha increases and estrogen receptor beta decreases apolipoprotein E expression in hippocampus in vitro and in vivo. Proc Natl Acad Sci U S A. 2006;103(45):16983–8.

[81] Bu G. Apolipoprotein E and its receptors in Alzheimer's disease: pathways, pathogenesis and therapy. Nat Rev Neurosci. 2009;10(5):333–44.

[82] Mahley RW, Weisgraber KH, Huang Y. Apolipoprotein E: structure determines function, from atherosclerosis to Alzheimer's disease to AIDS. J Lipid Res. 2009;50(Suppl):S183–8.

[83] Castellano JM, Kim J, Stewart FR, Jiang H, DeMattos RB, Patterson BW, et al. Human apoE isoforms differentially regulate brain amyloid-beta peptide clearance. Sci Transl Med. 2011;3(89):89ra57.

[84] Sanan DA, Weisgraber KH, Russell SJ, Mahley RW, Huang D, Saunders A, et al. Apolipoprotein E associates with beta amyloid peptide of Alzheimer's disease to form novel monofibrils. Isoform apoE4 associates more efficiently than apoE3. J Clin Invest. 1994;94(2):860–9.

[85] Shen N, Chen B, Jiang Y, Feng R, Liao M, Zhang L, et al. An updated analysis with 85,939 samples confirms the association between CR1 rs6656401 polymorphism and Alzheimer's disease. Mol Neurobiol. 2015;51(3):1017–23.

[86] Liu G, Wang H, Liu J, Li J, Li H, Ma G, et al. The CLU gene rs11136000 variant is significantly associated with Alzheimer's disease in Caucasian and Asian populations. Neuromolecular Med. 2014;16(1):52–60.

[87] Omoumi A, Fok A, Greenwood T, Sadovnick AD, Feldman HH, Hsiung GY. Evaluation of late-onset Alzheimer disease genetic susceptibility risks in a Canadian population. Neurobiol Aging. 2014;35(4):936 e5–12.

[88] Griciuc A, Serrano-Pozo A, Parrado AR, Lesinski AN, Asselin CN, Mullin K, et al. Alzheimer's disease risk gene CD33 inhibits microglial uptake of amyloid beta. Neuron. 2013;78(4):631–43.

[89] Guerreiro R, Wojtas A, Bras J, Carrasquillo M, Rogaeva E, Majounie E, et al. TREM2 variants in Alzheimer's disease. N Engl J Med. 2013;368(2):117–27.

[90] Jonsson T, Stefansson H, Steinberg S, Jonsdottir I, Jonsson PV, Snaedal J, et al. Variant of TREM2 associated with the risk of Alzheimer's disease. N Engl J Med. 2013;368(2): 107–16.

[91] Ruiz A, Heilmann S, Becker T, Hernandez I, Wagner H, Thelen M, et al. Follow-up of loci from the International Genomics of Alzheimer's Disease Project identifies TRIP4 as a novel susceptibility gene. Transl Psychiatry. 2014;4:e358.

[92] Singaraja RR. TREM2: a new risk factor for Alzheimer's disease. Clin Genet. 2013;83(6): 525–6.

[93] Sun M, Zhu M, Chen K, Nie X, Deng Q, Hazlett LD, et al. TREM-2 promotes host resistance against Pseudomonas aeruginosa infection by suppressing corneal inflammation via a PI3K/Akt signaling pathway. Invest Ophthalmol Vis Sci. 2013;54(5):3451–62.

[94] Hickman SE, El Khoury J. TREM2 and the neuroimmunology of Alzheimer's disease. Biochem Pharmacol. 2014;88(4):495–8.

[95] Fisher Y, Nemirovsky A, Baron R, Monsonego A. T cells specifically targeted to amyloid plaques enhance plaque clearance in a mouse model of Alzheimer's disease. PLoS One. 2010;5(5):e10830.

[96] Piccio L, Deming Y, Del-Aguila JL, Ghezzi L, Holtzman DM, Fagan AM, et al. Cerebrospinal fluid soluble TREM2 is higher in Alzheimer disease and associated with mutation status. Acta Neuropathol. 2016;131(6):925-33.

[97] Heslegrave A, Heywood W, Paterson R, Magdalinou N, Svensson J, Johansson P, et al. Increased cerebrospinal fluid soluble TREM2 concentration in Alzheimer's disease. Mol Neurodegener. 2016;11(1):3.

[98] Cruchaga C, Kauwe JS, Harari O, Jin SC, Cai Y, Karch CM, et al. GWAS of cerebrospinal fluid tau levels identifies risk variants for Alzheimer's disease. Neuron. 2013;78(2):256–68.

[99] Cirrito JR, Deane R, Fagan AM, Spinner ML, Parsadanian M, Finn MB, et al. P-glycoprotein deficiency at the blood-brain barrier increases amyloid-beta deposition in an Alzheimer disease mouse model. J Clin Invest. 2005;115(11):3285–90.

[100] Jeynes B, Provias J. An investigation into the role of P-glycoprotein in Alzheimer's disease lesion pathogenesis. Neurosci Lett. 2011;487(3):389–93.

[101] Lambert JC, Ibrahim-Verbaas CA, Harold D, Naj AC, Sims R, Bellenguez C, et al. Meta-analysis of 74,046 individuals identifies 11 new susceptibility loci for Alzheimer's disease. Nat Genet. 2013;45(12):1452–8.

[102] Cacabelos R. Epigenomic networking in drug development: from pathogenic mechanisms to pharmacogenomics. Drug Dev Res. 2014;75(6):348–65.

[103] Cacabelos R, Torrellas C. Epigenetic drug discovery for Alzheimer's disease. Expert Opin Drug Discov. 2014;9(9):1059–86.

[104] Bennett DA, Yu L, Yang J, Srivastava GP, Aubin C, De Jager PL. Epigenomics of Alzheimer's disease. Transl Res. 2015;165(1):200–20.

[105] Wang J, Yu JT, Tan MS, Jiang T, Tan L. Epigenetic mechanisms in Alzheimer's disease: implications for pathogenesis and therapy. Ageing Res Rev. 2013;12(4):1024–41.

[106] Veerappan CS, Sleiman S, Coppola G. Epigenetics of Alzheimer's disease and frontotemporal dementia. Neurotherapeutics. 2013;10(4):709–21.

[107] Mastroeni D, Grover A, Delvaux E, Whiteside C, Coleman PD, Rogers J. Epigenetic mechanisms in Alzheimer's disease. Neurobiol Aging. 2011;32(7):1161–80.

[108] Mill J. Toward an integrated genetic and epigenetic approach to Alzheimer's disease. Neurobiol Aging. 2011;32(7):1188–91.

[109] Graff J, Tsai LH. The potential of HDAC inhibitors as cognitive enhancers. Annu Rev Pharmacol Toxicol. 2013;53:311–30.

[110] Adwan L, Zawia NH. Epigenetics: a novel therapeutic approach for the treatment of Alzheimer's disease. Pharmacol Ther. 2013;139(1):41–50.

[111] Francis YI, Fa M, Ashraf H, Zhang H, Staniszewski A, Latchman DS, et al. Dysregulation of histone acetylation in the APP/PS1 mouse model of Alzheimer's disease. J Alzheimers Dis. 2009;18(1):131–9.

[112] Fang M, Wang J, Zhang X, Geng Y, Hu Z, Rudd JA, et al. The miR-124 regulates the expression of BACE1/beta-secretase correlated with cell death in Alzheimer's disease. Toxicol Lett. 2012;209(1):94–105.

[113] Walker MP, LaFerla FM, Oddo SS, Brewer GJ. Reversible epigenetic histone modifications and Bdnf expression in neurons with aging and from a mouse model of Alzheimer's disease. Age (Dordr). 2013;35(3):519–31.

[114] Ding H, Dolan PJ, Johnson GV. Histone deacetylase 6 interacts with the microtubule-associated protein tau. J Neurochem. 2008;106(5):2119–30.

[115] Ogawa O, Zhu X, Lee HG, Raina A, Obrenovich ME, Bowser R, et al. Ectopic localization of phosphorylated histone H3 in Alzheimer's disease: a mitotic catastrophe? Acta Neuropathol. 2003;105(5):524–8.

[116] Rao JS, Keleshian VL, Klein S, Rapoport SI. Epigenetic modifications in frontal cortex from Alzheimer's disease and bipolar disorder patients. Transl Psychiatry. 2012;2:e132.

[117] Tohgi H, Utsugisawa K, Nagane Y, Yoshimura M, Ukitsu M, Genda Y. The methylation status of cytosines in a tau gene promoter region alters with age to downregulate transcriptional activity in human cerebral cortex. Neurosci Lett. 1999;275(2):89–92.

[118] Wang SC, Oelze B, Schumacher A. Age-specific epigenetic drift in late-onset Alzheimer's disease. PLoS One. 2008;3(7):e2698.

[119] Fuso A, Seminara L, Cavallaro RA, D'Anselmi F, Scarpa S. S-adenosylmethionine/homocysteine cycle alterations modify DNA methylation status with consequent deregulation of PS1 and BACE and beta-amyloid production. Mol Cell Neurosci. 2005;28(1):195–204.

[120] Theuns J, Del-Favero J, Dermaut B, van Duijn CM, Backhovens H, Van den Broeck MV, et al. Genetic variability in the regulatory region of presenilin 1 associated with risk for Alzheimer's disease and variable expression. Hum Mol Genet. 2000;9(3):325–31.

[121] Tanzi RE, Bertram L. Twenty years of the Alzheimer's disease amyloid hypothesis: a genetic perspective. Cell. 2005;120(4):545–55.

[122] Rauhala HE, Porkka KP, Saramaki OR, Tammela TL, Visakorpi T. Clusterin is epigenetically regulated in prostate cancer. Int J Cancer. 2008;123(7):1601–9.

[123] Zhou XW, Gustafsson JA, Tanila H, Bjorkdahl C, Liu R, Winblad B, et al. Tau hyperphosphorylation correlates with reduced methylation of protein phosphatase 2A. Neurobiol Dis. 2008;31(3):386–94.

[124] Sontag E, Nunbhakdi-Craig V, Sontag JM, Diaz-Arrastia R, Ogris E, Dayal S, et al. Protein phosphatase 2A methyltransferase links homocysteine metabolism with tau and amyloid precursor protein regulation. J Neurosci. 2007;27(11):2751–9.

[125] Sanchez-Mut JV, Aso E, Panayotis N, Lott I, Dierssen M, Rabano A, et al. DNA methylation map of mouse and human brain identifies target genes in Alzheimer's disease. Brain. 2013;136(Pt 10):3018–27.

[126] Van den Hove DL, Kompotis K, Lardenoije R, Kenis G, Mill J, Steinbusch HW, et al. Epigenetically regulated microRNAs in Alzheimer's disease. Neurobiol Aging. 2014;35(4):731–45.

[127] Wu J, Li S, Jia W, Deng H, Chen K, Zhu L, et al. Reduced Let-7a Is Associated with chemoresistance in primary breast cancer. PLoS One. 2015;10(7):e0133643.

[128] Kumar P, Dezso Z, MacKenzie C, Oestreicher J, Agoulnik S, Byrne M, et al. Circulating miRNA biomarkers for Alzheimer's disease. PLoS One. 2013;8(7):e69807.

[129] Leidinger P, Backes C, Deutscher S, Schmitt K, Mueller SC, Frese K, et al. A blood based 12-miRNA signature of Alzheimer disease patients. Genome Biol. 2013;14(7):R78.

[130] Alexandrov PN, Dua P, Hill JM, Bhattacharjee S, Zhao Y, Lukiw WJ. microRNA (miRNA) speciation in Alzheimer's disease (AD) cerebrospinal fluid (CSF) and extracellular fluid (ECF). Int J Biochem Mol Biol. 2012;3(4):365–73.

[131] Long JM, Lahiri DK. MicroRNA-101 downregulates Alzheimer's amyloid-beta precursor protein levels in human cell cultures and is differentially expressed. Biochem Biophys Res Commun. 2011;404(4):889–95.

[132] Liu W, Liu C, Zhu J, Shu P, Yin B, Gong Y, et al. MicroRNA-16 targets amyloid precursor protein to potentially modulate Alzheimer's-associated pathogenesis in SAMP8 mice. Neurobiol Aging. 2012;33(3):522–34.

[133] Smith P, Al Hashimi A, Girard J, Delay C, Hebert SS. In vivo regulation of amyloid precursor protein neuronal splicing by microRNAs. J Neurochem. 2011;116(2):240–7.

[134] Zong Y, Wang H, Dong W, Quan X, Zhu H, Xu Y, et al. miR-29c regulates BACE1 protein expression. Brain Res. 2011;1395:108–15.

[135] Boissonneault V, Plante I, Rivest S, Provost P. MicroRNA-298 and microRNA-328 regulate expression of mouse beta-amyloid precursor protein-converting enzyme 1. J Biol Chem. 2009;284(4):1971–81.

[136] Zhu HC, Wang LM, Wang M, Song B, Tan S, Teng JF, et al. MicroRNA-195 downregulates Alzheimer's disease amyloid-beta production by targeting BACE1. Brain Res Bull. 2012;88(6):596–601.

[137] Caputo V, Sinibaldi L, Fiorentino A, Parisi C, Catalanotto C, Pasini A, et al. Brain derived neurotrophic factor (BDNF) expression is regulated by microRNAs miR-26a and miR-26b allele-specific binding. PLoS One. 2011;6(12):e28656.

[138] Mohamed JS, Lopez MA, Boriek AM. Mechanical stretch up-regulates microRNA-26a and induces human airway smooth muscle hypertrophy by suppressing glycogen synthase kinase-3beta. J Biol Chem. 2010;285(38):29336–47.

[139] Cogswell JP, Ward J, Taylor IA, Waters M, Shi Y, Cannon B, et al. Identification of miRNA changes in Alzheimer's disease brain and CSF yields putative biomarkers and insights into disease pathways. J Alzheimers Dis. 2008;14(1):27–41.

[140] Bilen J, Liu N, Burnett BG, Pittman RN, Bonini NM. MicroRNA pathways modulate polyglutamine-induced neurodegeneration. Mol Cell. 2006;24(1):157–63.

[141] Wang WX, Huang Q, Hu Y, Stromberg AJ, Nelson PT. Patterns of microRNA expression in normal and early Alzheimer's disease human temporal cortex: white matter versus gray matter. Acta Neuropathol. 2011;121(2):193–205.

[142] Farrer LA, Cupples LA, Haines JL, Hyman B, Kukull WA, Mayeux R, et al. Effects of age, sex, and ethnicity on the association between apolipoprotein E genotype and Alzheimer disease. A meta-analysis. APOE and Alzheimer Disease Meta Analysis Consortium. JAMA. 1997;278(16):1349–56.

[143] Payami H, Montee KR, Kaye JA, Bird TD, Yu CE, Wijsman EM, et al. Alzheimer's disease, apolipoprotein E4, and gender. JAMA. 1994;271(17):1316–7.

[144] Damoiseaux JS, Seeley WW, Zhou J, Shirer WR, Coppola G, Karydas A, et al. Gender modulates the APOE epsilon4 effect in healthy older adults: convergent evidence from functional brain connectivity and spinal fluid tau levels. J Neurosci. 2012;32(24):8254–62.

[145] Altmann A, Tian L, Henderson VW, Greicius MD. Alzheimer's disease neuroimaging initiative I. Sex modifies the APOE-related risk of developing Alzheimer disease. Ann Neurol. 2014;75(4):563–73.

[146] Reiman EM, Caselli RJ, Yun LS, Chen K, Bandy D, Minoshima S, et al. Preclinical evidence of Alzheimer's disease in persons homozygous for the epsilon 4 allele for apolipoprotein E. N Engl J Med. 1996;334(12):752–8.

[147] Corder EH, Ghebremedhin E, Taylor MG, Thal DR, Ohm TG, Braak H. The biphasic relationship between regional brain senile plaque and neurofibrillary tangle distributions: modification by age, sex, and APOE polymorphism. Ann N Y Acad Sci. 2004;1019:24–8.

[148] Ryan J, Carriere I, Carcaillon L, Dartigues JF, Auriacombe S, Rouaud O, et al. Estrogen receptor polymorphisms and incident dementia: the prospective 3C study. Alzheimers Dement. 2014;10(1):27–35.

[149] Stern Y, Gurland B, Tatemichi TK, Tang MX, Wilder D, Mayeux R. Influence of education and occupation on the incidence of Alzheimer's disease. JAMA. 1994;271(13):1004–10.

[150] Letenneur L, Gilleron V, Commenges D, Helmer C, Orgogozo JM, Dartigues JF. Are sex and educational level independent predictors of dementia and Alzheimer's disease? Incidence data from the PAQUID project. J Neurol Neurosurg Psychiatry. 1999;66(2):177–83.

[151] Fitzpatrick AL, Kuller LH, Ives DG, Lopez OL, Jagust W, Breitner JC, et al. Incidence and prevalence of dementia in the Cardiovascular Health Study. J Am Geriatr Soc. 2004;52(2):195–204.

[152] Tsvetanov KA, Henson RN, Tyler LK, Razi A, Geerligs L, Ham TE, et al. Extrinsic and intrinsic brain network connectivity maintains cognition across the lifespan despite accelerated decay of regional brain activation. J Neurosci. 2016;36(11):3115–26.

[153] Wilson RS, Scherr PA, Schneider JA, Tang Y, Bennett DA. Relation of cognitive activity to risk of developing Alzheimer disease. Neurology. 2007;69(20):1911–20.

[154] Akbaraly TN, Portet F, Fustinoni S, Dartigues JF, Artero S, Rouaud O, et al. Leisure activities and the risk of dementia in the elderly: results from the Three-City Study. Neurology. 2009;73(11):854–61.

[155] Fratiglioni L, Paillard-Borg S, Winblad B. An active and socially integrated lifestyle in late life might protect against dementia. Lancet Neurol. 2004;3(6):343–53.

[156] Abbott RD, White LR, Ross GW, Masaki KH, Curb JD, Petrovitch H. Walking and dementia in physically capable elderly men. JAMA. 2004;292(12):1447–53.

[157] Weuve J, Kang JH, Manson JE, Breteler MM, Ware JH, Grodstein F. Physical activity, including walking, and cognitive function in older women. JAMA. 2004;292(12):1454–61.

[158] Podewils LJ, Guallar E, Kuller LH, Fried LP, Lopez OL, Carlson M, et al. Physical activity, APOE genotype, and dementia risk: findings from the Cardiovascular Health Cognition Study. Am J Epidemiol. 2005;161(7):639–51.

[159] Larson EB, Wang L, Bowen JD, McCormick WC, Teri L, Crane P, et al. Exercise is associated with reduced risk for incident dementia among persons 65 years of age and older. Ann Intern Med. 2006;144(2):73–81.

[160] Ravaglia G, Forti P, Lucicesare A, Pisacane N, Rietti E, Bianchin M, et al. Physical activity and dementia risk in the elderly: findings from a prospective Italian study. Neurology. 2008;70(19 Pt 2):1786–94.

[161] Qiu C, Winblad B, Fratiglioni L. The age-dependent relation of blood pressure to cognitive function and dementia. Lancet Neurol. 2005;4(8):487–99.

[162] Launer LJ, Ross GW, Petrovitch H, Masaki K, Foley D, White LR, et al. Midlife blood pressure and dementia: the Honolulu-Asia aging study. Neurobiol Aging. 2000;21(1):49–55.

[163] Shobab LA, Hsiung GY, Feldman HH. Cholesterol in Alzheimer's disease. Lancet Neurol. 2005;4(12):841–52.

[164] Biessels GJ, Deary IJ, Ryan CM. Cognition and diabetes: a lifespan perspective. Lancet Neurol. 2008;7(2):184–90.

[165] Gillette Guyonnet S, Abellan Van Kan G, Andrieu S, Barberger Gateau P, Berr C, Bonnefoy M, et al. IANA task force on nutrition and cognitive decline with aging. J Nutr Health Aging. 2007;11(2):132–52.

[166] Heude B, Ducimetiere P, Berr C, Study EVA. Cognitive decline and fatty acid composition of erythrocyte membranes – the EVA study. Am J Clin Nutr. 2003;77(4):803–8.

[167] Barberger-Gateau P, Letenneur L, Deschamps V, Peres K, Dartigues JF, Renaud S. Fish, meat, and risk of dementia: cohort study. BMJ. 2002;325(7370):932–3.

[168] Barberger-Gateau P, Raffaitin C, Letenneur L, Berr C, Tzourio C, Dartigues JF, et al. Dietary patterns and risk of dementia: the Three-City cohort study. Neurology. 2007;69(20):1921–30.

Section 2

Clinical Section

Chapter 11

Normal Aging and Dementia

Michał Prendecki, Jolanta Florczak-Wyspianska,
Marta Kowalska, Margarita Lianeri,
Wojciech Kozubski and Jolanta Dorszewska

Additional information is available at the end of the chapter

http://dx.doi.org/10.5772/64203

Abstract

Normal aging begins after 60 years of age. According to Harman, the accumulation of free radicals, which results from weakening of repair and protective mechanisms, takes place in the aging brain. It is believed that especially in the population of the most elderly there is increased incidence of both dementia and depression. The causes of these central nervous system disorders in the aging human body are changes at the molecular level, such as changes in the biochemical parameters, the accumulation of mutations in nuclear and mitochondrial DNA, and epigenetic changes. Biomarkers associated with aging of the brain include accumulated deposits of β-amyloid (Aβ), disturbed cholesterol homeostasis, altered neuroimaging parameters, and impaired glucose metabolism. Genetic factors are also responsible for normal aging, for example, *SIRT1, AKT1*, and *CDKN1A*, and among them the longevity genes, such as *FOXO3A* and *CETP*. Dementia as well as cognitive decline may be modified by poly-T variants of *TOMM40* and *APOE* alleles via influencing the level of apolipoprotein E (apoE) in the brain and in the plasma as well as by its ability of Aβ clearance.

Identifying the molecular factors associated with aging and dementia may help introduce new approaches to preventing geriatric disorders, including depression and dementia.

Keywords: molecular factors, dementia, normal aging

1. Introduction

Currently, average life expectancy in the world is over 60 years. The world's longest life expectancy is in Japan, at 82.2 years, and in Australia, at 80.6 years. In Europe, the longest-lived people are the French, at 80.6 years, the Swedes, at 80.6 years, the Italians, at 79.9 years, the Greeks, at 79.3 years, the Dutch, at 79.1 years, and the Germans, at 78.9 years. It is predicted that in Europe from 2005 to 2050, the number of people following into their 80th year of life will increase by 43 million [1].

In psychological studies on the elderly, three subperiods were stratified among people over 60 years old; these included *young olds* (65–75 years of age), *old olds* (75–85 years old), and *eldest olds* (over 85 years of age). Deterioration of cognitive functions was visible in the *eldest olds* age group, while asymptomatic structural changes in the brain, such as cortical atrophy, poli- and leukoaraiosis (deterioration of white matter, present in 8–90% of the elderly with no signs of dementia), or decreased glucose metabolism and deteriorated subcortical and cortical flow, could be detected by neuroimaging even among the *young olds* [2].

Progressive aging of the population is one of the factors determining the increasingly frequent occurrence of cognitive impairment and dementia syndromes. Dementia, due to its prevalence in the population (it occurs in approximately 10% of those 65 years of age and in approximately 30–40% of those 90 years of age), requires great concern and clinical care. It is estimated that by 2040, the number of elderly people with dementia in the world will exceed 80 million [3].

According to the classification of mental disorders in the American Psychiatric Association's DSM – IV (Diagnostic and Statistical Manual of Mental Disorders) [4], there is no isolated, separate diagnostic category for "dementia," but the criteria for this diagnosis are contained in the various types of dementia, for example, Alzheimer's disease (AD), vascular dementia (VD), or in other diseases. According to these criteria, a diagnosis of dementia is necessary to determine the presence of multiple cognitive deficits that cause significant disturbances in the functioning of social exclusion and mental illness (depression) and delirium.

Dementia is a progressive impairment of the functional status and significantly reduces the quality of life of older people in all its dimensions, since physical disability and the loss of sphincter control coexist along with dementia. The most common cause of dementia in the oldest patients is the degenerative process that is underway in the brain in the course of AD. In old age, an important process associated with the degeneration of neurons in AD is cerebral arteriosclerosis. Dementia, with dying neurons, is caused by both pathologies. A high percentage of the causes of dementia in the elderly may develop depression. In these patients, the following is observed especially often: loss of interest, sleep disturbances, psychomotor disturbances, and problems with concentration. In turn, the use of multiple drugs in dementia complicates the diagnosis of depression [4].

Depression is defined as an emotional distress syndrome (states of depressed mood, depression), which is often co-morbid with somatic diseases and/or with intensifying their symptoms. Depression is a common and serious problem among the elderly and increases mortality. Approximately 15% of people over the age of 65 have symptoms of depression, which impede daily functioning [2, 4].

It is believed that the functional and cognition changes observed in older persons are associated with disturbances at the molecular level in the aging body. Molecular changes in the aging process may relate to genomic instability as a result of accumulation of mutations, telomere attrition and epigenetic alterations, and alteration in the level of brain biomarkers [2].

To select significant studies for this review, the authors conducted multiple searches through public databases, including PubMed and Scopus, by using the following search strategy: ("normal aging" or "aging") and ("dementia" or "cognitive decline") and ("biomarker" or "SNP" or "genetic polymorphism" or "mutation"). The last search was performed in February 2016. A subsequent data mining through review articles and references facilitated finding additional eligible studies.

2. Brain biomarkers and cognitive function in normal aging

Central changes leading to impaired brain and cognition functions have been reported in normal brain aging, but data are inconclusive [5, 6]. A study [5] using functional magnetic resonance imaging (MRI) with gadolinium contrast confirmed changes in the hippocampus associated with impairment of cognitive function in elderly people. Also, a study conducted on 564 cognitively normal individuals (average age was 78 years) using MRI and fluorodeoxyglucose positron emission tomography (FDG-PET) and Pittsburgh Compound B (PiB) PET indicated impairment of cognition and imaging biomarkers. The causes of these central changes in the brain of the aged subjects seem to have been increased β-amyloid (Aβ) levels [6]. In the senescent brain, accumulation of Aβ deposits is eminent, in the form of senile plaques as well as fibrillary tangles in the neurons. The lesions may develop in the human brain as late as in one's 80s (frequently with no signs of dementia). The slower the accumulation of lesions is, the longer the time period required to develop dementia [7, 8]. Cerebral amyloidosis has been associated not only with Aβ deposition but also with higher pulse pressure in the presence of neurodegeneration, which may lead to more rapid progression of dementia [9]. However, more recent data indicate that Aβ deposition may in time exceed brain structural changes, such as grey matter volume, as measured by MRI, and neuronal hypometabolism assessed using PET with 18F-fluorodeoxyglucose (FDG) [10]. Moreover, the cognitive decline in elderly patients is associated with brain infarcts [11]. Also dietary factors, such as ω-3 polyunsaturated fatty acids (PUFAs), were shown to be associated with normal brain function; the PUFA concentration remains in reverse correlation with brain atrophy in cognitively normal elders [10].

3. Molecular changes in normal aging and dementia

In the aging process, the epigenetic changes lead to expression alteration of genes associated with vital functions of cells, such as mitochondrial function, as well as protective and repair mechanisms, as shown in **Table 1**.

One of genetic hallmarks of aging is genomic instability which includes accumulation of genetic damage both in nuclear DNA (nDNA) and mitochondrial DNA (mtDNA). mtDNA is more susceptible to DNA damaging factors than nDNA due to its oxidative environment. Also DNA repair mechanisms are less efficient in mitochondria than in nucleus [23], although mitochondria have most of the DNA repair pathways existing in the nucleus [24]. The mitochondrial reactive oxygen species (ROS) theory of aging (mitochondrial free radical theory of aging [MFRTA]) proposed by Harman assumes that free radicals generated in normal metabolism cause mtDNA mutations and ageing is a result of oxidative damage accumulation. According to MFRTA, maximum life span can be decreased by mtDNA damage caused by oxidative stress [25]. Mitochondrial reactive oxygen species (mtROS) may play signaling role in mitochondrial stress during ageing [26]. It is also suggested that mtDNA mutation accumulation and mitochondrial dysfunction during aging are a result of decreased activity of autophagy and mitophagy [27]. Moreover, a study performed on 18 three-generation families of women shows decline in mtDNA copy number, mitochondrial protein expression, and oxidative function with age [28]. Oxidative DNA damage and mitochondrial dysfunction lead to neuronal loss and may play a role in the development of dementia. The decreased level of antioxidants was observed among dementia individuals [29, 30]. It was suggested that high levels of ROS and decline in neuronal DNA damage response may be associated with neuronal dysfunction and cognitive impairment characterized by lower Mini-Mental State Examination (MMSE) score [31]. Additionally, it is known that oxidative damage leads to frontal-executive dysfunction [32].

Gene/encoded product	Locus	Role in aging	References
SIRT1 sirtulin 1	10q21.3	Age-related decreased level of SIRT1 is associated with impaired oxidative stress response and changes in glucose metabolism. Indirectly may be involved in age-related diseases, for example, retinal degeneration, hypertension, and cardiovascular diseases.	[12]
AKT1 protein Kinase B	14q32.32	Decreased level of AKT1 with age alters regulation of glucose metabolism, apoptosis, cell proliferation and cell migration, and PI3K/AKT/mTOR pathway.	[13]
CDKN1A Cyclin-dependent kinase inhibitor 1 (p21)	6p21.2	Possible promoter of aging due to pro-aging activity of p53.Oxidative stress increases expression of CDKN1A and overexpression of p21 may be involved in age-related diseases such as atherosclerosis, amyloidosis, AD, and arthritis.	[14] [15]
CETP Cholesterol ester transfer protein	16q21	Responsible for cholesterol homeostasis in central nervous system. Decreased level of CETP results in healthier aging, slower memory decline, less frequency of dementia, and lower AD risk.	[16] [17]
FOXO3A Transcriptional factor FOXO3A	6q21	Involved in insulin metabolism and insulin/IGF1 signaling pathway. Protection from oxidative stress and reduction of age-related diseases.	[18] [19]
IGF-1 Insulin-like growth factor 1	12q23.2	Decreased level of IGF-1 with age leads to cell senescence.	[20]
PON1 Paraoxonase 1	7q21.3	Decreased level of PON1 with age impairs oxidative stress response and is a risk factor for cardiovascular diseases due to LDL oxidation.	[21] [22]

Table 1. The role of genes and their encoded products in aging.

http://dx.doi.org/10.5772/64203

Another mechanism involved in aging is epigenetic alterations. Epigenetics is defined as molecular traits that are "stably heritable phenotype resulting from changes in a chromosome without alterations in the DNA sequence." The epigenetic pathways include DNA methylation, histone modifications, and noncoding RNA [33].

The analyses of CpGs methylation changes show that genome-wide global levels of DNA methylation decrease during aging. Despite this, many promoters of genes which are unmethylated in young gain methylation in old individuals [34, 35]. Other authors [36] suggest that DNA methylation changes may result in age-associated immune deficiency. It is possible that hypermethylation is caused by programmed changes, while hypomethylation may be the result of environmental and stochastic processes. Multiple studies have identified genes undergoing hyper- and hypomethylation with age. The first group includes genes involved in process such as cell adhesion, cell-cell signaling, ion transport, neuron differentiation, and other genes associated with development. The hypermethylated genes are regulated by a common group of transcription factors, whereas hypomethylated genes are involved in metabolic process, RNA splicing, regulation of ligase activity and protein ubiquitination, transmission of nerve impulse, and many others. The hypomethylation in neurons may cause age-related memory deficits [36, 37]. The abnormal profile of methylation may contribute to dementia. It is shown that mutation in DNA methyltransferase 1 (*DNMT1*), gene encoding an enzyme crucial for methylation, leads to a condition called hereditary sensory and autonomic neuropathy (HSAN1) with early onset of dementia and hearing loss [38]. Other authors suggest [39] that changes in methylation may be involved in age-related cognitive functions decline.

Histone modification includes acetylation, methylation, phosphorylation, citrullination, ubiquitination, SUMOylation, adenosine diphosphate (ADP) ribosylation, deimination, and proline isomerization, in which the first three are the most-studied topics. Modifications can change the chromatin structure by histone-histone or histone-DNA interactions. The chromatin packaging affects many processes such as transcription, repair, replication, and chromosome condensation. Acetylation is associated with activation of transcription, while the result of lysine methylation can be either activation or repression [40]. Chromatin packaging changes during aging [41]. It is shown that higher level of histone acetylation facilitates memory and learning processes; therefore, acetylation decrement may lead to cognitive impairments and is associated with aging [42]. Also histone methylation may affect the life span; loss of H3K9 trimethylation which results in reduction of heterochromatin is the hallmark of aging [43]. The acetylation of H4K16 is necessary for maintaining the structure of chromatin and when impaired, the process of double-strand break repair is less efficient [44]. Subsequently, histone tail proteolytic cleavage, especially H3, may be involved in aging, but the exact mechanism remains unclear [45]. Additionally, the decline in histone chaperon levels is observed during aging and may be the answer for defective DNA repair mechanisms [46].

Both age-related changes in DNA methylation and histone modification alter the experience-dependent synaptic plasticity in hippocampus by changing the chromatin structure. Thus, it may be involved in memory loss and learning difficulties. Epigenetic changes may be possible brain biomarkers of cognitive aging [47].

4. Genes associated with age-dependent dementia

Several genes are involved in age-dependent dementia. Most of them, such as *ABCA7, APOE, APOC1, BIN1, CASS4, CELF1, CD33, CD2AP, CELF1, CLU, CR1, DSG2, EPHA1, FERMT2, HLA-DRB5/DBR1, IL1RAP, INPP5D, MEF2C, MS4A6A/MS4A4E, NME8, PCDH11X, PICALM, PLD3, PTK2B, TOMM40, TREM2, TRIP4, TRPC4AP, SLC24H4-RIN3, SORL1,* and *ZCWPW1*, are associated with AD, which is the most prevalent cause of dementia in elders [48]. AD affects 24 million people worldwide and accounts for 60–80% of dementia cases [49]. *APOE* cluster (*APOE, TOMM40*) and *CLU* gene of the genes mentioned above, as well as Aβ cascade genes (*APP, PSEN1, PSEN2*), have also been mentioned as linked to memory decline in cognitively normal adults.

4.1. *APP, PSEN1,* and *PSEN2*

Aβ is formed in a process called an amyloid cascade which involves the amyloid precursor protein (APP), encoded by the *APP* gene located on chromosome 21. APP is a transmembrane protein with high expression in developing human neurons. In normal conditions, APP is truncated by proteolytic enzymes such as α- and β-secretases. However, in individuals developing AD, APP is processed by an alternative pathway involving γ-secretase. This leads to the production of the 40–42 amino-acid Aβ peptide. The active subunits of γ-secretase presenilin 1 and/or 2 are encoded by genes *PSEN1* and *PSEN2*, respectively. So far, 230 clinically significant mutations have been described in *APP, PSEN1,* and *PSEN2* genes; however, these mutations are very rare and account for around 0.5% of dementia cases. Moreover, most of these mutations are considered to be associated with a familial form of AD. On the other hand, asymptomatic carriers of the mutations in Aβ cascade genes demonstrate significant changes in cognitive functions, advancing with age [48].

4.2. *TOMM40*, translocase of the outer mitochondrial membrane 40 homolog (TOM40)

TOMM40 is a gene encoding for translocase of the outer mitochondrial membrane 40 homolog (TOM40). The gene is located on chromosome 19 in a cluster with *APOE*. Both genes remain in linkage disequilibrium and are associated with dementia [50]. Most reports concerning the role of *TOMM40* in developing dementia have focused on a variable length poly-T sequence polymorphism (rs10524523) located in intron 6 [51–53]. The number of deoxythymidine residues in the rs10524523 polymorphism comprise the so-called "alleles" of the poly-T repeat as "short" (abbreviated here as S), "long" (L), or "very long" (VL). These remain in strong linkage with the *APOE* variants, as the *TOMM40* L allele is almost exclusively observed in the *APOE* E4 carriers, while *TOMM40* S and/or the VL variants are associated with *APOE* E3 [51–53]. The poly-T variation in *TOMM40* was shown to be significantly associated with the age of onset of dementia [52]. Moreover, as shown in [51], the *TOMM40* poly-T variant may facilitate the estimation of dementia progression in AD patients, independently from the status of other dementia loci. They also implied that the genome-wide association studies (GWAS) signals recorded in the *APOE* locus may indeed arise from *TOMM40*.

It has been suggested that Aβ may exert intracellular toxicity mediated by TOM40, for example, by affecting the function of cellular power plants—the mitochondria. According to [50], the mechanism underlying TOM40's role in dementia involves its ability to uptake Aβ to the mitochondrion, as Aβ has been found to be co-localized with cristae proteins in the mitochondria. Subsequently, after absorption the intracellular Aβ would cause increased production of ROS, thus leading to DNA damage and premature neuronal death.

Several studies have shown that poly-T *TOMM40* variation may influence cognitive performance in healthy elderly people. The authors of study [54] investigated a cohort of 1613 elderly volunteers whose cognitive decline was followed for a period of 14 years (range = 12–18 years). This study showed that the *TOMM40* S variant repressed the activity of luciferase assay. Correspondingly, expression of the S variant was half of that in the VL variant. Moreover, they observed that the S variant significantly reduced vocabulary ability, diminished age-dependent vocabulary decline, in subjects as compared to the VL variant carriers. Other authors [55] conducted longitudinal modeling of a cognitive aging study on a cohort of 639 subjects with no signs of dementia, aged 21 to 97 years with a known *TOMM40* and *APOE* status. The volunteers underwent neuropsychological testing every 2 years. This study [55] showed that the influence of *TOMM40* variation on memory decline was particularly visible in subjects before 60 years of age ($p = 0.009$), however only in *TOMM40* VL/VL carriers whose improvement after the test-retest was significantly less pronounced than in the S/S and S/VL carriers. Moreover, the authors performed a neuropsychological examination and testing using the human analog of the Morris water maze and brain MRI on 59 cognitively normal volunteers, stratified as S/S, S/VL, and VL/VL carriers. They found that the S/S group performed better on world-centered navigation ($p \leq 0.004$) and world-centered delayed recall ($p \leq 0.014$) but not on self-centered navigation tests. They also found that the *TOMM40* variants significantly influenced the brain structure. The S/S group had a thicker right entorhinal cortex ($p \leq 0.043$) than the S/VL and VL/VL groups, whereas significant thinning of the left entorhinal cortex and the left posterior cingulate cortex was present only in the VL/VL group ($p = 0.043$ and $p = 0.024$, respectively) as compared to the S/S group [55]. In another interesting study [56], the authors stratified 117 healthy adults (medium age: 55 years) with the *APOE* E3/E3 genotype according to the *TOMM40* status into three groups, S/S, S/VL, and VL/VL, and performed memory tests and structural brain imaging. They found that the asymptomatic carriers of the *TOMM40* VL/VL genotype performed worse on testing of episodic learning and had a smaller volume in the posterior cingulate as compared to the S/S and S/VL groups [56].

These studies suggest that the *TOMM40* role is not limited to decreasing age at the onset of dementia but may also influence the brain structure and hasten memory decline in cognitively normal, healthy individuals.

5. Cholesterol, lipoproteins, and dementia

Of the many lipids, cholesterol is believed to play a major role in brain function and development, as the brain contains as much as 23% of the total cholesterol deposits [57]. One of the most pronounced groups of genes described as dementia risk factors are involved in the transport of cholesterol and may be accounted for as apolipoproteins [58]. A misbalanced lipid metabolism may be associated with memory loss [59]. According to another paper [60], patients with higher levels of high-density lipoproteins (HDLs) had a decreased risk of developing dementia at the time of the study and in the future. For patients from the upper quartile (with a plasma HDL concentration higher than 55 mg/dL), the dementia hazard was decreased by 60%. Studies on the subjects were continued by several other teams; however, the obtained results seem to be rather inconsistent [61–67].

Generally, the HDL level is believed to negatively correlate with the prevalence of dementia in elderly people; however, many studies have implied that HDL influence may be characteristic of the VD development [58, 68].

5.1. *CLU*, apolipoprotein J (apoJ)

Apolipoprotein J (apoJ, also known as clusterin), encoded by the *CLU* gene, has been shown to probably be associated with dementia. Genome-wide association studies (GWAS) performed by authors [69] identified a genetic variation (rs11136000) which was a significant risk factor of dementia. The role of apoJ in the pathomechanism of AD is not fully understood. It has recently been shown that apoJ plasma levels positively correlate with the risk of dementia, as elevated apoJ levels have been reported in the plasma of AD patients as well as in their brain and cerebrospinal fluid (CSF). The study [70] showed that apoJ plasma, but not CSF, levels are elevated in AD patients and were a risk factor of dementia (HR 18.6). This biomarker was also shown to be significantly correlated with cognitive decline in AD patients and reversely correlated in individuals with mild cognitive impairment (MCI). Moreover, increased plasma apoJ levels in MCI indicated an amplified risk of further cognitive decline. Furthermore, it was shown that genetic variation in the *CLU* region may amplify the influence of personality type on the performance of declarative memory in older, non-demented adults [71].

5.2. *APOE*, apolipoprotein E (apoE)

ApoE is encoded by the *APOE* gene, which is located on the long arm of chromosome 19. It comprises four exons. Two frequent polymorphisms were described on the last exon: rs7412 and rs429358. These variants encode for three common alleles of *APOE*: E2, E3, and E4, encoding for apoE ε2, ε3, and ε4, respectively.

ApoE in physiological conditions is a major cholesterol carrier and one of the most vital proteins responsible for maintaining cholesterol homeostasis in the brain. ApoE is mostly synthesized by astrocytes and probably does not cross the blood-brain barrier [72].

A recent study [73] on transgenic rabbit *Apoe* knockouts (*Apoe* -/-) showed that apoE is essential for cholesterol homeostasis under stress conditions. Under normal conditions, the transgenic animals were able to maintain a stable, physiological level of plasma cholesterol. However, when the animals were transitioned to a diet with high cholesterol content, its level increased dramatically (1070 ± 61 mg/dL in apoE KO vs 169 ± 79 mg/dL in the wild type, $p < 0.001$). Another study [74] showed that increased content of fat and cholesterol in the diet increased apoE production, probably due to transcriptional and posttranscriptional mechanisms. This suggests that functional apoE is essential for cholesterol regulation in mammals and protects against diet-induced atherosclerosis. The various variants of *APOE* have a distinct influence on apoE function and effect. Studies on humans and in apoE transgenic mice suggest that lipidation of apoE depends strongly on the *APOE* genotype, and that apoE ε2 and ε3 are significantly more lipidated than apoE ε4. Interestingly, cholesterol and proper apoE lipidation are essential for apoE function in sustaining synapses [75].

A study [76] analyzing the association of plasma and CSF apoE concentrations showed that the CSF/serum ratios of apoE levels were associated with progression of dementia. Schmidt et al. observed that "the lower the ratio, the faster the deterioration," as measured by the MMSE, instrumental activities of daily living (iADL), or Geriatric Depression Scale (GDS). Subsequently, another study [77] showed that plasma apoE may be a biomarker of dementia, as patients suffering from memory decline had lowered concentrations of plasma apoE.

The first reports indicating that *APOE* may be associated with dementia were published more than 20 years ago. Detailed studies of this gene were carried out mainly in AD; however, the literature data support *APOE* influence on memory in people with no symptoms of dementia. It is believed that *APOE* E3 is the most common allele in the population and does not modify the risk of memory decline. The *APOE* E4 variant was shown to be overrepresented in dementia patients, especially those with AD [78]. So far, *APOE* E4 remains the most significant risk factor of sporadic AD and accounts for 30% of cases [79]. *APOE* E2 was shown to be associated with reduced age-dependent cognitive decline. This observation occurred independently of age-related neuroinflammation and synaptic changes or the Aβ burden [80]. The described effect may be explained by a higher apoE level in *APOE* E2 carriers as well as by more efficient Aβ clearance [81]. Moreover, according to study [75], the effects of *APOE* E2 and E4 counteract, and in transgenic mice the introduction of the E2 allele decreased Aβ deposition, while the E4 allele increased the Aβ burden.

According to [82], the most significant *APOE* effect on the onset of dementia may be observed in patients over the age of 60 ($p = 0.006$). This was visible as an accelerated memory decline in *APOE* E4 carriers. However, other authors [83] reported that characteristic changes in MRI may be observed even in healthy infants carrying the *APOE* E4 allele. According to authors of [84], the *APOE* E4 allele is not only responsible for a decline in episodic memory with age in cognitively normal adults but may also induce impaired olfaction due to deterioration of medial temporal lobe. This is consistent with the neuroimaging data, suggesting that in non-demented *APOE* E4 carriers, mediotemporal atrophy occurs prior to clinical dementia onset.

It is also interesting that multiple studies have confirmed that the *TOMM40/APOE* locus is associated not only with the risk of dementia but also with longevity. The GWAS confirmed that the rs4420638 polymorphism on chromosome 19q13.32 was significantly related to living longer than >85 years (OR = 0.72, $p = 3.40 \times 10^{-36}$) [85]. Similarly, according to a recent study [86], with the use of more sophisticated integrative GWAS (iGWAS) method to couple data from 14 meta-analyses, the locus housing *APOE* and *TOMM40* remained significantly associated with longevity, even when the false discovery rate (FDR) was set at 10%, which indicates that the *APOE*/*TOMM40* locus holds the key for healthy senescence without a pathological memory decline.

6. *APOE* in a healthy Polish population under 60 years of age

Despite the many years of research, AD remains a disease that is difficult to predict and diagnose, with few blood-derived biomarkers possible for use in routine clinical setting. As was stated before, *APOE* remains the most significant genetic risk factor of AD. This creates a need for the development of a novel, quick, and reliable method of analyzing the *APOE* genotype and the apoE plasma concentration. The role of *APOE* in the development of dementia and its influence on longevity in elderly people has been studied by [53]. As per our knowledge, *APOE* studies on a younger population in Poland have been neglected and there are no literature data on association of the *APOE* genotype and the apoE plasma level in non-demented Polish adults.

6.1. Aim of the study

In this study, we tried to assess the influence of the *APOE* genotype and the effect of demographic factors on the apoE level in a subset of Polish non-demented volunteers less than 60 years of age.

6.2. Subjects

A total of 83 healthy adults (70 females, mean age: 51.9 ± 7.2; 13 males, mean age: 44.9 ± 11.7) under 60 years of age with no signs of dementia or other neurological disorders were enrolled in the study. All participants provided signed, written consent. The research project was approved by the Bioethical Committee at the Poznan University of Medical Sciences, decision no. 1031/13, dated May 5, 2013.

6.3. Materials

Each volunteer's blood was collected on an anticoagulant—K_3EDTA (Monovette™ vacuum system, Sarstedt, USA). A total of 3 ml of blood was immediately aliquoted, then frozen and stored at −80°C upon nucleic acid isolation. Subsequently, the remaining blood was centrifuged (1400 relative centrifugal force [RCF], 10 min) and the collected plasma was aliquoted and stored at −80°C.

6.4. Methodology

6.4.1. APOE genotyping

First, a subject's DNA was extracted from frozen blood using gravity flow microcolumns (Genomic Micro AX Blood Gravity, A&A Biotechnology, Poland). The DNA concentration was measured by a microplate spectrophotometer (Take3, Epoch, BioTek, USA) and adjusted to 20 ng/µL with Milli-Q® water. Subsequently, genotyping was performed according to a modified mismatch primer method [87]. Briefly, three quantitative polymerase chain reaction (qPCR) specific to each *APOE* allele were performed with the use of four different primers (as shown in **Table 2**). The qPCR included two steps: primary pre-amplification (15 cycles) with annealing at 64°C followed by 30 cycles of secondary amplification with annealing at 62°C. The reactions were performed on a CFX Connect™ Real-Time PCR Detection System (Bio-rad, USA) in 10 µL volumes, with 250 nM primers and 50 ng of genomic DNA using 1× SsoFast™ EvaGreen® Supermix (Bio-rad, USA). The cycling conditions were: 30 s initial denaturation at 98°C followed by cycles of 98°C for 5 s and 64 and 62°C for 10 s. The reaction was considered positive once the products appeared before the 10th cycle of secondary qPCR. The method was validated by Sanger sequencing in an external laboratory.

Reaction	Starter	Sequence	Annealing temperature	Product melting point
APOE E2	APOE112C	CGGACATGGAGGACGTGT	62–64°C	91.4°C
	APOE158C	CTGGTACACTGCCAGGCA		
APOE E3	APOE112R	CGGACATGGAGGACGTGC		91.6°C
	APOE158C	CTGGTACACTGCCAGGCA		
APOE E4	APOE112R	CGGACATGGAGGACGTGC		91.8°C
	APOE158R	CTGGTACACTGCCAGGCG		

Table 2. Starters used for genotyping of *APOE*.

6.4.2. ApoE quantification

Determination of the plasma apoE concentration was performed by the enzyme-linked immunosorbent assay (ELISA) method. The analysis was performed according to the manufacturer's protocol (Human apoE ELISA Kit, Mabtech, Sweden) using 10,000× diluted plasma samples. Absorbance was measured by an EPOCH microplate reader (BioTek, USA). The concentrations were calculated from a four-parametric standard curve ($R = 0.998$) by Gen5 ver. 2.01 software (provided with the reader).

6.5. Results

Our study on Polish subjects showed that the observed genotype frequencies of *APOE* are in line with the Hardy-Weinberg equilibrium ($p = 0.9365$). The dominating allele was *APOE* E3 (83.7%) and the least common allele was *APOE* E2 (3.0%), as is shown in **Figure 1**. Interestingly, we did not observe any *APOE* E2/E2 homozygotes, as is shown in **Table 3**.

Our results indicate that the apoE plasma concentration depends on the *APOE* genotype (one-way analysis of variance [ANOVA], $p = 0.021$). Generally, in *APOE* E3/E3 carriers we recorded the highest mean concentrations of apoE, while in the *APOE* E4/E4 homozygotes we recorded the lowest mean concentrations. In females with the *APOE* E2/E3 allele, the concentration of apoE was slightly lower than in the E3 homozygotes. Interestingly, in a single case of an

E2/E4 carrier we observed an increased level of plasma apoE. Subsequently, the plasma apoE concentration in *APOE* E3/E3 carriers was higher in males than in females. Conversely, in *APOE* E3/E4 carriers the recorded apoE concentration was higher in females. Hence, the decrease in apoE due to the *APOE* E4 genotype was more pronounced in males than in females (41% vs 16%), as shown in **Table 3**. Overall, the apoE concentration was insignificantly higher in males than in females (2.54 vs 2.24 mg/dL; $p = 0.194$, Student's t-test). The observed positive trend of increasing apoE in older individuals did not reach statistical significance ($r = 0.201$, $p = 0.0687$; Pearson correlation coefficient). However, after stratification according to gender, we observed significant correlation of the apoE plasma level and age in females ($r = 0.348$, $p = 0.00128$; Pearson correlation coefficient). The concentrations of apoE stratified according to *APOE* status, gender, and age are shown in **Table 4** and **Figure 2**, respectively.

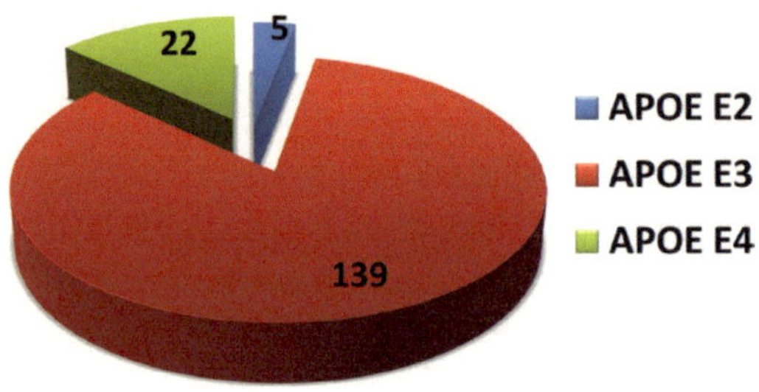

Figure 1. Frequencies of *APOE* alleles in Polish, cognitively normal volunteers under 60 years of age.

Genotypes	*APOE* E2/E2	*APOE* E2/E3	*APOE* E3/E3	*APOE* E3/E4	*APOE* E4/E4	*APOE* E2/E4
Observed frequencies	0	4	58	19	1	1
	0.0%	4.8%	69.9%	22.9%	1.2%	1.2%
Expected frequencies	0.08	4.19	58.20	18.42	1.40	0.66
	0.1%	5.0%	70.1%	22.2%	1.8%	0.8%

Note: Hardy-Weinberg equilibrium calculations, $p = 0.9365$, $n = 83$.

Table 3. Hardy-Weinberg equilibrium calculations of *APOE* variants in Polish, cognitively normal volunteers less than 60 years of age.

Gender	*APOE* E2/E3	*APOE* E2/E4	*APOE* E3/E3	*APOE* E3/E4	*APOE* E4/E4
Female	1.98 ± 0.67	2.91	2.35 ± 0.78	2.02 ± 0.52	0.69
Male	–	–	2.91 ± 0.63	1.72 ± 0.22	–
Combined	1.98 ± 0.67	2.91	2.43 ± 0.79	1.95 ± 0.49	0.69

Note: Mean concentration ± SD (mg/dL) or (single result).

Table 4. Mean plasma apoE concentration (mg/dL) in Polish, cognitively normal volunteers under 60 years of age stratified according to gender and *APOE* genotype.

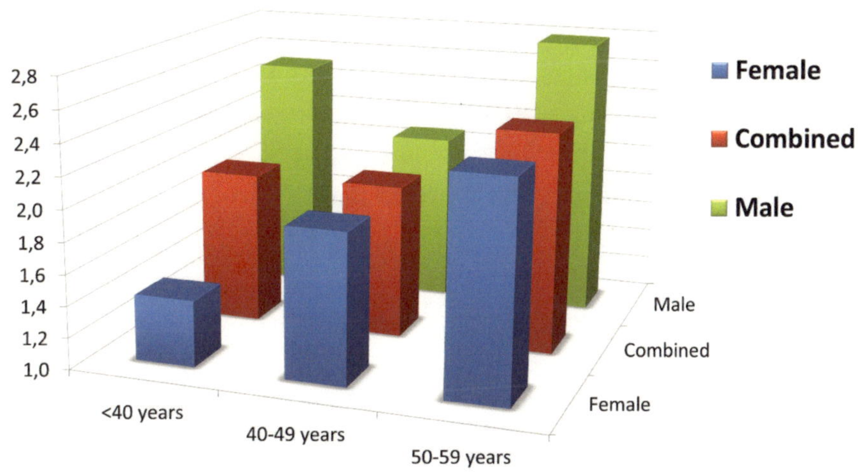

Figure 2. Mean apoE plasma concentration (mg/dL) in Polish, cognitively normal volunteers under 60 years of age stratified according to gender and age.

6.6. Discussion

As was stated before, the *APOE* E4 allele is associated with increased risk of developing dementia.

According to our results, the *APOE* E3 genotype was the most prevalent genotype in the studied group, while the E2 genotype was the least common. Similar results were reported in the Polish population [53].

Our study shows that *APOE* E4 variant is associated with a decreased concentration of plasma apoE in cognitively normal Polish volunteers less than 60 years of age. Our results are supported by the results of other authors [77], who analyzed plasma apoE concentrations and *APOE* status in a cohort of 75,708 participants in the Copenhagen General Population Study and the Copenhagen City Heart Study. The authors also showed that apoE is dependent on the *APOE* genotype, as they found substantial differences in plasma apoE concentrations between carriers of distinct *APOE* genotypes. However, contrary to our results, in their study the highest level of apoE was observed in *APOE* E2 homozygotes and decreased in E4 carriers in a dose-dependent manner: E2/E2 > E2E3 > E2/E4 > E3/E3 > E3/E4 > E4/E4. The plasma concentration of apoE in E4/E4 homozygotes was up to 65% lower as compared to *APOE* E2/E2 carriers. This partial incompatibility with our results may be explained by the utilization of various methods: the authors used the nephelometry and turbidimetry methods, whereas we used the well-established ELISA method. In another study [88], the authors showed that apoE concentrations in plasma apoE increased with age in a healthy population. We observed a similar trend; however, it was significant only in the female group.

The plasma concentration of apoE may be a valuable dementia biomarker because it is easily available and, according to literature data, decreased apoE may be a risk factor for developing dementia. The above-mentioned Australian follow-up cohort study, comprising mostly

Caucasian subjects, showed that the reduced apoE plasma level may be a predictor of a transition from MCI to AD. Moreover, the plasma apoE concentration correlates positively with cognitive function, and patients with a lower apoE level tend to perform worse in neuropsychological tests assessing spatial memory and language abilities [89].

Hence, the assessment of the plasma apoE concentration and the *APOE* status may give valuable information to physicians trying to predict the rate of cognitive decline in the course of dementive disease as well as in normally ageing adults and elderly persons.

7. Summary

The appearance of dementia in old age is influenced by both biochemical and genetic factors leading to structural disorders in the brain of elderly persons. The level of Aβ is mentioned among the other biochemical factors associated with dementia. The deposition of Aβ in the brain is controlled by *APOE* and by genes associated with the amyloid cascade (*APP, PSEN1,* and *PSEN2*). Subsequently, Aβ toxicity is modified by the *TOMM40*. In the elderly, also abnormal cholesterol, glucose levels, and the weakening of protective and repair mechanisms leading to the generation of ROS (mediated, e.g. by *PON1*) may cause a reduction in cognitive functions. However, the role of genes associated with longevity (e.g. *FOXO3A, CETP*) and normal aging (e.g. *SIRT1, AKT1, CDKN1A*) is not clearly defined in the occurrence of diseases typical for this age group, as shown in **Figure 3**.

Finding a way to control the genetic factors and their protein products may contribute to the prevention of diseases of old age, including depression and dementia, and to improve the quality of life of elderly people.

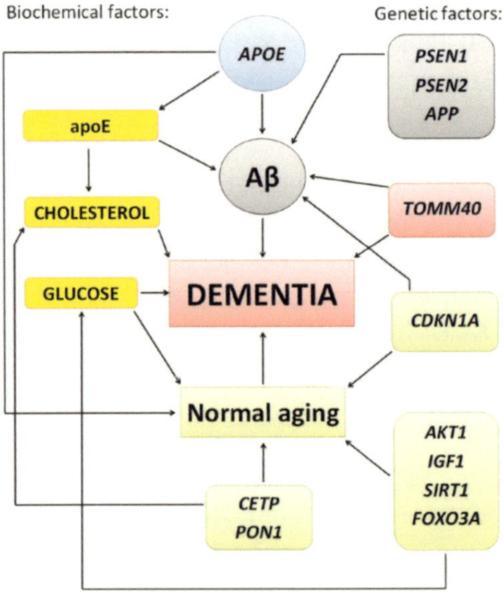

Figure 3. The genetic and biochemical factors associated with normal aging and dementia; β-amyloid—Aβ.

Acknowledgements

This study was supported by the Poznan University of Medical Sciences grant no. 502-14-01111677-10342.

Author details

Michał Prendecki[1], Jolanta Florczak-Wyspianska[2], Marta Kowalska[1], Margarita Lianeri[1], Wojciech Kozubski[2] and Jolanta Dorszewska[1*]

*Address all correspondence to: dorszewskaj@yahoo.com

1 Laboratory of Neurobiology, Department of Neurology, Poznan University of Medical Sciences, Poznan, Poland

2 Chair and Department of Neurology, Poznan University of Medical Sciences, Poznan, Poland

References

[1] Robertson R. Weight loss in elderly. (in) Rosenthal T, Naughton R, Williams M. Geriatria, Czelej, Lublin 2009:131–145.(Article in Polish)

[2] Dorszewska J. Cell biology of normal brain aging: Synaptic plasticity – Cell death. Aging Clin Exp Res. 2013; 25:25–34. DOI: 10.1007/s40520-013-0004-2

[3] Holle R, Grässel E, Ruckdäschel S, Wunder S, Mehlig H, Marx P, Pirk O, Butzlaff M, Kunz S, Lauterberg J. Dementia care initiative in primary practice: Study protocol of a cluster randomized trial on dementia management in a general practice setting. BMC Health Serv Res. 2009; 6:9, 91. DOI: 10.1186/1472-6963-9-91

[4] Jóźwiak A. Dementia in the elderly. Geriatria 2008; 2:237–246.(Article in Polish)

[5] Montagne A, Pa J, Zlokovic BV. Vascular plasticity and cognition during normal aging and dementia. JAMA Neurol. 2015; 72:495–496. DOI: 10.1001/jamaneurol

[6] Petersen RC, Wiste HJ, Weigand SD, Rocca WA, Roberts RO, Mielke MM, Lowe VJ, Knopman DS, Pankratz VS, Machulda MM, Geda YE, Jack CR Jr. Association of elevated amyloid levels with cognition and biomarkers in cognitively normal people from the community. JAMA Neurol. 2016; 73:85–92. DOI: 10.1001/jamaneurol.2015.3098

[7] Dickstein DL, Kabaso D, Rocher AB, Luebke JI, Wearne SL, Hof PR. Changes in the structural complexity of the aged brain. Aging Cell. 2007; 6:275–284.

[8] Bishop NA, Lu T, Yankner BA. Neural mechanisms of ageing and cognitive decline. Nature. 2010; 464:529–535. DOI: 10.1038/nature08983

[9] Nation DA, Edmonds EC, Bangen KJ, Delano-Wood L, Scanlon BK, Han SD, Edland SD, Salmon DP, Galasko DR, Bondi MW, Alzheimer's Disease Neuroimaging Initiative Investigators. Pulse pressure in relation to tau-mediated neurodegeneration, cerebral amyloidosis, and progression to dementia in very old adults. JAMA Neurol. 2015; 72:546–553. DOI: 10.1001/jamaneurol.2014.4477

[10] Berti V, Murray J, Davies M, Spector N, Tsui WH, Li Y, et al. Nutrient patterns and brain biomarkers of Alzheimer's disease in cognitively normal individuals. J Nutr Health Aging. 2015; 19:413–423. DOI: 10.1007/s12603-014-0534-0

[11] Torralva T, Sposato LA, Riccio PM, Gleichgerrcht E, Roca M, Toledo JB, Trojanowski JQ, Kukull WA, Manes F, Hachinski V. Role of brain infarcts in behavioral variant frontotemporal dementia: Clinicopathological characterization in the National Alzheimer's Coordinating Center database. Neurobiol. Aging. 2015; 36:2861–2868. DOI: 10.1016/j.neurobiolaging.2015.06.026

[12] Kida Y, Goligorsky MS. Sirtuins, Cell Senescence, and Vascular Aging. Can J Cardiol, 2016; 32:634–641.DOI: 10.1016/j.cjca.2015.11.022

[13] Morris BJ, Willcox DC, Donlon TA, Willcox BJ. FOXO3: A major gene for human longevity – a mini-review. Gerontology. 2015; 61:515–525. DOI: 10.1159/000375235

[14] Vijg J, Hasty P. Aging and p53: Getting it straight. A commentary on a recent paper by Gentry and Venkatachalam. Aging Cell. 2005; 4:331–338.

[15] Gravina S, Lescai F, Hurteau G, Brock GJ, Saramaki A, Salvioli S, Franceschi C, Roninson IB. Identification of single nucleotide polymorphisms in the p21 (CDKN1A) gene and correlations with longevity in the Italian population. Aging (Albany, NY). 2009; 1:470–480.

[16] Gudnason V, Kakko S, Nicaud V, Savolainen MJ, Kesäniemi YA, Tahvanainen E, Humphries S. Cholesteryl ester transfer protein gene effect on CETP activity and plasma high-density lipoprotein in European populations. The EARS Group. Eur J Clin Invest. 1999; 29:116–128.

[17] Sanders AE, Wang C, Katz M, Derby CA, Barzilai N, Ozelius L, Lipton RB. Association of a functional polymorphism in the cholesteryl ester transfer protein (CETP) gene with memory decline and incidence of dementia. JAMA. 2010; 303:150–158. DOI: 10.1001/jama.2009.1988

[18] Brooks-Wilson AR. Genetics of healthy aging and longevity. Hum Genet. 2013; 132:1323–1338. DOI: 10.1007/s00439-013-1342-z

[19] Forte G, Grossi V, Celestini V, Lucisano G, Scardapane M, Varvara D, Patruno M, Bagnulo R, Loconte D, Giunti L, Petracca A, Giglio S, Genuardi M, Pellegrini F, Resta N, Simone C. Characterization of the rs2802292 SNP identifies FOXO3A as a modifier locus predicting cancer risk in patients with PJS and PHTS hamartomatous polyposis syndromes. BMC Cancer. 2014; 14:661. DOI: 10.1186/1471-2407-14-661

[20] López-Otín C, Blasco MA, Partridge L, Serrano M, Kroemer G. The hallmarks of aging. Cell. 2013; 153:1194–1217. DOI: 10.1016/j.cell.2013.05.039

[21] Kilic U, Gok O, Erenberk U, Dundaroz MR, Torun E, Kucukardali Y, Elibol-Can B, Uysal O, Dundar T. A remarkable age-related increase in SIRT1 protein expression against oxidative stress in elderly: SIRT1 gene variants and longevity in human. PLoS One. 2015; 10:e0117954. DOI: 10.1371/journal.pone.0117954

[22] Lescai F, Marchegiani F, Franceschi C. PON1 is a longevity gene: Results of a meta-analysis. Ageing Res Rev. 2009; 8:277–284. DOI: 10.1016/j.arr.2009.04.001

[23] Blasiak J, Glowacki S, Kauppinen A, Kaarniranta K. Mitochondrial and nuclear DNA damage and repair in age-related macular degeneration. Int J Mol Sci. 2013; 14:2996–3010. DOI: 10.3390/ijms14022996

[24] Alexeyev M, Shokolenko I, Wilson G, LeDoux S. The maintenance of mitochondrial DNA integrity – critical analysis and update. Cold Spring Harb Perspect Biol. 2013; 5:a012641. DOI: 10.1101/cshperspect.a012641

[25] Harman D. A theory based on free radical and radical chemistry. J Gerontol. 1956; 11:298–300.

[26] Sanz A, Stefanatos RK. The mitochondrial free radical theory of aging: A critical view. Curr Aging Sci. 2008; 1:10–21.

[27] Gaziev AI, Abdullaev S, Podlutsky A. Mitochondrial function and mitochondrial DNA maintenance with advancing age. Biogerontology. 2014; 15:417–438. DOI: 10.1007/s10522-014-9515-2

[28] Hebert SL, Marquet-de Rougé P, Lanza IR, McCrady-Spitzer SK, Levine JA, Middha S, Carter RE, Klaus KA, Therneau TM, Highsmith EW, Nair KS. Mitochondrial aging and physical decline: Insights from three generations of women. J Gerontol A Biol Sci Med Sci. 2015; 70:1409–1417. DOI: 10.1093/gerona/glv086

[29] Gackowski D, Rozalski R, Siomek A, Dziaman T, Nicpon K, Klimarczyk M, Araszkiewicz A, Olinski R. Oxidative stress and oxidative DNA damage is characteristic for mixed Alzheimer disease/vascular dementia. J Neurol Sci. 2008; 266:57–62.

[30] Hatanaka H, Hanyu H, Fukasawa R, Sato T, Shimizu S, Sakurai H. Peripheral oxidative stress markers in diabetes-related dementia. Geriatr Gerontol Int. 2015. DOI: 10.1111/ggi.12645.

[31] Simpson JE, Ince PG, Matthews FE, Shaw PJ, Heath PR, Brayne C, Garwood C, Higginbottom A, Wharton SB; MRC Cognitive Function and Ageing Neuropathology

Study Group. A neuronal DNA damage response is detected at the earliest stages of Alzheimer's neuropathology and correlates with cognitive impairment in the Medical Research Council's Cognitive Function and Ageing Study ageing brain cohort. Neuropathol Appl Neurobiol. 2015; 41:483–496. DOI: 10.1111/nan.12202

[32] Newton DF, Naiberg MR, Goldstein BI. Oxidative stress and cognition amongst adults without dementia or stroke: Implications for mechanistic and therapeutic research in psychiatric disorders. Psychiatry Res. 2015; 227(2–3):127–134. DOI: 10.1016/j.psychres.2015.03.038

[33] Berger SL, Kouzarides T, Shiekhattar R, Shilatifard A. An operational definition of epigenetics. Genes Dev. 2009; 23:781–783. DOI: 10.1101/gad.1787609

[34] Jones MJ, Goodman SJ, Kobor MS. DNA methylation and healthy human aging. Aging Cell. 2015; 14:924–932. DOI: 10.1111/acel.12349

[35] Zampieri M, Ciccarone F, Calabrese R, Franceschi C, Bürkle A, Caiafa P. Reconfiguration of DNA methylation in aging. Mech Ageing Dev. 2015; 151:60–70. DOI: 10.1016/j.mad.2015.02.002

[36] Marttila S, Kananen L, Häyrynen S, Jylhävä J, Nevalainen T, Hervonen A, Jylhä M, Nykter M, Hurme M. Ageing-associated changes in the human DNA methylome: Genomic locations and effects on gene expression. BMC Genomic. 2015; 16:179. DOI: 10.1186/s12864-015-1381-z

[37] Sun D, Yi SV. Impacts of chromatin states and long-range genomic segments on aging and DNA methylation. PLoS One. 2015; 10:e0128517.

[38] Klein CJ, Botuyan MV, Wu Y, Ward CJ, Nicholson GA, Hammans S, Hojo K, Yamanishi H, Karpf AR, Wallace DC, Simon M, Lander C, Boardman LA, Cunningham JM, Smith GE, Litchy WJ, Boes B, Atkinson EJ, Middha S, B Dyck PJ, Parisi JE, Mer G, Smith DI, Dyck PJ. Mutations in DNMT1 cause hereditary sensory neuropathy with dementia and hearing loss. Nat Genet. 2011; 43:595–600. DOI: 10.1038/ng.830

[39] Xu X. DNA methylation and cognitive aging. Oncotarget. 2015; 6:13922–13932.

[40] Kouzarides T. Chromatin modifications and their function. Cell. 2007; 128(4):693–705.

[41] Di Bernardo G, Cipollaro M, Galderisi U. Chromatin modification and senescence. Curr Pharm Des. 2012; 18:1686–1693.

[42] Gräff J, Tsai LH. Histone acetylation: Molecular mnemonics on the chromatin. Nat Rev Neurosci. 2013; 14:97–111. DOI: 10.1038/nrn3427

[43] Scaffidi P, Misteli T. Lamin A-dependent nuclear defects in human aging. Science. 2006; 312:1059–1063.

[44] Krishnan V, Liu B, Zhou Z. 'Relax and Repair' to restrain aging. Aging (Albany, NY). 2011; 3:943–954.

[45] Zhou P, Wu E, Alam HB, Li Y. Histone cleavage as a mechanism for epigenetic regulation: Current insights and perspectives. Curr Mol Med. 2014; 14:1164–1172.

[46] Das C, Tyler JK. Histone exchange and histone modifications during transcription and aging. Biochim Biophys Acta. 2013; 1819:332–342.

[47] Spiegel AM, Sewal AS, Rapp PR. Epigenetic contributions to cognitive aging: Disentangling mindspan and lifespan. Learn Mem. 2014; 21:569–574. DOI: 10.1101/lm.033506.113

[48] Dorszewska J, Prendecki M, Oczkowska A, Dezor M, Kozubski W. Molecular basis of familial and sporadic Alzheimer's disease. Curr Alzheimer Res. 2016; 13:1–12. e-pub

[49] Fargo K. Alzheimer's Association Report: 2014 Alzheimers disease facts and figures. Alzheimer's Dement. 2014; 10:e47–e92.

[50] Hansson Petersen CA, Alikhani N, Behbahani H, Wiehager B, Pavlov PF, Alafuzoff I, et al. The amyloid beta-peptide is imported into mitochondria via the TOM import machinery and localized to mitochondrial cristae. Proc Natl Acad Sci U S A. 2008; 105:13145–13150. DOI: 10.1073/pnas.0806192105

[51] Roses AD, Lutz MW, Amrine-Madsen H, Saunders AM, Crenshaw DG, Sundseth SS, et al. A TOMM40 variable-length polymorphism predicts the age of late-onset Alzheimer's disease. Pharmacogenomics J. 2010; 10(5):375–384. DOI: 10.1038/tpj.2009.69

[52] Lutz MW, Crenshaw DG, Saunders AM, Roses AD. Genetic variation at a single locus and age of onset for Alzheimer's disease. Alzheimers Dement. 2010; 6:125–131. DOI: 10.1016/j.jalz.2010.01.011

[53] Maruszak A, Pepłońska B, Safranow K, Chodakowska-Żebrowska M, Barcikowska M, Zekanowski C. TOMM40 rs10524523 polymorphism's role in late-onset Alzheimer's disease and in longevity. J Alzheimers Dis. 2012; 28:309–322. DOI: 10.3233/JAD-2011-110743

[54] Payton A, Sindrewicz P, Pessoa V, Platt H, Horan M, Ollier W, et al. A TOMM40 poly-T variant modulates gene expression and is associated with vocabulary ability and decline in nonpathologic aging. Neurobiol Aging. 2015; 39:217.e1–7. DOI: 10.1016/j.neurobiolaging.2015.11.017

[55] Laczó J, Andel R, Vyhnalek M, Matoska V, Kaplan V, Nedelska Z, et al. The effect of TOMM40 on spatial navigation in amnestic mild cognitive impairment. Neurobiol Aging. 2015; 36:2024–2033. DOI: 10.1016/j.neurobiolaging.2015.03.004

[56] Johnson SC, La Rue A, Hermann BP, Xu G, Koscik RL, Jonaitis EM, et al. The effect of TOMM40 poly-T length on gray matter volume and cognition in middle-aged persons with APOE ε3/ε3 genotype. Alzheimer's Dement. 2011; 7:456–465. DOI: 10.1016/j.jalz.2010.11.012

[57] Dietschy JM. Central nervous system: Cholesterol turnover, brain development and neurodegeneration. Biol Chem. 2009; 390:287–293. DOI: 10.1515/BC.2009.035

[58] Koch M, Jensen MK. HDL-cholesterol and apolipoproteins in relation to dementia. Curr Opin Lipidol. 2016; 27:76–87. DOI: 10.1097/MOL.0000000000000257

[59] Ettcheto M, Petrov D, Pedrós I, de Lemos L, Pallàs M, Alegret M, et al. Hypercholesterolemia and neurodegeneration. Comparison of hippocampal phenotypes in LDLr knockout and APPswe/PS1dE9 mice. Exp Gerontol. 2015; 65:69–78. DOI: 10.1016/j.exger.2015.03.010

[60] Reitz C, Tang M-X, Schupf N, Manly JJ, Mayeux R, Luchsinger JA. Association of higher levels of high-density lipoprotein cholesterol in elderly individuals and lower risk of late-onset Alzheimer disease. Arch Neurol. 2010; 67:1491–1497. DOI: 10.1001/archneurol.2010.297

[61] Ancelin M-L, Ripoche E, Dupuy A-M, Barberger-Gateau P, Auriacombe S, Rouaud O, et al. Sex differences in the associations between lipid levels and incident dementia. J Alzheimers Dis. 2013; 34:519–528. DOI: 10.3233/JAD-121228

[62] Mielke MM, Bandaru VVR, Haughey NJ, Xia J, Fried LP, Yasar S, et al. Serum ceramides increase the risk of Alzheimer disease: The Women's Health and Aging Study II. Neurology. 2012; 79:633–641. DOI: 10.1212/WNL.0b013e318264e380

[63] Gupta VB, Laws SM, Villemagne VL, Ames D, Bush AI, Ellis KA, et al. Plasma apolipoprotein E and Alzheimer disease risk: The AIBL study of aging. Neurology. 2011; 76:1091–1098. DOI: 10.1212/WNL.0b013e318211c352

[64] Ghebranious N, Mukesh B, Giampietro PF, Glurich I, Mickel SF, Waring SC, et al. A pilot study of gene/gene and gene/environment interactions in Alzheimer disease. Clin Med Res. 2011; 9:17–25. DOI: 10.3121/cmr.2010.894

[65] Dias IHK, Polidori MC, Li L, Weber D, Stahl W, Nelles G, et al. Plasma levels of HDL and carotenoids are lower in dementia patients with vascular comorbidities. J Alzheimers Dis. 2014; 40:399–408. DOI: 10.3121/cmr.2010.894

[66] Czapski GA, Maruszak A, Styczyńska M, Żekanowski C, Safranow K, Strosznajder JB. Association between plasma biomarkers, CDK5 polymorphism and the risk of Alzheimer's disease. Acta Neurobiol Exp (Wars). 2012; 72:397–411.

[67] Warren MW, Hynan LS, Weiner MF. Lipids and adipokines as risk factors for Alzheimer's disease. J Alzheimers Dis. 2012; 29:151–157. DOI: 10.3233/JAD-2012-111385

[68] Tai LM, Thomas R, Marottoli FM, Koster KP, Kanekiyo T, Morris AWJ, et al. The role of APOE in cerebrovascular dysfunction. Acta Neuropathol. 2016; 131:709–723

[69] Lambert J-C, Heath S, Even G, Campion D, Sleegers K, Hiltunen M, et al. Genome-wide association study identifies variants at CLU and CR1 associated with Alzheimer's disease. Nat Genet. 2009; 41:1094–1099. DOI: 10.1038/ng.439.

[70] Jongbloed W, van Dijk KD, Mulder SD, van de Berg WDJ, Blankenstein MA, van der Flier W, et al. Clusterin levels in plasma predict cognitive decline and progression to Alzheimer's disease. J Alzheimers Dis. 2015; 46:1103–1110. DOI: 10.3233/JAD-150036

[71] Sapkota S, Wiebe SA, Small BJ, Dixon RA. Apolipoprotein E and Clusterin can magnify effects of personality vulnerability on declarative memory performance in non-demented older adults. Int J Geriatr Psychiatry. 2016; 31:502–509. DOI: 10.1002/gps.4355

[72] Liu C-C, Liu C-C, Kanekiyo T, Xu H, Bu G. Apolipoprotein E and Alzheimer disease: Risk, mechanisms and therapy. Nat Rev Neurol. 2013; 9:106–118. DOI: 10.1038/nrneurol.2012.263

[73] Niimi M, Yang D, Kitajima S, Ning B, Wang C, Li S, et al. ApoE knockout rabbits: A novel model for the study of human hyperlipidemia. Atherosclerosis. 2016; 245:187–193. DOI: 10.1016/j.atherosclerosis.2015.12.002

[74] Srivastava RA. Regulation of the apolipoprotein E by dietary lipids occurs by transcriptional and post-transcriptional mechanisms. Mol Cell Biochem. 1996; 155:153–162.

[75] Hu J, Liu C-C, Chen X-F, Zhang Y-W, Xu H, Bu G. Opposing effects of viral mediated brain expression of apolipoprotein E2 (apoE2) and apoE4 on apoE lipidation and Aβ metabolism in apoE4-targeted replacement mice. Mol Neurodegener. 2015; 10:6. DOI: 10.1186/s13024-015-0001-3

[76] Schmidt C, Gerlach N, Schmitz M, Thom T, Kramer K, Friede T, et al. Baseline CSF/serum-ratio of apolipoprotein e and rate of differential decline in Alzheimer's disease. J Alzheimer's Dis. 2015; 48:189–196. DOI: 10.3233/JAD-150286

[77] Rasmussen KL, Tybjaerg-Hansen A, Nordestgaard BG, Frikke-Schmidt R. Plasma levels of apolipoprotein E and risk of dementia in the general population. Ann Neurol. 2015; 77:301–311. DOI: 10.1002/ana.24326. DOI: 10.1002/ana.24326

[78] Corder EH, Saunders AM, Strittmatter WJ, Schmechel DE, Gaskell PC, Small GW, et al. Gene dose of apolipoprotein E type 4 allele and the risk of Alzheimer's disease in late onset families. Science. 1993; 261:921–923.

[79] Seshadri S, Fitzpatrick AL, Ikram MA, DeStefano AL, Gudnason V, Boada M, et al. Genome-wide analysis of genetic loci associated with Alzheimer disease. JAMA. 2010; 303:1832–1840. DOI: 10.1001/jama.2010.574

[80] Shinohara M, Kanekiyo T, Yang L, Linthicum D, Shinohara M, Fu Y, et al. APOE2 eases cognitive decline during aging: clinical and preclinical evaluations. Ann Neurol. 2016; 79:758–774. DOI: 10.1002/ana.24628

[81] Arold S, Sullivan P, Bilousova T, Teng E, Miller CA, Poon WW, et al. Apolipoprotein E level and cholesterol are associated with reduced synaptic amyloid beta in Alzheimer's disease and apoE TR mouse cortex. Acta Neuropathol. 2012; 123:39–52. DOI: 10.1007/s00401-011-0892-1

[82] Caselli RJ, Dueck AC, Huentelman MJ, Lutz MW, Saunders AM, Reiman EM, et al. Longitudinal modeling of cognitive aging and the TOMM40 effect. Alzheimer's Dement. 2012; 8:490–495. DOI: 10.1016/j.jalz.2011.11.006

[83] Dean DC, Jerskey BA, Chen K, Protas H, Thiyyagura P, Roontiva A, et al. Brain differences in infants at differential genetic risk for late-onset Alzheimer disease: A cross-sectional imaging study. JAMA Neurol. 2014; 71:11–22. DOI: 10.1001/jamaneurol.2013.4544

[84] Olofsson JK, Josefsson M, Ekström I, Wilson D, Nyberg L, Nordin S, et al. Long-term episodic memory decline is associated with olfactory deficits only in carriers of ApoE-ϵ4. Neuropsychologia. 2016; 85:1–9. DOI: 10.1016/j.neuropsychologia.2016.03.004

[85] Deelen J, Beekman M, Uh HW, Broer L, Ayers KL, Tan Q, et al. Genome-wide association meta-analysis of human longevity identifies a novel locus conferring survival beyond 90 years of age. Hum Mol Genet. 2014; 23:4420–4432. DOI: 10.1093/hmg/ddu139

[86] Fortney K, Dobriban E, Garagnani P, Pirazzini C, Monti D, Mari D, et al. Genome-wide scan informed by age-related disease identifies loci for exceptional human longevity. Li H, editor. PLoS Genet. 2015; 11:e1005728. DOI: 10.1371/journal.pgen.1005728

[87] Calero O, Hortigüela R, Bullido MJ, Calero M. Apolipoprotein E genotyping method by real time PCR, a fast and cost-effective alternative to the TaqMan and FRET assays. J Neurosci Methods. 2009; 183:238–240. DOI: 10.1016/j.jneumeth.2009.06.033

[88] Rasmussen KL, Tybjærg-Hansen A, Nordestgaard BG, Frikke-Schmidt R. Plasma levels of apolipoprotein E and risk of ischemic heart disease in the general population. Atherosclerosis. 2016; 246:63–70. DOI: 10.1016/j.atherosclerosis.2015.12.038

[89] Gupta VB, Wilson AC, Burnham S, Hone E, Pedrini S, Laws SM, et al. Follow-up plasma apolipoprotein E levels in the Australian Imaging, Biomarkers and Lifestyle Flagship Study of Ageing (AIBL) cohort. Alzheimers Res Ther. 2015; 7:16. DOI: 10.1186/s13195-015-0105-6

Chapter 12

Changes in Visual Cortex in Healthy Aging and Dementia

Alyssa A. Brewer and Brian Barton

Additional information is available at the end of the chapter

http://dx.doi.org/10.5772/64562

Abstract

This chapter reviews the differences in specific structural and functional characteristics of human visual cortex among young adults, healthy aging adults, and patients with dementia, with a primary focus on those with Alzheimer's disease (AD). Such visual cortex changes have been shown to underlie many of the behavioral deficits that develop in healthy aging and AD. Measurements of disordered visual cortex in dementia patients may be possible early in the course of neurodegeneration and thus may be useful for improving early diagnosis of these devastating diseases.

Keywords: visual cortex, visual field mapping, dementia, healthy aging, functional neuroimaging

1. Introduction

1.1. Overview of visual cortex characteristics

Human visual cortex can be partitioned into distinct topographical representations of visual space called visual field maps (VFMs), each of which subserves separate perceptual functions spanning the hierarchical stages of visual processing [1–3]. The organization of a VFM follows the organization of the retina; hence, retinotopic VFMs are cortical regions in which nearby neurons analyze the properties of nearby points of an image on the retina, and thus of visual space. This VFM organization is one of the more important, larger-scale, organizing principles of visual cortex. Such topographic organization is thought to allow for efficient connectivity among neurons that represent nearby aspects of visual space, likely necessary for such processes as lateral inhibition and to compactly organize neural signals ranging from the molecular level to that of the cerebral hemisphere [4–7]. In addition, measurements of the characteristics of these VFMs, together with an understanding of the stimulus selectivity of the neurons within them, is the foundation for understanding the specific visual computations carried out in particular cortical regions. Not only are such *in vivo* measurements of VFMs essential for the study of visual processing in healthy subjects, but they also are very effective for tracking changes in visual cortex in response to changes in visual inputs such as those that arise from retinal or cortical damage [8–12].

Although historically the organization and function of visual cortex have been primarily well characterized in healthy young adults or young patient populations [1–3, 8, 12–16], many behavioral studies [17–38] and more recent neuroimaging studies [36, 37, 39–55] are suggesting that several changes occur within visual pathways during what is considered otherwise healthy aging. These studies specifically describe retinal and cortical changes, rather than optical changes in the eye, that primarily contribute to the decreases in visual acuity and related issues that have been measured in healthy aging subjects [19, 33, 46, 50, 54]. These healthy aging changes are also now starting to be compared to pathophysiological changes in visual cortex in age-related disorders like dementia, including diseases such as Alzheimer's disease (AD), posterior cortical atrophy (PCA), and dementia with Lewy bodies (DLB), in the hopes of both improving our understanding of these diseases and aiding improvements in potential therapies [37, 56].

Visual deficits are reported surprisingly often as one of the first symptoms of AD, the most common form of dementia. These deficits can include problems with visual-spatial attention, visual-spatial tasks, and visual-processing speed [37, 40, 47, 57–75]. A subset of dementia patients presents with prominent visual symptoms such as problems with visual field defects, contrast sensitivity, color discrimination, and feature recognition of complex objects, but little initial decline in memory. These patients have increased neuropathology in visual cortex, as compared to typical AD patients [76–84]. Dementia with these characteristics was initially often referred to as visual variant AD, but it is now usually termed PCA. DLB, the second most common type of dementia, also often presents with visual complaints [85]. Like in AD and PCA, the central features of DLB include progressive cognitive decline, typically with impairments in memory, visual-spatial abilities, and attention. However, unlike AD and PCA, one of the earliest visual symptoms in this disease is commonly visual hallucination [86].

Early detection and accurate diagnosis are keys in the hope for a cure for such dementias, as early, precise diagnosis would allow for more timely initiation of treatments. As visual symptoms can occur early in these diseases, studies are beginning to demonstrate that measurements of related changes in visual cortex in these patients could aid early detection of neurodegeneration. The highly structured representations within VFMs afford a fundamental measurement that might be used to detect subtle effects of neurodegeneration early in the disease process. Clear measures of the progression of the pathology within visual cortex might also help to target drug research for therapeutic interventions, especially by differentiating among different types of dementia [62]. The information reviewed in this chapter will serve as a foundation for subsequent use of this knowledge in our evaluation, interpretation, and treatment of these diseases. As little has been studied regarding VFMs in patients with PCA or DLB, this chapter will focus on measurements from patients with AD.

http://dx.doi.org/10.5772/64562

1.2. Review methodology

We performed a systematic review to investigate whether there are changes in early VFMs V1, V2, V3, and hV4 characteristics to healthy aging subjects and patients with AD or related dementias that can be measured using functional magnetic resonance imaging (fMRI). In order to include as many relevant citations as possible, we searched a comprehensive range of scientific databases including CogPrints, FreeFullPDF, Google Scholar, IngentaConnect, JSTOR, Mendeley, Microsoft Academic Search, PubMed, PubPsych, ResearchGate, and Web of Science. In addition, the Google search engine was used to find institutional, professional, and personal webpages hosting potentially relevant PDFs or citation links. Searches were performed from November 2015, to May 2016. Search queries included the following terms in various combinations: visual cortex, visual field map, visual area, primary visual cortex, V1, V2, V3, hV4, occipital cortex, visual changes, fMRI, pRF modeling/modeling, neuroimaging, aging, healthy aging, human, dementia, neurodegeneration, mild cognitive impairment, Alzheimer's disease, dementia with Lewy bodies, Lewy body dementia, and posterior cortical atrophy. Related citation links available for the various database searches were routinely evaluated to investigate additional potential citations of interest. All potential study designs were included, and potentially relevant citations spanned the dates 1925–2016; note that visual field mapping with fMRI was relatively recently introduction in 1994 [87].

Ultimately, 317 potentially relevant citations were downloaded to EndNote for further evaluation. The full papers of these citations were assessed and selected to only include studies that directly related to comparing fMRI measures of visual cortex or visual field maps in healthy young adults (aged 18–40 years) to changes in visual cortex or visual field maps in healthy aging subjects with no known age-related diseases or specific, clinically recognized deficits in vision (aged 55–80 years) and/or to patients with mild-to-moderate AD with no known visual deficits unrelated to dementia (aged 55–80 years). No studies of VFM changes in DLB or PCA were found during the initial database searches, which was not unexpected given the very recent emergence of interest in visual field mapping in dementia. Additional studies of visual field mapping methodology and of visual symptoms associated with healthy aging, AD, DLB, and PCA were also retained for methods discussion and hypothesis development, respectively. Studies were further evaluated for quality and were excluded if they lacked statistical analysis or if they did not use accurate cortical field mapping techniques with individual subject analysis (for further discussion of these criteria, see [1, 3, 88]).

Of the 317 downloaded studies, 165 papers were directly relevant to this review, of which 88 focused on visual changes in aging or dementia. Of these, 24 studies measured changes specifically in visual cortex related to aging and/or dementia, and three studies explicitly investigated VFM changes in aging and/or dementia, as appropriate with respect to the inclusion and exclusion criteria [36, 37, 39]. Here, we provide both a narrative discussion of all 165 sources as well as graphical examples drawn from the three key visual field mapping studies. We discuss what is known regarding changes in early visual cortex during healthy aging and AD, how these findings relate to visual symptoms in these conditions, and what remains to be studied, and we recommend directions for future research.

2. The measurement and organization of visual cortex in healthy young adults

In order to carefully evaluate alterations of visual cortex in healthy aging and age-related neurodegenerative diseases such as AD, we must first have an accurate and detailed understanding of the characteristics of visual cortex in healthy young adults. Visual cortex encompasses nearly 20% of the human cortical sheet, and studies are demonstrating that nearly all of it is organized into VFMs [1, 3]. Because many calculations are necessary to produce our visual world, our brains have many specialized VFMs which perform one or more of those calculations [3, 89]. Most—if not all—of these calculations are performed across the entire visual scene; color perception, for example, occurs throughout the visual field, not just in the lower right quadrant. Ultimately, it will be very interesting to investigate changes in visual cortex among all levels of the cortical visual hierarchy, from low-level visual processing in primary visual cortex (V1) to mid-level specialization like motion processing to higher-level processing like face recognition and visual-spatial attention [2, 90]. For now, studies of plasticity and neurodegeneration primarily investigate the lower level visual areas like V1, V2, V3, and hV4, as these VFMs are particularly well established in healthy young adults, relatively uncontroversial, and typically easily measured across most types of patients [1, 3, 8, 12, 14, 15, 37, 91].

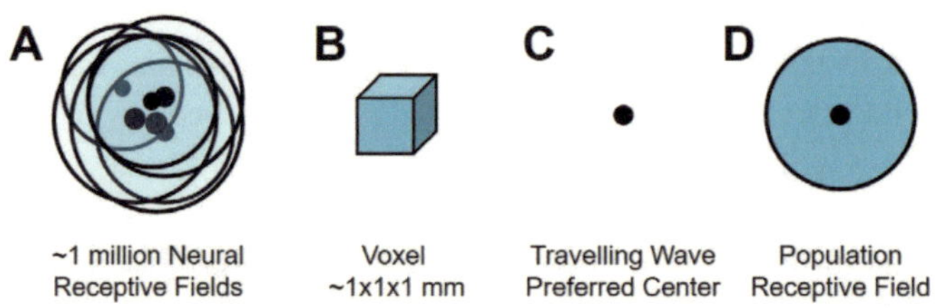

Figure 1. Schematic of measurements of an individual voxel. (A) Within a typical voxel measured with a standardly used 3T MRI scanner, there are on the order of ~1 million neurons, depending on the size of the voxel. For voxels in retinotopic visual cortex, the neurons each have similarly located spatial receptive fields (*teal circles with black outlines*) with preferred centers (*black dots*). Note how the overlapping receptive fields concentrate coverage in one region of visual space (*darker teal*) corresponding to the average receptive field of the group, as shown in **(D)**. **(B)** Each typical voxel is on the order of 1 × 1 × 1 mm for structural measurements and 1 × 1 × 3 mm for visual field mapping functional experiments, though voxels are often slightly larger (e.g., 3 × 3 × 3 mm) for other types of functional MR studies. **(C)** Traveling wave retinotopy (TWR) utilizes the organization of retinotopic cortex, in which neighboring neurons have preferred centers (*black dot*) representing similar portions of visual space, to estimate the average preferred representation (center) for the population of neurons in a given voxel (e.g., [1, 3]). **(D)** Population receptive field (pRF) modeling similarly utilizes retinotopic organization to estimate not only the preferred center (*black dot*) in a given voxel, but also the average receptive field—the population receptive field (*teal circle*)—for the voxel's population of neurons (e.g., [1, 3, 92]).

2.1. Human visual field map measurements use simple stimuli and tasks, but provide exquisite detail of cortical organization

We briefly review here two of the most powerful fMRI techniques for very detailed measurements of VFMs in individual subjects, traveling wave retinotopy (TWR) [87] and population receptive field (pRF) modeling [92], to demonstrate what types of measurements are possible and how to interpret the existing literature regarding changes in aging or damaged visual cortex (**Figures 1–4**).

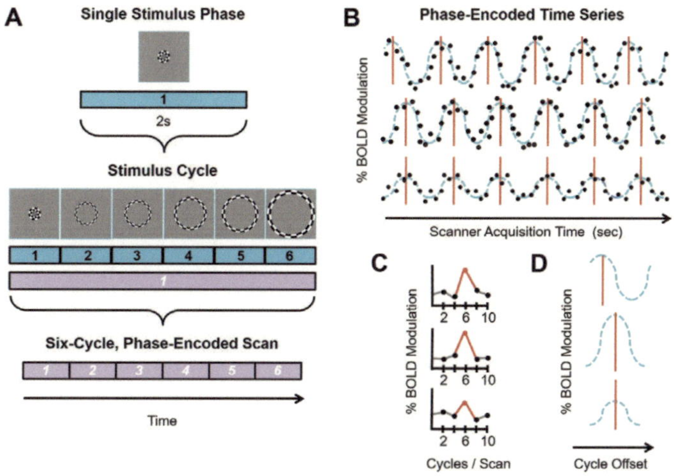

Figure 2. Phase-encoded fMRI paradigm for visual field map measurements. (A) An example phase-encoded experimental design [87]. Top diagram shows the components of a single block of one stimulus presentation (*teal*) for one position (i.e., stimulus phase) of an expanding ring stimulus composed of a black and white moving checkerboard pattern. Middle diagram shows six blocks (*teal*) grouped together into one stimulus cycle (*purple*). The progressively larger ring stimulus is shown above each block. Each block in one cycle presents a specific stimulus in the "phase-encoded"—or "traveling wave"—sequence. Each cycle then repeats the same set of blocks. Lower diagram shows a full, single scan comprising six cycles; each cycle is one purple block. **(B)** Schematic diagram of three example phase-encoded time series with different stimulus responses. Each row depicts the time series measurement for a single voxel arising from a single, six-cycle scan using one experimental stimulus (e.g., polar angle). Simulated raw data points showing percent blood-oxygen-level-dependent (BOLD) modulation (i.e., response amplitude) are denoted by the black dots. The teal dotted lines represent sinusoidal fits of the simulated data points; each teal line characterizes the average BOLD activation in a different example voxel. The red lines indicate the peak activations per cycle for this imaginary set of voxels. Top and middle rows represent time series of voxels with the same %BOLD modulation, but different timing of peak responses, which indicates different stimulus selectivity (i.e., responses to different "phases" of the stimulus). Note the offset of the red lines between the two rows. For example, the top row might represent a voxel with a preferred eccentricity tuning of 2° eccentric to fixation, whereas the middle row might have a preferred tuning of 5° eccentric to fixation. Middle and bottom rows represent time series of voxels with the same timing of peak responses, indicating matching stimulus selectivity; i.e., both might have a preferred eccentricity tuning of 5° eccentric to fixation. However, the bottom row has much lower %BOLD modulation than the middle row. Such a difference in response amplitude can be due to several factors, such as differences in local vasculature or receptive field tuning. **(C)** Diagram of three example Fourier power spectra corresponding to the schematic time series in **(B)**. In the phase-encoded paradigm, only BOLD responses that match the stimulus frequency of six cycles per scan (*red peak*) are considered as data. The responses must also be above a predetermined statistical threshold, typically measured in coherence or percentage variance explained [3, 87, 92]. **(D)** Diagram of three example averaged stimulus cycles corresponding to the schematic Fourier spectra in **(C)** and to averages of the time series in **(B)**. Each teal dotted line represents the sinusoidal fit for the average, while the peak activation is again marked by the red line. The timing of the peak of each averaged cycle is used to calculate the phase of the preferred stimulus independently for each voxel. Typical pseudocolor overlays on 3D or flattened brain renderings as shown in **Figures 6** and **12** use color to denote cortical responses to this peak activation. Note how the top measurement has an earlier peak (*red line*) that corresponds to an earlier phase of the stimulus (i.e., an earlier presentation time in the cycle) while the middle and bottom measurements' peaks are shifted to later in time (e.g., [3]). The bottom example has a lower %BOLD modulation than the other two schematics, but the same peak activation as the middle example. For additional discussion, see [1, 3, 87, 91, 92].

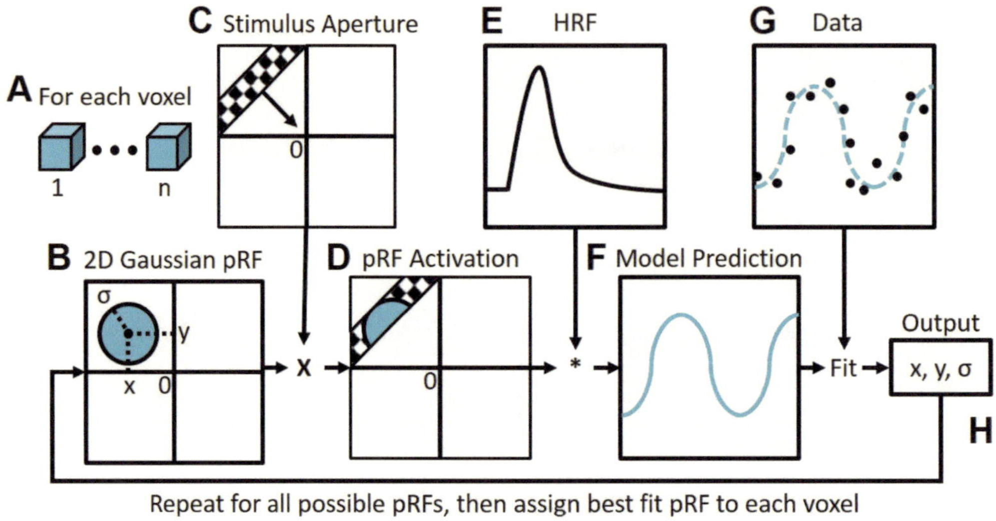

Figure 3. Population receptive field modeling. The parameter estimation procedure for the population receptive field (pRF) model is shown as a flow chart [92]. The pRF parameters are estimated from time series measurements using a linear spatiotemporal model of the fMRI response, which is a reasonable approximation over a wide range of spatio-temporal conditions [94–96]. The neuronal model is estimated by finding the model parameters that best predict the fMRI measurements. **(A)** The pRF modeling analysis is applied to all voxels (1:*n*) within the defined region of interest (ROI; e.g., occipital lobe, V1). **(B)** Multiple models of the expected average receptive field of the neuronal population may be used. Most commonly, a two-dimensional Gaussian is estimated, which is defined by three parameters, x, y, and σ, where (x, y) denotes the pRF center within the visual field, and σ is the Gaussian spread (i.e., pRF radius). Note that these parameters are stimulus-referred in degrees of visual angle. **(C)** The example moving bar stimulus composed of a black and white moving checkerboard pattern moves systematically across visual space. **(D)** The overlap between the pRF and effective stimulus is determined. **(E, F)** Next, the predicted pRF response is calculated for a given pRF model and effective stimulus location. The time series model prediction **(F)** is estimated by convolving the pRF activation with a model of the hemodynamic response function (HRF) as in **(E)** [94, 97]. The goodness-of-fit is estimated by computing the residual sum of squares (RSS) between this prediction and the data (*black dots*) **(G)**. **(H)** 100,000 different fMRI time series predictions are iteratively tested by varying the pRF model parameters across a wide range of plausible values (e.g., locations across visual space covered by the stimulus; varying pRF sizes). Ultimately, the optimal pRF parameters (x, y, σ) are found for each voxel independently by minimizing the RSS using a two-stage, coarse-to-fine search. Adapted from **Figure 2** in [92].

2.1.1. Traveling wave retinotopy

Developed in the 1990s, TWR is still the primary fMRI paradigm used to measure early VFMs like V1–3 (**Figures 1** and **2**) [13, 15, 87, 91, 93]. This technique uses two types of periodic stimuli that move smoothly across a contiguous region of visual space to measure the orthogonal dimensions of polar angle (i.e., "around the clock") and eccentricity (i.e., center to periphery; **Figure 5**). These stimuli are typically composed of a set of high-contrast, flickering checkerboard patterns that are designed to maximally stimulate primary visual cortex and generally elicit an fMRI signal modulation on the order of 1–3% (**Figure 2A**). This modulation is typically 15–20 standard deviations above the background noise. Each voxel's preferred polar angle representation is measured by a rotating wedge stimulus, which extends from the central fovea to more peripheral regions and covers a small section of polar angles (**Figure 6C**, *central* *inset*). This wedge stimulus revolves either counterclockwise or clockwise in discrete steps around the central fixation point, successively stimulating distinct polar angle representations of visual space [3]. Each voxel's preferred eccentricity representation is measured by an expanding ring stimulus, which expands in discrete even steps between the central fovea and the periphery of the visual field (**Figure 6B**, *central inset*). These functional data are represented as color-coded overlays on anatomical data that demark the voxel's preferred polar angle or eccentricity (**Figure 6B** and **C**). The accurate delineation of VFMs relies upon the measurement of these two, orthogonal dimensions—polar angle and eccentricity, which produce a unique mapping between a location in visual space and the preferred responses of the neurons within a single voxel in cortex. If only a single measurement is obtained (e.g., of only polar angle or only eccentricity), the representation in cortex could only be associated with a wide section of visual space and would not lead to the correct definition of VFM boundaries (**Figure 5**) [3].

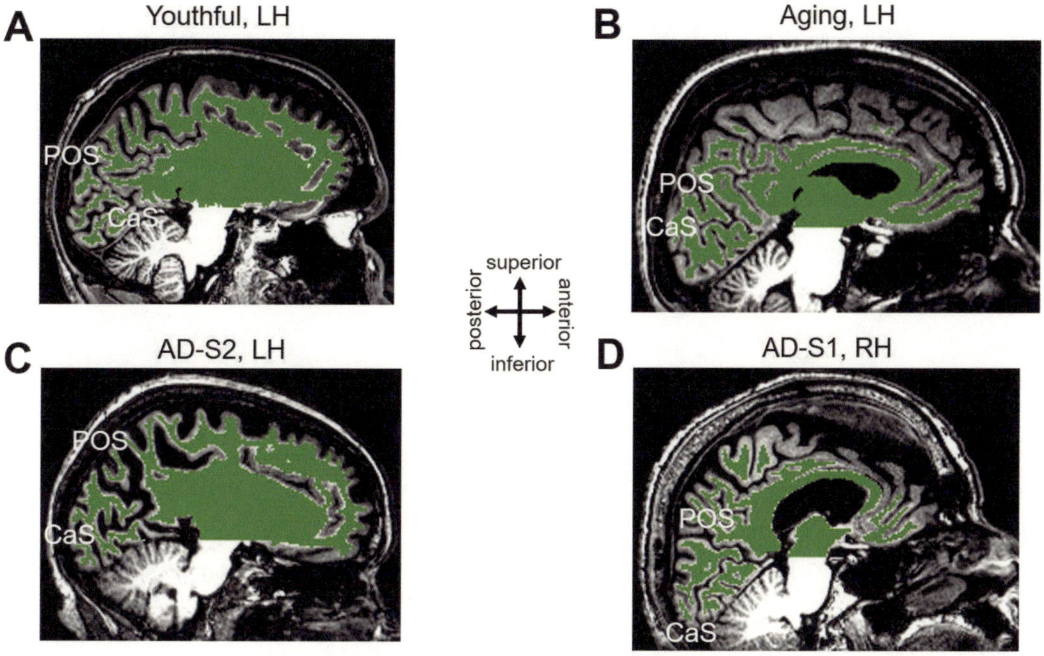

Figure 4. White/gray matter segmentation for young, healthy aging, and mild Alzheimer's disease subjects. Each panel is a T1-weighted 3D MPRAGE image showing a sagittal slice near the midline of the brain. Green-colored overlay represents white matter identified by an automated algorithm [104] and adjusted by hand-editing to minimize segmentation errors [1, 3, 92]. White regions below the green overlay represent unsegmented white matter within the cerebellum. Gray matter is shown as the gray regions along the surface of the green overlay and adjacent to the black cerebral spinal fluid (CSF; *black regions within the skull*). Middle inset displays approximate anatomical directions. CaS: calcarine sulcus; POS: parietal-occipital sulcus. **(A)** Left hemisphere of healthy young subject. **(B)** Left hemisphere of healthy aging subject. **(C)** Left hemisphere of a subject with mild Alzheimer's disease (AD-S2). **(D)** Right hemisphere of a second subject with mild Alzheimer's disease (AD-S1). Note how AD-S1's anatomy is relatively intact, but the visual field map measurements from this subject shown in **Figure 12** are perceptibly abnormal. Also compare the strikingly increased CSF-filled space in this T1 image of AD-S2 to the relatively normal visual field map organization for this subject in **Figure 12**. Data were adapted from [36, 37].

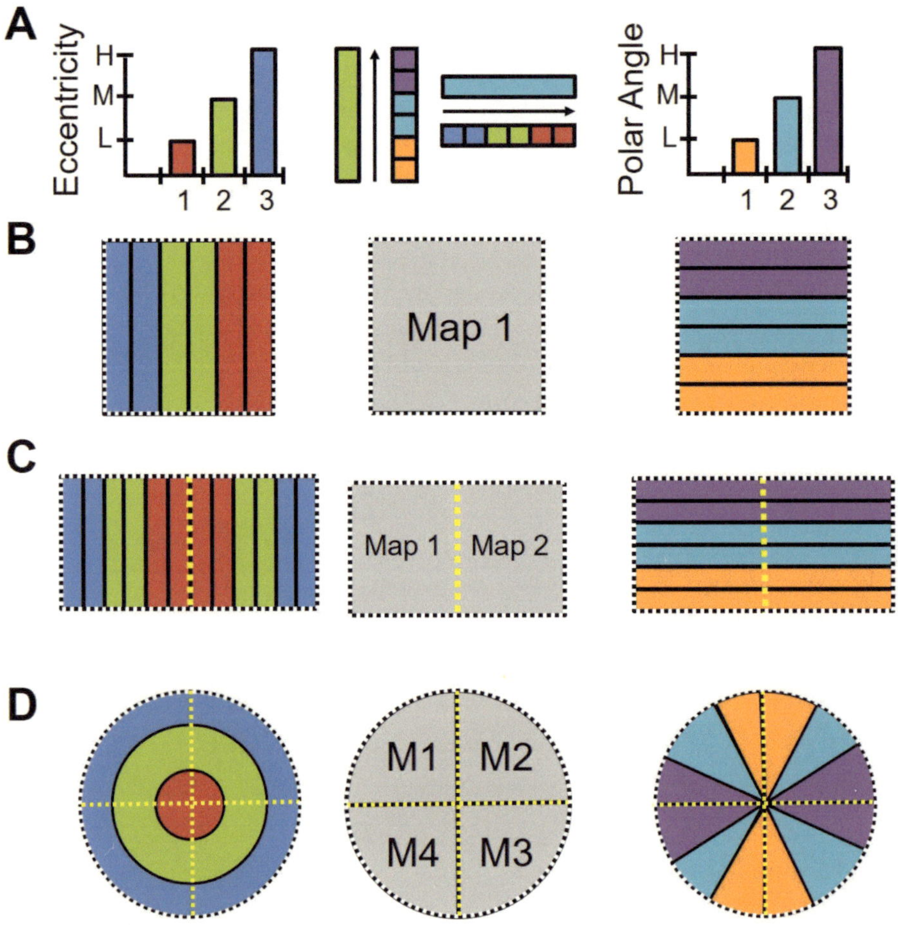

Figure 5. Two orthogonal gradients are required to define a cortical field map. (A)*Left:* The graph demonstrates measurements of three stimulus values—1: low (L, *red*); 2: medium (M, *green*); 3: high (H, *blue*)—for one sensory dimension (e.g., eccentricity). *Right:* The graph demonstrates measurements of three stimulus values—1: low (L, *orange*); 2: medium (M, *aqua*); 3: high (H, *purple*) for a second sensory dimension (e.g., polar angle). *Middle:* Schematic of the orthogonal gradients defining a cortical field map shows how measurements of the cortical representation of dimension 2 change along measurements of the representation of a single value of dimension 1, and vice versa. **(B)** Diagrams demonstrate how a single set of orthogonal gradients (one for each dimension) defines a single cortical field map. Black dotted lines demark the edge of the gradient representations. **(C)** Diagrams here demonstrate how a reversal in the dimension 1 gradient representations (*left*) divides up the single representation of the dimension 2 gradient (*right*) into two cortical field maps (*middle*). Yellow dotted lines demark a boundary defined by a gradient reversal, and black dotted lines again denote the edge of the gradient representations. A reversal in the dimension 2 gradient representations would similarly divide up a single representation of the dimension 1 gradient (*not shown*). **(D)** Cloverleaf cluster organization of multiple cortical field maps. *Left:* Schematic of an example macrostructural organization of dimension 1 (e.g., eccentricity) across a region of the cortical surface, with low (*red*) to medium (*green*) to high (*blue*) stimulus values represented in concentric circles. *Right:* Schematic of an example macrostructural organization of orthogonal dimension 2 (e.g., polar angle) across the same region of the cortical surface, with low (*orange*) to medium (*aqua*) to high (*purple*) stimulus values represented in wedges running "around the clock". *Middle:* Schematic shows the four cortical field maps defined by these orthogonal gradients and arranged in a cloverleaf cluster [3, 111–113]. Black dotted lines demark the edge of the gradient representations. Yellow dotted lines demark boundaries defined by a gradient reversal. For additional discussions, see [1, 3, 88].

http://dx.doi.org/10.5772/64562

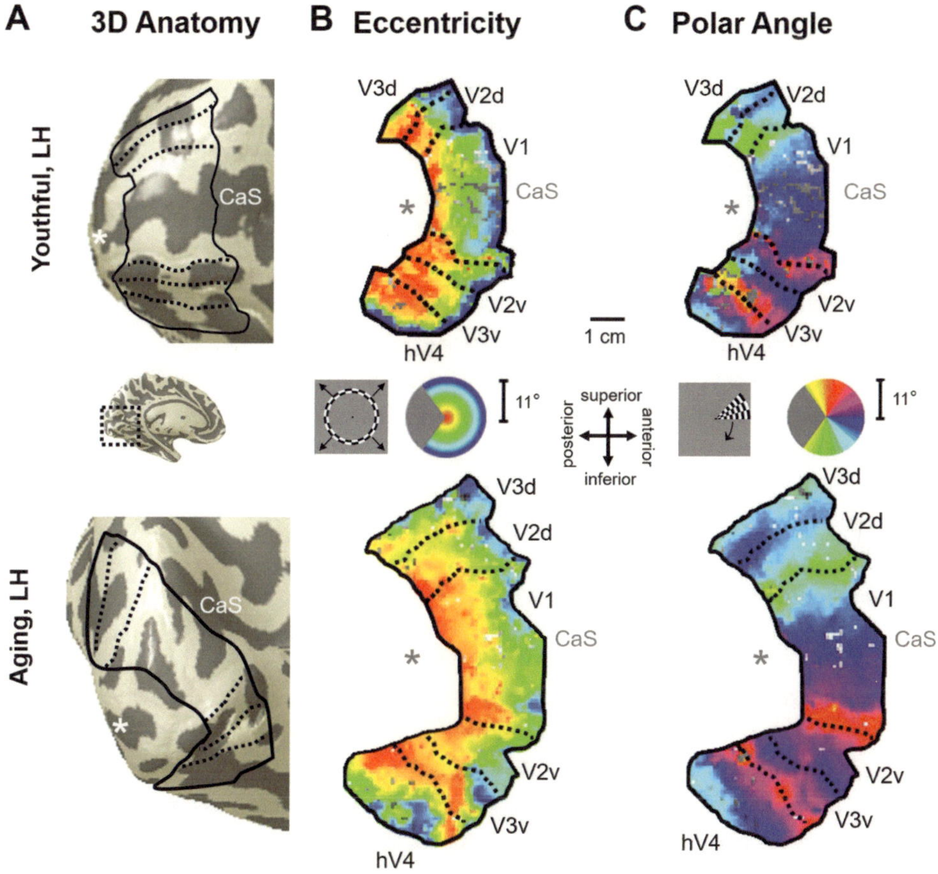

Figure 6. Visual field map measurements in healthy young and aging subjects. The images show example measurements of VFMs V1, V2, V3, and hV4 from a healthy young adult's left hemisphere (*top row*) and from a healthy aging adult's left hemisphere (*bottom row*). **(A)** Cortical locations of VFMs (black lines) are show on 3D renderings of each subject's left hemisphere. Central inset shows the approximate location of the cropped sections of the hemispheres. For cortical surfaces, dark gray represents sulci, and light gray represents gyri. "*" denotes the approximate location of the occipital pole; CaS: calcarine sulcus. **(B, C)** Flattened views of the cortical surfaces surrounding CaS are shown for the measurements of eccentricity **(B)** and polar angle **(C)** in each subject. The pseudocolor overlay on each flattened section of cortex signifies the location in visual space that creates the highest activity at each cortical position (see colored legend insets, *middle*). The wedge and ring stimuli each maximally spanned the central 11° radius of visual space. For simplicity, cortical representations are only shown for V1, V2, V3, and hV4—the VFMs of interest. Also note that functional data are only shown for voxels with a strong response at a coherence ≥0.20. Flattened renderings are scaled to the same size (see 1 cm scale bar, *middle inset*). Approximate anatomical directions for the flattened representations are shown in the central inset. Data were adapted from [36, 37].

The term "traveling wave" arises from the repeating pattern of cortical activity that is activated from one end of the VFM to the other along iso-angle or iso-eccentricity lines in response to these periodic stimuli (**Figure 2B**) [87, 91]. Thus, the time, or phase, of the peak modulation induced by the stimulus varies smoothly across the cortical surface. This phase defines the most effective stimulus eccentricity (i.e., ring) and polar angle (i.e., wedge) to activate that region of cortex, giving TWR its description as "phase-encoded retinotopy" (**Figure 2D**). This paradigm only produces activity in regions that are retinotopically organized and is excellent for measuring early VFMs such as V1, V2, and V3.

In neuroimaging experiments, cortical activity driven by a particular stimulus is typically differentiated from unrelated activity and noise by setting well-defined statistical thresholds [94]. The statistical threshold for cortical activity arising from the TWR paradigm is commonly determined by coherence, which is equal to the amplitude of the blood-oxygen-level-dependent (BOLD) signal modulation at the frequency of stimulus presentation (e.g., six stimulus cycles per scan), divided by the square root of the power over all other frequencies except the first and second harmonics. Note that the activity must be correlated with the stimulus modulation frequency; unrelated activity at other frequencies is not included in the coherence measure. For each stimulus condition (e.g., wedge or ring), each voxel is independently assigned a coherence value, which denotes the strength of the BOLD response of that voxel for that particular stimulus (**Figure 2C**). Only voxels with a coherence above a chosen threshold —typically a coherence of 0.15–0.30—are further evaluated to determine the organization of cortical visual-spatial representations into specific VFMs [1, 3].

2.1.2. *Population receptive field modeling*

A newer method of measuring VFMs called population receptive field (pRF) modeling has been introduced not only for measurements of early visual cortex (e.g., V1–3), but also to improve measurements of the visual-spatial organization of higher-order regions that contain larger RFs (**Figures 1** and **3**) [92]. This model relies on the fact that the population of RFs in each voxel of retinotopically organized regions of cortex is expected to have similar preferred centers (i.e., location in visual space driving the peak neural responses) and sizes (i.e., the degrees of visual angle driving significant neural responses), allowing their combined pRF to be estimated as a single, two-dimensional Gaussian RF (**Figure 3B**). The pRF method does not require two distinct stimuli to measure orthogonal dimensions of visual space as in TWR, but can use any stimulus that systematically traverses the entire field of view. Most commonly in current measurements, this is a moving bar composed of the same checkerboard pattern with neutral gray blocks inserted at a nonstimulus frequency (**Figure 3C**). The neutral gray blocks allow for an estimation of a voxel's response to any visual stimulus versus just the preferred visual stimulus, which is necessary for the accurate measurement of pRF sizes.

For the first part of the analysis, the pRF model generates a database of many possible pRF centers and sizes within the field of view covered by the stimulus. The analysis then convolves the standard hemodynamic response function (HRF) with each of the possible pRFs (**Figure 3E**). Lastly, a least-squares fitting method is used to iteratively test the actual data collected against each of the possible pRFs for each voxel independently. The best-fit pRF position and size is then allocated as the pRF parameters for that voxel. As in TWR, further analysis is only performed on voxels with responses above a specific threshold of variance explained—which can be converted to coherence—as determined by the model are included for further analysis (for additional discussions, see [1, 3, 92]).

http://dx.doi.org/10.5772/64562

2.1.3. *VFMs are defined using data from individual subjects*

It is vital to correctly localize common functional areas across subjects in order to then study which specific computations are carried out by each area and how these functions change with damage and disease; however, the size of functional regions across the cortical surface varies significantly across individuals, complicating measurements across subject groups [14, 92, 98–102]. The surface area of primary visual cortex (V1) can differ across subjects by a factor of 3 or more; this variation in VFM size is independent of the total brain size [14]. Consequently, the position of each VFM with respect to the underlying structural anatomy varies across individuals. In addition, the amount of variation tends to increase from V1 to regions of visual cortex involved in higher-order computations (e.g., object recognition). Therefore, the common fMRI approach of averaging measurements across subjects does not work in the case of VFM data, as this approach will problematically blur the VFM boundaries to an unusable degree and may even destroy all traces of VFM organization in some regions [3]. Likewise, standardized brain-template coordinates (e.g., Talairach or Montreal Neurological Institute—MNI—coordinates) cannot be used to accurately estimate the position of any VFMs beyond area V1 in group-averaged or individual-subject data. Furthermore, issues like cortical degeneration introduce even greater variability into the match between cortical function and structure. The only accurate approach is to measure VFMs in individual subjects. Functional or structural measurements from each VFM—each region of interest (ROI) —can be obtained from individual subjects and then averaged across the subject group by VFM.

For analysis of such functional imaging data for individual subjects, several neuroimaging software packages are available. We use a signal-processing, Matlab-based software package called *mrVista*, which was originally developed by the Wandell lab at Stanford University and is now commonly available for neuroimaging analysis (http://white.stanford.edu/software/) [103, 104]. Using this software, each subject's cortical white matter is determined—"segmented"—in that subject's high-resolution anatomical scan, first with an automated algorithm and then by hand-editing to minimize errors for individual-subject analyses (**Figure 4**) [104]. Then a 3–4 mm layer of gray matter is automatically formed arising from the segmented white matter surface. Only data drawn from this identified gray matter are analyzed, in order to reduce extraneous measurements arising in the white matter or noise outside the head. The gray matter of the cortical sheet can then be visualized in three dimensions or as a flat sheet to allow analysis of functional activity within the sulci. For analysis of the functional data, linear trends are removed from the time series during preprocessing. Individual scans are inspected for motion artifacts; issues with motion between individual scans or across scan sessions can be corrected using mutual-information algorithms [105]; however, motion-correction algorithms should not be routinely applied if not needed, as they themselves may create artifacts. Once the preprocessed functional dataset is registered to the high-resolution anatomical scan, the VFM activity can be viewed along the cortical sheet to allow for optimal definition of VFM boundaries (e.g., **Figures 5** and **6**; for detailed discussions, see [1, 3, 88]). Importantly, we never apply spatial smoothing to the data, as smoothing will destroy key details of VFM organization, much like averaging data across subjects.

The description of a cortical "map" is frequently used nonspecifically for topographical gradients or other related cortical representations; however, it is advantageous for research into visual processing to explicitly define a "visual field map" in accordance with very exact criteria: (i) a VFM comprises two (or more) orthogonal, nonrepeating topographical representations of fundamental sensory dimensions (e.g., eccentricity and polar angle); (ii) each of these topographical representations must be organized as an generally contiguous, orderly gradient; (iii) each VFM should represent a substantial portion of sensory space (e.g., a hemifield of the visual field); and (iv) the general features of each VFM should be consistent across individuals (**Figure 5**) [1, 3, 13, 15, 88, 106–111]. For additional discussion, see *A Brief Primer on Cortical Field Mapping* in the supplemental material of [88].

2.2. Characteristics of V1, V2, V3, and hV4 in healthy young adults

Three VFMs known as V1, V2, and V3 occupy the medial wall of occipital cortex in humans and participate in the first stages of visual processing (for detailed reviews, see [1, 3]). Each represents a full hemifield of the opposite—i.e., contralateral—visual field in each hemisphere; the left hemisphere VFMs represent the right visual field, and vice versa (**Figure 6**).

V1 is very reliably located along the calcarine sulcus, bounded on either side by the unique split-hemifield representations of V2 and V3 on the cuneus and lingual gyri. V1, V2, and V3 each contain a representation of the center of visual space located at the occipital pole. Increasingly more peripheral representations form complete eccentricity gradients extending into more anteromedial cortex forming complete eccentricity gradients (**Figure 6A** and **B**; e.g., [1, 3, 13, 15, 91]). The position at which the central—i.e., foveal—representations of these three VFMs come together at the occipital pole is called the foveal confluence [114]. The boundaries between each map are delineated by reversals in polar angle gradients (**Figure 6A** and **C**). The polar angle gradient of V1 represents a contiguous hemifield of visual space. In contrast, the polar angle representations of V2 and V3 each consist of a split-hemifield representation (i.e., a quarterfield of visual space). The separate quarterfield sections are denoted by their positions ventral or dorsal to V1 (e.g., V2d, V2v, V3d, and V3v). For each of these three VFMs, the upper visual quarterfield is represented on the ventral surface, and the lower visual quarterfield is represented on the dorsal surface. The V2 and V3 quarterfields each meet at the fovea, but are otherwise separate [3]. Due to their relatively consistent anatomical locations and unique concentric organization, these three VFMs form the easiest landmarks to be identified in visual field mapping analyses [13–15, 87]. An additional VFM is adjacent to V3v along the ventral occipital surface: human V4, designated hV4 because of the unclear homology to macaque V4 [106]. The eccentricity representation of hV4 merges with the foveal confluence of V1, V2, and V3, and the polar angle representation moves smoothly from the boundary at the upper visual field representation of the V3v quarterfield into a full hemifield representation.

V1 is labeled as primary visual cortex, because it receives direct input from the retinal-thalamic pathway and is the first place along this pathway where information from the two eyes is combined [115]. In addition, V1 is an important site of initial basic calculations for such visual processing as orientation, color, and motion [116–120]. Beyond V1, perceptual calculations become more specialized, with V2 subserving relatively simple color and form perception and

V3 more selectively supporting motion processing [118, 119, 121–124]. hV4 serves as the next stage of the V1–V2 processing pathway with specialized neuronal populations for somewhat more complicated color and form visual perception [106, 125, 126]. Damage to part of the retina or V1 produces a complete loss of visual perception within the region normally processed by the damaged tissue in most cases [9], while damage to VFMs beyond V1 can produce more selective visual deficits like loss of color vision (i.e., achromatopsia; damage to hV4) or loss of motion perception (i.e., akinetopsia; damage to hMT+) [121, 127–131].

3. Specific changes occur in early visual cortex during otherwise healthy aging

In order to carefully evaluate alterations of visual cortex in the age-related neurodegenerative destruction of AD, we must investigate what changes occur across visual cortex during healthy aging [57, 132, 133]. To do so, studies have typically measured healthy visual aging in subjects over the age of 55 with no known age-related diseases or specific, clinically recognized deficits in vision. Major lesions along the retino-cortical visual pathways are not expected to occur in healthy aging, unlike in AD, but subtle retinal and cortical lesions as described below likely contribute to the variations in visual behavior associated with aging.

Lesion studies in young adult human subjects and animal models have outlined general expectations for changes in cortex that underlie the behavioral deficits arising from the loss of or alterations to the retina or visual pathways (**Figure 7**). Consider a retinal lesion that destroys function in the center of vision (i.e., the fovea). In this case, neurons with a pRF entirely within the cortical region to which the lesion projects (i.e., the lesion projection zone, LPZ) will be silenced, causing the cortical activity—and thus the corresponding BOLD signal—to drop to near zero and the distribution of the central eccentricity representation across the surface area of a VFM to shift to be more peripheral, as activity in the foveal representation would be lost (**Figure 7A** and **B**, *top row*). A second set of neurons would have RF centers located within the LPZ, but would have some of the spread of the pRF remain activated by still-healthy retinal regions. Here, the BOLD signal may drop somewhat but not completely, the surface area distribution would still shift toward the periphery, and the pRF centers of these neurons would also be measured as shifting toward the periphery (**Figure 7A** and **B**, *middle row*). Finally, a third set of neurons would have pRF centers outside of the LPZ, but would have some of the spread of the pRF still within the LPZ. Measurements of these neurons would likely show little drop in BOLD signal, a small shift of surface area distributions to the periphery, and also a small shift of pRF centers toward the periphery (**Figure 7A** and **B**, *bottom row*).

Anatomical and neuroimaging measurements from the few studies to date examining VFM changes in healthy aging have demonstrated several such changes in aging visual pathways that may contribute to such age-related behavioral changes as a decline in visual acuity, deficits in contrast sensitivity, and changes in color vision and visual-spatial attention. Next, we examine how such cortical changes may contribute to these healthy-aging behavioral deficits.

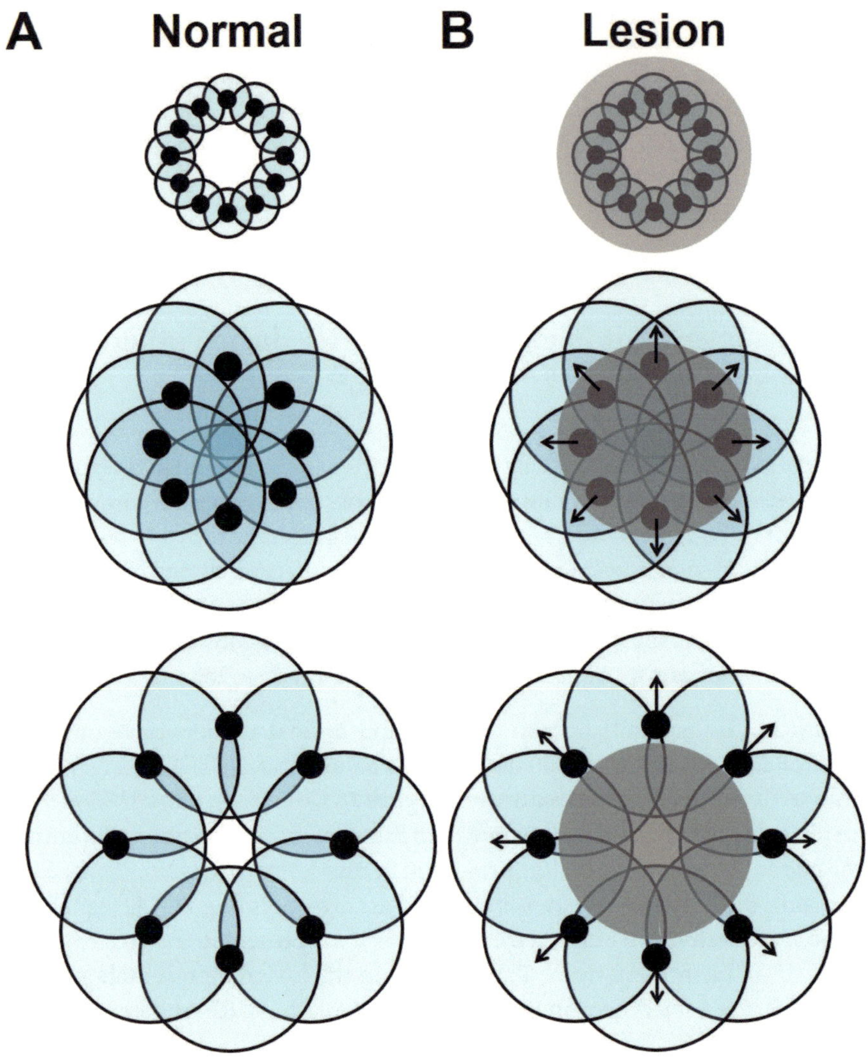

Figure 7. Schematic of the predicted effects of a retinal or cortical lesion on receptive field responses. (A) Solid black disks and the black-outlined teal circles around them indicate the preferred center and spread of a neuron's receptive field, respectively. Each row represents neurons with preferred centers at one specific eccentricity under normal conditions. **(B)** The gray-shaded regions indicate the lesion projection zone (LPZ) arising from retinal or cortical neuronal loss. The interaction of the LPZ with a neuron's receptive field is expected to shift the receptive field center more peripherally relative to normal conditions, as indicated by the black arrows. *Top:* RFs of these neurons are completely obscured by the LPZ. *Middle:* RFs of these neurons are partially obscured by the LPZ, and the RF centers fall within the LPZ. *Bottom:* RFs of these neurons are partially obscured by the LPZ, and the RF centers fall outside the LPZ. For additional discussions, see [8, 9, 12, 16].

3.1. Reductions in cortical activity

A change in cortical activity, whether from a change in peripheral inputs to a particular region (**Figure 7B**, *top row*) or from general changes in cortical responsivity with aging, is a likely component of such aging deficits as a decrease in effective peripheral vision and problems with color discrimination. Given the increase in our knowledge of the role of certain cortical regions with specific behaviors, it is particularly interesting to examine changes in the level of activity of individual VFMs between healthy young adult and aging subjects.

3.1.1. Shrinkage of the useful field of view

Decrease in sensitivity across the visual field and a shrinkage of the useful field of view have been measured in behavioral studies of healthy aging subjects, with greater impairments in peripheral vision [28, 29, 38, 134]. The useful field of view is defined as the visual area in which information can be acquired while the eyes are held steady on a single fixation point. Within the useful field of view, a subject is able to detect, identify and discriminate visual stimuli without making an eye movement away from central fixation.

Measurements of visual search, in which the subject seeks a visual target (e.g., a single "T") hidden among distractors (e.g., many "L"s) demonstrated that there is a reduction as a function of increasing age in the size of the visual field used in the visual search task [38]. This reduction in the useful visual field size arises from a decrease in useful peripheral vision, but can be seen in healthy aging subjects without any clinical conditions affecting the optics of the eye. Although relative lens density increases with age and average pupil size is reduced, these changes do not account for the loss of useful peripheral vision or for the decrease in visual field sensitivity, which suggests that age-related visual field sensitivity changes are primarily due to neural losses rather than preretinal issues.

Evidence for how these changes may arise in cortex has been found with fMRI measurements of the BOLD signal modulation (measured as coherence) in early VFMs. In our recent study that used fMRI with pRF modeling to measure healthy aging VFM characteristics, the coherence of the peripheral 7–10° representation in V1 was found to be significantly lower in aging subjects than in youthful subjects (**Figure 8A**) [36, 37]. No significant differences in more peripheral regions of V2, V3, or hV4 were measured between subject groups (**Figure 8B–D**), so it is possible that the decrease in V1 alone—the primary visual cortex through which the majority of visual inputs pass—is sufficient to drive the behavioral changes. Due to the difficulty in setting up an fMRI paradigm to measure the visual periphery beyond 15–20°, no studies have yet investigated whether additional changes occur in this region across these VFMs.

Similarly, electrophysiology measurements of normally aging macaque monkeys have shown a significant decrease in the response-to-noise ratio and an increase in the neural-response variability in V1 and in the motion-selective medial temporal area (MT, also known as V5) in aging macaque monkeys [43]. These changes in cortical signals have been suggested to possibly arise from a degradation of inhibitory intra-cortical circuits in aging. With such degradations, the selectivity of particular neurons likely decreases, leading to greater activity arising from noise in a particular visual pathway and a consequent decrease in accurate signal-to-noise visual discrimination. In addition, anatomical studies of the visual pathway changes in normal aging humans demonstrate a decline in the retinal-nerve-fiber-layer thickness [46, 54] and a loss of retinal rod photoreceptors [49, 50, 53], both of which could cause a decrease in coherence in peripheral V1 and subsequent VFMs as well as a reduction in the general visual field sensitivity.

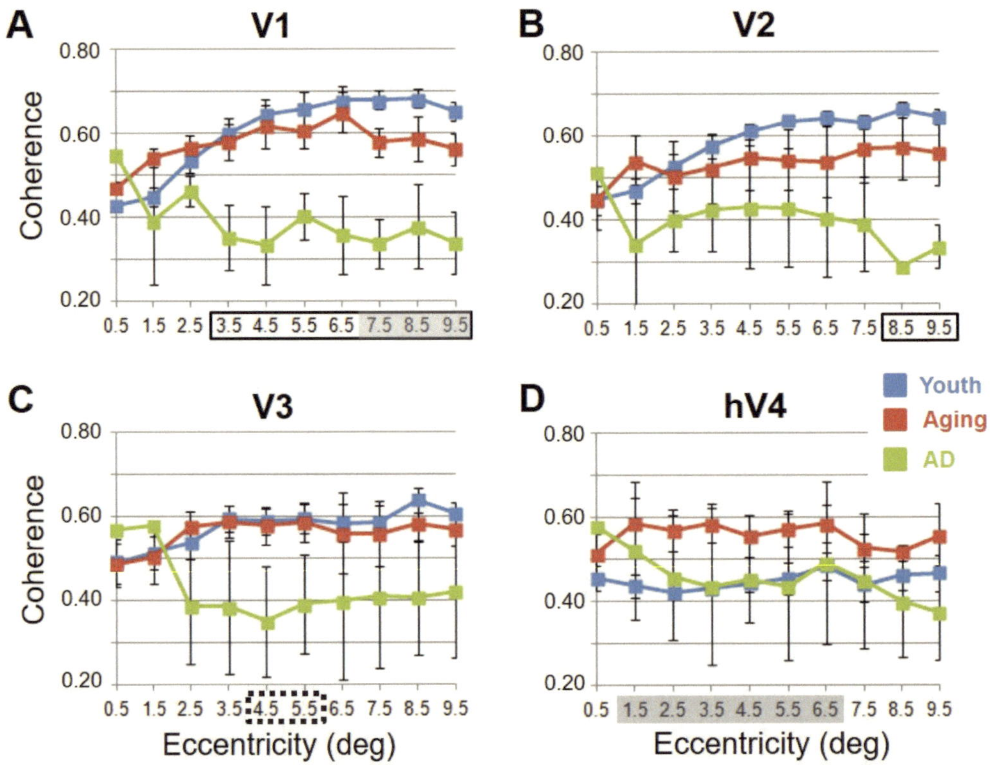

Figure 8. Average measurements of BOLD response in coherence for visual field maps in young, healthy aging, and mild Alzheimer's disease subjects. Blue lines represent data from healthy young subjects, red lines represent data from healthy aging subjects, and green lines represent data from AD subjects. Each line represents data measured in individual subjects and then averaged by iso-eccentricity band across hemispheres. Regions for each measurement shown to be significant are shown along the *x*-axis with shaded gray regions for comparisons between aging and youthful subjects and solid black lines for comparisons between AD and aging subjects. Dotted black lines represent regions shown to be marginally significant for comparisons between AD and aging subjects. Error bars indicate S.E.M. **(A)** V1; **(B)** V2; **(C)** V3; **(D)** hV4. Note the consistency for the youthful subjects and the somewhat greater variability for the healthy aging subjects. Also note both the decreased coherence and increased measurement variability for the AD subjects. Data were collected from [36, 37, 39].

3.1.2. Problems with color discrimination

Aging subjects frequently demonstrate losses in color discrimination—the ability to tell color hues apart—especially along the blue-yellow axis. While these issues can be partially attributed to changes in the aging lens [35] or to a loss of retinal S-cone (short wavelength) photoreceptors, which have a peak selectivity for shorter wave lengths of light [29, 30, 135], growing evidence points to additional concurrent neural changes underlying these deficits (e.g., [27, 37, 136]). For example, after corrections for preretinal losses, the decrease in the sensitivity of

S-cone pathways was found to be approximately 0.09 log units per decade in central vision, and these reductions became larger with measurements across the peripheral visual field to 30° [27]. M-cone (middle wavelength) and L-cone (long wavelength) pathways showed similar but not as severe age-related losses, with a decrease per decade of approximately 0.06–0.70 log units. Only some of this loss can be attributed to retinal changes, with the rest arising in central visual pathways.

Along these lines, fMRI measurements of cortical activity suggest that changes in the cortical color processing pathways may reflect issues with S-cone sensitivity and may further contribute to problems with color discrimination in normally aging subjects. Interestingly, our measurements of the BOLD coherence in hV4 demonstrated an increase in cortical activity over the central 1–7° of eccentricity in healthy aging relative to youthful subjects (**Figure 8D**) [37]. This coherence increase was consistent across all hemispheres in all subjects. It is possible that aging changes specific to the ventral visual color and form pathway involving V1, V2, and hV4 culminate in increased hV4 activity. In addition, although the total surface areas of V1–3 spanning the tested fields of view did not significantly change with age, the total surface area of hV4 was significantly smaller in the healthy aging subjects, perhaps due to losses in color pathway inputs (**Figure 9**) [36, 37, 39, 45]. Similar increases in occipital activity in healthy aging subjects in studies of visual working memory have been suggested to be a sign of a form of compensatory cognitive activity [55]; perhaps the increased hV4 activity in healthy aging similarly reflects a cognitive attempt to compensate for the reduced size of hV4 and/or for issues with color processing elsewhere in the visual pathways.

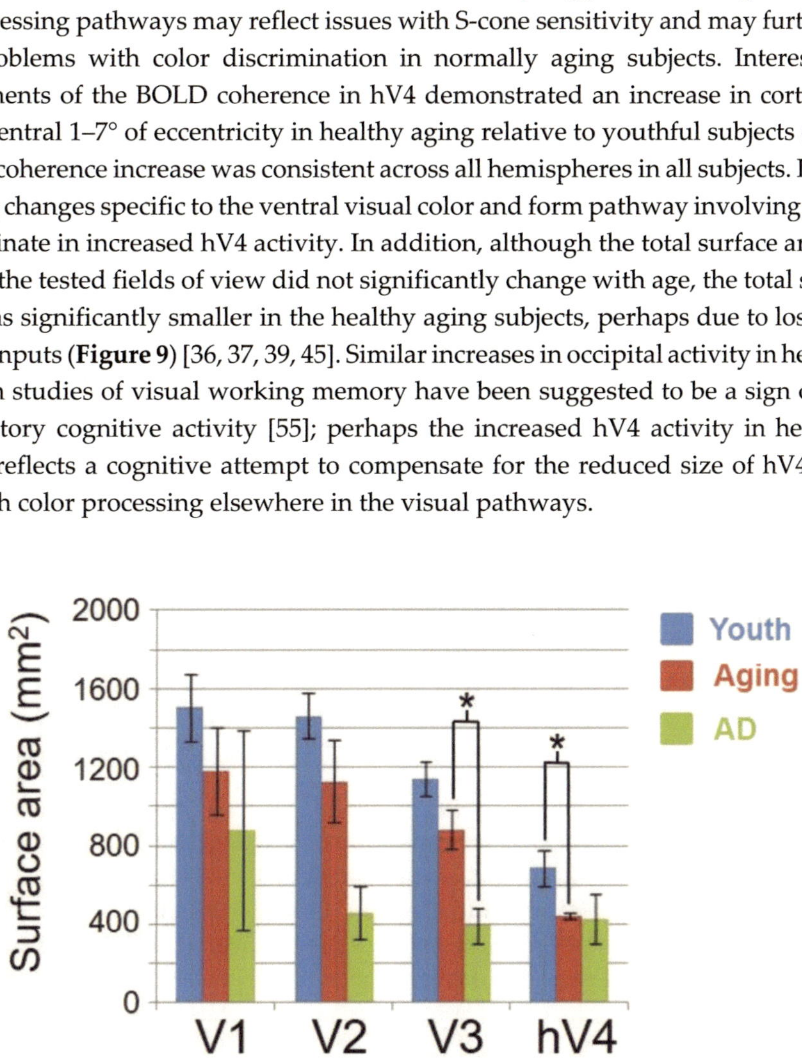

Figure 9. Total surface area measurements for visual field maps in young, healthy aging, and mild Alzheimer's disease subjects. Blue shading again indicates youthful subjects, red shading indicates normal aging subjects, and green shading indicates AD subjects. Total surface area in mm^2 for each visual field map was averaged across the individual subject measurements within in each group. "*" marks statistically significant differences ($p < 0.05$). Error bars indicate S.E.M. Data were collected from [36, 37].

3.2. Decreases in the cortical magnification of foveal representations

Cortical magnification is a common property of sensory systems that may arise from the increased cortical representation of a particular region of sensory space important for behavior. A change in the size of a specific part of a cortical representation between species or subject groups would suggest a related change in the functional properties of that region of cortex and possibly in behavior. For example, if the foveal representation of V1 is significantly reduced in extent for a particular patient group, then it is likely that there is a difference between those patients' central visual processing and that of healthy subjects with normally sized foveal representations (e.g., [8, 10, 12, 36, 37]).

Current measurements of cortical magnification usually consider only one dimension of visual space (e.g., position along eccentricity axis) and disregard the other dimension (e.g., position along polar angle axis) [14]. Thus, the cortical magnification factor as a function of position along the eccentricity axis does not reflect the magnification of representation along an iso-eccentricity line (i.e., across polar angles). We have recently altered such measurements to provide a measure that takes this "width" across polar angles into account by determining the surface-area-percent distributions for each VFM [3, 36, 37, 88, 111]. This is a measurement of what percentage of the total surface area of a VFM (spanning the tested field of view) is the surface area of the representation of a 1° band of eccentricity. As in cortical magnification, changes in the surface-area-percent distribution within a VFM can propose likely changes in function; for example, decreases in the foveal surface area may correlate with deficits in central vision (**Figure 7B**).

3.2.1. Decline in visual acuity

Our static visual acuity determines the smallest detail that we can distinguish in a stationary visual target. Such acuity has been shown to decline after 50 years of age, even in healthy aging subjects with good visual correction through glasses or contact lenses [24, 29, 41, 50, 137]. This loss in visual acuity is exacerbated by low contrast or low luminance in the visual scene [29]. As we rely on our central, foveal vision for our highest acuity, changes in foveal representations would be expected as part of a cortical contribution to this age-related decline in visual acuity.

Our pRF measurements of cortical surface area demonstrated just such a change, measuring a significant decrease in the foveal surface-area-percent distributions of early VFMs V1–hV4 for healthy aging subjects relative to young subjects (**Figure 10**, *red* and *blue lines*, respectively) [36, 37]. A second study by Crossland et al. [39] similarly measured a comparable decrease in the proportion of V1 representing the fovea, by comparing foveal eccentricity activations within polar angle measurements. These aging foveal-representation decreases are consistent with the decline in visual acuity seen normally in aging [24, 29, 41, 50, 137]. These measurements of foveal changes are unlikely to have arisen from unstable eye position, as Crossland et al. [39] demonstrated that aging has no effect on fixation stability, and models of improper fixation do not predict such results [12, 138]. Such a decrease in the size of the aging foveal representations across multiple early VFMs would be expected to lead to a loss in the resolution of cortical processing of visual information within the fovea, thus diminishing visual acuity.

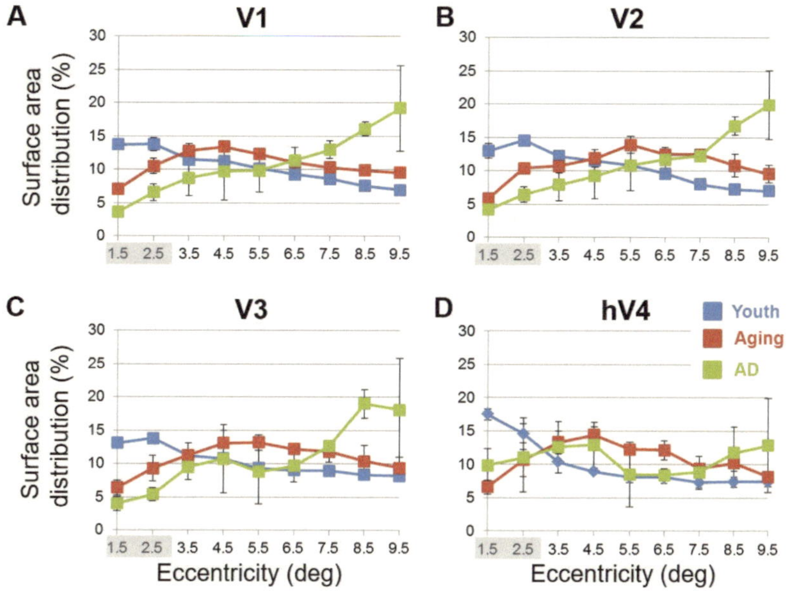

Figure 10. Surface area distribution as the percentage of total surface area. Graphs display average surface-area-percent-distribution measurements for visual field maps in young (*blue lines*), healthy aging (*red lines*), and AD (*green lines*) subjects. Each line represents data measured in individual subjects and then averaged by iso-eccentricity band across hemispheres. Regions for each measurement shown to be significantly different are shown with shaded gray regions for comparisons between aging and youthful subjects **(A)** V1; **(B)** V2; **(C)** V3; **(D)** hV4. Note the relatively increased foveal distribution in the youthful subjects, and the relatively increased peripheral distribution in AD subjects. Error bars indicate S.E.M. Data were collected from [36, 37].

3.2.2. Deficits in spatial and temporal contrast sensitivity

Spatial contrast is the difference in luminance (i.e., brightness) or color that makes an object within a visual scene distinguishable from the rest of the scene. Spatial contrast sensitivity, then, is a measure of a subject's ability to distinguish bright and dark aspects of a scene. This ability is a very important part of visual function, especially in situations of low light or glare (e.g., as in night driving), when the contrast between objects and their background is reduced. Spatial contrast sensitivity is commonly measured by a patient's ability to distinguish light and dark gratings, and age-related declines are most notable for gratings of intermediate and high spatial frequency [139, 140]. This problem cannot be eliminated by optimal lens correction [141, 142] or by elevated luminance [18, 141]. Along these lines, Elliot et al. [19, 33] demonstrated that the decrease in spatial contrast sensitivity at medium and high spatial frequencies with increasing age is mostly due to retinal and cortical changes rather than optical changes in the eye. The decreases in the surface-area-percent distributions of the V1–hV4 foveal representations in healthy aging compared with young adult subjects are likely to play a role in these spatial-contrast-sensitivity impairments, in addition to the decline in visual acuity described above (**Figure 10**) [36, 37, 39]. As the cortical territory devoted to central visual processing decreases, fewer neurons will be available to subserve behavioral discrimination of differences in spatial contrast.

The visual system also is sensitive to temporal contrast; temporal contrast sensitivity is a measure of the light-level difference (i.e., contrast modulation) required for an observer to be able discriminate a light source as flickering versus steady. Temporal contrast sensitivity is typically measured using a spatially uniform, randomly flickering stimulus. If the stimulus changes too slowly, an observer cannot detect the change, and if the stimulus changes too quickly, it is seen as a steady rather than flickering image. Similar to the problems with spatial contrast, aging subjects have decreased temporal contrast sensitivity at intermediate and high temporal frequencies [22, 25], as well as problems with motion discrimination [21, 32]. As human V1 and V3 have been implicated in motion processing [118, 143], the decreased foveal surface areas of aging V1 and V3 may similarly play a role in these temporal-contrast-sensitivity and motion-discrimination deficits (**Figure 10A** and **C**) [141].

3.2.3. Difficulties with visual-spatial attention

Visual-spatial attention is our ability to focus on a specific stimulus in our visual environment. When we look at a visual scene, our attention is drawn to a handful of locations that contain critical pieces of information. Normal visual processing relies on accurate and efficient use of visual-spatial attention, calibrated over a lifetime of visual experiences. Deficits in visual-spatial attention are associated with many neurological and neuropsychiatric disorders (e.g., hemispatial neglect [144], autism [145], schizophrenia [146]), and subtle problems with attention are thought to contribute to issues in healthy aging such as increased difficulty with driving [147, 148].

Measurements in macaque and human visual areas V1, V2, and V4 have demonstrated neural mechanisms in these VFMs possibly subserving selective visual-spatial attention [125, 149–151]. In humans, the significantly smaller surface areas of V2 from 1° to 7° and from 0° to 3° in V1 and hV4 in aging subjects likely denote issues in the processing of high acuity central vision in these regions. Such changes could then contribute to these deficits in visual-spatial attention, (**Figure 10A, B,** and **D**). In addition, the shrinkage of the useful field of view in aging described above may arise from issues correctly deploying visual-spatial attention to the periphery [28, 29, 31, 134].

3.3. Increases in the size of population receptive fields (pRFs)

As seen for cortical magnification, the receptive field sizes of sensory neurons suggest sensitivity to key aspects of sensory space. Smaller receptive fields can produce a higher resolution of sensory processing and suggest improved behavioral discrimination. For VFMs V1–hV4 in healthy subjects, the foveal representations are relatively magnified and also contain the smallest receptive fields [3, 14, 36, 92]. As inputs to visual areas are degraded, as from lesions to the retina or earlier visual pathways, these receptive fields tend to change in size (e.g., [8, 10, 12, 16, 152]). Changes can either be an increase in size, as, for example, normal lateral inhibition—which tends to refine and narrow receptive fields—is lost, or be a decrease in size, as inputs to that receptive field drop out (**Figure 7B**).

3.3.1. *Enlargement of foveal pRFs likely contributes to many of the behavioral deficits associated with healthy aging*

Further cortical changes that may contribute to the decreased visual acuity in normal aging include the differences in pRF sizes measured across the early VFMs of healthy aging subjects (**Figure 11**) [19, 26, 33, 36, 50]. Significant increases in pRF sizes are present in the foveal representations across V1, V2, V3, and hV4 from 0° to at least 3° of eccentricity [36, 37]. The ~2° foveal pRF size in the V1 of aging subjects is near that of the more peripheral pRF sizes (e.g., 5–7° of eccentricity) in young adults [36, 92]. Similarly, V2, V3, and hV4 of the healthy aging subjects contain foveal pRFs comparable in size to the pRF sizes of the more peripheral regions of these VFMs in healthy young subjects [37]. The increased foveal pRF sizes in these VFMs may reflect the decrease in visual acuity seen in healthy aging subjects. The decreased foveal surface area in the VFMs of aging subjects may drive these increases in pRF sizes as a compensatory mechanism, but we do not yet know whether such changes in pRF sizes arise directly within these VFMs during healthy aging or reflect other variations such as loss of retinal ganglion cells or alterations in feedback from higher-order VFMs.

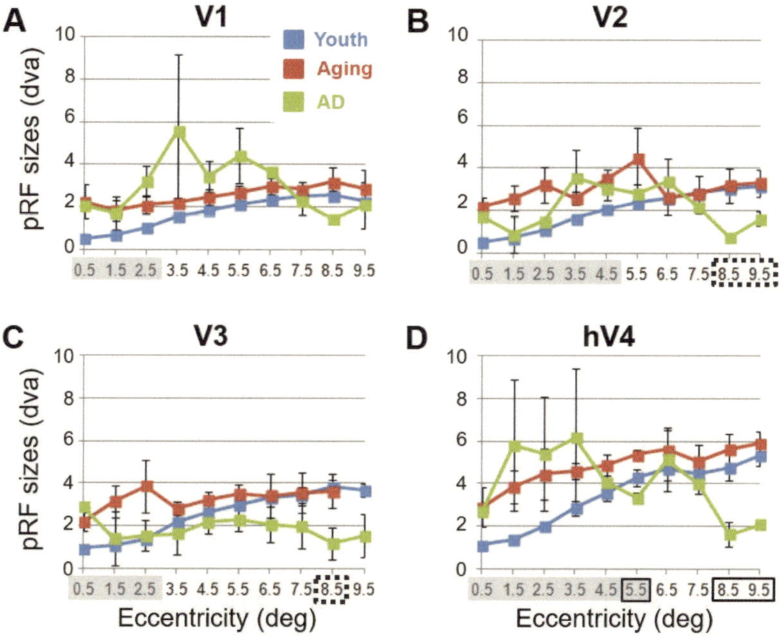

Figure 11. Average population receptive field size measurements for visual field maps in young, healthy aging, and mild Alzheimer's disease subjects. Average pRF radius in degrees of visual angle (dva) across each visual field map is shown for young (*blue lines*), healthy aging (*green lines*), and AD (*red lines*) subjects. Each line again represents data measured in individual subjects and then averaged by iso-eccentricity band across hemispheres. Regions for each measurement shown to be significantly different are shown with shaded gray regions for comparisons between aging and youthful subjects and solid black lines for comparisons between AD and aging subjects. Dotted black lines represent regions shown to be marginally significant for comparisons between AD and aging subjects **(A)** V1; **(B)** V2; **(C)** V3; **(D)** hV4. Note the generally increased pRF sizes and variability for measurements in aging and AD subjects relative to the youthful subjects. Data were collected from [36, 37].

In addition, the broadening of pRF sizes in the aging foveae of these four early VFMs is also consistent with the other behavioral deficits discussed in the sections above. Loss of resolution through these increased foveal pRF sizes likely underlies the decrease in spatial contrast sensitivity (**Figure 11**). The increased pRF sizes of aging V1 and V3 may similarly play a role in temporal-contrast-sensitivity and motion-discrimination deficits (**Figure 11A** and **C**). With respect to issues with color discrimination [27, 29, 30, 35], we have measured significant differences in pRF sizes in V2 and hV4 out to 5° and 6°, respectively, as well as foveal changes in V1 from 0° to 3° (**Figure 11A, B,** and **D**). It is possible that these greater regions of expanded pRFs in aging subjects are associated with aging changes specific to a ventral visual color and form pathway involving V1, V2, and hV4. Finally, V2 and hV4 both showed increases in pRF sizes across larger foveal and parafoveal regions (**Figure 11B** and **D**). These larger pRF sizes could reflect deficits in the proper tuning of visual-spatial attention and less ability to attend across the entire visual field.

4. Alzheimer's disease can present with additional changes in visual cortex

AD is characterized by progressive cognitive deficits including disturbances in memory, language, executive function, and vision [57, 84]. Somewhat surprisingly, it is not uncommon for visual deficits to be reported as one of the first symptoms of AD. However, despite many descriptions of visual symptoms in AD, only a very few studies have begun to examine the extent of changes in the organization, functionality, and connectivity of visual cortex that underlie these visual deficits.

4.1. Patterns of neurodegeneration in the visual cortex of AD patients

AD can present with a variety of visual symptoms across subjects, from lower-level deficits such as changes in visual acuity, contrast sensitivity, color discrimination, visual-spatial perception, and visual-processing speed [40, 73, 85, 132, 153, 154] to higher-level deficits such as problems in visual-spatial attention and in feature recognition of complex objects such as faces [40, 61, 63, 65, 69, 76, 78, 155, 156]. The neuropathology of AD results in gray matter lesions of varying density within regions of visual cortex [48, 57, 76, 84], and the visual symptoms could be attributed in part to a random pattern of neurodegeneration across regions of visual cortex [132]. However, there is also evidence for a more precise distribution of neurodegeneration in the AD visual pathways [48, 84], with some studies showing neurofibrillary tangles and neuritic senile plaques increasing steadily from primary to associative visual cortex and degenerative changes in both the retina ganglion cells and optic nerves [58, 59, 64, 66–68, 70]. The role that such changes may play in the visual symptoms of AD is discussed in the following sections.

Although AD is primarily a disorder of cortical gray matter, some studies have also shown a decreased density of the connections through the splenium of the corpus callosum, the region of the major interhemispheric white matter pathway that connects left and right visual cortex [47, 79, 157]. The changes in the white matter tracts in dementia may result from Wallerian

http://dx.doi.org/10.5772/64562

degeneration following retinal and cortical lesions or may be the product of a primary neuropathological process within the white matter itself. In the first case, we expect such white matter changes to reflect the behavioral deficits associated with the related gray matter or retinal lesion. In the latter, the direct loss of white matter connectivity may itself further contribute to these visual symptoms. Future studies tying functional MRI measurements of VFM organization and function together with diffusion tensor imaging (DTI) MR measurements of white matter tracts in the same subjects should help to clarify the presence and extent of each option in dementia with visual symptoms.

4.2. Visual deficits may arise in AD from both random and precise degenerative changes in cortex

fMRI measurements of cortical gray matter in AD subjects point to a combination of patterns of neurodegeneration, with some specific changes within cortical representations like VFMs seen consistently across subjects (e.g., **Figures 8–11**) in addition to variable alterations in gross

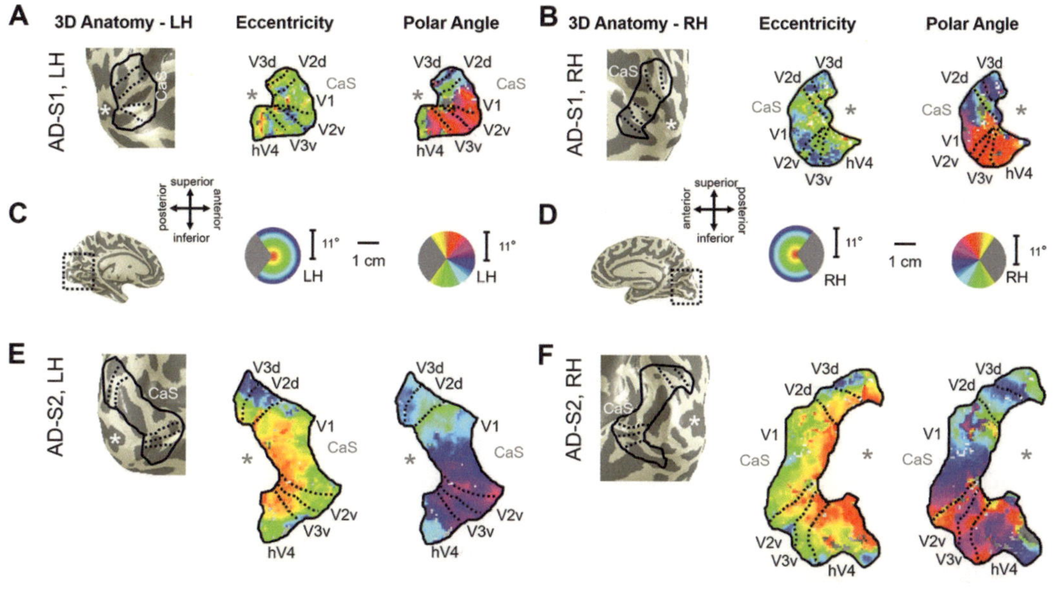

Figure 12. Visual field map measurements in mild Alzheimer's disease subjects. (A, B) Examples of VFMs V1, V2, V3, and hV4 are shown for the left **(A)** and right **(B)** hemispheres of a single subject with mild AD (AD-S1). For clarity, the visual responses are only shown for the VFMs of interest—V1, V2, V3, and hV4—and only voxels with a powerful response at a coherence ≥0.20 are colored. Note the visibly smaller size of these VFMs in this subject compared to those shown for young and healthy aging subjects in **Figure 6**. While the polar angle gradients still contain the expected representations of contralateral visual space with orderly reversals between VFMs, the eccentricity measurements, drawn from the same fMRI scans using the moving bar stimulus, are more disorganized. For cortical surfaces, dark gray represents sulci, and light gray represents gyri. "*" denotes the approximate location of the occipital pole. CaS: calcarine sulcus. **(C, D)** Images depict the full 3D cortical renderings, approximate anatomical orientations for each hemisphere, the color legends for the respective measurements, and the 1 cm scale bar. Note that all flattened hemispheres have been adjusted to the same scale; scale bar is duplicated for ease of comparison. **(E, F)** A second set of examples is shown for the left **(E)** and right **(F)** hemispheres from a second subject with mild AD (AD-S2). This AD subject displays more normal VFM sizes and foveal eccentricity representations, but also has visible changes in the peripheral eccentricity representations. Other details are as described in **Figure 6**. Data were collected from [37].

cortical organization (e.g., **Figure 12**). Measurements of both aspects of distributed neurodegeneration in the visual pathways can be useful in the diagnosis of AD in a specific individual and for understanding the progression this disease across cortex generally.

To date, the only neuroimaging study of VFM changes in AD patients that we are aware of is our Brewer and Barton (2014) study [36, 37], which used fMRI and pRF modeling to measure VFMs in a small number of patients with mild-to-moderate AD. Our results did not demonstrate simply a worsening of the deficits we measured in healthy aging subjects; rather, we observed both the visual deficits we found in healthy aging and additional changes in extrastriate VFMs (V2, V3, and hV4) unique to our AD subjects. Differences among our measurements of the hemispheres of each AD subject were likely primarily due to individual variations in the pattern and progression of neurodegeneration in each subject, revealed by detailed individual-subject data analysis. In addition, there were consistent patterns of changes across the cortical hemispheres that also likely reflected more uniform effects of AD on the visual pathways.

These measurements both demonstrated the feasibility of examining VFM changes in patients with dementia—despite the potentially difficult requirements of maintaining fixation and visual-spatial attention for several consecutive minutes—and emphasized the need for such detailed analyses in individual subjects for these types of investigations. Cortical changes seen consistently across AD patients may underlie the visual symptoms seen early in the disease [67] and may prove to be a useful tool for early and accurate diagnosis of AD. We review here some of the basic trends of VFM changes in AD patients, and, as above for healthy aging subjects, we suggest how these cortical changes may relate to specific deficits in visual behavior.

4.2.1. Declines in visual acuity and contrast sensitivity

Psychophysical studies have observed decreases in both visual acuity and contrast sensitivity in AD subjects beyond that expected for age-matched controls [71, 75]. In particular, psychophysical measures in AD patients showed a decrease in spatial contrast sensitivity for lower spatial frequencies than measured in the healthy aging population [40, 63]. Our measurements of significantly decreased BOLD coherence in regions of V1 and V2, with a marginally significant decrease in coherence in V3, could underlie these deficits (**Figure 8A–C**) [37]. Similarly, we found that the AD subjects significantly differed from healthy aging subjects in terms of total surface area of V3, with a general trend for decreased total surface area across V1–3 (**Figure 9**). While there were no significant differences in the surface area of V1 between healthy aging and AD subjects, the higher variability of these measurements highlights individual differences in neurodegenerative patterns in primary visual cortex as well as the need for additional studies of VFMs in a large number of AD subjects. On average, our AD subjects had no further decline in the surface-area-percent distribution of the foveal representation from 0° to 3° than that seen in the healthy aging subjects compared to youth (**Figure 10**). However, there was a trend for shifts from foveal to peripheral representations, which could point to a variable but important loss of central visual processing.

A striking feature of our AD measurements was the much-reduced total surface areas of V1–hV4 in one subject (AD-S1; **Figure 12A** and **B**). The shrunken VFMs additionally displayed very disorganized eccentricity representations with little foveal representation, likely due to an idiosyncratic pattern of neurodegeneration around the occipital pole. It is important to note that the polar angle representation, drawn from the same scan as the eccentricity representation, remained normal; thus the disorganization seen in the eccentricity representations cannot be simply attributed to a problem with that particular scan, but rather likely reflects alterations in visual function in this individual. Such a dramatic change in early VFM sizes would be expected to result in at least a significant decline in visual acuity and likely reflects changes in multiple aspects of visual processing; even so, the clinical examination of visual function in this subject reported no issues.

4.2.2. Deficiencies in color and form processing

Our measurements of VFM changes in AD were also consistent with the deficiencies in color and form processing frequently described in AD [73, 85, 153]. As suggested by Chan et al. [153], the degeneration of excitatory neurons in AD with the relative sparing of inhibitory interneurons in V1 may result in the color vision disorders reported by a subset of AD patients. This process could also drive the significant decrease we observed in pRF sizes in more peripheral hV4, a key region for color vision processing (**Figure 11D**). Patients with idiosyncratic foveal loss—as seen in our AD subject with greatly reduced VFM surface areas—might also present with these deficiencies in color and form processing.

4.2.3. Problems in the visual-spatial attentional network

Finally, the commonly reported changes in visual-spatial attention in AD patients may be related to the coherence changes we observed in V1 and V2 (**Figure 8**) [40, 63]. The marginally significant decreases in pRF sizes in the periphery of V2 and V3 and the significant pRF size decreases in the periphery of hV4 may also be involved in the deficiencies in the visual-spatial attentional network in AD and could contribute to the shrinkage of useful visual field that is often be even worse in AD patients than in healthy aging (**Figure 11B–D**) [72]. These cortical changes again may reflect degenerative disease in the retina and optic nerves or variations in feedback from higher-order VFMs [37]; some studies have shown that these regions contain more lesions in mild-to-moderate AD than V1 [48, 132]. In addition, V1, V2, and V4 both have been shown to play major roles in the visual-spatial attentional network, as described above [125, 149–151]. Future studies will be needed to examine whether similar changes in VFMs can be measured in the higher-order visual-spatial attention regions of parietal and frontal cortex (e.g., [158–161]).

4.3. These visual field map measurements may be able to improve the early diagnosis of specific types of dementia

Investigations into the early diagnosis of AD include such a wide range of methods as biochemical markers, cognitive testing, and structural and functional neuroimaging [47, 162,

163]. The ability to identify changes in cortical structure or function very early in the development of AD would increase the efficacy of treatments that stop the progression of the neurodegeneration before a significant amount of cortex is lost [62]. Neuroimaging measurements of VFM changes in patients with mild AD may provide an avenue for such early diagnosis, as these measurements can reveal subtle and highly detailed cortical changes using non-invasive fMRI [37]. In addition, these measurements in individual subjects also provide the opportunity to follow neurodegenerative changes in specific individuals over the course of their dementia progression (e.g., [9]). Further research into VFM characteristics in AD should include not only a larger population of AD patients, but also should examine the potential onset of visual symptoms in patients with mild cognitive impairment (MCI), which may provide an even earlier diagnostic tool [37, 55, 154, 164].

Disagreement also persists regarding the categorization of neurodegenerative symptoms into specific types of dementia. We do not yet have a complete understanding of how the different types of dementia—e.g., AD, PCA, DLB, etc.—vary with respect to the start of their associated neurodegenerative changes. Criteria have been outlined to differentiate AD from other dementias, but there still remains significant overlap across the symptoms associated with each dementia (e.g., [56, 78, 85, 86, 165]). The ability to distinguish a patient's particular type of dementia at an early time point in the disease may be vital for the identifying the correct treatment. Such comprehensive measurements of alterations in VFM characteristics as discussed here may assist in this early identification and diagnosis, as the onset and severity of changes in visual cortex are expected to follow patterns specific to each particular dementia [37].

5. Conclusion

Systematic changes in visual cortex likely occur as part of both the normal aging process and the pathophysiology of AD. A better understanding of the alteration of visual representations during healthy aging would both help reveal the effects of healthy aging on visual processing and enhance the use of age-matched controls in studies of visual symptoms in age-related diseases [57, 132]. Our hope is that such data will contribute to earlier and more definitive detection of these forms of dementia and a better understanding of the differences between AD and related dementias.

Acknowledgements

This work was supported in part by the National Institutes of Health Loan Repayment Program award #L30 EY019249 to A.A.B. and by the pilot grant to A.A.B. from the MIND Institute and Alzheimer's Disease Research Center at the University of California, Irvine, supported by the National Institutes of Health grant #AG16573.

Author details

Alyssa A. Brewer* and Brian Barton

*Address all correspondence to: aabrewer@uci.edu

Department of Cognitive Sciences, University of California, Irvine, CA, USA

References

[1] Wandell BA, Dumoulin SO, Brewer AA. Visual field maps in human cortex. Neuron. 2007;56(2):366–83. DOI: 10.1016/j.neuron.2007.10.012.

[2] Felleman DJ, Van Essen DC. Distributed hierarchical processing in the primate cerebral cortex. Cereb Cortex. 1991;1(1):1–47.

[3] Brewer AA, Barton B. Visual field map organization in human visual cortex. In: Molotchnikoff S, Rouat J, editors. Visual Cortex – Current Status and Perspectives. Rijeka, Croatia: InTech; 2012. pp. 29–60. DOI: 10.5772/51914.

[4] Mitchison G. Neuronal branching patterns and the economy of cortical wiring. Proc Biol Sci. 1991;245(1313):151–8. DOI: 10.1098/rspb.1991.0102.

[5] Chklovskii DB, Koulakov AA. Maps in the brain: what can we learn from them? Annu Rev Neurosci. 2004;27:369–92. DOI: 10.1146/annurev.neuro.27.070203.144226.

[6] Shapley R, Hawken M, Xing D. The dynamics of visual responses in the primary visual cortex. Prog Brain Res. 2007;165:21–32. DOI: 10.1016/S0079-6123(06)65003-6.

[7] Moradi F, Heeger DJ. Inter-ocular contrast normalization in human visual cortex. J Vis. 2009;9(3):13, 1–22. DOI: 10.1167/9.3.13.

[8] Baseler HA, Gouws A, Haak KV, Racey C, Crossland MD, Tufail A, et al. Large-scale remapping of visual cortex is absent in adult humans with macular degeneration. Nat Neurosci. 2011;14(5):649–55. DOI: 10.1038/nn.2793.

[9] Smirnakis SM, Brewer AA, Schmid MC, Tolias AS, Schuz A, Augath M, et al. Lack of long-term cortical reorganization after macaque retinal lesions. Nature. 2005;435(7040): 300–7. DOI: 10.1038/nature03495.

[10] Brewer AA, Barton B. Developmental plasticity: fMRI investigations into human visual cortex. In: Papageorgiou TD, Christopoulos G, Smirnakis S, editors. Advanced Brain Neuroimaging Topics in Health and Disease – Methods and Applications. Rijeka, Croatia: InTech; 2014. pp. 305–34. DOI: 10.5772/58256.

[11] Fine I, Wade AR, Brewer AA, May MG, Goodman DF, Boynton GM, et al. Long-term deprivation affects visual perception and cortex. Nat Neurosci. 2003;6(9):915–6. DOI: 10.1038/nn1102.

[12] Baseler HA, Brewer AA, Sharpe LT, Morland AB, Jagle H, Wandell BA. Reorganization of human cortical maps caused by inherited photoreceptor abnormalities. Nat Neurosci. 2002;5(4):364–70. DOI: 10.1038/nn817.

[13] DeYoe EA, Carman GJ, Bandettini P, Glickman S, Wieser J, Cox R, et al. Mapping striate and extrastriate visual areas in human cerebral cortex. Proc Natl Acad Sci USA. 1996;93:2382–6.

[14] Dougherty RF, Koch VM, Brewer AA, Fischer B, Modersitzki J, Wandell BA. Visual field representations and locations of visual areas V1/2/3 in human visual cortex. J Vis. 2003;3(10):586–98. DOI: 10:1167/3.10.1.

[15] Sereno MI, Dale AM, Reppas JB, Kwong KK, Belliveau JW, Brady TJ, et al. Borders of multiple visual areas in humans revealed by functional magnetic resonance imaging. Science. 1995;268(5212):889–93.

[16] Barton B, Brewer AA. fMRI of the rod scotoma elucidates cortical rod pathways and implications for lesion measurements. Proc Natl Acad Sci USA. 2015;112(16):5201–6. DOI: 10.1073/pnas.1423673112.

[17] Sloane ME, Owsley C, Alvarez SL. Aging, senile miosis and spatial contrast sensitivity at low luminance. Vision Res. 1988;28(11):1235–46.

[18] Sloane ME, Owsley C, Jackson CA. Aging and luminance-adaptation effects on spatial contrast sensitivity. J Opt Soc Am A. 1988;5(12):2181–90.

[19] Whitaker D, Elliott DB. Simulating age-related optical changes in the human eye. Docum Ophthalmol. 1992;82(4):307–16.

[20] Whitaker D, Elliott DB, MacVeigh D. Variations in hyperacuity performance with age. Ophthalmic Physiol Opt. 1992;12(1):29–32.

[21] Wojciechowski R, Trick GL, Steinman SB. Topography of the age-related decline in motion sensitivity. Optom Vis Sci. 1995;72(2):67–74.

[22] Wright CE, Drasdo N. The influence of age on the spatial and temporal contrast sensitivity function. Docum Ophthalmol. 1985;59(4):385–95.

[23] Wright CE, Williams DE, Drasdo N, Harding GF. The influence of age on the electroretinogram and visual evoked potential. Docum Ophthalmol. 1985;59(4):365–84.

[24] Pitts DG. The effects of aging on selected visual functions: dark adaptation, visual acuity, stereopsis, and brightness contrast. In: Sekuler R, Kline D, Dismukes K, editors. Aging and Human Visual Function. New York: Alan R. Liss; 1982. pp. 131–59.

[25] Mayer MJ, Kim CB, Svingos A, Glucs A. Foveal flicker sensitivity in healthy aging eyes. I. Compensating for pupil variation. J Opt Soc Am A. 1988;5(12):2201–9.

[26] Kline DW, Culham JC, Bartel P, Lynk L. Aging effects on vernier hyperacuity: a function of oscillation rate but not target contrast. Optom Vis Sci. 2001;78(9):676–82.

[27] Johnson CA, Adams AJ, Twelker JD, Quigg JM. Age-related changes in the central visual field for short-wavelength-sensitive pathways. J Opt Soc Am A. 1988;5(12):2131–9.

[28] Johnson CA, Adams AJ, Lewis RA. Evidence for a neural basis of age-related visual field loss in normal observers. Invest Ophthalmol Vis Sci. 1989;30(9):2056–64.

[29] Haegerstrom-Portnoy G, Schneck ME, Brabyn JA. Seeing into old age: vision function beyond acuity. Optom Vis Sci. 1999;76(3):141–58.

[30] Haegerstrom-Portnoy G, Hewlett SE, Barr SAN. S-cone loss with aging. In: Verriest G, editor. Colour vision deficiencies IX. The Hague: Junk Publisher; 1988. pp. 349–56.

[31] Haas A, Flammer J, Schneider U. Influence of age on the visual fields of normal subjects. Am J Ophthalmol. 1986;101(2):199–203.

[32] Gilmore GC, Wenk HE, Naylor LA, Stuve TA. Motion perception and aging. Psychol Aging. 1992;7(4):654–60.

[33] Elliott DB. Contrast sensitivity decline with ageing: a neural or optical phenomenon? Ophthal Physiolog Opt. 1987;7(4):415–9.

[34] Burton KB, Owsley C, Sloane ME. Aging and neural spatial contrast sensitivity: photopic vision. Vis Res. 1993;33(7):939–46.

[35] Bron AJ, Vrensen GF, Koretz J, Maraini G, Harding JJ. The ageing lens. Ophthalmologica. 2000;214(1):86–104.

[36] Brewer AA, Barton B. Effects of healthy aging on human primary visual cortex. Health. 2012;4(9A):695–702. DOI: 10.4236/health.2012.429109.

[37] Brewer AA, Barton B. Visual cortex in aging and Alzheimer's disease: changes in visual field maps and population receptive fields. Front Psychol. 2014;5:74. DOI: 10.3389/fpsyg.2014.00074.

[38] Ball KK, Beard BL, Roenker DL, Miller RL, Griggs DS. Age and visual search: expanding the useful field of view. J Opt Soc Am A. 1988;5(12):2210–9.

[39] Crossland MD, Morland AB, Feely MP, von dem Hagen E, Rubin GS. The effect of age and fixation instability on retinotopic mapping of primary visual cortex. Invest Ophthalmol Vis Sci. 2008;49(8):3734–9. DOI: 10.1167/iovs.07-1621.

[40] Thiyagesh SN, Farrow TF, Parks RW, Accosta-Mesa H, Young C, Wilkinson ID, et al. The neural basis of visuospatial perception in Alzheimer's disease and healthy elderly

comparison subjects: an fMRI study. Psychiatry Res. 2009;172(2):109–16. DOI: 10.1016/j.pscychresns.2008.11.002.

[41] Weale RA. Senile changes in visual acuity. Trans Ophthalmol Soc UK. 1975;95(1):36–8.

[42] Yang Y, Zhang J, Liang Z, Li G, Wang Y, Ma Y, et al. Aging affects the neural representation of speed in Macaque area MT. Cereb Cortex. 2009;19(9):1957–67. DOI: 10.1093/cercor/bhn221.

[43] Yang Y, Liang Z, Li G, Wang Y, Zhou Y. Aging affects response variability of V1 and MT neurons in rhesus monkeys. Brain Res. 2009;1274:21–7. DOI: 10.1016/j.brainres.2009.04.015.

[44] Raemaekers M, Vink M, van den Heuvel MP, Kahn RS, Ramsey NF. Effects of aging on BOLD fMRI during prosaccades and antisaccades. J Cogn Neurosci. 2006;18(4):594–603. DOI: 10.1162/jocn.2006.18.4.594.

[45] Raz N, Gunning-Dixon F, Head D, Rodrigue KM, Williamson A, Acker JD. Aging, sexual dimorphism, and hemispheric asymmetry of the cerebral cortex: replicability of regional differences in volume. Neurobiol Aging. 2004;25(3):377–96. DOI: 10.1016/S0197-4580(03)00118-0.

[46] Parikh RS, Parikh SR, Sekhar GC, Prabakaran S, Babu JG, Thomas R. Normal age-related decay of retinal nerve fiber layer thickness. Ophthalmology. 2007;114(5):921–6. DOI: 10.1016/j.ophtha.2007.01.023.

[47] Naggara O, Oppenheim C, Rieu D, Raoux N, Rodrigo S, Dalla Barba G, et al. Diffusion tensor imaging in early Alzheimer's disease. Psychiatry Res. 2006;146(3):243–9. DOI: 10.1016/j.pscychresns.2006.01.005.

[48] Lewis DA, Campbell MJ, Terry RD, Morrison JH. Laminar and regional distributions of neurofibrillary tangles and neuritic plaques in Alzheimer's disease: a quantitative study of visual and auditory cortices. J Neurosci. 1987;7(6):1799–808.

[49] Jackson GR, Owsley C, Curcio CA. Photoreceptor degeneration and dysfunction in aging and age-related maculopathy. Ageing Res Rev. 2002;1(3):381–96.

[50] Gao H, Hollyfield JG. Aging of the human retina. Differential loss of neurons and retinal pigment epithelial cells. Invest Ophthalmol Vis Sci. 1992;33(1):1–17.

[51] D'Esposito M, Zarahn E, Aguirre GK, Rypma B. The effect of normal aging on the coupling of neural activity to the bold hemodynamic response. Neuroimage. 1999;10(1):6–14. DOI: 10.1006/nimg.1999.0444.

[52] D'Esposito M, Deouell LY, Gazzaley A. Alterations in the BOLD fMRI signal with ageing and disease: a challenge for neuroimaging. Nat Rev Neurosci. 2003;4(11):863–72. DOI: 10.1038/nrn1246.

[53] Curcio CA, Millican CL, Allen KA, Kalina RE. Aging of the human photoreceptor mosaic: evidence for selective vulnerability of rods in central retina. Invest Ophthalmol Vis Sci. 1993;34(12):3278–96.

[54] Balazsi AG, Rootman J, Drance SM, Schulzer M, Douglas GR. The effect of age on the nerve fiber population of the human optic nerve. Am J Ophthalmol. 1984;97(6):760–6.

[55] Alichniewicz KK, Brunner F, Klunemann HH, Greenlee MW. Structural and functional neural correlates of visuospatial information processing in normal aging and amnestic mild cognitive impairment. Neurobiol Aging. 2012. DOI: 10.1016/j.neurobiolaging.2012.02.010.

[56] Armstrong RA, Lantos PL, Cairns NJ. Overlap between neurodegenerative disorders. Neuropathology. 2005;25(2):111–24.

[57] Yankner BA, Lu T, Loerch P. The aging brain. Ann Rev Pathol. 2008;3:41–66. DOI: 10.1146/annurev.pathmechdis.2.010506.092044.

[58] Danesh-Meyer HV, Birch H, Ku JY, Carroll S, Gamble G. Reduction of optic nerve fibers in patients with Alzheimer disease identified by laser imaging. Neurology. 2006;67(10):1852–4. DOI: 10.1212/01.wnl.0000244490.07925.8b.

[59] Berisha F, Feke GT, Trempe CL, McMeel JW, Schepens CL. Retinal abnormalities in early Alzheimer's disease. Invest Ophthalmol Vis Sci. 2007;48(5):2285–9. DOI: 10.1167/iovs.06-1029.

[60] Teipel SJ, Stahl R, Dietrich O, Schoenberg SO, Perneczky R, Bokde AL, et al. Multivariate network analysis of fiber tract integrity in Alzheimer's disease. Neuroimage. 2007;34(3):985–95. DOI: 10.1016/j.neuroimage.2006.07.047.

[61] van Rhijn SJ, Glosser G, de Vries JJ, Clark CM, Newberg AB, Alavi A. Visual processing impairments and decrements in regional brain activity in Alzheimer's disease. J Clin Exp Neuropsychol. 2004;26(1):11–23. DOI: 10.1076/jcen.26.1.11.23931.

[62] Rosen PN. Vision screening for Alzheimer's disease: prevention from an ophthalmologist's perspective (there is more to vision than meets the eye). Permanente J. 2004;8(1):15–21.

[63] Parasuraman R, Greenwood PM, Haxby JV, Grady CL. Visuospatial attention in dementia of the Alzheimer type. Brain. 1992;115(Pt 3):711–33.

[64] Paquet C, Boissonnot M, Roger F, Dighiero P, Gil R, Hugon J. Abnormal retinal thickness in patients with mild cognitive impairment and Alzheimer's disease. Neurosci Lett. 2007;420(2):97–9. DOI: 10.1016/j.neulet.2007.02.090.

[65] Pache M, Smeets CH, Gasio PF, Savaskan E, Flammer J, Wirz-Justice A, et al. Colour vision deficiencies in Alzheimer's disease. Age Ageing. 2003;32(4):422–6.

[66] Katz B, Rimmer S, Iragui V, Katzman R. Abnormal pattern electroretinogram in Alzheimer's disease: evidence for retinal ganglion cell degeneration? Ann Neurol. 1989;26(2):221–5. DOI: 10.1002/ana.410260207.

[67] Katz B, Rimmer S. Ophthalmologic manifestations of Alzheimer's disease. Surv Ophthalmol. 1989;34(1):31–43.

[68] Iseri PK, Altinas O, Tokay T, Yuksel N. Relationship between cognitive impairment and retinal morphological and visual functional abnormalities in Alzheimer disease. J Neuroophthalmol. 2006;26(1):18–24. DOI: 10.1097/01.wno.0000204645.56873.26.

[69] Holroyd S, Shepherd ML. Alzheimer's disease: a review for the ophthalmologist. Surv Ophthalmol. 2001;45(6):516–24.

[70] Hinton DR, Sadun AA, Blanks JC, Miller CA. Optic-nerve degeneration in Alzheimer's disease. N Engl J Med. 1986;315(8):485–7. DOI: 10.1056/NEJM198608213150804.

[71] Gilmore GC, Whitehouse PJ. Contrast sensitivity in Alzheimer's disease: a 1-year longitudinal analysis. Optom Vis Sci. 1995;72(2):83–91.

[72] Duchek JM, Hunt L, Ball K, Buckles V, Morris JC. Attention and driving performance in Alzheimer's disease. J Gerontol B Psychol Sci Soc Sci. 1998;53(2):P130–41.

[73] Cronin-Golomb A, Sugiura R, Corkin S, Growdon JH. Incomplete achromatopsia in Alzheimer's disease. Neurobiol Aging. 1993;14(5):471–7.

[74] Cronin-Golomb A, Rizzo JF, Corkin S, Growdon JH. Visual function in Alzheimer's disease and normal aging. Ann NY Acad Sci. 1991;640:28–35.

[75] Cronin-Golomb A, Corkin S, Rizzo JF, Cohen J, Growdon JH, Banks KS. Visual dysfunction in Alzheimer's disease: relation to normal aging. Ann Neurol. 1991;29(1): 41–52. DOI: 10.1002/ana.410290110.

[76] Giannakopoulos P, Gold G, Duc M, Michel JP, Hof PR, Bouras C. Neuroanatomic correlates of visual agnosia in Alzheimer's disease: a clinicopathologic study. Neurology. 1999;52(1):71–7.

[77] Giannakopoulos P, Gold G, Duc M, Michel JP, Hof PR, Bouras C. Neural substrates of spatial and temporal disorientation in Alzheimer's disease. Acta Neuropathol. 2000;100(2):189–95.

[78] Tang-Wai DF, Graff-Radford NR, Boeve BF, Dickson DW, Parisi JE, Crook R, et al. Clinical, genetic, and neuropathologic characteristics of posterior cortical atrophy. Neurology. 2004;63(7):1168–74.

[79] Yoshida T, Shiga K, Yoshikawa K, Yamada K, Nakagawa M. White matter loss in the splenium of the corpus callosum in a case of posterior cortical atrophy: a diffusion tensor imaging study. Eur Neurol. 2004;52(2):77–81. DOI: 10.1159/000079750.

[80] Whitwell JL, Jack CR, Jr., Kantarci K, Weigand SD, Boeve BF, Knopman DS, et al. Imaging correlates of posterior cortical atrophy. Neurobiol Aging. 2007;28(7):1051–61. DOI: 10.1016/j.neurobiolaging.2006.05.026.

[81] Schmidtke K, Hull M, Talazko J. Posterior cortical atrophy: variant of Alzheimer's disease? A case series with PET findings. J Neurol. 2005;252(1):27–35. DOI: 10.1007/s00415-005-0594-5.

[82] Mendez MF, Ghajarania M, Perryman KM. Posterior cortical atrophy: clinical characteristics and differences compared to Alzheimer's disease. Dement Geriatr Cogn Disord. 2002;14(1):33–40.

[83] Charles RF, Hillis AE. Posterior cortical atrophy: clinical presentation and cognitive deficits compared to Alzheimer's disease. Behav Neurol. 2005;16(1):15–23.

[84] Black SE. Focal cortical atrophy syndromes. Brain Cogn. 1996;31(2):188–229. DOI: 10.1006/brcg.1996.0042.

[85] Sauer J, ffytche DH, Ballard C, Brown RG, Howard R. Differences between Alzheimer's disease and dementia with Lewy bodies: an fMRI study of task-related brain activity. Brain. 2006;129(Pt 7):1780–8. DOI: 10.1093/brain/awl102.

[86] Harding AJ, Broe GA, Halliday GM. Visual hallucinations in Lewy body disease relate to Lewy bodies in the temporal lobe. Brain. 2002;125(Pt 2):391–403.

[87] Engel SA, Rumelhart DE, Wandell BA, Lee AT, Glover GH, Chichilnisky EJ, et al. fMRI of human visual cortex. Nature. 1994;369(6481):525. DOI: 10.1038/369525a0.

[88] Brewer AA, Barton B. Maps of auditory cortex. Annu Rev Neurosci. 2016;39(1):385–407. DOI: 10.1146/annurev-neuro-070815-014045.

[89] Bartels A, Zeki S. The theory of multistage integration in the visual brain. Proc R Soc Lond B Biol Sci. 1998;265(1412):2327–32. DOI: 10.1098/rspb.1998.0579.

[90] VanEssen D. Organization of visual areas in Macaque and human cerebral cortex. In: Chalupa L, Werner J, editors. The Visual Neurosciences. Boston: Bradford Books; 2003. pp. 507–21.

[91] Engel SA, Glover GH, Wandell BA. Retinotopic organization in human visual cortex and the spatial precision of functional MRI. Cereb Cortex. 1997;7(2):181–92.

[92] Dumoulin SO, Wandell BA. Population receptive field estimates in human visual cortex. Neuroimage. 2008;39(2):647–60. DOI: 10.1016/j.neuroimage.2007.09.034.

[93] Wandell BA, Winawer J. Imaging retinotopic maps in the human brain. Vision Res. 2011;51(7):718–37. DOI: 10.1016/j.visres.2010.08.004.

[94] Boynton GM, Engel SA, Glover GH, Heeger DJ. Linear systems analysis of functional magnetic resonance imaging in human V1. J Neurosci. 1996;16(13):4207–21.

[95] Birn RM, Saad ZS, Bandettini PA. Spatial heterogeneity of the nonlinear dynamics in the FMRI BOLD response. Neuroimage. 2001;14(4):817–26. DOI: 10.1006/nimg.2001.0873.

[96] Hansen KA, David SV, Gallant JL. Parametric reverse correlation reveals spatial linearity of retinotopic human V1 BOLD response. Neuroimage. 2004;23(1):233–41. DOI: 10.1016/j.neuroimage.2004.05.012.

[97] Friston KJ, Fletcher P, Josephs O, Holmes A, Rugg MD, Turner R. Event-related fMRI: characterizing differential responses. Neuroimage. 1998;7(1):30–40. DOI: 10.1006/nimg.1997.0306.

[98] Leonard CM, Puranik C, Kuldau JM, Lombardino LJ. Normal variation in the frequency and location of human auditory cortex landmarks. Heschl's gyrus: where is it? Cereb Cortex. 1998;8(5):397–406.

[99] Rademacher J, Caviness VS, Jr., Steinmetz H, Galaburda AM. Topographical variation of the human primary cortices: implications for neuroimaging, brain mapping, and neurobiology. Cereb Cortex. 1993;3(4):313–29.

[100] Rademacher J, Morosan P, Schormann T, Schleicher A, Werner C, Freund HJ, et al. Probabilistic mapping and volume measurement of human primary auditory cortex. Neuroimage. 2001;13(4):669–83. DOI: 10.1006/nimg.2000.0714.

[101] Amunts K, Schleicher A, Burgel U, Mohlberg H, Uylings HB, Zilles K. Broca's region revisited: cytoarchitecture and intersubject variability. J Comp Neurol. 1999;412(2):319–41.

[102] Clarke S, Morosan P. Architecture, connectivity, and transmitter receptors of human auditory cortex. In: Poeppel D, Overath T, Popper A, Richard R, editors. The Human Auditory Cortex. New York: Springer; 2012. pp. 11–38.

[103] Wandell BA, Chial S, Backus BT. Visualization and measurement of the cortical surface. J Cogn Neurosci. 2000;12(5):739–52.

[104] Teo PC, Sapiro G, Wandell BA. Creating connected representations of cortical gray matter for functional MRI visualization. IEEE Trans Med Imaging. 1997;16(6):852–63. DOI: 10.1109/42.650881.

[105] Nestares O, Heeger DJ. Robust multiresolution alignment of MRI brain volumes. Magn Reson Med. 2000;43(5):705–15.

[106] Brewer AA, Liu J, Wade AR, Wandell BA. Visual field maps and stimulus selectivity in human ventral occipital cortex. Nat Neurosci. 2005;8(8):1102–9. DOI: 10.1038/nn1507.

[107] Van Essen DC. Organization of visual areas in Macaque and human cerebral cortex. In: Chalupa LM, Werner JS, editors. The Visual Neurosciences. Boston: Bradford Books; 2003. pp. 507–21.

[108] Zeki S. Improbable areas in the visual brain. Trends Neurosci. 2003;26(1):23–6.

[109] Press WA, Brewer AA, Dougherty RF, Wade AR, Wandell BA. Visual areas and spatial summation in human visual cortex. Vision Res. 2001;41(10–11):1321–32.

[110] Baumann S, Griffiths TD, Sun L, Petkov CI, Thiele A, Rees A. Orthogonal representation of sound dimensions in the primate midbrain. Nat Neurosci. 2011;14(4):423–5. DOI: 10.1038/nn.2771.

[111] Barton B, Venezia JH, Saberi K, Hickok G, Brewer AA. Orthogonal acoustic dimensions define auditory field maps in human cortex. Proc Natl Acad Sci USA. 2012;109(50): 20738–43. DOI: 10.1073/pnas.1213381109.

[112] Kolster H, Mandeville JB, Arsenault JT, Ekstrom LB, Wald LL, Vanduffel W. Visual field map clusters in macaque extrastriate visual cortex. J Neurosci. 2009;29(21):7031–9. DOI: 10.1523/JNEUROSCI.0518-09.2009.

[113] Kolster H, Peeters R, Orban GA. The retinotopic organization of the human middle temporal area MT/V5 and its cortical neighbors. J Neurosci. 2010;30(29):9801–20. DOI: 10.1523/JNEUROSCI.2069-10.2010.

[114] Schira MM, Tyler CW, Breakspear M, Spehar B. The foveal confluence in human visual cortex. J Neurosci. 2009;29(28):9050–8. DOI: 10.1523/JNEUROSCI.1760-09.2009.

[115] Adams DL, Sincich LC, Horton JC. Complete pattern of ocular dominance columns in human primary visual cortex. J Neurosci. 2007;27(39):10391–403. DOI: 10.1523/JNEUROSCI.2923-07.2007.

[116] Bartfeld E, Grinvald A. Relationships between orientation-preference pinwheels, cytochrome oxidase blobs, and ocular-dominance columns in primate striate cortex. Proc Natl Acad Sci USA. 1992;89(24):11905–9.

[117] Livingstone MS, Hubel DH. Anatomy and physiology of a color system in the primate visual cortex. J Neurosci. 1984;4(1):309–56.

[118] Smith AT, Greenlee MW, Singh KD, Kraemer FM, Hennig J. The processing of first- and second-order motion in human visual cortex assessed by functional magnetic resonance imaging (fMRI). J Neurosci. 1998;18(10):3816–30.

[119] Zeki S. The distribution of wavelength and orientation selective cells in different areas of monkey visual cortex. Proc R Soc Lond B Biol Sci. 1983;217(1209):449–70.

[120] Zeki S. The relationship between wavelength and color studied in single cells of monkey striate cortex. Prog Brain Res. 1983;58:219–27. DOI: 10.1016/S0079-6123(08)60023-0.

[121] Bartels A, Zeki S. The architecture of the colour centre in the human visual brain: new results and a review. Eur J Neurosci. 2000;12(1):172–93.

[122] Zeki S, Watson JD, Lueck CJ, Friston KJ, Kennard C, Frackowiak RS. A direct demonstration of functional specialization in human visual cortex. J Neurosci. 1991;11(3):641–9.

[123] Amano K, Wandell BA, Dumoulin SO. Visual field maps, population receptive field sizes, and visual field coverage in the human MT+ complex. J Neurophysiol. 2009;102(5):2704–18. DOI: 10.1152/jn.00102.2009.

[124] Huk AC, Dougherty RF, Heeger DJ. Retinotopy and functional subdivision of human areas MT and MST. J Neurosci. 2002;22(16):7195–205.

[125] Gallant JL, Shoup RE, Mazer JA. A human extrastriate area functionally homologous to macaque V4. Neuron. 2000;27(2):227–35.

[126] Wade AR, Brewer AA, Rieger JW, Wandell BA. Functional measurements of human ventral occipital cortex: retinotopy and colour. Philos Trans R Soc Lond B Biol Sci. 2002;357(1424):963–73. DOI: 10.1098/rstb.2002.1108.

[127] Zeki S, Bartels A. The autonomy of the visual systems and the modularity of conscious vision. Philos Trans R Soc Lond B Biol Sci. 1998;353(1377):1911–4. DOI: 10.1098/rstb.1998.0343.

[128] Zeki S. A century of cerebral achromatopsia. Brain. 1990;113(Pt 6):1721–77.

[129] Meadows JC. Disturbed perception of colours associated with localized cerebral lesions. Brain. 1974;97(4):615–32.

[130] Vaina LM. Functional segregation of color and motion processing in the human visual cortex: clinical evidence. Cereb Cortex. 1994;4(5):555–72.

[131] Beckers G, Homberg V. Cerebral visual motion blindness: transitory akinetopsia induced by transcranial magnetic stimulation of human area V5. Philos Trans R Soc Lond B Biol Sci. 1992;249(1325):173–8. DOI: 10.1098/rspb.1992.0100.

[132] Jackson GR, Owsley C. Visual dysfunction, neurodegenerative diseases, and aging. Neurol Clin. 2003;21(3):709–28.

[133] Raz N, Rodrigue KM, Head D, Kennedy KM, Acker JD. Differential aging of the medial temporal lobe: a study of a five-year change. Neurology. 2004;62(3):433–8.

[134] Ball K, Owsley C. The useful field of view test: a new technique for evaluating age-related declines in visual function. J Am Optom Assoc. 1993;64(1):71–9.

[135] Werner JS, Steele VG. Sensitivity of human foveal color mechanisms throughout the life span. J Opt Soc Am A. 1988;5(12):2122–30.

[136] Schefrin BE, Werner JS, Plach M, Utlaut N, Switkes E. Sites of age-related sensitivity loss in a short-wave cone pathway. J Opt Soc Am A. 1992;9(3):355–63.

[137] Elliott DB, Yang KC, Whitaker D. Visual acuity changes throughout adulthood in normal, healthy eyes: seeing beyond 6/6. Optom Vis Sci. 1995;72(3):186–91.

[138] Levin N, Dumoulin SO, Winawer J, Dougherty RF, Wandell BA. Cortical maps and white matter tracts following long period of visual deprivation and retinal image restoration. Neuron. 2010;65(1):21–31. DOI: 10.1016/j.neuron.2009.12.006.

[139] Elliott D, Whitaker D, MacVeigh D. Neural contribution to spatiotemporal contrast sensitivity decline in healthy ageing eyes. Vis Res. 1990;30(4):541–7.

[140] Kline DW, Schieber F, Abusamra LC, Coyne AC. Age, the eye, and the visual channels: contrast sensitivity and response speed. J Gerontol. 1983;38(2):211–6.

[141] Owsley C, Sekuler R, Siemsen D. Contrast sensitivity throughout adulthood. Vis Res. 1983;23(7):689–99.

[142] Scialfa CT, Adams EM, Giovanetto M. Reliability of the Vistech Contrast Test System in a life-span adult sample. Optom Vis Sci. 1991;68(4):270–4.

[143] McKeefry DJ, Watson JD, Frackowiak RS, Fong K, Zeki S. The activity in human areas V1/V2, V3, and V5 during the perception of coherent and incoherent motion. Neuroimage. 1997;5(1):1–12. DOI: 10.1006/nimg.1996.0246.

[144] Hillis AE, Newhart M, Heidler J, Barker PB, Herskovits EH, Degaonkar M. Anatomy of spatial attention: insights from perfusion imaging and hemispatial neglect in acute stroke. J Neurosci. 2005;25(12):3161–7. DOI: 10.1523/JNEUROSCI.4468-04.2005.

[145] Mundy P, Sullivan L, Mastergeorge AM. A parallel and distributed-processing model of joint attention, social cognition and autism. Autism Res. 2009;2(1):2–21. DOI: 10.1002/aur.61.

[146] Maruff P, Hay D, Malone V, Currie J. Asymmetries in the covert orienting of visual spatial attention in schizophrenia. Neuropsychologia. 1995;33(10):1205–23.

[147] Ball K, Owsley C, Sloane ME, Roenker DL, Bruni JR. Visual attention problems as a predictor of vehicle crashes in older drivers. Invest Ophthalmol Vis Sci. 1993;34(11):3110–23.

[148] Owsley C, Ball K. Assessing visual function in the older driver. Clin Geriatr Med. 1993;9(2):389–401.

[149] Luck SJ, Chelazzi L, Hillyard SA, Desimone R. Neural mechanisms of spatial selective attention in areas V1, V2, and V4 of macaque visual cortex. J Neurophysiol. 1997;77(1):24–42.

[150] Reynolds JH, Pasternak T, Desimone R. Attention increases sensitivity of V4 neurons. Neuron. 2000;26(3):703–14.

[151] Serences JT, Yantis S. Selective visual attention and perceptual coherence. Trends Cogn Sci. 2006;10(1):38–45. DOI: 10.1016/j.tics.2005.11.008.

[152] Haak KV, Cornelissen FW, Morland AB. Population receptive field dynamics in human visual cortex. PLoS One. 2012;7(5):e37686. DOI: 10.1371/journal.pone.0037686.

[153] Chan D, Crutch SJ, Warrington EK. A disorder of colour perception associated with abnormal colour after-images: a defect of the primary visual cortex. J Neurol, Neurosurg Psych. 2001;71(4):515–7.

[154] Mapstone M, Steffenella TM, Duffy CJ. A visuospatial variant of mild cognitive impairment: getting lost between aging and AD. Neurology. 2003;60(5):802–8.

[155] Giannakopoulos P, Gold G, Duc M, Michel JP, Hof PR, Bouras C. Impaired processing of famous faces in Alzheimer's disease is related to neurofibrillary tangle densities in the prefrontal and anterior cingulate cortex. Dement Geriatr Cogn Disord. 2000;11(6): 336–41.

[156] Bokde AL, Lopez-Bayo P, Meindl T, Pechler S, Born C, Faltraco F, et al. Functional connectivity of the fusiform gyrus during a face-matching task in subjects with mild cognitive impairment. Brain. 2006;129(Pt 5):1113–24. DOI: 10.1093/brain/awl051.

[157] Takahashi S, Yonezawa H, Takahashi J, Kudo M, Inoue T, Tohgi H. Selective reduction of diffusion anisotropy in white matter of Alzheimer disease brains measured by 3.0 Tesla magnetic resonance imaging. Neurosci Lett. 2002;332(1):45–8.

[158] Silver MA, Kastner S. Topographic maps in human frontal and parietal cortex. Trends Cogn Sci. 2009;13(11):488–95. DOI: 10.1016/j.tics.2009.08.005.

[159] Swisher JD, Halko MA, Merabet LB, McMains SA, Somers DC. Visual topography of human intraparietal sulcus. J Neurosci. 2007;27(20):5326–37. DOI: 10.1523/JNEUROSCI.0991-07.2007.

[160] Sereno MI, Pitzalis S, Martinez A. Mapping of contralateral space in retinotopic coordinates by a parietal cortical area in humans. Science. 2001;294(5545):1350–4. DOI: 10.1126/science.1063695.

[161] Silver MA, Ress D, Heeger DJ. Topographic maps of visual spatial attention in human parietal cortex. J Neurophysiol. 2005;94(2):1358–71. DOI: 10.1152/jn.01316.2004.

[162] Ringman JM, Younkin SG, Pratico D, Seltzer W, Cole GM, Geschwind DH, et al. Biochemical markers in persons with preclinical familial Alzheimer disease. Neurology. 2008;71(2):85–92. DOI: 10.1212/01.wnl.0000303973.71803.81.

[163] Graham DP, Cully JA, Snow AL, Massman P, Doody R. The Alzheimer's Disease Assessment Scale-Cognitive subscale: normative data for older adult controls. Alzheimer Dis Assoc Disord. 2004;18(4):236–40.

[164] Tabert MH, Manly JJ, Liu X, Pelton GH, Rosenblum S, Jacobs M, et al. Neuropsychological prediction of conversion to Alzheimer disease in patients with mild cognitive impairment. Arch Gen Psychiatry. 2006;63(8):916–24. DOI: 10.1001/archpsyc.63.8.916.

[165] Saygin AP, Sereno MI. Retinotopy and attention in human occipital, temporal, parietal, and frontal cortex. Cereb Cortex. 2008;18(9):2158–68. DOI: 10.1093/cercor/bhm242.

Chapter 13

Clusterin (APOJ) in Alzheimer's Disease: An Old Molecule with a New Role

Sarah K. Woody and Liqin Zhao

Additional information is available at the end of the chapter

http://dx.doi.org/10.5772/64233

Abstract

Clusterin (CLU), initially identified in 1983 as a "clustering factor" in ram rete testis fluid, is a multifaceted protein that was re-discovered and subsequently renamed eight times from 1983 to 1992. CLU exists as multiple protein isoforms including the 80 kDa glycosylated mature/secreted form of CLU (mCLU) and the smaller non-modified nuclear and intracellular forms of CLU (nCLU and icCLU, respectively). These isoforms, which are expressed at the highest levels in the brain, are suggested to play distinct roles in various disease processes such as those involving inflammation and apoptosis. Currently, CLU, also known as apolipoprotein J (APOJ) which belongs to the same protein family as apolipoprotein E (APOE), is the third most significant genetic risk factor for the development of late-onset Alzheimer's disease (LOAD); however, an extensive gap exists in the literature in understanding the physiological roles of CLU in normal brain and the pathogenic mechanisms conferred by CLU polymorphisms in the onset of LOAD. In this chapter, we discuss the status of the current knowledge regarding the generation and regulation of CLU protein isoforms, the clinical evidence and possible mechanisms involved in LOAD, and provide our perspectives for future studies.

Keywords: late-onset Alzheimer's disease (LOAD), genetic risk factors, clusterin (CLU), apolipoprotein J (APOJ), apolipoprotein E (APOE)

1. Introduction

1.1. Alzheimer's disease: current status and challenges

Alzheimer's disease (AD) currently affects 35 million people worldwide, including 5.4 million Americans; a number that is estimated to triple by the year 2050 [1]. As the prevalence of AD increases, the AD-associated economic burden will also increase. In 2015, the direct costs associated with the care of AD patients in the United States reached $226 billion. This number is predicted to reach $1.1 trillion by the year 2050 making AD one of the most costly chronic illnesses in the world [1]. At present, AD is the sixth leading cause of death in the United States and is the only leading cause of death that cannot be prevented or cured. There are currently five FDA-approved drugs available to treat AD; however, these drugs do not address the underlying cause of AD and provide only temporary therapeutic relief in a fraction of the patients to whom they are administered. An extensive amount of clinical trials aimed at treating AD have been performed in the last 15 years; all of which have failed [2, 3]. These unanticipated challenges combined with the estimated rapid increases in AD prevalence stress the importance of identifying the underlying AD risk mechanisms that would allow prevention, risk reduction, and early intervention in the preclinical stage of AD.

1.2. Late-onset AD: complex etiology and risk factors

There are two types of AD: early-onset familial AD (FAD) and late-onset sporadic AD (LOAD). FAD is rare and mostly caused by inherited genetic mutations that result in abnormal overproduction of neurotoxic β-amyloid (Aβ) peptides. LOAD, the most common form of AD representing 95% of human cases, develops after age 60 and involves a heterogeneous and multifactorial etiology. It is now widely accepted that a person's risk for developing LOAD is primarily influenced by a combination of complex interactions between genetic and environmental risk factors. At present, age remains the most predominant risk factor for LOAD. It is estimated that one in nine (11.1%) senior citizens aged 65 or older have been diagnosed with LOAD; a ratio that increases to one in three (33.3%) by age 85 [1]. The National Institute on Aging (NIA) indicates that the risk of developing LOAD doubles every 5 years past the age of 65 [4]. Additionally, epidemiologic studies from the NIA estimate that the total percentage of senior citizens in the United States will increase by 7% by 2030 making senior citizens the fastest-growing age group in the United States and consequently the most at-risk population [4].

Sex also plays a significant role in the development of LOAD. Of the 5.4 million Americans currently living with AD, approximately 65% are women [1]. It was originally postulated that the higher percentage of women living with AD was due to the increased life span of the female population; however, as the average worldwide life expectancy of men and women differs by only 4 years, this presumption is invalid. A meta-analysis of seven sex-specific clinical studies revealed that women are 1.5 times more likely to develop AD than age-matched men, indicating that the female sex confers AD risk independent of age [5]. In addition to a higher incidence of AD, it is now well established that sex influences both the development and progression of LOAD. For example, female AD patients have been shown to exhibit more severe cognitive decline than men during the progression of AD pathology [6–8]. While the exact mechanisms underlying this sex bias are currently unknown, mounting evidence suggests that female vulnerability to AD is largely associated with the irreversible decline of female sex hormones during the onset of menopause [9–11]. However, despite these findings, the precise molecular mechanisms underlying female vulnerability remain uncharacterized.

Genetic predisposition is another prominent risk factor associated with the development of AD. A long-standing observation in the field of LOAD research is the significantly increased AD risk associated with possession of the human apolipoprotein E ε4 allele (APOE ε4) [12], the most predominant genetic risk factor for LOAD. Possession of the ε4 allele is clinically associated with an increased rate and severity of cognitive decline, a younger age of onset, and altered response to AD treatments [13–16]. Moreover, the ε4 allele has been shown to reduce brain glucose utilization [17], increase neuronal inflammation [18], and is associated with increased Aβ dyshomeostasis [19, 20]. In addition to these data, studies have demonstrated that the APOE ε4-associated AD risk is significantly more pronounced in the female population. For example, a recent clinical study conducted in a cohort of 8084 elderly individuals (healthy controls: $n = 5496$; MCI cases: $n = 2588$) demonstrated that the risk of clinical conversion from healthy aging to MCI or from MCI to AD conferred by the ε4 allele was significantly greater in women than in men, a finding that corresponds with several earlier reports [21–25].

In addition to APOE ε4, two of the largest genome-wide association (GWA) studies ever conducted to date have recently identified several other genetic risk factors that confer a significantly increased risk of developing LOAD [26, 27]. Of the genetic risk factors identified, clusterin (CLU), also known as apolipoprotein J (APOJ), was established as the third most predominant genetic risk factor for LOAD. CLU, which belongs to the same protein family as APOE, has been shown to regulate inflammation, oxidative stress, and amyloid homeostasis in the brain. Moreover, a recent study conducted by our laboratory indicated that CLU mRNA and protein expression levels are significantly reduced specifically in female brain during a time period that likely corresponds to the onset of reproductive senescence. These data suggest that, similar to APOE ε4, CLU is also influenced by sex in the brain aging process and the pathogenesis of LOAD [28]. In the following sections, we summarize the current understanding of CLU protein isoforms and their biological functions with specific emphasis on the neuroprotective potential of CLU protein isoforms in the brain.

2. Clusterin: from form to function

2.1. CLU: discovery and nomenclature

In 1983, Blaschuk et al. identified a high-molecular weight protein in ram rete testis fluid [29]. Further analyses indicated that this unknown protein was capable of eliciting the "clustering" of Sertoli cells, mouse testis TM-4 cells, and erythrocytes resulting in the name clusterin. In 1984, Griswold and colleagues purified a dimeric acidic glycoprotein (DAG) from the Sertoli cells of rat testes [30]. This abundantly expressed but uncharacterized protein was detected at several molecular weights via reducing chromatography (41 and 29 kDa), western blot (27 and 21 kDa), and immunoprecipitation (70 kDa) [30]. In 1988, another study identified a "novel" protein in human serum. This heterodimeric protein had a molecular mass of 80 kDa, was composed of two 40-kDa chains, and was sequentially unique to all other proteins. Furthermore, it was concluded that this protein, which was deposited in the renal glomeruli of patients with glomerulonephritis, was integrally involved in kidney health [31]. As a result of these observations, Murphy and colleagues named this protein serum protein 40 kDa,40 kDa (SP-40,40) [31]. In 1990 and the years following, Harmony and colleagues identified and extensively characterized a component of high-density lipoproteins in human plasma which was referred to as apolipoprotein J (APOJ) [32]. However, upon the advent of DNA sequencing technology, it was determined that clusterin, DAG, SP-40,40, and APOJ were in fact the same protein. In the following decade, clusterin was "re-discovered" and subsequently re-labeled with other alternative names including testosterone-repressed prostrate message-2 (TRPM-2) [33], KU70-binding protein 1 (KUB1) [34], complement lysis inhibitor (CLI) [35], and sulphated glycoprotein-2 (SGP2) [36]. In 1992, a forum conducted at Cambridge University officially deemed this diverse protein clusterin (CLU).

2.2. CLU: from gene to protein

CLU is a single-copy gene located on the short arm of chromosome 8 (8p21-12) [37, 38] where it spans approximately 18,115 base pairs (bp). Upon the splicing of eight introns, this nine-exon product spans approximately 2877 bp, and is transcribed into at least two distinct mRNA transcripts. CLU mRNA transcript 1 (NM_001831.3), the most extensively characterized transcript, is translated into the mature/secreted isoform of CLU (mCLU) that has been predominantly identified and studied in the field of CLU research. CLU mRNA transcript 1 is initially translated into a 449-amino-acid precursor protein (pCLU, 60 kDa) beginning at a canonical translational start site located at base pair 187 in exon 2. This pCLU protein contains an N-terminal 22-amino-acid endoplasmic reticulum (ER)-targeted signaling peptide (amino acids 1–22 or bp 187–252) and two nuclear localization sequences in exon 3 (amino acids 78–81 or bp 418–429) and exons 8–9 (amino acids 443–447 or bp 1513–1528). The translated pCLU protein is then targeted to the ER where the 22-amino-acid leader sequence (LS) is cleaved. Following LS cleavage, the peptide bond between R227 and S228 is cleaved resulting in the formation of two individual CLU subunits: the alpha subunit (CLUα, 34–37 kDa) and the beta subunit (CLUβ, 36–39 kDa). These two subunits are subsequently linked by five disulphide bonds to form an anti-parallel heterodimer [39]. N-glycosylation at six glycosylation sites is the final step in the generation of mCLU which, under nonreducing conditions, has a molecular weight of 75–80 kDa (**Figure 1A**) [40]. Alternatively, complete removal of exon 2 via alternative splicing results in the fusion of exons 1 and 3, thereby creating CLU mRNA transcript 2. In this secondary transcript, translation is initiated at a canonical translational start site located in exon 3. This results in the production of a CLU protein isoform that lacks the ER LS but retains the nuclear localization sequences. This alternative CLU isoform, which is non-ER targeted and unglycosylated, is shuttled between the cytoplasm and the nucleus and is referred to as "nuclear" CLU (nCLU, 49 kDa, **Figure 1B**). In addition to mCLU and nCLU, emerging evidence indicates that several different splicing variants of CLU also exist. These splicing variants, which are relatively uncharacterized, are suggested to lack portions of exon 2 and/or exon 5 and are generally referred to as "intracellular" isoforms (icCLU, 45, 50, and 53–55 kDa) [41–43].

Initial characterization by Harmony et al. indicated the expression of CLU mRNA in liver, lung, spleen, heart, reproductive tissues, and brain with predominant expression in brain and reproductive tissues [44]. Since this initial characterization, several other research groups,

http://dx.doi.org/10.5772/64233

including our own, have detected CLU mRNA and protein expression in many cell lines and tissue types tested. Moreover, CLU appears to be ubiquitously expressed on the subcellular level with multiple studies demonstrating CLU expression in the cytosol [45], nucleus [41], ER, and Golgi apparatus. Within the brain, CLU expression has been detected within neurons [46], astrocytes [46–48], microglia [49], and within the extracellular space [50]. While initial reports indicated that CLU was solely synthesized and secreted from the astrocytes in a manner similar to APOE [51], our recent findings demonstrate that pure cultures of primary neurons express

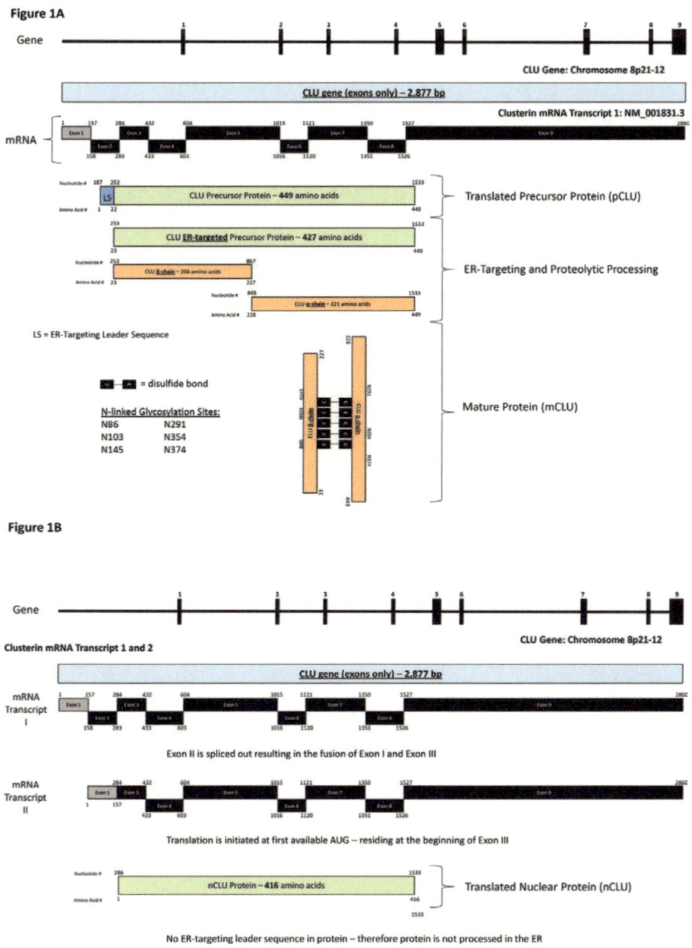

Figure 1. CLU transcription and translation. In humans, CLU is a single-copy gene located on the short arm of chromosome 8 that is comprised of nine exons spanning approximately 2.8 kb. (**A**) The mCLU isoform is generated from mRNA transcript 1 from a canonical translational start site in exon 2. The resulting precursor protein (pCLU), which contains an N-terminal ER-targeting leader sequence (LS), is transported to the ER where the 22-amino-acid LS is removed. CLU is then cleaved into the alpha and beta subunits and rapidly disulfide bonded and glycosylated to form an anti-parallel, heterodimeric glycoprotein: mCLU. (**B**) Alternatively, the nCLU isoform is generated from mRNA transcript 2. In this transcript, a splicing event removes exon 2 resulting in the fusion of exons 1 and 3. Translation is initiated at the beginning of exon 3 resulting in a truncated CLU isoform that lacks the ER-targeting LS. Therefore, the nCLU isoform, which retains the nuclear localization sequence, bypasses the ER/Golgi apparatus and is shuttled between the cytosol and the nuclear compartment.

mCLU, nCLU, and to a lesser extent icCLU isoforms indicating that neurons are also capable of generating de novo CLU. Though the exact physiological functions of CLU remain a mystery, the nearly ubiquitous nature of CLU indicates the significance of this protein in cellular homeostasis.

2.3. CLU: transcriptional regulation

Though the gene promoter of CLU is highly conserved across species, the transcriptional regulation of CLU is complex as the predominant CLU transcriptional regulators appear to differ between tissue and cell type. However, despite the controversy in the literature, it is generally agreed that CLU is primarily upregulated by cellular injury, cytotoxic insult, and various stress stimuli [52–54]. For instance, Loisen and colleagues demonstrated that the CLU gene promoter contains an MG132 responsive region and a heat-shock element (HSE) indicating that proteasomal stress directly influences CLU transcription [52]. Another study demonstrated that the CLU gene promoter contains both HSEs and an activator protein-1 (AP-1) response element indicating direct transcriptional regulation by stimuli derived from cellular proliferation and differentiation [54]. In addition to these data, alternative stress-related transcription factor response elements have been identified in the CLU gene promoter including a cAMP response element (CRE), an AP-2 response element, a specificity protein-1 (SP1) response element, and a glucocorticoid response element (GRE) [33, 53]. It has also been demonstrated that apoptotic stimuli modulates CLU transcription, specifically in cancer. An early study from Cervellera et al. identified a MYB binding site in the 5′ flanking region of CLU and that B-MYB, a MYB family member that regulates cellular proliferation and apoptosis, directly bound to and transactivated the CLU gene [55]. CLU transcription is also regulated by several different growth factors including nerve growth factor (NGF) and transforming growth factor beta (TGFβ) [56–58]. For instance, it has been demonstrated that TGFβ induces the upregulation of CLU gene expression by stimulating the interaction between the CLU gene promoter and AP-1 [57]. An extension of these studies demonstrated that TGFβ deficiency resulted in the repression of CLU gene expression via interaction between c-Fos and the CLU gene promoter; an interaction that was abrogated upon cellular stimulation with TGFβ [58].

2.4. CLU: posttranslational modification

CLU is regulated by several types of posttranslational modification (PTM), the most predominant type being N-linked glycosylation. As previously indicated, mCLU is N-glycosylated at six different asparagine residues (N86, N103, N145, N291, N354, and N374) during ER-Golgi processing: a modification that comprises approximately 20–25% of the total mass of mCLU [59]. While glycosylation status was originally thought to have little to no impact on CLU function [40, 60], a recent study demonstrated that the chaperone activity of mCLU is dependent upon mCLU glycosylation [61]. This study also demonstrated that the glycosylation of nCLU did not result in chaperone activity indicating that glycosylation-mediated effects are specific to the mCLU isoform. It has also been established that complete deglycosylation of mCLU results in a 70–90% decrease in mCLU chaperone activity and a significant decrease in

http://dx.doi.org/10.5772/64233

the number of α-helices in the secondary structure of CLU. These data suggest that the lack of chaperone activity in deglycosylated mCLU could be, in part, due to the significant changes in secondary structure. Additionally, this study indicates that partially glycosylated mCLU retains chaperone activity suggesting that "core" glycosylation sites are crucial for mCLU function, while peripheral glycosylation may be dispensable [61]. Parallel to these findings, a study by Kang et al. indicated that ER stress, which inhibits protein glycosylation, resulted in rapid retro-translocation of mCLU from the ER yielding several hypo-glycosylated CLU isoforms. These hypo-glycosylated isoforms, which are misfolded and generally nonfunctional, are rapidly poly-ubiquitinated under normal conditions and cleared through proteasomal degradation. However, if the proteasome is chemically inhibited following ER stress, hypo-glycosylated CLU accumulates in the cytosolic compartment resulting in cytotoxicity [62]. Collectively, these studies indicate that, contrary to what was originally postulated, glycosylation is crucial for mCLU chaperone activity.

In addition to N-linked glycosylation, CLU is also a primary target for ubiquitination and phosphorylation. It has been demonstrated that nCLU is a target for K63 ubiquitination through the ubiquitin E3 ligase, a product of von Hippel-Lindau (pVHL). However, contrary to the canonical function of protein ubiquitination, K63-linked ubiquitination of nCLU does not target nCLU for destruction, rather it promotes nCLU nuclear translocation for reasons that are currently unknown [63]. Pertaining to CLU phosphorylation, a recent proteomics study which focused on the identification of the serum phospho-proteome has identified three different phosphorylation sites at residues Thr393, Ser394, and Ser39 within the CLU protein. Additionally, a more recent study indicated that treatment of hepatocytes with 10-mM glucose and fructose significantly increased the levels of mCLU serine phosphorylation. This same study demonstrated increased mCLU serine phosphorylation in both the skeletal muscle and the liver of rats that were orally administered high doses of glucose and/or fructose indicating that phosphorylated CLU may interact with or respond to the activation of glucose-sensitive cellular bioenergetic pathways. In addition to ubiquitination and phosphorylation, an early report indicated that CLU is iodinated at 1 of the 12 tyrosine residues within the CLU protein. This iodination occurs within the apical plasma membrane of thyrocytes and is suggested to serve as a mechanism by which the thyroid gland can conserve iodine, which is relatively rare in the body [64]. It is also suggested that CLU activity is regulated by both sialylation [65] and acetylation [66]; however, definitive acetylation or sialylation sites have not been identified.

3. CLU in Alzheimer's disease: clinical findings

3.1. CLU polymorphisms in LOAD

Since the initial determination of CLU SNP-associated AD risk by Harold et al. and Lambert et al. [26, 27], there have been approximately 40 independent follow-up meta-analyses and case-control studies that have examined the association between CLU SNPs and AD risk (**Table 1**). These reports were located through a PubMed search focused on topics pertaining to CLU SNPs in AD. Resulting articles were reviewed and those studies which provided a listing of the CLU SNP(s) studied, population demographics, and a thorough description of cognitive assessment and statistical analysis were included in **Table 1**. Though conflicting evidence exists, the majority of the studies indicate that genetic variation in CLU increases the risk of developing AD and that this association is independent of APOE ε4 status. There are approximately 355 identified SNPs in the CLU gene [67]; however, it appears that the primary risk-conferring CLU SNP is rs11136000. Of the 33 studies summarized in **Table 1**, 25 studies either include or exclusively focus on the impact of the rs11136000 SNP on AD risk; however, the results are inconsistent. Thirteen studies conclude that possession of rs11136000 does confer increased AD risk [26, 27, 68–77], while ten studies conclude no significant association between rs11136000 and AD [78–85]. Moreover, two studies conclude that possession of the rs11136000 SNP reduces risk of AD development [86, 87]. A possible explanation for these discrepancies may be found by examining the population ethnicities. Of the 13 studies that conclude rs11136000 confers AD risk, 11 studies are performed in a predominantly or exclusively western European or American Caucasian population. Alternatively, nine of the 10 studies that conclude no significant association (NSA) between rs11136000 and AD were performed in Asian, eastern European and Russian, Middle Eastern, or Hispanic populations indicating that the risk associated with the rs11136000 SNP may vary based on population ethnicity. Contrary to these data, two separate studies performed in exclusively German and American Caucasian populations found NSA between rs11136000 and AD risk. Moreover, the notion that rs11136000 does not confer AD risk in Asian populations is contradicted by two independent studies that indicate rs11136000-mediated AD risk in exclusively Chinese populations. As all the presented studies performed in Asian populations are adjusted for age, gender, and APOE status, and are comprised of numerically similar sample sizes, it is difficult to identify the exact reason underlying these discrepancies. One observation is that some studies have divided study populations into much smaller groups based upon the specific nucleotide substitution located at the rs11136000 SNP site (i.e. C,T,A substitution), while others have examined only rs11136000 carriers vs. non-carriers. The failure to stratify study populations based on the rs11136000 allele/genotype would have a significant impact on study outcome as the C allele of rs11136000 is considered the risk-conferring allele, while the A allele and T allele are considered normal and neuroprotective, respectively (i.e. C = risk allele, A = normal, and T = protective). Specifically, studies have indicated that the C allele confers a 1.16-fold increased chance of developing LOAD and that 36% of Caucasians carry two copies of this AD-risk variant [26, 27]. Moreover, the C allele is associated with faster cognitive decline in preclinical AD [66] and lower memory scores in healthy elderly controls and elderly AD patients [67]. Young healthy carriers of the C allele exhibit neural hyperactivation in memory-associated brain regions during working memory tasks [73], neural inefficiency in memory-related prefrontal and limbic areas during working memory [88], and reduced coupling between hippocampus and prefrontal cortex during memory processing [89]. Structurally, possession of the C allele is associated with diminished white matter integrity in several brain regions [90] and increased longitudinal ventricular expansion in elderly patients independent of APOE ε4 and dementia status [91]. Taken together, these data indicate that the rs11136000 SNP is significantly associated with the development of AD in predominantly Caucasian populations and that the rs11136000 AD-associated risk may be initiated several decades prior to the onset of AD.

In addition to rs11136000, another CLU SNP, rs9331888, which was also identified by Lambert and colleagues in the original GWA studies, has also been repeatedly investigated as an AD risk SNP. Of the 33 studies presented in **Table 1**, seven clinical studies and two meta-analyses examined the association of rs9331888 with AD risk [27, 69, 81, 83, 84, 92–95]. However, similar to that of rs11136000, the results vary and appear to be dependent upon population ethnicity. For instance, two separate meta-analyses conclude that rs9331888 confers AD risk in Caucasian but not Asian populations [92, 95]. However, two separate case-control studies performed in exclusively Chinese populations both indicate that rs9331888 is significantly associated with AD risk [84, 94]. In addition to differing and/or small sample sizes, one possible confounding factor could be sex of the study population. As sex modulates an individual's risk for LOAD, it is likely that stratification of study populations by sex will have a significant impact on the study results.

CLU gene variant	**Study and year of publication**	**Study design and subjects**	**Diagnoses criteria**	**Major findings**
rs11136000	Harold et al. (2009)	GWA study in European and US population: *Stage 1 population:* AD cases: n = 3941, control cases: n = 7848 *Stage 2 population:* AD cases: n = 2023, control cases: n=2340	*AD diagnoses:* DSM-IV and NINCDS criteria for probable AD or CERAD criteria for definite AD	- rs11136000 SNP was significantly associated with the development of LOAD but not the age of onset.
rs2279590 *rs9331888* *rs11136000*	Lambert et al. (2009)	GWA study in French, Finnish, Italian, Spanish, and Belgian population: *Stage 1 population:* AD cases: *n* = 2032, control cases: *n* = 5328 *Stage 2 population:* AD cases: *n* = 3978, control cases: *n* = 3297	*AD diagnoses:* DSM-III-R and NINCDS-ADRDA criteria for probable AD *Control criteria:* Subjects without DMS-III-R dementia criteria and with integrity of their cognitive functions (MMSE >25)	- All CLU polymorphisms examined showed a significant association with AD development.
rs2279590 *rs9331888* *rs11136000*	Yu et al. (2010)	Case-control study in Han Chinese population: *AD cases:* *n* = 324, AOO > 65 years, 181 females: age = 76.87 ± 5.58 *Control cases:* *n* = 388, 211 females: age = 75.93 ± 4.69	*AD diagnoses:* NINCDS-ADRDA criteria for probable AD; no family history of dementia *Control criteria:* Healthy and neurologically normal individuals as determined by medical records	- -rs9331888 SNP was significantly associated with increased AD risk. - rs2279590 showed significant association only in APOE ε4 carriers. - rs11136000 was not significantly associated with increased AD risk in

CLU gene variant	Study and year of publication	Study design and subjects	Diagnoses criteria	Major findings
			and examination and MMSE score > 28 Subjects with CHF, MI, T2DM, and AS were excluded from study	Han Chinese population.
rs11136000	Seshadri et al. (2010)	Three-stage GWA study in a white population: *Stage 1 population:* Dementia-free subjects at start: $n = 8935$, AD cases: $n = 2033$, dementia-free control cases: $n = 14{,}642$ *Stage 2 population:* AD cases: $n = 2032$, control cases: $n = 5328$ *Stage 3 population:* AD cases: $n = 3333$, control cases: $n = 6995$ *Independent case-control replication population:* Ethnicity—Spanish, AD cases: $n = 1140$, age = 78.8 ± 7.9, 69.9% female; control cases: $n = 1209$, age = 49.9 ± 9.2, 58.2% female	*Dementia diagnoses:* DSM-IV criteria *AD diagnoses*: NINCDS-ADRDA criteria for definite, probable, or possible AD; AD pathology confirmed at autopsy	- rs11136000 was significantly associated with increased risk for LOAD in all study populations analyzed. - Presence of the rs11136000 risk allele did not improve ability to predict AD onset.
rs7982 *rs7012010* *rs11136000*	Jun et al. (2010)	Meta-analysis in nine European white cohorts and five non-European cohorts (African American, Israeli-Arab, and Caribbean Hispanic): *AD cases:* $n = 7070$ *Control cases:* $n = 8169$	Not provided	- All CLU polymorphisms examined demonstrated a significant association with AD in only white cohorts.
rs11136000	Corneveaux et al. (2010)	GWA study of a European population *AD cases:* $n = 1019$, 652 females, 367 males *Control cases:*	*AD diagnoses:* Clinically diagnosable dementia at time of death and neuropathological confirmation of AD (Braak stage V or VI) upon autopsy	- rs11136000 SNP was significantly associated with LOAD.

CLU gene variant	Study and year of publication	Study design and subjects	Diagnoses criteria	Major findings
		n = 591, 285 females, 306 males	*Control criteria:* Without clinically diagnosable dementia at time of death; autopsy confirmation of an absence of neuropathological hallmarks (Braak stage < III)	
rs11136000	Jessen et al. (2010)	Longitudinal cohort study in German population: *No memory impairment:* 685 females, 342 males, age = 79.4 ± 3.4 *Memory impairment without worry:* 591 females, 415 males, age = 79.8±3.6 *Memory impairment with worry:* 273 females, 109 males, age = 79.8±3.5	*AD diagnoses:* NINCDS-ADRDA criteria for probable AD	- The rs1113600 AD-risk variant is associated with low plasma CLU levels in cognitively intact healthy controls and numerically (but non-significantly) associated with lowered plasma CLU in AD cases.
rs11136000	Lancaster et al. (2011)	fMRI study in young Caucasian cohort: *Subjects:* n = 43, 22 males, 21 females, age 18–51 Subjects were genotyped for rs11136000 SNP and pooled according to genotype: CC = risk group (n = 13) and CT/TT = non-risk group (n = 24/6)	*Inclusion criteria:* No personal or family history of neuropsychiatric, neurological, or neurodegenerative disease; no chronic somatic illnesses or history of substance abuse	- Carriers of the CLU risk genotype (CC) exhibited neural hyperactivity during working memory tasks in the frontal and posterior cingulate cortex and the hippocampus compared to participants in the non-risk group.
rs11136000	Schurmann et al. (2011)	GWA study on a subset of participants from the German Study on Aging Cognition and Dementia: *AD cases:* n = 67, 47 females, 20 males, age = 85.3±3.7 *Control cases:* n = 191, 134 females, 57 males, age = 83.7±3.2	Not provided	- rs11136000 AD-risk variant was associated with low plasma CLU levels.

CLU gene variant	Study and year of publication	Study design and subjects	Diagnoses criteria	Major findings
Rs7982 *Rs572844* *rs1532277* *rs2279590* *Rs9331888* *rs10503814*	Komatsu et al. (2011)	Case-control study in Japanese population: *AD cases:* *n* = 180, 101 females, 79 males, age = 67.4±6.7 *Control cases:* *n* = 130, 67 females, 63 males, age = 64.4±6.7	*AD diagnoses:* NINCDS-ADRDA criteria; subjects had no family history of AD *Control criteria:* No history of dementia or other neuropsychiatric disorders	- No association was detected between CLU SNPs and AD in a Japanese population.
rs11136000	Golenkina et al. (2010)	Cohort study in a Russian population: *AD cases:* Early-onset— *n* = 214, AOO = 56.9 ± 5.38 Late-onset— *n* = 320, AOO 72.2 ± 5.04 *Control cases:* Moscow region: *n* = 343, age range = 35–85, age = 60.96 ± 7.94 Ural region: *n* = 160, age range = 69–89, age = 73.87 ± 3.87 Siberian region: *n* = 199, age range = 41–96, age = 61 ± 15.34	*AD diagnoses:* NINCDS-ADRDA criteria, ICD-10 criteria, and DSM-IV criteria *Control criteria:* Cognitively intact individuals	- No significant association was detected between rs11136000 SNP and the development of AD in a Russian population.
rs881146 *rs11136000* *rs17057441* *rs70120100*	Lee et al. (2011)	Nested case-control GWAS in a cohort of Caribbean Hispanic subjects: *AD cases*: *n* = 549, age of onset = 79.98 ± 8.0 *Control cases*: *n* = 544	*Dementia diagnoses:* Diagnoses established on the basis of all available information gathered from initial and follow-up studies *AD diagnoses:* NINDS-ADRDA criteria	- rs881146 SNP was significantly associated with LOAD - rs11136000 and other SNPs were not significantly associated with LOAD in a Caribbean Hispanic population.
rs11136000	Ma et al. (2011)	Case-control study in Chinese Han population: *AD cases:* *n* = 127, 73 females, 54 males, age = 73.12 ± 8.58 *Control cases:* *n* = 143, 79 females, 64 males, age = 73.80 ± 6.30	*AD diagnoses:* 2007 revised AD diagnoses criteria *Control criteria:* No history of neurological disease and MMSE score > 29	- rs11136000 was significantly associated with LOAD in Chinese Han population.

CLU gene variant	Study and year of publication	Study design and subjects	Diagnoses criteria	Major findings
rs11136000	Braskie et al (2011)	Brain imaging study of Australian Caucasian population: *Subjects:* *n* = 398, age range = 20–29, mean age = 23.6 ± 2.2	*Subject criteria:* Healthy, young, right-handed Australian Caucasian twins containing the rs11136000 genotype and ventricle size consistent with a healthy adult	- Young healthy carriers of the CLU AD-risk SNP exhibit lower white matter integrity in the corpus callosum, fornix, cingulum, and superior and inferior longitudinal fasciculi.
rs11136000	Ferrari et al. (2012)	Case-control study in a Caucasian-American population: *AD cases:* *n* = 342, age = 76.78 ± 8.6 *Control cases:* *n* = 277, age = 70.21 ± 8.6	*AD diagnoses:* NINCDS-ADRDA criteria *Control criteria:* Subject within cognitively normal limits on a standard psychometric test	- rs11136000 was significantly associated with LOAD.
rs2279590rs11136000	Kamboh et al. (2012)	Case-control study in Caucasian-American population: *AD cases:* *n* = 1348, AOO = 72.6 ± 6.4, 65.6% female *Control cases:* *n* = 1359, age = 74.7 ± 6.5, 60.8% female	*AD diagnoses:* NINCDS-ADRDA criteria for probable or definite AD *Control criteria:* Non-demented Caucasian-American over 60 years of age	- No significant association was observed between CLU SNPs and AD in case-control study.
rs7982	Karch et al. (2012)	GWA study in Euro-American population: *AD cases:* *n* = 73, age = 87 ± 7, 42% male *Control cases:* *n* = 39, age = 86 ± 9, 44% male	*AD diagnoses:* Autopsy confirmed AD *Control criteria:* Age-matched cognitively normal controls	- rs7982 was associated with disease status. - Elevated CLU levels are associated with AD brains. - CLU is altered at the mRNA level in AD brain.
rs3087554 *rs9331942* *rs9331949* *rs11136000*	Lin et al. (2012)	Case-control study in Taiwanese population: *AD cases:* *n* = 268, *Control cases:* *n* = 389	*AD diagnoses:* DSM-IV criteria and NINCDS-ADRDA criteria *Control cases:* Assessed via Short Portable Mental Status Questionnaire	- rs11136000 was associated with significantly reduced risk for AD.
rs2279590 *rs9331888*	Chen et al. (2012)	Case-control study in southern Chinese population:	*AD diagnoses:* NINCDS-ADRDA criteria and no family history of AD	- rs2279590 and rs11136000 SNPs confer susceptibility to AD in

CLU gene variant	Study and year of publication	Study design and subjects	Diagnoses criteria	Major findings
rs11136000		*AD cases:* *n* = 462 *Control cases:* *n* = 350	*Control criteria:* Cognitively normal individuals as indicated by CDR scale	southern Chinese population.
rs9331888	Xing et al. (2012)	Case-control study: *AD cases:* *n* = 104, AOO = ≥65, age = 80.20 ± 5.57, 63 females, 41 males *Control cases:* *n* = 104, age = 79.32 ± 5.37, 58 females, 46 males	*AD diagnoses:* NINCDS-ADRDA criteria for probable AD *Control criteria:* Confirmed healthy by medical history, medical examination, and MMSE score > 28	- Subjects who were homozygous for the AD-risk allele exhibited a significant decrease in CLU protein and mRNA levels.
rs11136000	Klimkowicz-Mrowiec et al. (2012)	Case-control study in a Polish population: *AD cases:* *n* = 253, age = 73.9 ± 5.8, 173 females *Control cases:* *n* = 240, age = 73.8 ± 6.9, 138 females	*AD diagnoses:* NINCDS-ADRDA criteria for probable AD—no family history of AD *Control criteria:* MMSE > 26, no family history of dementia, no apparent neurological, psychiatric, or cerebrovascular disease	- No significant association between rs11136000 and the AD in a Polish population.
18 CLU SNPS	Yu et al. (2013)	Case-control study in Han Chinese population: *AD cases:* *n* = 796, AOO = ≥65, age = 74.3 ± 7.0, 396 females *Control cases:* *n* = 796, age = 73.9 ± 6.5, 388 females	*AD diagnoses:* NINCDS-ADRDA criteria for probable AD. No family history of neurodegenerative disorders or dementia *Control criteria:* Free of cognitive impairment as indicated by neurophysiological and medical exams	- Of the 18 SNPs tested, only the C allele (major allele) of rs9331949 was significantly associated with AD in the Han Chinese population.
rs11136000	Thambisetty et al. (2013)	Two-part longitudinal study from Baltimore Longitudinal Aging Study: *Study 1 population:* *n* = 88, age = 69, age range = 56–86 *Study 2 population:* *n* = 599, age = 67.5, age range = 60–93	*Inclusion criteria:* No history of clinical stroke, head trauma, or CNS inflammation; Subject without cognitive impairment as indicated by NINCDS-ADRDA criteria	- Cognitively normal subjects carrying the CLU risk allele exhibit increased rCBF in brain regions intrinsic to memory processes. - Risk allele carriers who converted to MCI exhibit increased rates of

CLU gene variant	Study and year of publication	Study design and subjects	Diagnoses criteria	Major findings
				memory decline over non-carriers.
rs11136000	Pedroza et al. (2014)	Association study in a white and black population: *AD cases:* $n = 44$ black, $n = 432$ white, age = 78.9, age range = 52.2–91.2 *Control cases:* $n = 224$ black, $n = 2219$ white, age = 78.7, age range = 60.5–96.4	*AD diagnoses:* NINCDS-ADRDA criteria for probable AD *Control criteria:* CDR score of 0	- The minor allele of rs11136000 may confer enhanced memory in whites.
rs1532278 *rs2279590* *rs9331888* *Rs11136000*	Lu et al. (2014)	Case-control study in southern Han Chinese population: *AD cases:* $n = 499$, age = 69.990 ± 9.961 *Control cases:* $n = 592$, age = 68.930 ± 9.390	Not provided	- No significant association was detected between CLU SNPs and LOAD in southern Han Chinese population.
rs1532278	Patel et al. (2014)	Prospective cohort study in a British Caucasian cohort with Down syndrome: *Subjects:* $n = 304$ Down syndrome patients, age > 16	*Dementia diagnoses:* ICD-10 research criteria	- No significant association between rs1532278 and the development of dementia in a cohort of Caucasian Down syndrome patients.
rs11136000	Lancaster et al. (2015)	fMRI study in young Caucasian population: *Subjects:* $n = 85$, age range = 19–47	*Inclusion criteria:* Healthy, right-handed, young Caucasians with no history of mental illness or drug abuse	- Carriers of the rs11136000 risk variant exhibit higher activation levels in memory-related pre-frontal and limbic areas during working memory tasks.
rs11136000	Sen et al. (2015)	Case-control study in a Turkish population: *AD cases:* $n = 112$, age range = 65–98, age = 73.59 ± 7.59 *Control cases:* $n = 106$, age = 74.04 ± 5.29	*AD diagnoses:* NINCDS-ADRDA criteria for probable AD—no family history of dementia *Control criteria:* Cognitively intact	- No significant association was observed between rs11136000 and AD in the entire Turkish population. - Turkish females carrying the rs11136000 TT genotype exhibited increased BEHAVE-AD scores

CLU gene variant	Study and year of publication	Study design and subjects	Diagnoses criteria	Major findings
				suggesting a possible association between the TT genotype and female Turkish subjects.
rs11136000	Sohrabifar et al. (2015)	Case-control study in an Iranian population: *AD cases:* *n* = 160 *Control cases:* *n* = 163	Not provided	- No significant association between rs11136000 and AD in an Iranian population.
rs9331888	Toral-Rios et al. (2015)	Case-control study in a Mexican population: *AD cases:* *n* = 94, age > 60 *Control cases:* *n* = 100, age > 60	*AD diagnoses:* NINCDS-ADRDA criteria *Control criteria:* MMSE ≥ 24, no memory complaints, no acute or severe chronic illness	- No significant association between rs9331888 and AD in a Mexican population.
rs9331888	Shuai et al. (2015)	Meta-analysis of 11 case-control studies: *Ethnicities:* Caucasian and Asian populations *AD cases:* *n* = 8766 *Control cases:* *n* = 11,366	*Study inclusion criteria:* (1) Study evaluated rs9331888 SNP and AD risk (2) Case-control design (3) Sufficient study population was provided	-Significant association between rs9331888 and AD in Caucasian population among allelic, additive, and recessive models. - No association in combined population or only Asian population.
rs2279590	Zhang et al. (2015)	Meta-analysis of 11 case-control studies: *Ethnicities:* Caucasian and Asian populations *AD cases:* *n* = 8605 *Control cases:* *n* = 12,050	*Study inclusion criteria:* (1) Study evaluated rs2279590 SNP and AD risk (2) Case-control design (3) Study provided the number of rs2279590 genotypes (4) Study provided OR with a 95% CI	- Significant association detected between rs2279590 and AD in Asian population among additive and recessive models.
rs9331888	Zhang et al. (2015)	Meta-analysis of 12 case-control studies: *Ethnicities:* Caucasian and Asian populations *AD cases:* *n* = 16,876 *Control cases:* *n* = 19,295	*Study inclusion criteria:* (1) Study evaluated rs9331888 SNP and AD risk (2) Case-control design (3) Study provided the number of SNP genotypes (4) Study provided OR with a 95% CI	- Significant association detected in pooled population. - Subgroup analysis demonstrates a significant association between rs9331888 and AD in Caucasian

CLU gene variant	Study and year of publication	Study design and subjects	Diagnoses criteria	Major findings
				population but not Asian population.

Abbreviations: Age of onset (AOO), behavioural pathology in Alzheimer's disease (BEHAVE-AD), the Consortium to Establish a Registry for Alzheimer's Disease (CERAD), Clinical Dementia Rating (CDR), congestive heart failure (CHF), Diagnostic and Statistical Manual of Mental Disorders, Third Edition, Revised (DSM-III-R), Diagnostic and Statistical Manual of Mental Disorders, Fourth Edition (DSM-IV), functional magnetic resonance imaging (fMRI), genome-wide association (GWA), mini-mental state examination (MMSE), National Institute of Neurological and Communicative Disorders and Stroke and the Alzheimer's Disease and Related Disorders Association (NINCDS-ADRDA), odds ratio (OR), type 2 diabetes mellitus (T2DM).

Table 1. CLU polymorphisms in AD (2009–2016).

3.2. CLU as an AD biomarker

In 1992, it was suggested that peripheral CLU (then referred to as SGP-2) expression may serve as a potential biomarker for predicting the onset and/or severity of neurodegenerative disorders such as LOAD [96]. Though this concept was proposed over 20 years ago, the possibility of CLU as an AD biomarker is only recently being examined. Since 2010, 10 different studies have been performed with the aim of determining the validity of CLU as an AD biomarker (**Table 2**). However, the conclusions of these studies are contradictory at best. Of the 10 studies presented in **Table 2**, six studies conclude that increased plasma CLU levels are associated with increased rate of cognitive decline [97], increased white matter atrophy [98], increased risk for AD [99], and were indicative of greater fibrillar Aβ burden [100]. However, contrary to these findings, four studies conclude that CLU levels are not significantly different between control subjects and subjects with MCI, AD, or dementia, suggesting that peripheral CLU is unreliable as an AD biomarker [101–105]. One primary difference between these studies is the fluid that was analyzed for CLU concentration. The six studies concluding that CLU would be a reliable biomarker utilize plasma samples for analysis, whereas the three of the four studies indicating no difference between control and AD subjects measure serum or platelets. Another key difference between these conflicting reports is the sample size. In three of the four studies concluding that CLU would not be a reliable AD biomarker, the sample size per group is less than 70 subjects, whereas most of the studies indicating the possibility of CLU as a peripheral biomarker contain several hundred subjects per group. Therefore, it is also possible that these differences are the result of inadequate sample size. Despite these discrepancies, these studies collectively suggest that at least plasma CLU could provide a predictive biomarker for determining the risk for AD.

Study and year of publication	Fluid analyzed	Study design and subjects	Diagnoses criteria	Major findings
Thambisetty et al. (2010)	Plasma	Prospective cohort study: *Subjects:* $n = 844$	*AD diagnoses:* NINCDS-ADRDA criteria for probable AD	-Increased plasma concentration of CLU was

Study and year of publication	Fluid analyzed	Study design and subjects	Diagnoses criteria	Major findings
		Ethnicity: White European (UK, France, Italy, Finland, Poland, Greece) derived from the KLC-ART and AddNeuroMed cohort studies and the Baltimore Longitudinal Study of Aging	*MCI diagnoses:* Subjective memory complaints, CDR scores of less than 1, and evidence of objective memory impairment using the CERAD criteria *Control criteria:* Subjects with no MCI and MMSE ≥ 28	predictive of greater fibrillar Aβ burden.
Schrijvers et al. (2011)	Plasma	Case-cohort study from the Rotterdam Study in the Netherlands: *Subjects:* 60 individuals with prevalent AD at baseline, a sub-cohort of 926 subjects, and an additional 156 subjects diagnosed with AD throughout follow-up time	*Study outcome:* Prevalent AD *AD diagnoses:* Severity of AD measured by the MMSE score, and the risk of developing AD during follow-up examinations	- In AD patients, higher plasma CLU was associated with more severe AD. - The likelihood of prevalent AD increased with increasing plasma CLU levels.
Ijsselstijn et al. (2011)	Serum	Case-control study derived from the Rotterdam Scan Study: *AD cases:* $n = 43$, age = 78 ± 6.5, 32 females *Control cases:* $n = 43$, age = 78 ± 6.8, 32 females	*AD diagnoses:* DSM-III R criteria *Control criteria:* MMSE ≥ 28	- No significant difference in serum CLU levels between pre-symptomatic AD and controls (p-value = 0.54).
Thambisetty et al. (2012)	Plasma	Longitudinal cohort study: 139 cognitively intact subjects, age = 70.5	*Baseline criteria:* Free of clinical diagnosis of dementia at evaluation *MCI diagnoses:* Petersen criteria *Dementia diagnoses:* DSM III criteria	- Higher baseline concentration of plasma was associated with slower rates of brain atrophy. - Peripheral concentrations of CLU appear to reflect concentrations in AD-vulnerable brain regions.
Mukaetova-Ladinska et al. (2012)	Platelets	Case-control study: *AD cases:* n =25, age = 78.08 ± 1.0, 10 females *Control cases:* n = 26, age = 70.81 ± 1.98, 18 females	*AD diagnoses:* NINCDS-ADRDA criteria for probable AD *Control criteria:* Subjects with no cognitive and/or neurological problems	- No significant difference in platelet CLU levels between control and AD patients.
Silajdzic et al. (2012)	Plasma	Quantitative ELISA assessment of plasma	*AD diagnoses:* DSM-IIIR criteria and NINCDS-	- No significant difference in plasma CLU levels

Study and year of publication	Fluid analyzed	Study design and subjects	Diagnoses criteria	Major findings
		CLU levels: *AD cases:* *n* = 127 *Dementia cases:* *n* = 82 *Depression cases:* *n* = 30 *Control cases:* *n* = 171	ADRDA criteria for probable AD *VaD diagnoses:* DSM-IIIR criteria and NINDS-AIREN criteria for probable dementia *DLB diagnoses:* Consensus criteria by McKeith and McKhann Control criteria: No memory complaints	between control cases and AD, dementia or depression cases.
Song et al. (2012)	Plasma	Longitudinal cohort study—Sydney Memory and Aging Study: *MCI cases:* *n* = 257 *Control cases:* *n* = 407	*MCI diagnoses:* International consensus criteria and CDR > 0.5	- CLU plasma levels were negatively correlated with gray matter volume and positively correlated with CSF volume. - Higher plasma CLU levels predict white matter atrophy over 2 years in elderly subjects.
Sattlecker et al. (2014)	Whole blood	Prospective cohort study—AddNeuroMed Biomarker Study: *AD cases:* *n* = 331 *MCI cases:* *n* = 149 *Control cases:* n = 211	Not provided	- Increased plasma CLU is significantly associated with increased rate of cognitive decline.
Jongbloed et al. (2015)	CSF and plasma	Quantitative diagnostic study: *AD cases:* *n* = 107 *MCI cases:* *n* = 50 *Control cases:* *n* = 67	*AD diagnoses:* NINCDS-ADRDA criteria for probable AD *MCI diagnoses:* Petersen's criteria *Control criteria:* Cognitively healthy spouses or relatives of AD group	- Elevated plasma CLU was associated with increased risk for AD and related to cognitive decline in MCI patients. - Plasma CLU is inversely related to cognitive decline in AD patients.
Dukic et al. (2016)	Serum	Quantitative comparison of serum CLU levels: *AD cases:* *n* = 70 *Dementia cases:* *n* = 67 *MCI cases:* *n* = 48	*AD diagnoses:* NINCDS-ADRDA criteria *VaD diagnoses:* NINCS-AIREN criteria *MCI diagnoses:* Peterson's criteria	- Serum concentrations of CLU did not differ between groups.

Study and year of publication	Fluid analyzed	Study design and subjects	Diagnoses criteria	Major findings
		Control cases: $n = 50$	*Control criteria:* Cognitively healthy spouses of AD and VaD patients	

Table 2. CLU as an AD biomarker (2010–2016).

4. CLU in the brain: mechanisms of action

Of the known CLU isoforms, mCLU is by far the most studied and has been described as a chaperone-like protein that clears misfolded proteins, cellular debris, and protein aggregates from the cytosol and extracellular space [106–113]. However, the nCLU and icCLU isoforms remain relatively uncharacterized. Several reports have suggested that nCLU and icCLU exhibit solely proapoptotic characteristics; however, results vary across laboratories and are inconsistent [41, 42, 114–116]. This section reviews the available literature pertaining to CLU isoforms in the brain with particular emphasis on the molecular mechanisms by which CLU protein isoforms regulate amyloid homeostasis, inflammation, and apoptosis.

4.1. CLU and Aβ homeostasis

In the early 1990s, CLU mRNA and protein levels were found to be significantly elevated in AD brain, specifically in the frontal cortex and hippocampus of post-mortem AD brain tissue [117, 118]. Shortly after these discoveries, McGeer et al. demonstrated robust CLU immunoreactivity within senile plaques [119]. It was further demonstrated that mCLU-bound soluble Aβ proteins in the cerebral spinal fluid (CSF) [120] and that CLU expression increased the solubility of Aβ and prevented Aβ aggregation [121]. These data strongly suggested that CLU may play an important role in the pathogenesis of AD via regulation of brain amyloid burden. However, contrary to these findings, it has also been demonstrated that increased CLU expression exacerbated Aβ-induced neurotoxicity [122]. Moreover, DeMattos et al. demonstrated that Aβ plaque formation was facilitated by CLU in an animal model of AD suggesting that CLU exerts a negative impact on the brain in the development of AD pathology [123]. These literary contradictions continued to persist until 2007 when a study by Yerbery and colleagues provided a possible explanation for the simultaneously pro- and anti-amyloidogenic effects associated with mCLU [124]. This study indicated that the pro-amyloidogenic effects of mCLU were restricted to conditions in which Aβ was present in a very large molar excess. Under these conditions, mCLU, which functions as a chaperone-like protein to temporarily stabilize misfolded proteins [125], bound to and stabilized Aβ thereby facilitating Aβ aggregation. Alternatively, when mCLU was present at much higher but still substoichiometric levels (i.e. a molar ratio of clusterin:Aβ = 1:10), mCLU provided substantial anti-amyloidogenic effects by inhibiting plaque formation [124]. These data suggest that CLU may exhibit neuroprotective characteristics in preclinical or early stages of AD when brain amyloid burden is significantly lower. Alternatively, CLU may exert a negative impact during later stages of AD when brain amyloid burden is extensive, though this hypothesis is yet to be tested. Parallel to this notion, a more recent study performed in rat brains indicated that mCLU prevented Aβ42-induced learning and memory impairments, reduced Aβ42-induced glia inflammation, and reduced Aβ42-mediated neuronal degeneration when Aβ42 oligomers were incubated with mCLU prior to brain injection. However, these effects were not observed in rats injected with pre-formed Aβ42 oligomers and mCLU without pre-incubation indicating that mCLU does prevent Aβ42-induced neurotoxicity prior to extensive Aβ42 oligomerization [126]. In addition to these studies, mCLU has been shown to impact the rate of Aβ42 clearance. A study by Bell and colleagues demonstrated that the rate of Aβ clearance was increased by as much as 83% when bound to CLU. This same study further demonstrated that CLU-bound Aβ is transported across the blood-brain barrier specifically through LRP2-mediated transport, while APOE-bound Aβ was transported through LRP-1 [127]. While the regulation of Aβ by mCLU is relatively well characterized, one question that remains unanswered is whether alternative CLU isoforms exert some impact on amyloid homeostasis. It has been demonstrated that Aβ toxicity induces the expression of intracellular CLU (icCLU) in neurons; however, the physiological impact of increased icCLU expression was not determined in this study [128]. At present, no literature specifically implicates a role for nCLU/icCLU isoforms in the regulation of Aβ; however, as nCLU/icCLU isoforms are reportedly induced by cellular stress in multiple peripheral cell lines and nCLU is induced upon treatment with exogenous Aβ, it is likely that nCLU/icCLU isoforms mediate some effect on amyloid homeostasis in the brain; however, more research is needed before a conclusion can be made.

4.2. CLU and inflammation

It is well established that persistent inflammation likely caused by the deposition of neurotoxic protein aggregates in the brain is a key component of LOAD [129]. Early studies suggest that CLU inhibits the activation of the complement system in the brain [31, 130–132]. For instance, several early publications indicated that CLU (then referred to as SP-40,40) prevented the formation of the membrane attack complex (MAC), suggesting that increased CLU would suppress initiation of acute inflammation. However, these data were contradicted by a more recent study that demonstrated CLU-mediated activation of the major histocompatibility complex class II (MHC II) antigen in primary cultures of rat microglia. This same study showed that administration of exogenous CLU resulted in the direct activation of microglia in the brain and the subsequent secretion of pro-inflammatory cytokines such as tumour necrosis factor alpha (TNF-α) indicating that increased CLU expression induces the acute inflammatory response [49]. These findings were corroborated by another study that demonstrated increased CLU staining within reactive microglia in the cortices of rats following cerebral ischemia [133]. Collectively, these studies suggest that increased CLU expression results in the activation of glial cells and the subsequent secretion of pro-inflammatory mediators. Therefore, it is possible that the increased secretion of cytokines such as TNF-α could contribute to chronic inflammation in AD brain; however, this hypothesis requires further testing.

4.3. CLU and apoptosis

Several studies performed in human cancer cell lines have demonstrated that mCLU and nCLU exhibit opposing effects on cell death pathways. mCLU has been shown to protect cells from oxidative stress and inhibit intrinsic apoptosis by interacting with and stabilizing the KU-70-Bax protein complex [134–138]. In contrast, nCLU is suggested to initiate intrinsic apoptotic pathways resulting in rapid cell death [115, 136]. The contrasting functions of mCLU and nCLU appear to also exist in the brain; however, unlike cancer-focused studies, relatively few brain-based investigations have included an examination of the apoptotic characteristics of nCLU. An early study by Schreiber et al. demonstrated that CLU (then referred to as SGP-2) mRNA expression was rapidly and transiently increased in astrocytes, but not CA3 and CA1 neurons, following administration of kainic acid (KA), a neurotoxic seizure-inducing compound [139]. Another study performed in WT, human CLU overexpressing (hCLU-OE) mice and Clu-knockout (Clu-/-) mice subjected to middle cerebral artery occlusion (MCAO) indicated that CLU overexpression resulted in reduced brain injury. Specifically, this study demonstrated a 30–50% increase in CLU mRNA expression 7 days post-ischemia in the ischemic brain hemisphere specifically in the penumbral area (the area that separates necrotic from normal brain tissue). Morphometric analysis of the ischemic hemisphere revealed that the penumbra was significantly thinner in hCLU-OE mice and significantly thicker in Clu-/- mice when compared with WT mice indicating an inverse relationship between CLU mRNA expression and brain injury [140]. Collectively, these two studies strongly support a neuroprotective role for CLU in the brain following significant brain injury. In contrast, ethanol-mediated toxicity has been shown to significantly increase CLU expression in the cortex and amygdala. This upregulated CLU, which was shown to interact with Bcl-XL, was translocated to the nucleus upon exposure to ethanol, and was associated with increased cell death suggesting that these effects were mediated by nCLU [135]. Another study performed in neonatal mice subjected to hypoxic-ischemic brain injury indicated that CLU accumulated in dying neurons following brain injury. Moreover, this study indicated that CLU-deficient mice exhibited 50% less brain injury when compared to wild-type controls indicating that CLU expression exacerbates neuronal cell death following brain injury [141]. Collectively, these studies indicate that nCLU protein expression may be associated with increased cell death following traumatic brain injury or in response to cytotoxic stimuli.

5. Future perspectives

CLU is currently the third most significant genetic risk factor for the development of LOAD; however, an extensive gap exists in the literature in understanding the neurophysiological and neuropathological functions of CLU. Moreover, the bulk of brain-based CLU research refers to CLU as a single protein with few studies including a characterization of its isoforms. As CLU isoforms appear to mediate different physiological processes, the tendency to focus on the effects of CLU as a singular protein could lead to conflicting reports in the literature that are currently unresolved. Therefore, before researchers can fully ascertain the therapeutic potential of CLU from a clinical perspective, it is vital that these key deficiencies are addressed at the molecular level.

First, it is crucial that current and future studies strive to examine CLU isoforms individually, with particular emphasis on separating the nCLU and mCLU isoforms. Of the studies published pertaining to CLU in the brain, approximately five studies include an examination of nCLU. While it is possible that nCLU does function to regulate apoptosis, recent findings from our laboratory indicate roughly equivalent expression levels of both mCLU and nCLU in healthy primary cortical neurons suggesting that nCLU may be integrally involved in cellular homeostasis. Moreover, our recent data indicate that a nCLU or icCLU isoform is localized to the mitochondria suggesting that these alternative CLU isoforms may play an important role in the regulation of brain mitochondria function. While these studies are still underway, future work should focus on identifying the exact CLU isoforms expressed in other types of brain cells including astrocytes and microglia. Moreover, these studies should examine the cellular distribution, key protein modulators, and the neurophysiological function of each nCLU/icCLU isoform.

An emerging topic in the study of AD is the impact of sex on the development and progression of LOAD. As previously discussed, the female population is more susceptible to developing LOAD and the risk conferred by genetic factors, such as APOE, is greater in females. Moreover, our recent analyses have demonstrated that CLU expression is significantly reduced in the early aging of female but not male brain during a time that corresponds with the onset of reproductive senescence [28]. These data strongly suggest that CLU expression is modulated, in part, by sex hormone signaling pathways in the brain. Parallel to these findings, our recent studies have revealed that brain CLU isoform expression is regulated via estrogen receptor (ER) signaling. Additionally, we find that testosterone (TT) differentially regulates mCLU and nCLU expression; TT increases mCLU expression and decreases nCLU expression. An extension of these studies revealed that TT-mediated upregulation of mCLU expression results from the aromatization of TT to 17β-estradiol (E2). These data are particularly interesting when considered in the context of sex hormone changes between men and women throughout the aging process. It is well established that menopausal onset results in a significant and irreversible decline in ovarian sex hormones, such as E2. However, TT levels in males gradually decline with age at a rate of approximately 2% per year [142]. Therefore, it is possible that TT-mediated upregulation of the neuroprotective mCLU isoform may, in part, contribute to the reduced incidence of AD in men. Likewise, the significant reduction in E2 levels in menopausal and/or postmenopausal women may result in significantly reduced mCLU levels thereby contributing to female vulnerability. While more research is needed to fully elucidate the interactions between sex hormones and neuronal CLU isoforms, these data underscore the importance of including sex as a variable in the study of risk factors that mediate the development of LOAD.

It is particularly interesting that two of the top five genetic risk factors associated with the development of LOAD are members of the apolipoprotein family: APOE and CLU. Therefore, another avenue of research to be considered in the AD field is the possibility of intersecting or overlapping risk pathways mediated by these two genetic factors. Studies have shown that

APOE and CLU share a number of important physiological properties. For instance, they are among the few proteins associated with brain lipoproteins [143, 144]. They interact with a shared set of cell-surface receptors [108] and both APOE and CLU promote neurite outgrowth [145, 146]. Moreover, elimination of either protein in an AD mouse model results in increased accumulation of Aβ [147]. Furthermore, presence of the C allele of the CLU AD-risk SNP has been shown to exacerbate the APOE ε4-mediated decrease in brain activity during executive attention tasks in young healthy dementia-free adults [148]. In addition, the genetic variance that results in increased AD risk from both genes is also associated with compromised or reduced protein expression and/or binding capabilities. Our data indicate that APOE protein expression levels are significantly increased in 6-month-old female Clu-/- mice. However, mCLU expression levels are significantly reduced in 6-month-old female human APOE ε4 gene targeted-replacement mice when compared to APOE ε3 mice indicating that reduced CLU expression may contribute to APOE ε4-mediated AD risk. Collectively, these studies indicate that APOE and CLU could share common risk pathways that contribute to the development of LOAD. Delineation of such pathways will potentially provide valuable insights for an increased understanding of the etiology of LOAD and ultimately help to devise therapeutic strategies to prevent or reduce the risk of developing the disease.

Author details

Sarah K. Woody[1] and Liqin Zhao[1,2*]

*Address all correspondence to: lzhao@ku.edu

1 Department of Pharmacology and Toxicology, School of Pharmacy, University of Kansas, Lawrence, KS, USA

2 Neuroscience Graduate Program, University of Kansas, Lawrence, KS, USA

References

[1] Alzheimer's A. 2015 Alzheimer's disease facts and figures. Alzheimer's & Dementia: The Journal of the Alzheimer's Association. 2015;11(3):332–84.

[2] Why Do All the Large Alzheimer's Drug Trials Fail? [press release]. http://www.dana.org/News/Why_Do_All_the_Large_Alzheimer_s_Drug_Trials_Fail_/: The Dana Foundation, July 8, 2013.

[3] Pharma counts just 3 Alzheimer's drug wins in 13 years (101 losses!) [press release]. http://www.fiercebiotech.com/story/pharma-counts-just-3-alzheimers-drug-wins-13-years-101-losses/2012-09-14: FierceBiotech, September 14, 2012.

[4] National Institute on Aging. Alzheimer's Disease. 2015; 1–8 https://www.nia.nih.gov/alzheimers/publication/alzheimers-disease-fact-sheet.

[5] Gao S, Hendrie HC, Hall KS, Hui S. The relationships between age, sex, and the incidence of dementia and Alzheimer disease: a meta-analysis. Archives of General Psychiatry. 1998;55(9):809–15.

[6] Irvine K, Laws KR, Gale TM, Kondel TK. Greater cognitive deterioration in women than men with Alzheimer's disease: a meta analysis. Journal of Clinical and Experimental Neuropsychology. 2012;34(9):989–98.

[7] Chapman RM, Mapstone M, Gardner MN, Sandoval TC, McCrary JW, Guillily MD, et al. Women have farther to fall: gender differences between normal elderly and Alzheimer's disease in verbal memory engender better detection of Alzheimer's disease in women. Journal of International Neuropsychology Society. 2011;17(4):654–62.

[8] Schmidt R, Kienbacher E, Benke T, Dal-Bianco P, Delazer M, Ladurner G, et al. Sex differences in Alzheimer's disease. Neuropsychiatry. 2008;22(1):1–15.

[9] Zhao L, Mao Z, Brinton RD. A select combination of clinically relevant phytoestrogens enhances estrogen receptor beta-binding selectivity and neuroprotective activities in vitro and in vivo. Endocrinology. 2009;150(2):770–83.

[10] Zhao L, Brinton RD. Structure-based virtual screening for plant-based ERbeta-selective ligands as potential preventative therapy against age-related neurodegenerative diseases. Journal of Medicinal Chemistry. 2005;48(10):3463–6.

[11] Zhao L, Wu TW, Brinton RD. Estrogen receptor subtypes alpha and beta contribute to neuroprotection and increased Bcl-2 expression in primary hippocampal neurons. Brain Research. 2004;1010(1–2):22–34.

[12] Saunders AM, Schmader K, Breitner JC, Benson MD, Brown WT, Goldfarb L, et al. Apolipoprotein E epsilon 4 allele distributions in late-onset Alzheimer's disease and in other amyloid-forming diseases. Lancet. 1993;342(8873):710–1.

[13] Blacker D, Haines JL, Rodes L, Terwedow H, Go RC, Harrell LE, et al. ApoE-4 and age at onset of Alzheimer's disease: the NIMH genetics initiative. Neurology. 1997;48(1): 139–47.

[14] Corder EH, Saunders AM, Risch NJ, Strittmatter WJ, Schmechel DE, Gaskell PC, Jr., et al. Protective effect of apolipoprotein E type 2 allele for late onset Alzheimer disease. Nature Genetics. 1994;7(2):180–4.

[15] Corder EH, Saunders AM, Strittmatter WJ, Schmechel DE, Gaskell PC, Small GW, et al. Gene dose of apolipoprotein E type 4 allele and the risk of Alzheimer's disease in late onset families. Science. 1993;261(5123):921–3.

[16] Liu CC, Kanekiyo T, Xu H, Bu G. Apolipoprotein E and Alzheimer disease: risk, mechanisms and therapy. Nature Reviews Neurology. 2013;9(2): 106–18.

[17] Langbaum JB, Chen K, Lee W, Reschke C, Bandy D, Fleisher AS, et al. Categorical and correlational analyses of baseline fluorodeoxyglucose positron emission tomography images from the Alzheimer's disease neuroimaging initiative (ADNI). NeuroImage. 2009;45(4):1107–16.

[18] Lynch JR, Tang W, Wang H, Vitek MP, Bennett ER, Sullivan PM, et al. APOE genotype and an ApoE-mimetic peptide modify the systemic and central nervous system inflammatory response. The Journal of Biological Chemistry. 2003;278(49): 48529–33.

[19] Drzezga A, Grimmer T, Henriksen G, Muhlau M, Perneczky R, Miederer I, et al. Effect of APOE genotype on amyloid plaque load and gray matter volume in Alzheimer disease. Neurology. 2009;72(17):1487–94.

[20] Drzezga A, Riemenschneider M, Strassner B, Grimmer T, Peller M, Knoll A, et al. Cerebral glucose metabolism in patients with AD and different APOE genotypes. Neurology. 2005;64(1):102–7.

[21] Altmann A, Tian L, Henderson VW, Greicius MD, Alzheimer's Disease Neuroimaging Initiative I. Sex modifies the APOE-related risk of developing Alzheimer disease. Annals of Neurology. 2014;75(4):563–73.

[22] Farrer LA, Cupples LA, Haines JL, Hyman B, Kukull WA, Mayeux R, et al. Effects of age, sex, and ethnicity on the association between apolipoprotein E genotype and Alzheimer disease. A meta-analysis. APOE and Alzheimer disease meta analysis consortium. JAMA. 1997;278(16):1349–56.

[23] Fleisher A, Grundman M, Jack CR, Jr., Petersen RC, Taylor C, Kim HT, et al. Sex, apolipoprotein E epsilon 4 status, and hippocampal volume in mild cognitive impairment. Archives of Neurology. 2005;62(6):953–7.

[24] Payami H, Montee KR, Kaye JA, Bird TD, Yu CE, Wijsman EM, et al. Alzheimer's disease, apolipoprotein E4, and gender. JAMA. 1994;271(17):1316–7.

[25] Payami H, Zareparsi S, Montee KR, Sexton GJ, Kaye JA, Bird TD, et al. Gender difference in apolipoprotein E-associated risk for familial Alzheimer disease: a possible clue to the higher incidence of Alzheimer disease in women. American Journal of Human Genetics. 1996;58(4):803–11.

[26] Harold D, Abraham R, Hollingworth P, Sims R, Gerrish A, Hamshere ML, et al. Genome-wide association study identifies variants at CLU and PICALM associated with Alzheimer's disease. Nature Genetics. 2009;41(10):1088–93.

[27] Lambert JC, Heath S, Even G, Campion D, Sleegers K, Hiltunen M, et al. Genome-wide association study identifies variants at CLU and CR1 associated with Alzheimer's disease. Nature Genetics. 2009;41(10):1094–9.

[28] Zhao L, Mao Z, Woody SK, Brinton RD. Sex differences in metabolic aging of the brain: insights into female suceptibility to Alzheimer's disease. Neurobiology of Aging. 2016;42:69–79.

[29] Fritz IB, Burdzy K, Setchell B, Blaschuk O. Ram rete testis fluid contains a protein (clusterin) which influences cell-cell interactions in vitro. Biology of Reproduction. 1983;28(5):1173–88.

[30] Sylvester SR, Skinner MK, Griswold MD. A sulfated glycoprotein synthesized by Sertoli cells and by epididymal cells is a component of the sperm membrane. Biology of Reproduction. 1984;31(5):1087–101.

[31] Murphy BF, Kirszbaum L, Walker ID, d'Apice AJ. SP-40,40, a newly identified normal human serum protein found in the SC5b-9 complex of complement and in the immune deposits in glomerulonephritis. The Journal of Clinical Investigation. 1988;81(6):1858–64.

[32] de Silva HV, Stuart WD, Park YB, Mao SJ, Gil CM, Wetterau JR, et al. Purification and characterization of apolipoprotein J. The Journal of Biological Chemistry. 1990;265(24): 14292–7.

[33] Wong P, Pineault J, Lakins J, Taillefer D, Leger J, Wang C, et al. Genomic organization and expression of the rat TRPM-2 (clusterin) gene, a gene implicated in apoptosis. The Journal of Biological Chemistry. 1993;268(7):5021–31.

[34] Yang CR, Yeh S, Leskov K, Odegaard E, Hsu HL, Chang C, et al. Isolation of Ku70-binding proteins (KUBs). Nucleic Acids Research. 1999;27(10):2165–74.

[35] Jenne DE, Tschopp J. Molecular structure and functional characterization of a human complement cytolysis inhibitor found in blood and seminal plasma: identity to sulfated glycoprotein 2, a constituent of rat testis fluid. Proceedings of the National Academy of Sciences of the United States of America. 1989;86(18):7123–7.

[36] Purrello M, Bettuzzi S, Di Pietro C, Mirabile E, Di Blasi M, Rimini R, et al. The gene for SP-40,40, human homolog of rat sulfated glycoprotein 2, rat clusterin, and rat testosterone-repressed prostate message 2, maps to chromosome 8. Genomics. 1991;10(1): 151–6.

[37] Dietzsch E, Murphy BF, Kirszbaum L, Walker ID, Garson OM. Regional localization of the gene for clusterin (SP-40,40; gene symbol CLI) to human chromosome 8p12→p21. Cytogenetics and Cell Genetics. 1992;61(3):178–9.

[38] Tobe T, Minoshima S, Yamase S, Choi NH, Tomita M, Shimizu N. Assignment of a human serum glycoprotein SP-40,40 gene (CLI) to chromosome 8. Cytogenetics and Cell Genetics. 1991;57(4):193–5.

[39] Burkey BF, deSilva HV, Harmony JA. Intracellular processing of apolipoprotein J precursor to the mature heterodimer. The Journal of Lipid Research. 1991;32(6):1039–48.

[40] Stewart EM, Aquilina JA, Easterbrook-Smith SB, Murphy-Durland D, Jacobsen C, Moestrup S, et al. Effects of glycosylation on the structure and function of the extracellular chaperone clusterin. Biochemistry. 2007;46(5):1412–22.

[41] Leskov KS, Klokov DY, Li J, Kinsella TJ, Boothman DA. Synthesis and functional analyses of nuclear clusterin, a cell death protein. The Journal of Biological Chemistry. 2003;278(13):11590–600.

[42] Prochnow H, Gollan R, Rohne P, Hassemer M, Koch-Brandt C, Baiersdorfer M. Non-secreted clusterin isoforms are translated in rare amounts from distinct human mRNA variants and do not affect Bax-mediated apoptosis or the NF-kappaB signaling pathway. PloS One. 2013;8(9):e75303.

[43] Reddy KB, Jin G, Karode MC, Harmony JA, Howe PH. Transforming growth factor beta (TGF beta)-induced nuclear localization of apolipoprotein J/clusterin in epithelial cells. Biochemistry. 1996;35(19):6157–63.

[44] de Silva HV, Harmony JA, Stuart WD, Gil CM, Robbins J. Apolipoprotein J: structure and tissue distribution. Biochemistry. 1990;29(22):5380–9.

[45] Nizard P, Tetley S, Le Drean Y, Watrin T, Le Goff P, Wilson MR, et al. Stress-induced retrotranslocation of clusterin/APOJ into the cytosol. Traffic. 2007;8(5):554–65.

[46] Pasinetti GM, Johnson SA, Oda T, Rozovsky I, Finch CE. Clusterin (SGP-2): a multifunctional glycoprotein with regional expression in astrocytes and neurons of the adult rat brain. The Journal of Comparative Neurology. 1994;339(3):387–400.

[47] Cordero-Llana O, Scott SA, Maslen SL, Anderson JM, Boyle J, Chowhdury RR, et al. Clusterin secreted by astrocytes enhances neuronal differentiation from human neural precursor cells. Cell Death and Differentiation. 2011;18(5):907–13.

[48] Zwain IH, Grima J, Cheng CY. Regulation of clusterin secretion and mRNA expression in astrocytes by cytokines. Molecular and Cellular Neurosciences. 1994;5(3):229–37.

[49] Xie Z, Harris-White ME, Wals PA, Frautschy SA, Finch CE, Morgan TE. Apolipoprotein J (clusterin) activates rodent microglia in vivo and in vitro. Journal of Neurochemistry. 2005;93(4):1038–46.

[50] Kumita JR, Poon S, Caddy GL, Hagan CL, Dumoulin M, Yerbury JJ, et al. The extracellular chaperone clusterin potently inhibits human lysozyme amyloid formation by interacting with prefibrillar species. Journal of Molecular Biology. 2007;369(1):157–67.

[51] DeMattos RB, Brendza RP, Heuser JE, Kierson M, Cirrito JR, Fryer J, et al. Purification and characterization of astrocyte-secreted apolipoprotein E and J-containing lipopro-

teins from wild-type and human apoE transgenic mice. Neurochemistry International. 2001;39(5–6):415–25.

[52] Loison F, Debure L, Nizard P, le Goff P, Michel D, le Drean Y. Up-regulation of the clusterin gene after proteotoxic stress: implication of HSF1-HSF2 heterocomplexes. The Biochemical Journal. 2006;395(1):223–31.

[53] Michel D, Chatelain G, North S, Brun G. Stress-induced transcription of the clusterin/APOJ gene. The Biochemical Journal. 1997;328 (Pt 1):45–50.

[54] Trougakos IP, Gonos ES. Regulation of clusterin/apolipoprotein J, a functional homologue to the small heat shock proteins, by oxidative stress in ageing and age-related diseases. Free Radical Research. 2006;40(12):1324–34.

[55] Cervellera M, Raschella G, Santilli G, Tanno B, Ventura A, Mancini C, et al. Direct transactivation of the anti-apoptotic gene apolipoprotein J (clusterin) by B-MYB. The Journal of Biological Chemistry. 2000;275(28):21055–60.

[56] Gutacker C, Klock G, Diel P, Koch-Brandt C. Nerve growth factor and epidermal growth factor stimulate clusterin gene expression in PC12 cells. The Biochemical Journal. 1999;339 (Pt 3):759–66.

[57] Jin G, Howe PH. Regulation of clusterin gene expression by transforming growth factor beta. The Journal of Biological Chemistry. 1997;272(42): 26620–6.

[58] Jin G, Howe PH. Transforming growth factor beta regulates clusterin gene expression via modulation of transcription factor c-Fos. European Journal of biochemistry/FEBS. 1999;263(2):534–42.

[59] Kapron JT, Hilliard GM, Lakins JN, Tenniswood MP, West KA, Carr SA, et al. Identification and characterization of glycosylation sites in human serum clusterin. Protein Science: A Publication of the Protein Society. 1997;6(10):2120–33.

[60] Dunker AK, Lawson JD, Brown CJ, Williams RM, Romero P, Oh JS, et al. Intrinsically disordered protein. Journal of Molecular Graphics & Modelling. 2001;19(1):26–59.

[61] Rohne P, Prochnow H, Wolf S, Renner B, Koch-Brandt C. The chaperone activity of clusterin is dependent on glycosylation and redox environment. Cellular Physiology and Biochemistry : International Journal of Experimental Cellular Physiology, Biochemistry, and Pharmacology. 2014;34(5):1626–39.

[62] Kang SW, Yoon SY, Park JY, Kim DH. Unglycosylated clusterin variant accumulates in the endoplasmic reticulum and induces cytotoxicity. The International Journal of Biochemistry & Cell Biology. 2013;45(2):221–31.

[63] Xue J, Lv DD, Jiao S, Zhao W, Li X, Sun H, et al. pVHL mediates K63-linked ubiquitination of nCLU. PloS One. 2012;7(4):e35848.

[64] Lemansky P, Brix K, Herzog V. Subcellular distribution, secretion, and posttranslational modifications of clusterin in thyrocytes. Experimental Cell Research. 1999;251(1):147–55.

[65] Ghosh P, Hale EA, Lakshman MR. Plasma sialic-acid index of apolipoprotein J (SIJ): a new alcohol intake marker. Alcohol. 2001;25(3):173–9.

[66] Nuutinen T, Suuronen T, Kyrylenko S, Huuskonen J, Salminen A. Induction of clusterin/APOJ expression by histone deacetylase inhibitors in neural cells. Neurochemistry International. 2005;47(8):528–38.

[67] Masoodi TA, Al Shammari SA, Al-Muammar MN, Alhamdan AA, Talluri VR. Exploration of deleterious single nucleotide polymorphisms in late-onset Alzheimer disease susceptibility genes. Gene. 2013;512(2):429–37.

[68] Braskie MN, Jahanshad N, Stein JL, Barysheva M, McMahon KL, de Zubicaray GI, et al. Common Alzheimer's disease risk variant within the CLU gene affects white matter microstructure in young adults. The Journal of Neuroscience: The Official Journal of the Society for Neuroscience. 2011;31(18):6764–70.

[69] Chen LH, Kao PY, Fan YH, Ho DT, Chan CS, Yik PY, et al. Polymorphisms of CR1, CLU and PICALM confer susceptibility of Alzheimer's disease in a southern Chinese population. Neurobiology of Aging. 2012;33(1):210 e1–7.

[70] Corneveaux JJ, Myers AJ, Allen AN, Pruzin JJ, Ramirez M, Engel A, et al. Association of CR1, CLU and PICALM with Alzheimer's disease in a cohort of clinically characterized and neuropathologically verified individuals. Human Molecular Genetics. 2010;19(16):3295–301.

[71] Ferrari R, Moreno JH, Minhajuddin AT, O'Bryant SE, Reisch JS, Barber RC, et al. Implication of common and disease specific variants in CLU, CR1, and PICALM. Neurobiology of Aging. 2012;33(8):1846 e7–18.

[72] Jun G, Naj AC, Beecham GW, Wang LS, Buros J, Gallins PJ, et al. Meta-analysis confirms CR1, CLU, and PICALM as alzheimer disease risk loci and reveals interactions with APOE genotypes. Archives of Neurology. 2010;67(12):1473–84.

[73] Lancaster TM, Baird A, Wolf C, Jackson MC, Johnston SJ, Donev R, et al. Neural hyperactivation in carriers of the Alzheimer's risk variant on the clusterin gene. European Neuropsychopharmacology: The Journal of the European College of Neuropsychopharmacology. 2011;21(12):880–4.

[74] Ma JF, Liu LH, Zhang Y, Wang Y, Deng YL, Huang Y, et al. Association study of clusterin polymorphism rs11136000 with late onset Alzheimer's disease in Chinese Han

population. American Journal of Alzheimer's Disease and Other Dementias. 2011;26(8): 627–30.

[75] Schurmann B, Wiese B, Bickel H, Weyerer S, Riedel-Heller SG, Pentzek M, et al. Association of the Alzheimer's disease clusterin risk allele with plasma clusterin concentration. Journal of Alzheimer's Disease : JAD. 2011;25(3):421–4.

[76] Seshadri S, Fitzpatrick AL, Ikram MA, DeStefano AL, Gudnason V, Boada M, et al. Genome-wide analysis of genetic loci associated with Alzheimer disease. JAMA. 2010;303(18):1832–40.

[77] Thambisetty M, Beason-Held LL, An Y, Kraut M, Nalls M, Hernandez DG, et al. Alzheimer risk variant CLU and brain function during aging. Biological Psychiatry. 2013;73(5):399–405.

[78] Golenkina SA, Gol'tsov A, Kuznetsova IL, Grigorenko AP, Andreeva TV, Reshetov DA, et al. Analysis of clusterin gene (CLU/APOJ) polymorphism in Alzheimer's disease patients and in normal cohorts from Russian populations. Molekuliarnaia Biologiia. 2010;44(4):620–6.

[79] Kamboh MI, Minster RL, Demirci FY, Ganguli M, Dekosky ST, Lopez OL, et al. Association of CLU and PICALM variants with Alzheimer's disease. Neurobiology of Aging. 2012;33(3):518–21.

[80] Klimkowicz-Mrowiec A, Sado M, Dziubek A, Dziedzic T, Pera J, Szczudlik A, et al. Lack of association of CR1, PICALM and CLU gene polymorphisms with Alzheimer disease in a Polish population. Neurologia i Neurochirurgia Polska. 2013;47(2):157–60.

[81] Komatsu M, Shibata N, Kuerban B, Ohnuma T, Baba H, Arai H. Genetic association between clusterin polymorphisms and Alzheimer's disease in a Japanese population. Psychogeriatrics : The Official Journal of the Japanese Psychogeriatric Society. 2011;11(1):14–8.

[82] Lee JH, Cheng R, Barral S, Reitz C, Medrano M, Lantigua R, et al. Identification of novel loci for Alzheimer disease and replication of CLU, PICALM, and BIN1 in Caribbean Hispanic individuals. Archives of Neurology. 2011;68(3):320–8.

[83] Lu SJ, Li HL, Sun YM, Liu ZJ, Yang P, Wu ZY. Clusterin variants are not associated with southern Chinese patients with Alzheimer's disease. Neurobiology of Aging. 2014;35(11):2656 e9–11.

[84] Yu JT, Li L, Zhu QX, Zhang Q, Zhang W, Wu ZC, et al. Implication of CLU gene polymorphisms in Chinese patients with Alzheimer's disease. Clinica Chimica Acta: International Journal of Clinical Chemistry. 2010;411(19–20):1516–9.

[85] Yu JT, Ma XY, Wang YL, Sun L, Tan L, Hu N, et al. Genetic variation in clusterin gene and Alzheimer's disease risk in Han Chinese. Neurobiology of Aging. 2013;34(7):1921 e17–23.

[86] Lin YL, Chen SY, Lai LC, Chen JH, Yang SY, Huang YL, et al. Genetic polymorphisms of clusterin gene are associated with a decreased risk of Alzheimer's disease. European Journal of Epidemiology. 2012;27(1):73–75.

[87] Pedraza O, Allen M, Jennette K, Carrasquillo M, Crook J, Serie D, et al. Evaluation of memory endophenotypes for association with CLU, CR1, and PICALM variants in black and white subjects. Alzheimer's & Dementia: The Journal of the Alzheimer's Association. 2014;10(2):205–13.

[88] Lancaster TM, Brindley LM, Tansey KE, Sims RC, Mantripragada K, Owen MJ, et al. Alzheimer's disease risk variant in CLU is associated with neural inefficiency in healthy individuals. Alzheimer's & Dementia: The Journal of the Alzheimer's Association. 2015;11(10):1144–52.

[89] Erk S, Meyer-Lindenberg A, Opitz von Boberfeld C, Esslinger C, Schnell K, Kirsch P, et al. Hippocampal function in healthy carriers of the CLU Alzheimer's disease risk variant. The Journal of Neuroscience: The Official Journal of the Society for Neuroscience. 2011;31(49):18180–4.

[90] Thambisetty M, An Y, Kinsey A, Koka D, Saleem M, Guntert A, et al. Plasma clusterin concentration is associated with longitudinal brain atrophy in mild cognitive impairment. NeuroImage. 2012;59(1):212–7.

[91] Roussotte FF, Gutman BA, Madsen SK, Colby JB, Thompson PM, Alzheimer's Disease Neuroimaging I. Combined effects of Alzheimer risk variants in the CLU and ApoE genes on ventricular expansion patterns in the elderly. The Journal of Neuroscience: The Official Journal of the Society for Neuroscience. 2014;34(19):6537–45.

[92] Shuai P, Liu Y, Lu W, Liu Q, Li T, Gong B. Genetic associations of CLU rs9331888 polymorphism with Alzheimer's disease: a meta-analysis. Neuroscience Letters. 2015;591:160–5.

[93] Toral-Rios D, Franco-Bocanegra D, Rosas-Carrasco O, Mena-Barranco F, Carvajal-Garcia R, Meraz-Rios MA, et al. Evaluation of inflammation-related genes polymorphisms in Mexican with Alzheimer's disease: a pilot study. Frontiers in Cellular Neuroscience. 2015;9:148.

[94] Xing YY, Yu JT, Cui WZ, Zhong XL, Wu ZC, Zhang Q, et al. Blood clusterin levels, rs9331888 polymorphism, and the risk of Alzheimer's disease. Journal of Alzheimer's Disease: JAD. 2012;29(3):515–9.

[95] Zhang S, Li X, Ma G, Jiang Y, Liao M, Feng R, et al. CLU rs9331888 Polymorphism contributes to Alzheimer's disease susceptibility in Caucasian but not East Asian populations. Molecular Neurobiology. 2015.

[96] Michel D, Chabot JG, Moyse E, Danik M, Quirion R. Possible functions of a new genetic marker in central nervous system: the sulfated glycoprotein-2 (SGP-2). Synapse. 1992;11(2):105–11.

[97] Sattlecker M, Kiddle SJ, Newhouse S, Proitsi P, Nelson S, Williams S, et al. Alzheimer's disease biomarker discovery using SOMAscan multiplexed protein technology. Alzheimer's & Dementia: The Journal of the Alzheimer's Association. 2014;10(6):724–34.

[98] Song F, Poljak A, Crawford J, Kochan NA, Wen W, Cameron B, et al. Plasma apolipoprotein levels are associated with cognitive status and decline in a community cohort of older individuals. PloS One. 2012;7(6):e34078.

[99] Jongbloed W, van Dijk KD, Mulder SD, van de Berg WD, Blankenstein MA, van der Flier W, et al. Clusterin levels in plasma predict cognitive decline and progression to Alzheimer's disease. Journal of Alzheimer's Disease: JAD. 2015;46(4): 1103–10.

[100] Schrijvers EM, Koudstaal PJ, Hofman A, Breteler MM. Plasma clusterin and the risk of Alzheimer disease. JAMA. 2011;305(13):1322–6.

[101] Dukic L, Simundic AM, Martinic-Popovic I, Kackov S, Diamandis A, Begcevic I, et al. The role of human kallikrein 6, clusterin and adiponectin as potential blood biomarkers of dementia. Clinical Biochemistry. 2016;49(3):213–8.

[102] IJ L, Dekker LJ, Koudstaal PJ, Hofman A, Sillevis Smitt PA, Breteler MM, et al. Serum clusterin levels are not increased in presymptomatic Alzheimer's disease. Journal of Proteome Research. 2011;10(4):2006–10.

[103] Mukaetova-Ladinska EB, Abdel-All Z, Andrade J, Alves da Silva J, O'Brien JT, Kalaria RN. Plasma and platelet clusterin ratio is altered in Alzheimer's disease patients with distinct neuropsychiatric symptoms: findings from a pilot study. International Journal of Geriatric Psychiatry. 2015;30(4):368–75.

[104] Mukaetova-Ladinska EB, Abdel-All Z, Dodds S, Andrade J, Alves da Silva J, Kalaria RN, et al. Platelet immunoglobulin and amyloid precursor protein as potential peripheral biomarkers for Alzheimer's disease: findings from a pilot study. Age and Ageing. 2012;41(3):408–12.

[105] Silajdzic E, Minthon L, Bjorkqvist M, Hansson O. No diagnostic value of plasma clusterin in Alzheimer's disease. PloS One. 2012;7(11):e50237.

[106] Bailey RW, Dunker AK, Brown CJ, Garner EC, Griswold MD. Clusterin, a binding protein with a molten globule-like region. Biochemistry. 2001;40(39): 11828–40.

[107] Bartl MM, Luckenbach T, Bergner O, Ullrich O, Koch-Brandt C. Multiple receptors mediate APOJ-dependent clearance of cellular debris into nonprofessional phagocytes. Experimental Cell Research. 2001;271(1):130–41.

[108] Kounnas MZ, Loukinova EB, Stefansson S, Harmony JA, Brewer BH, Strickland DK, et al. Identification of glycoprotein 330 as an endocytic receptor for apolipoprotein J/clusterin. The Journal of Biological Chemistry. 1995;270(22):13070–5.

[109] Lakins JN, Poon S, Easterbrook-Smith SB, Carver JA, Tenniswood MP, Wilson MR. Evidence that clusterin has discrete chaperone and ligand binding sites. Biochemistry. 2002;41(1):282–91.

[110] Law GL, Griswold MD. Activity and form of sulfated glycoprotein 2 (clusterin) from cultured Sertoli cells, testis, and epididymis of the rat. Biology of Reproduction. 1994;50(3):669–79.

[111] Leeb C, Eresheim C, Nimpf J. Clusterin is a ligand for apolipoprotein E receptor 2 (ApoER2) and very low density lipoprotein receptor (VLDLR) and signals via the Reelin-signaling pathway. The Journal of Biological Chemistry. 2014;289(7): 4161–72.

[112] Poon S, Rybchyn MS, Easterbrook-Smith SB, Carver JA, Pankhurst GJ, Wilson MR. Mildly acidic pH activates the extracellular molecular chaperone clusterin. The Journal of Biological Chemistry. 2002;277(42):39532–40.

[113] Wyatt A, Yerbury J, Poon S, Dabbs R, Wilson M. Chapter 6: The chaperone action of Clusterin and its putative role in quality control of extracellular protein folding. Advances in Cancer Reserch. 2009;104:89–114.

[114] Debure L, Vayssiere JL, Rincheval V, Loison F, Le Drean Y, Michel D. Intracellular clusterin causes juxtanuclear aggregate formation and mitochondrial alteration. Journal of Cell Science. 2003;116(Pt 15):3109–21.

[115] Dia VP, Mejia EG. Lunasin promotes apoptosis in human colon cancer cells by mitochondrial pathway activation and induction of nuclear clusterin expression. Cancer Letters. 2010;295(1):44–53.

[116] Kimura K, Asami K, Yamamoto M. Effect of heat shock treatment on the production of variant testosterone-repressed prostate message-2 (TRPM-2) mRNA in culture cells. Cell Biochemistry and Function. 1997;15(4):251–7.

[117] Lidstrom AM, Bogdanovic N, Hesse C, Volkman I, Davidsson P, Blennow K. Clusterin (apolipoprotein J) protein levels are increased in hippocampus and in frontal cortex in Alzheimer's disease. Experimental Neurology. 1998;154(2):511–21.

[118] May PC, Lampert-Etchells M, Johnson SA, Poirier J, Masters JN, Finch CE. Dynamics of gene expression for a hippocampal glycoprotein elevated in Alzheimer's disease and in response to experimental lesions in rat. Neuron. 1990;5(6):831–9.

[119] McGeer PL, Klegeris A, Walker DG, Yasuhara O, McGeer EG. Pathological proteins in senile plaques. The Tohoku Journal of Experimental Medicine. 1994;174(3):269–77.

[120] Ghiso J, Matsubara E, Koudinov A, Choi-Miura NH, Tomita M, Wisniewski T, et al. The cerebrospinal-fluid soluble form of Alzheimer's amyloid beta is complexed to SP-40,40 (apolipoprotein J), an inhibitor of the complement membrane-attack complex. The Biochemical Journal. 1993;293(Pt 1):27–30.

[121] Matsubara E, Soto C, Governale S, Frangione B, Ghiso J. Apolipoprotein J and Alzheimer's amyloid beta solubility. The Biochemical Journal. 1996;316(Pt 2):671–9.

[122] Oda T, Wals P, Osterburg HH, Johnson SA, Pasinetti GM, Morgan TE, et al. Clusterin (APOJ) alters the aggregation of amyloid beta-peptide (A beta 1-42) and forms slowly sedimenting A beta complexes that cause oxidative stress. Experimental Neurology. 1995;136(1):22–31.

[123] DeMattos RB, O'Dell M A, Parsadanian M, Taylor JW, Harmony JA, Bales KR, et al. Clusterin promotes amyloid plaque formation and is critical for neuritic toxicity in a mouse model of Alzheimer's disease. Proceedings of the National Academy of Sciences of the United States of America. 2002;99(16):10843–8.

[124] Yerbury JJ, Poon S, Meehan S, Thompson B, Kumita JR, Dobson CM, et al. The extracellular chaperone clusterin influences amyloid formation and toxicity by interacting with prefibrillar structures. FASEB J. 2007;21(10):2312–22.

[125] Poon S, Easterbrook-Smith SB, Rybchyn MS, Carver JA, Wilson MR. Clusterin is an ATP-independent chaperone with very broad substrate specificity that stabilizes stressed proteins in a folding-competent state. Biochemistry. 2000;39(51):15953–60.

[126] Cascella R, Conti S, Tatini F, Evangelisti E, Scartabelli T, Casamenti F, et al. Extracellular chaperones prevent Abeta42-induced toxicity in rat brains. Biochimica et Biophysica Acta. 2013;1832(8):1217–26.

[127] Bell RD, Sagare AP, Friedman AE, Bedi GS, Holtzman DM, Deane R, et al. Transport pathways for clearance of human Alzheimer's amyloid beta-peptide and apolipoproteins E and J in the mouse central nervous system. Journal of Cerebral Blood Flow and Metabolism: Official Journal of the International Society of Cerebral Blood Flow and Metabolism. 2007;27(5):909–18.

[128] Killick R, Ribe EM, Al-Shawi R, Malik B, Hooper C, Fernandes C, et al. Clusterin regulates beta-amyloid toxicity via Dickkopf-1-driven induction of the wnt-PCP-JNK pathway. Molecular Psychiatry. 2014;19(1):88–98.

[129] Akiyama H, Barger S, Barnum S, Bradt B, Bauer J, Cole GM, et al. Inflammation and Alzheimer's disease. Neurobiology of Aging. 2000;21(3):383–421.

[130] Choi NH, Mazda T, Tomita M. A serum protein SP40,40 modulates the formation of membrane attack complex of complement on erythrocytes. Molecular Immunology. 1989;26(9):835–40.

[131] Choi NH, Nakano Y, Tobe T, Mazda T, Tomita M. Incorporation of SP-40,40 into the soluble membrane attack complex (SMAC, SC5b-9) of complement. International Immunology. 1990;2(5):413–7.

[132] Kirszbaum L, Bozas SE, Walker ID. SP-40,40, a protein involved in the control of the complement pathway, possesses a unique array of disulphide bridges. FEBS Letters. 1992;297(1–2):70–6.

[133] Van Beek J, Chan P, Bernaudin M, Petit E, MacKenzie ET, Fontaine M. Glial responses, clusterin, and complement in permanent focal cerebral ischemia in the mouse. Glia. 2000;31(1):39–50.

[134] Jun HO, Kim DH, Lee SW, Lee HS, Seo JH, Kim JH, et al. Clusterin protects H9c2 cardiomyocytes from oxidative stress-induced apoptosis via Akt/GSK-3beta signaling pathway. Experimental and Molecular Medicine. 2011;43(1): 53–61.

[135] Kim N, Han JY, Roh GS, Kim HJ, Kang SS, Cho GJ, et al. Nuclear clusterin is associated with neuronal apoptosis in the developing rat brain upon ethanol exposure. Alcoholism, Clinical and Experimental Research. 2012;36(1):72–82.

[136] Miyake H, Chi KN, Gleave ME. Antisense TRPM-2 oligodeoxynucleotides chemosensitize human androgen-independent PC-3 prostate cancer cells both in vitro and in vivo. Clinical Cancer Research: An Official Journal of the American Association for Cancer Research. 2000;6(5):1655–63.

[137] Trougakos IP, Lourda M, Antonelou MH, Kletsas D, Gorgoulis VG, Papassideri IS, et al. Intracellular clusterin inhibits mitochondrial apoptosis by suppressing p53-activating stress signals and stabilizing the cytosolic Ku70-Bax protein complex. Clinical Cancer Research: An Official Journal of the American Association for Cancer Research. 2009;15(1):48–59.

[138] Zhang H, Kim JK, Edwards CA, Xu Z, Taichman R, Wang CY. Clusterin inhibits apoptosis by interacting with activated Bax. Nature Cell Biology. 2005;7(9):909–15.

[139] Schreiber SS, Tocco G, Najm I, Baudry M. Seizure activity causes a rapid increase in sulfated glycoprotein-2 messenger RNA in the adult but not the neonatal rat brain. Neuroscience Letters. 1993;153(1):17–20.

[140] Wehrli P, Charnay Y, Vallet P, Zhu G, Harmony J, Aronow B, et al. Inhibition of post-ischemic brain injury by clusterin overexpression. Nature Medicine. 2001;7(9):977–9.

[141] Han BH, DeMattos RB, Dugan LL, Kim-Han JS, Brendza RP, Fryer JD, et al. Clusterin contributes to caspase-3-independent brain injury following neonatal hypoxia-ischemia. Nature Medicine. 2001;7(3):338–43.

[142] Brawer MK. Testosterone replacement in men with andropause: an overview. Reviews in urology. 2004;6(Suppl 6):S9–15.

[143] Elliott DA, Weickert CS, Garner B. Apolipoproteins in the brain: implications for neurological and psychiatric disorders. Clinical Lipidology. 2010;51(4):555–73.

[144] Koch S, Donarski N, Goetze K, Kreckel M, Stuerenburg HJ, Buhmann C, et al. Characterization of four lipoprotein classes in human cerebrospinal fluid. Journal Lipid Research. 2001;42(7):1143–51.

[145] Kang SW, Shin YJ, Shim YJ, Jeong SY, Park IS, Min BH. Clusterin interacts with SCLIP (SCG10-like protein) and promotes neurite outgrowth of PC12 cells. Experimental Cell Research. 2005;309(2):305–15.

[146] Nathan BP, Bellosta S, Sanan DA, Weisgraber KH, Mahley RW, Pitas RE. Differential effects of apolipoproteins E3 and E4 on neuronal growth in vitro. Science. 1994;264(5160):850–2.

[147] DeMattos RB, Cirrito JR, Parsadanian M, May PC, O'Dell MA, Taylor JW, et al. ApoE and clusterin cooperatively suppress Abeta levels and deposition: evidence that ApoE regulates extracellular Abeta metabolism in vivo. Neuron. 2004;41(2):193–202.

[148] Green AE, Gray JR, Deyoung CG, Mhyre TR, Padilla R, Dibattista AM, et al. A combined effect of two Alzheimer's risk genes on medial temporal activity during executive attention in young adults. Neuropsychologia. 2014;56:1–8.

Chapter 14

New Targets for Diagnosis and Treatment Against Alzheimer's Disease: The Mitochondrial Approach

María José Pérez, Claudia Jara,
Ernesto Muñoz-Urrutia and Rodrigo A. Quintanilla

Additional information is available at the end of the chapter

http://dx.doi.org/10.5772/64327

Abstract

Alzheimer's disease (AD) is a neurodegenerative disorder and the most common form of dementia. AD is characterized by brain presence of senile plaques, which are formed by aggregates of Aβ peptide and neurofibrillary tangles (NFTs), formed by pathological forms of tau protein. Evidence suggests that these elements affect neurons compromising energy supply, antioxidant response and synaptic activity. AD principally affects the memory and cognitive functions of the patients, and currently, successful strategies for diagnosis and early treatment are lacking. In this scenario, accumulative evidence suggests that mitochondrial dysfunction precedes the establishment of tau and Aβ pathology and contributes to synaptic degeneration observed in AD. Therefore, reducing mitochondrial injury may have beneficial effects for neuronal dysfunction and cognitive decline observed in AD patients. Interestingly, the examination of peripheral cells from AD patients also presents mitochondrial dysfunction, suggesting that tracking these mitochondrial defects in peripheral cells could be a potential mechanism of early diagnosis of AD. In this chapter, we analyse current evidence that suggests that mitochondrial injury is an important factor in the pathogenesis of AD and how studying this process could reveal new strategies to mitigate neurodegeneration and to develop new diagnostic methods for an early detection of AD.

Keywords: Alzheimer's disease, mitochondria, oxidative stress, tau, Aβ, synaptic dysfunction

1. Introduction

Alzheimer's disease (AD) is a complex and irreversible neurodegenerative disorder characterized by a progressive memory and cognitive impairment. AD patients present a deficiency in short-term memory and problem-solving skills, affecting his daily activities and quality of life [1]. According to the World Alzheimer's report, this pathology comprises over the 60% of all causes of dementia, and they estimate that there are around 46.8 million people living with the disease at 2015. Because of their importance in public health, it is necessary to study the causes, diagnosis methods and possible treatments of this pathology [1]. AD is pathologically characterized by the presence of extracellular deposition of Aβ in the brain called senile plaques and intracellular neurofibrillary tangles (NFTs) containing pathological forms of tau protein [2]. Several studies had shown that these aggregates and its precursors induce neuronal dysfunction, leading to the memory and cognitive impairment [3]. Interestingly, in cellular and animal models of AD in which Aβ, tau or both pathological aggregates have been induced, impairment of mitochondrial function even prior to the characteristic establishment of NFTs and Aβ plaques [4] is shown.

Mitochondria are cellular organelles required for energy and bioenergetics processes and it is also involved in amino acid and lipid metabolism, calcium homeostasis, free radical production and apoptosis [5]. In the brain, mitochondria are involved in energy supply, antioxidant defences, vesicle transport and synaptic communication [4]. These defects could lead to the memory and cognitive impairment seen in AD patients [4].

In this chapter, we discuss the pathways involved in mitochondrial dysfunction observed in different animal and cellular models of AD. These alterations in mitochondrial function include: mitochondrial dynamics, bioenergetics and mitochondrial axonal transport [4]. All these mitochondrial defects lead to an impaired neuronal communication and that could explain the cognitive and memory failure seen in AD [2]. Also in this chapter, we discuss new strategies to diminish mitochondrial injury in AD, in order to ameliorate the pathology progression of this disease.

The references and articles utilized in the development of this chapter were obtained using online compressive search engines like PUBMED and MEDLINE. Scientific articles were obtained from the online subscription services provided by Universidad Autónoma de Chile.

1.1. Defects of mitochondrial dynamics in AD

Mitochondria is a versatile organelle that forms an intracellular network that undergoes continuous fission and fusion processes named mitochondrial dynamics [6]. This process plays a crucial role in the control of mitochondrial shape, size and number, which influences important mitochondrial properties including bioenergetics and quality control [7]. Mitochondrial fusion serves to unify the mitochondrial compartment, and mitochondrial fission contributes to the removal of damaged organelle via mitophagy and may facilitate apoptosis in conditions of cellular stress [8]. Generally, mitophagy is initiated when mitochondrial membrane potential is compromised [9]. Under this condition, the phosphatase and tensin homolog induced protein kinase 1 (PINK1) and Parkin complex ubiquitinates the mitochondrial outer membrane proteins called, mitofusins, leading to mitochondrial fragmentation and recruitment of optineurin [9]. This process induces recruitment of the autophagy-related binding protein LC3 (microtubule-associated protein light chain 3) that promotes nucleation of the autophagosome leading to mitochondrial degradation [9]. Defects in mitochondrial dynamics have been linked to several diseases, and particularly important is the process in neurons [10]. Neurons' requirements are extremely unique, because of their dependence on energy production from mitochondria, which are needed in the synaptic process [8].

Mitochondrial biogenesis occurs to supply cellular energy through the fission of preexisting mitochondria followed by growth [11]. Little is known about the regulatory mechanisms of mitochondrial biogenesis in mammalian neurons under physiological or pathological conditions. However, these processes quickly respond to changes due to mitochondrial damage or increased stimulation of PGC-1 α, Nrf1/2 and TFAM pathways [5]. Interestingly, expression levels of those proteins were significantly decreased in both AD hippocampal tissue and a neuronal cell line with overexpression of Swedish mutant forms of APP protein (APPswe), suggesting that mitochondrial biogenesis was affected during neurodegeneration and contributes to mitochondrial dysfunction in AD [12].

On the other hand, mitochondrial dynamics depends on the interaction of different proteins within the mitochondrial membranes [13, 14]. Mitochondrial fission depends on dynamin-related protein 1 (Drp1) and mitochondrial fission protein 1 (Fis1) [6]. Drp1 is mainly located in cytoplasm and is recruited by Fis1 that is in the mitochondrial outer membrane [14]. Then Drp1 by its guanosine triphosphatase (GTPase) activity assembles itself constricting mitochondrial membrane until the formation of two daughter mitochondrias [15]. Moreover, fusion of the mitochondria is control by optic atrophy protein (Opa1) and both, mitofusins 1 and 2 (Mfn1 and Mfn2) [16]. This fusion of outer mitochondrial membrane is mediated by the concerted GTPases actions of Mfn 1 and Mfn 2, and fusion of the inner membranes are mediated by Opa1 through its proteolytic processing [4, 7].

Several studies showed that mitochondrial morphological changes are present in AD [17, 18]. Brain-derived mitochondria from AD patients are smaller and more fragmented compared to age-matched individuals [19], and reduced mitochondrial density in synaptic structures and shorter mitochondria in brain axons were found in mouse overexpressing APP/Aβ (mAPP transgenic mouse) [20]. In different neuronal cell models treated with Aβ or with overexpression of Swedish mutant forms of APP protein, mitochondria present changes in their structure: a fragmented and punctiform form and a reduction of mitochondrial density in neurites [19–21]. On the other hand, tau also has a role on the Aβ-induced mitochondrial impairment. In mature neurons, it has been shown that truncated and pseudo-phosphorylated forms of tau mediates mitochondrial shortening, reducing mitochondrial movement and mitochondrial potential and increasing superoxide levels induced by Aβ [22–24]. All this morphological changes are related to changes in mitochondrial dynamics.

An increase in Fis1 protein expression and a reduced expression of Drp1, Mfn1, Mfn2 and Opa1 in the cytosolic fraction was found in post-mortem brain tissue and neuroblastoma cell line M17 treated with amyloid-β-derived diffusible ligands (ADDLs) [19]. However, Drp1 expression was increased in brain frontal cortex from AD patients [25], suggesting a deregulation of Drp1 activity associated with mitochondria [25]. Furthermore, it has been shown that oxidative stress-mediated S-nitrosylation of Drp1 induced by Aβ triggers mitochondrial fragmentation [26]. Interestingly, in another model of AD, N2a cells that expressed APP Swedish mutation, Aβ accumulation induced a decrease in both Mfn1 and Mfn2 levels, with a subsequent fragmentation of mitochondria [27]. On the other hand, in transgenic mouse models of AD a direct interaction between Drp1 and hyperphosphorylated tau has been found, suggesting a direct effect of tau on the mitochondrial dynamics dysfunction [28].

All these data suggest that tau pathology and Aβ impairs mitochondrial morphology even before the NFTs and senile plaques establishment. These are important features because a regulated fusion-fission cycle is needed to maintain a healthy mitochondrial pool. In AD, mitochondrial biogenesis is impaired, mitophagy process is reduced and alterations in cycle of mitochondria dynamics generate mitochondrial fragmentation [9, 29]. Overall, these defects could be the cause of an increase in the number of damaged organelles in AD neurons and the source of mitochondrial bioenergetics dysfunction that this disease presents.

1.2. Reduction of mitochondrial bioenergetics performance in AD

The main function of the mitochondria is generating ATP [30]. In the organelles, the electron transport chain (ETC) is responsible for oxidative phosphorylation, which is the biochemical pathway that produces ATP by consuming oxygen [30]. The electrons pass through the respiratory complexes I–IV of the ETC and as a consequence, a membrane potential is generated for the electrochemical force of a proton gradient [30]. This process generates ATP by complex V, and this energetic molecule would help, among other things, to regulate the intracellular calcium homeostasis [4]. This process normally generates reactive oxygen species (ROS); however, oxidative stress occurs when the balance between the production of oxidants molecules and the endogenous antioxidant defences in cells is deregulated [31].

Bioenergetics damage includes low ATP production, failure in ETC, mitochondria depolarization, defects in calcium buffering capacity and increase of ROS [10, 18]. Mitochondria are the primary source of oxidative species, and mitochondria-linked oxidative stress has been found to be a major factor associated with the development and progression of AD [31–33]. In fact, excessive generation of ROS contributes to neuronal dysfunction and bioenergetics failure in AD even before the appearance of Aβ plaques and NFTs [32, 34], thus supporting the hypothesis that mitochondrial failure is an early event in the AD progression.

In animal models of AD, several data suggest that the Aβ pathology is an important participant in mitochondrial bioenergetics dysfunction [35, 36]. Brain slices from APP/Aβ transgenic mice shows Aβ localization in mitochondria and increased levels of oxidative markers, carbonylated proteins and reduced cytochrome c oxidase (CoxIV or Complex IV) activity, suggesting increased oxidative stress and impaired mitochondrial metabolism in this AD model [32]. Besides, several experiments with neuronal cell lines treated with different forms of the Aβ peptide indicated that the treatment generate impairment of ETC, mitochondrial depolarization and also, opening of mitochondrial permeability transition pore (mPTP) with the resulting calcium leaking and ROS production [36, 37].

Interestingly, studies have shown that the increased oxidative stress seen in AD could generate a vicious circle in which ROS promotes Aβ generation in in vitro and in vivo models [38]. For example, in brain mitochondria from a variant of APPswe mouse, mitochondrial depolarization, low ATP levels and decreased cytochrome c oxidase activity have been found prior to Aβ plaque deposition [39]. Similar results were found in triple Tg (PS1M146V/APPSwe/TauP301L) mice [40], suggesting that both Aβ and tau pathology present mitochondrial dysfunction prior to the formation of toxic protein aggregates [41, 42].

As we already discussed, neurons are particularly sensitive to mitochondrial dysfunction since they are extremely energy dependent with many cellular activities, such as synaptic transmission and axonal and dendritic transport [43, 44]. Therefore, it is proposed that mitochondrial bioenergetics defects could be considered as a hallmark in AD, since there is evidence that is an early event in the progression of the disease.

1.3. Mitochondria are not properly transported in AD

Defects in axonal transport of mitochondria in AD have been reviewed by our group and others [4, 45]. The axonal transport comprises the action of motor proteins that carry organelles, vesicles and other proteins through microtubules [46]. Kinesins family protein commands anterograde transport (from cell body to terminals) and dynein-dynactin complexes are responsible for the retrograde transport (from terminals to cell body) [46]. Also, each cargo proteins need adaptor proteins to bring specificity to the transport process such the Miro GTPase and trafficking kinesin (TRAK) family of proteins [46]. By the other hand, the docking protein syntaphilin helps mitochondria to stay at zones of higher energy demand, such as synaptic terminals, in a way to modulate the energy requirements of the neurons [47].

Studies on APPswe mice show reduced axonal transport in vivo [48]. Neurons from human APP Tg mice showed reduced moving mitochondria when they were treated with Aβ, and interestingly, knocking down of tau protein prevented this effect [49]. Inversely, neurons of tau knock out mouse transfected with wild-type tau protein make these cells sensitive to Aβ, showing deficits in axonal transport [49, 50]. Also this group has suggested that GSK-3β is involved in this mechanism due to its interaction with presenilin 1 (PS1) a transmembrane protein related with Aβ production [50]. Furthermore, in neurons from $PS1^{-/-}$ [51] and $PS1_{M146v}$, mutation related to familiar AD [52], mice show impaired anterograde axonal transport [53]. Also, in SH-SY5Y neuroblastoma cells, it has been found that tau directly interacts with dynactin complexes suggesting a potential effect on retrograde axonal transport in tau pathology [54]. Complementary to these studies, the TPR50 transgenic mice that contain a human P301S tau, a tau gene mutant form found in frontotemporal dementia and parkinsonism linked to chromosome 17 (FTDP-17) [55], exhibited early cognitive impairment, reduced retrograde transport and increased kinesin protein expression [56].

Interestingly, Guo and coworkers found that reduction of cyclophilin D (CycD) prevented axonal transport impairment induced by Aβ [57]. CycD is a component of the mPTP located through the outer and inner mitochondrial membranes [58]. mPTP plays a key role in cell death inducing the release of cytochrome c, collapsing mitochondrial membrane potential and releasing calcium at the cytosol [58]. Furthermore, defects of mitochondrial dynamics and axonal transport induced by Aβ were prevented in CycD-depleted neurons obtained from CycD knockout mice ($Ppif^{-/-}$). In addition, restoration of mitochondrial dynamics was replicated using the CycD inhibitor cyclosporin A in the same neuronal model [57].

Overall, defects of mitochondrial transport through axons include the reduced anterograde or/and retrograde movement, increased stationary mitochondria and reduced mitochondrial density in synaptic terminals [45]. These alterations affect neuronal function including autophagy, vesicle transport and energy supply leading to synaptic failure [45].

Mitochondrial defects in dynamics, bioenergetics and transport are tightly related (**Figure 1**). Morphology alterations impair mitochondrial bioenergetics, and this deficiency generates fragmented and dysfunctional mitochondria. Also, defects in both transport and dysfunctional mitochondria could affect the energy and bioavailability of fresh mitochondria in demand zones such as nervous terminals. Together with an increased oxidative stress and reduced mitophagy may affect synaptic communication. Altogether, these alterations in mitochondrial health suggest the possibility that modulating mitochondrial function could be a key strategy to prevent or retard the progression of AD (**Figure 1**).

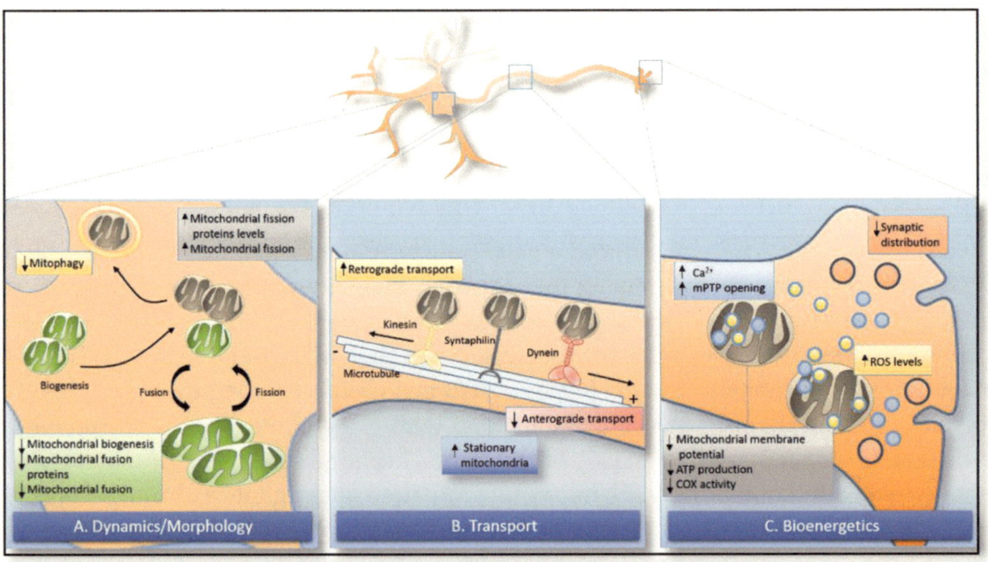

Figure 1. Mitochondrial function defects in AD. (**A**). **Dynamics/morphology**. The regulation of mitochondrial dynamics, such as fusion, fission, biogenesis and mitophagy, represents an important mechanism that control neuronal fate. Mitochondrial morphological alterations are present in all levels in AD, and the consequence is the accumulation of fragmented and dysfunctional mitochondria in all the cell body (**B**). **Transport**. Kinesin and dynein proteins mediate axonal transport of mitochondria. Generally, this movement is bidirectional in an anterograde (kinesin) and retrograde direction (dynein). In several models of AD, a deregulated mitochondrial movement together with an increase of immobile mitochondria population associated with syntaphilin has been reported. This alteration generates a decrease in the total mitochondria movement and their distribution to the synaptic space (**C**) **Bioenergetics**. Neuronal models of AD present a severe mitochondrial dysfunction with an increase in oxidative stress. This alteration leads to a bioenergetic imbalance that affects ATP levels in the presynaptic neuron, with an increase in calcium overload and a consequent synaptic dysfunction.

2. Improving mitochondrial health as a valid therapy for AD

AD is one of the most common forms of dementia in elderly and one of the biggest health problems worldwide [59, 60]. This disease represents a high monetary, personal and family cost, and despite the large number of investigations and tremendous progress that has been made in understanding the molecular mechanism underlying the disease progression, currently there are no available therapies to cure AD. Nowadays, existing treatments for AD are only symptomatic [60]. The current therapies are palliatives that focus on reducing symptoms, but they do not delay the progression of the disease [60].

Currently, the most used drugs to treat AD are the inhibitors of the enzyme acetylcholinesterase [61, 62], as donepezil [62–66], which acts by increasing the availability of acetylcholine in the synaptic space of cholinergic neurons [62, 67, 68]. Another drug used is memantine, which is a pharmacological antagonist of glutamatergic receptor N-methyl-D-aspartate (NMDA) [62, 69, 70]. Both drugs protect neurons against glutamate excitotoxicity, which is considered a major player in the neuronal damage observed in AD progression [70]. However, the approval of these drugs has not been based on their ability to slow down the disease progression but to improve the clinical symptomatology [62]. Therefore, only symptomatic drugs with transient benefits have been approved for clinical use in AD patients by the US Food and Drug Administration (FDA) [62].

Today, multiple therapies for AD are being studied [62, 70, 71]. The progress in the knowledge of the molecular characteristics of the disease and the availability of several animal models for study, it has open the boundaries to test and develop new therapies [61, 62, 72], for example, strategies for modifying AD progression include reducing neuroinflammation, metabolic approaches such as lipid-lowering agents, estrogen, antioxidants, anti-Aβ immunotherapy and recent neurotrophin-based approaches [62, 69, 72, 73]. In this scenario, and given the importance and the temporality of mitochondrial damage in AD, we believe that mitochondrial-targeted therapeutic strategies are one of the most promising areas of interest.

Mitochondria-targeted protective compounds that prevent or minimize mitochondrial dysfunction represent a potential target in the prevention and treatment of the pathogenesis of ageing-related diseases [4, 10, 74–79]. Recently, it have been reported several progresses in the use of mitochondrial therapies against several neurodegenerative diseases [44]. These strategies include preventing mitochondrial fragmentation, reducing ROS levels and increasing ATP production in the brain [4, 10, 36, 79].

2.1. Reducing defects of mitochondrial dynamics as a therapeutic target against AD

As mentioned earlier, mitochondrial dynamics is an essential mitochondrial process for the maintenance of cell viability [20, 59, 79], and apparently, it is involved in the development of many neurodegenerative diseases [44, 80]. Mitochondrial dynamics defects may result in an impaired bioenergetics and reduced mitochondrial localization in the synaptic area [20, 78, 80]. In AD, extensive researches based on the analysis of post-mortem brains, cell and animal models have reported several defects in mitochondrial dynamics [44, 81]. Therefore, increasing mitophagy and mitochondrial biogenesis may represent a promising therapeutic strategy in the treatment and prevention of common neurodegenerative diseases [82].

Preventing defects in mitochondrial dynamics reduce neuronal injury in neurodegenerative diseases [83]. For example, in Parkinson's disease (PD) the use of different compounds that regulate mitochondrial dynamics as Mdivi-1 (mitochondrial division inhibitor-1), an inhibitor of Drp1 activity, restored dopamine release, reduced mitochondrial fragmentation and prevented cell death in dopaminergic neurons [78]. In C57BL/6 mice hippocampal neurons incubated with $A\beta_{25-35}$, the use of the antioxidant peptide SS31 decreased the levels of both mitochondrial fissions proteins, Drp1 and Fis1, and managed to increase the number of healthy and intact mitochondria [44, 78]. Mitochondria plays several key roles in synaptic communication [81, 84], and to exert their synaptic roles, mitochondria must be actively transported from the soma to distal synapses zones through cytoskeleton [80, 85–87]. Interestingly, the treatment with SS31 peptide was able to reverse both the trafficking deficit and the occurrence of excess mitochondrial fission [88], restoring mitochondrial transport defects and increasing mitophagy of defective mitochondria in dopaminergic neurons [78].

Stimulation of mitophagy can also equilibrate the dysfunctional mitochondria in AD; in fact, the use of candidate drugs that increase mitophagy appears to be a promising target against many neurodegenerative diseases [89]. PINK1 is a key molecule in the signal transduction of mitophagy [90], and drugs enhancing the activity of this pathway increase the elimination of depolarizing mitochondria, which seems to be an interesting alternative for mitochondrial therapy [89, 91]. Also, the use of autophagy inducers such as rapamycin presents another tool to increase the mitophagy [90, 91]. For example, treatment with rapamycin prevented from mitochondrial fragmentation and bioenergetics defects in a rat model of PD [92].

Mitochondrial biogenesis seems to be an interesting alternative to reduce or prevent mitochondrial dynamics defects in AD. Peroxisome proliferators-activated receptors gamma (PPARγ) are nuclear receptors that, together with PGC1-alpha, participate in lipid metabolism, and they are key players in the control of energy metabolism and mitochondrial biogenesis [93, 94]. PPARγ are significantly reduced in AD as the severity of the disease increases. [93, 95] and, interestingly, improvement of neuronal mitochondrial biogenesis through PPARγ activation has been suggested to be a potential therapeutic target to reduce mitochondrial dysfunction in AD [94]. In fact, activation of those receptors using antidiabetic drugs called thiazolidinediones (TZDs) reduced mitochondrial dysfunction, decreased oxidative stress and improved memory impairment in AD mice models and patients with mild to moderate AD [22, 96, 97].

2.2. Improving mitochondrial bioenergetics in AD

Neurodegeneration and synaptic damage in AD are primarily mediated by defective mitochondrial function [31, 57, 59, 98]. This mitochondrial alteration, together with the progressive accumulation of Aβ and pathological tau, affects mitochondrial membrane potential, respiration and energy metabolism and calcium homeostasis; promotes mPTP opening; and increase oxidative stress [57, 99]. Because the bioenergetics functions are closely related to each other, overall treatments of mitochondrial-targeted compounds will generate a general improvement in several aspects of this organelle performance [79].

Several groups have reported that enhanced antioxidant capacity lowers the risk of development and progression of neurodegenerative diseases [60, 100–102]. At the same time, other studies have explored the use of mitochondrial antioxidants in order to reduce neurodegeneration in AD [4, 10, 103, 104]. Mitochondrial-targeted antioxidants have been developed in this regard and they are currently undergoing preclinical testing [106]. For example, treatment with CoQ10 decreased oxidative stress, Aβ42 levels and β-amyloid burden, and improved cognitive impairment in AD transgenic mice [4, 10, 105]. CoQ10 is an essential biologic factor of the ETC, where it accepts electrons from complexes I and II, and also serves as an important antioxidant molecule in mitochondrial lipid membranes [10, 103].

Another example of mitochondrial targeted antioxidant is the MitoQ drug, a lipophilic cation compound with strong antioxidant actions that has been successfully targeted to mitochondria, where it reduce ROS levels, leading to the protection of neurons in AD [78, 106]. MitoQ and MitoE, both are mito-targeted compounds and they accumulate in the mitochondria, enhancing ETC function and preventing oxidation of an important lipidic component of the mitochondrial membrane called cardiolipin [78, 107].

Also, in experiments with AD mice models and neuronal cultures treated with MitoQ, it was shown that mitochondria maintain their integrity and function, decrease CycD expression and prevent mitochondrial depolarization, with an additional prevention of the caspases activation [105]. In addition, in N2a cells treated with Aβ, MitoQ decreased abnormal expression of mitochondrial structural genes and reduced mitochondrial population [106]. Other studies showed that in primary cortical neurons treated with Aβ and in the 3xTg-AD mice, MitoQ showed prevention of Aβ-induced oxidative stress, reduced Aβ accumulation, improved synaptic loss and caspase activation in the brain [105]. Additionally, in a PD pharmacological model, treatment with MitoQ inhibited the activation of mitochondrial apoptotic pathway, decreasing the levels of Bax and Drp1 protein, which suggests a possible role in the control of mitochondrial dynamics [78, 108].

Another bioenergetics feature that is significantly affected in AD mitochondria is the calcium homeostasis and the opening of mPTP [99, 109, 110]. Research has demonstrated that mitochondria isolated from the hippocampus of AD patients showed elevated levels of CypD [109, 110]. CypD is a necessary component of mPTP formation, triggering the opening of mPTP by translocation of CypD to the inner membrane [57]. Studies of the genetic deletion of CypD showed a decrease in the probability of mPTP opening and a great increase in mitochondrial capacity to buffer calcium [57, 87, 110–112].

Evidence indicates that the use of CypD inhibitors may improve mitochondrial function, and even if these inhibitors can cross the blood-brain barrier, it can have considerable potential as prevention and treatment drugs against AD [57]. Additionally, it has been shown that the treatment with CsA could have mitochondrial protective effects in neurons [99, 113]. That is, because treatment with this drug enhances mitochondrial transmembrane potential, the releasing of cytochrome c outside the mitochondria is prevented and superoxide dismutase activity is increased [113], suggesting an important role of the mPTP in mitochondrial injury in AD [113, 114].

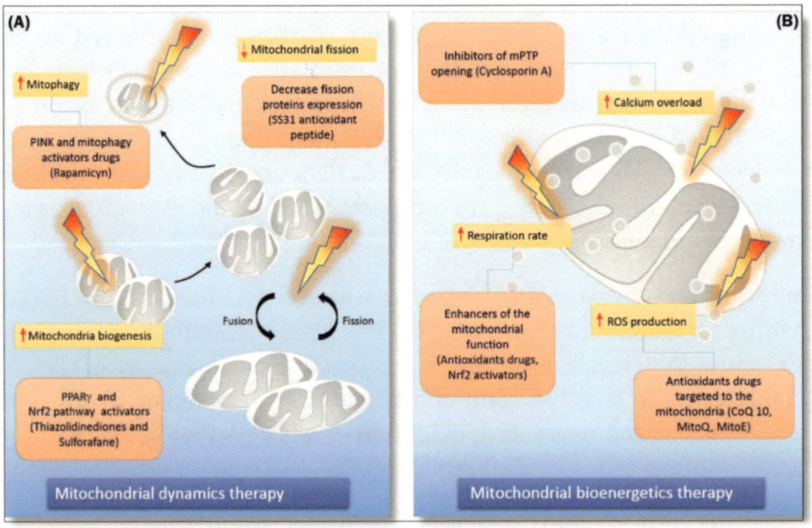

Figure 2. Improving mitochondrial health as a valid therapy for AD. (**A**) **Mitochondrial morphology therapy**. Manipulating the processes of mitochondrial dynamics has a considerable potential for treating neurodegenerative diseases. Therapies that increase mitochondrial biogenesis and fission/fusion cycle may improve mitochondrial function and decreased oxidative stress. Mitophagy is a selective autophagy process that removes dysfunctional mitochondria and maintains adequate mitochondria quality control. Increasing PINK1-mediated mitophagy improves mitochondrial integrity and function. (**B**) **Mitochondrial bioenergetics therapy**. Several agents that boost bioenergetics could have efficacy in improving mitochondrial function. These compounds show neuroprotective effects, which may be a useful target for treating neurodegenerative diseases. Treatment with CoQ10, MitoQ and MitoE prevented oxidative stress; cyclosporine A, a substance that blocks the opening of mPTP, prevented mitochondrial depolarization, blocks cytochrome c release and increased superoxide dismutase activity. Drugs that mediate the activation of Nrf2 induce the expression of antioxidant enzymes and improve mitochondrial function and biogenesis.

In that context, several groups have found that some compounds not only improve one aspect of mitochondrial damage but also improve several alterations at once by the activation of several pathways like nuclear factor E2-related factor 2 (Nrf2) [10, 101, 102]. The Nfr2 and the Nrf2-Are pathways have been studied in mitochondrial dysfunction and neurodegeneration [10, 115]. In response to oxidative stress, the Nrf2 translocate from the cytoplasm into the nucleus and activates the expression of several antioxidant genes [116]. Nrf2 is the principal regulator of the antioxidant cellular response and seems to be a promising target in the treatment of age-related neurodegenerative diseases [10, 101, 102, 117]. Nrf2 activation induces changes in mitochondrial structure and function, which is of particular importance under conditions of oxidative stress [10, 102, 118]. In primary murine cortical cultures, neurons lacking Nrf2 are more susceptible to oxidative stress induced by H_2O_2 and glutamate [116, 119] and overexpression of Nrf2, totally prevented these changes [116]. Furthermore, overexpression of Nrf2 can rescue neurons from mitochondrial complex II inhibition and ischemic insult in animal models of Huntington disease and stroke [116, 120, 121].

Interestingly, it has been suggested that Nrf2 may play a role in the pathogenesis of AD [102, 116]. Positive outcomes of Nrf2 activation include decreasing oxidative stress, reducing inflammation and increasing autophagy [115, 122]. Studies from human AD brains showed a decrease in Nrf2 levels in the cytoplasm of hippocampal neurons [115, 116]. In addition, studies in neuronal cultures derived from Nrf2 knockout mice show increased susceptibility to oxidative damage, as well as damage produced by mitochondrial electron transport gene complex inhibitors such as MPP+ and rotenone [10, 102]. Interestingly, small food-derived molecule such as sulforaphane (SFN) is a nutritional and natural activator of Nrf2 and presented neuroprotective effects and attenuated oxidative damage induced by $A\beta_{25-35}$ [102].

Overall, improving mitochondrial defects using the strategies mentioned above could have a potential impact reducing neurodegeneration in AD (**Figure 2**).

3. Mitochondrial dysfunction can help us to predict AD?

In 2011, the National Institute of Aging (NIA) and the Alzheimer's Association proposed a revised criteria and new guidelines for diagnosing Alzheimer's disease [123]. They proposed three stages of progression of AD, preclinical AD, mild cognitive impairment (MCI) due to AD and dementia due to AD. Also, they incorporated the use of biomarker tests to corroborate the presence or absence of AD or the risk to develop it [124]. Biomarker tests will be essential to identify which individuals are in the early stages of the disease and if they should receive some disease-modifying treatment. They are also critical for monitoring the effects of treatment against AD [123, 124].

AD mainly affects memory and cognitive functions and to this date, there is no early biomarker that shows the reliability and accuracy needed to diagnose the disease [125]. Currently, AD can be diagnosed with over 90% of confidence but with invasive and expensive tools based on cerebrospinal fluid (CSF) analysis and neuroimaging with positron emission tomography, with Pittsburgh compound-B radiotracer (PET/PiB) [126]. For this reason, the diagnosis is based on neuropsychological surveys and in the exclusion of other age-related dementias only when there is an advanced cognitive impairment [127]. The conclusive diagnosis of AD is only possible in autopsy with the presence of characteristic pathological brain lesions [125, 127].

Despite that AD early treatment can slow down the progression of the disease, the ability to diagnose AD at early stages is currently limited. In the search for potential biomarkers for early diagnosis of AD, several studies have shown that a significant number of peripheral tissues, both in animal models and patients, showed from early stages of the disease an abnormal presence of markers normally associated with nerve tissue [128].

For example, deposits of Aβ have been reported in skin, blood vessels, glandular structures and fibroblasts in human tissue [129–131], and the presence of total and phosphorylated tau protein were detected in plasma of AD and healthy patients [132, 133]. These facts suggest that the use of peripheral tissues as a source of inexpensive and minimally invasive samples is taking force in the diagnosis of AD. Interestingly, several studies have shown that there is an important relationship between the peripheral tissue in patients and animal models that develop AD and mitochondrial damage. Here, we show that AD peripheral tissues present different mitochondrial alterations that include mitochondrial defects in morphology, dynamics and bioenergetics.

3.1. Evidence for mitochondrial dynamics defects in AD peripheral tissues.

Mitochondrial dynamics is a complex cellular process that controls the shape, localization, turnover and function of mitochondria. As we previously discussed, several findings in patients and animal models of AD suggest that the deregulation of mitochondrial dynamics is a common feature in the disease, but may vary from case to case [134]. In the case of peripheral tissue of patients with AD, different studies indicated an altered mitochondrial morphology that could be related with changes in mitochondrial dynamics [21, 140, 141].

Several studies had proposed that the platelets could be a promising peripheral surrogate to detect AD [135], which is because these cell fragments express high levels of APP [136], tau protein [137, 138] and they have an increased GSK3β activity, a kinase responsible for tau hyperphosphorylation [139]. More important, in studies with cytoplasmic hybrid (cybrid) cells created from human neuroblastoma cells repopulated with mitochondria from platelets obtained from sporadic AD and control donors, it was shown that cybrid cells from AD patients contained a significantly increased percentage of enlarged or swollen mitochondria, and they also present a reduced mitochondrial membrane potential [140].

Using another blood cell component, the analysis of peripheral blood lymphocytes from AD patients showed an increase in SNO-Drp1 and Fis1 and reduced Drp1 levels compared with healthy controls, PD patients and vascular dementia patients [141]. The protein expression pattern observed here suggests the presence of morphological alterations of mitochondria [141].

On the other hand, in a study with fibroblasts of sporadic AD patients, an abnormal mitochondrial distribution characterized by elongated mitochondria that are accumulated in perinuclear areas with a significant decreased in Drp1 levels was found [21]. These findings are very relevant because several publications suggest that the basic pathogenic mechanism of amyloidogenesis is similar in brain and skin fibroblasts, with an increase in the production and depositions of Aβ [128, 142]. Therefore, a mitochondrial deregulation in the fibroblasts of AD patients could be indicative of the neurological progression of the disease [143, 144].

3.2. Mitochondrial bioenergetics is altered in AD peripheral tissues.

Evidence of a primary role for mitochondrial damage in AD development has also been provided through post-mortem examination of AD brains, revealing oxidative stress, mitochondrial DNA damage and bioenergetic deficiencies in MCI and AD patients [145–147]. In contrast, studies on peripheral tissues of AD patients have generated inconsistent findings [135, 140, 148–174].

Different studies reviewed by Cervellati's group have reported changes in the hydroperoxide levels, a biomarker of oxidative stress, in plasma and serum of AD patients [148]. In addition,

http://dx.doi.org/10.5772/64327

these studies revealed that the levels of the oxidant damage markers, MDA and 4-HNE, were increased in plasma and serum of AD and MCI patients compared to controls [148]. Complementary, in blood samples of individuals with mild cognitive impairment and AD, there are evidence of mitochondrial dysfunction with decreased expression of respiratory complex genes, TOMM40, and subunits of the core mitochondrial ribosome complex [149, 150]. In addition, in human peripheral blood mononuclear cells was found an increase in oxidative stress and phosphorylated levels of Nrf2 [151].

On the other hand, several studies had shown that blood platelets from AD patients also present an increase in markers related to mitochondrial bioenergetics damage [135]. Platelets presented intracellular calcium deregulation [152, 153], an increase in oxidative damage [152, 153], a decrease in CoxIV and ATP synthase activities [154–158], and as we previously mentioned, a reduced mitochondrial potential in the cybrid condition [140]. Interestingly, in a study with cognitively normal individuals with maternal history of late onset of AD was found a reduced activity of platelet CoxIV compared to those with paternal or negative family history [159]. These findings suggest not only a possible mitochondrial peripheral biomarker but also an exclusively maternally inherited marker in humans [159].

Mitochondria isolated from AD lymphocytes showed an increase in several markers of oxidative stress [160, 161], increased susceptibility to oxidative death [162, 163], and the extent of this oxidative damage inversely correlated with dementia severity [161, 162, 164]. Also, this cell type presented alterations in proteins levels of mitochondrial-related factors categorized as energetic, structural and antioxidants such as glyceraldehyde 3-phosphate dehydrogenase (GAPDH), lactate dehydrogenase B chain and ATP synthase [164]. Furthermore, analysis of mitochondrial function in lymphocytes of AD patients showed a reduction in basal respiration and a lower ATP turnover that could finally lead to accumulate mutations in mitochondrial DNA [161].

Furthermore, a recent study determined that mitochondrial population, ATP production and respiratory function are altered in fibroblasts of patients with genetic type of AD [165]. While genetic forms of the disease do not account for the majority of cases, these observations marks an important precedent that directly links mitochondrial dysfunction in peripheral tissue of AD patients [165]. Also, in this cell type, mitochondrial dysfunction is associated with high levels of ROS and oxidative damage [166–168]. This alterations could be explained because of the lower levels of antioxidant defences observed in AD patients [169], and more interesting is the fact that these fibroblasts exhibit an alteration of the calcium buffering capacity compared to control cells [170, 171].

Based on that, recent studies have shown that fibroblasts of sporadic and familial AD present an enhanced link between the endoplasmic reticulum (ER) and mitochondria, through the mitochondria-associated ER membranes structures (MAMs) [172]. This alteration in the communication between these organelles could affect the mitochondrial dynamics and function, calcium homoeostasis and production of ROS [172]. This is an interesting observation, since a recent study showed that nanomolar concentrations of oligomeric Aβ regulated MAM and mitochondrial calcium in neuronal cells of human AD cortical tissue, as well as in

AD mouse models [173]. These findings suggest that these subcellular structures are affected in AD and this would not be considered an isolated effect of fibroblasts culture.

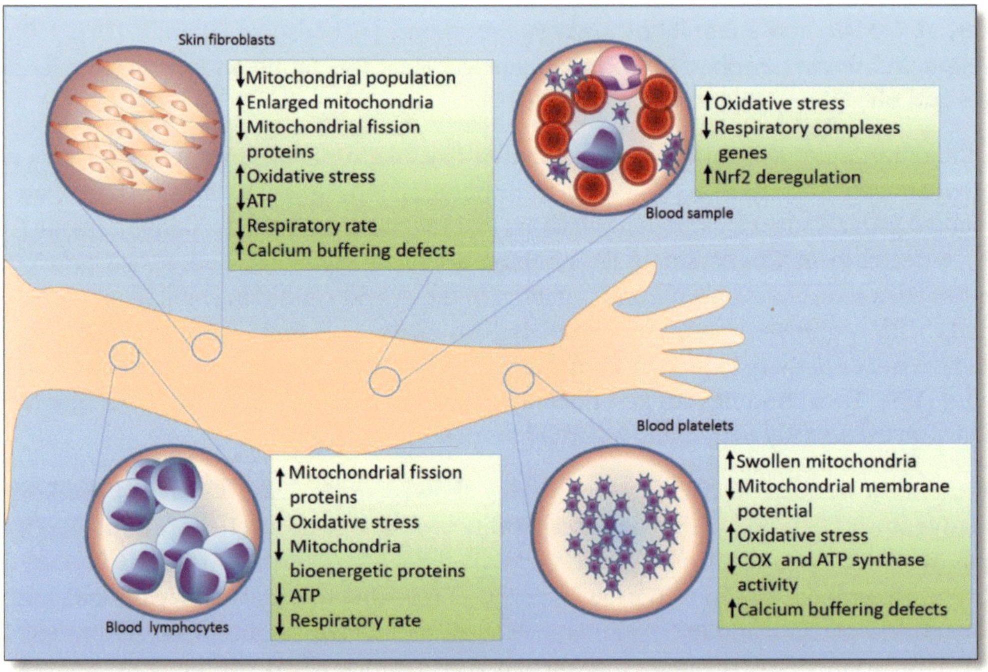

Figure 3. Mitochondrial impairment as a potential biomarker for early diagnosis of AD. Diagram shows that possible markers of mitochondrial damage could be present in blood plasma, blood cells and skin fibroblasts from AD patients. The compressive evaluation of mitochondrial health in these tissues could early detect neurodegenerative changes reported in AD.

Interestingly, a recent study with fibroblasts from an AD patient demonstrated that is possible to induce the differentiation of dermal fibroblasts into neuronal cells [174]. This study demonstrated that those neurons derived from fibroblasts expressed significant levels of phosphorylated tau and presented significant changes in the expression of genes associated with AD [174]. These studies indicate that the fibroblasts of patients could be a reliable tool for obtaining physiological information that reflects the neurological state of the patients.

Peripheral biomarkers with effective action in the early detection of Alzheimer's pathology are currently unknown, but the evidence of possible markers of mitochondrial damage in blood plasma, blood cells and skin fibroblasts represents an important step in the search for an AD biomarker (**Figure 3**). Although the fact that these tissues may provide less invasive and inexpensive sources to investigate AD progression, the finding of a new biomarker would not only be important for early diagnosis but also be an opportunity to prove direct and personalized therapies in patients with AD. Future research should focus not only in search for therapies of the disease but also in the search for a good and safe model to test the effectiveness of these pathways proposed.

http://dx.doi.org/10.5772/64327

4. Conclusions

The focus of this chapter is to discuss the principal pathways involved in mitochondrial dysfunction seen in different models of AD. We present clear evidence that showed defects in mitochondrial morphology, bioenergetics and mitochondrial axonal transport, and how these alterations lead to an impaired neuronal communication in AD. Also, we discussed different therapeutic that reduce mitochondrial damage in AD. It is important to say that several of these therapies had probe to improve not only mitochondrial health but also the neuropathological damage in AD. Finally, we showed that those mitochondrial alterations are also present in several peripheral tissues. This is a relevant aspect to consider because it could represent a promising diagnostic method, and also an easy and accessible tool for measuring the progression and development of AD.

Acknowledgements

This work was supported by Fondecyt #1140968 (RAQ) and Anillo ACT #1411 (RAQ).

Author details

María José Pérez, Claudia Jara, Ernesto Muñoz-Urrutia and Rodrigo A. Quintanilla*

*Address all correspondence to: rodrigo.quintanilla@uautonoma.cl

Laboratory of Neurodegenerative Diseases, Centro de Investigación Biomédica, Universidad Autónoma de Chile, Santiago, Chile

References

[1] Prince M, Wimo A, Guerchet M, Ali G, Gu Y, M. P. World Alzheimer Report 2015. [Internet]. 2015. 92. Available from: http://www.alz.co.uk/research/WorldAlzheimer-Report2015.pdf [Accessed: 2016-04-01].

[2] Selkoe DJ. Alzheimer's disease: genes, proteins, and therapy. Physiological reviews. 2001;81(2):741–66.

[3] Raskin J, Cummings J, Hardy J, Schuh K, Dean RA. Neurobiology of Alzheimer's disease: integrated molecular, physiological, anatomical, biomarker, and cognitive dimensions. Current Alzheimer research. 2015;12(8):712–22.

[4] Cabezas-Opazo FA, Vergara-Pulgar K, Perez MJ, Jara C, Osorio-Fuentealba C, Quintanilla RA. Mitochondrial dysfunction contributes to the pathogenesis of Alzheimer's

disease. Oxidative medicine and cellular longevity. 2015;2015:509654. DOI: 10.1155/2015/509654.

[5] Picone P, Nuzzo D, Caruana L, Scafidi V, Di Carlo M. Mitochondrial dysfunction: different routes to Alzheimer's disease therapy. Oxidative medicine and cellular longevity. 2014;2014:780179. DOI: 10.1155/2014/780179.

[6] Mishra P, Chan DC. Mitochondrial dynamics and inheritance during cell division, development and disease. Nature reviews molecular cell biology. 2014;15(10):634–46. DOI: 10.1038/nrm3877.

[7] Chen H, Chan DC. Mitochondrial dynamics—fusion, fission, movement, and mitophagy—in neurodegenerative diseases. Human molecular genetics. 2009;18(R2):R169–76. DOI: 10.1093/hmg/ddp326.

[8] Cagalinec M, Safiulina D, Liiv M, Liiv J, Choubey V, Wareski P, et al. Principles of the mitochondrial fusion and fission cycle in neurons. Journal of cell science. 2013;126(Pt 10):2187–97. DOI: 10.1242/jcs.118844.

[9] Edens BM, Miller N, Ma YC. Impaired autophagy and defective mitochondrial function: converging paths on the road to motor neuron degeneration. Frontiers in cellular neuroscience. 2016;10:44. DOI: 10.3389/fncel.2016.00044.

[10] Johri A, Beal MF. Mitochondrial dysfunction in neurodegenerative diseases. The Journal of pharmacology and experimental therapeutics. 2012;342(3):619–30. DOI: 10.1124/jpet.112.192138.

[11] Schrepfer E, Scorrano L. Mitofusins, from mitochondria to metabolism. Molecular cell. 2016;61(5):683–94. DOI: 10.1016/j.molcel.2016.02.022.

[12] Sheng B, Wang X, Su B, Lee HG, Casadesus G, Perry G, et al. Impaired mitochondrial biogenesis contributes to mitochondrial dysfunction in Alzheimer's disease. Journal of neurochemistry. 2012;120(3):419–29. DOI: 10.1111/j.1471-4159.2011.07581.x.

[13] Patrushev MV, Mazunin IO, Vinogradova EN, Kamenski PA. Mitochondrial fission and fusion. Biochemistry Biokhimiia. 2015;80(11):1457–64. DOI: 10.1134/S0006297915110061.

[14] Pernas L, Scorrano L. Mito-morphosis: mitochondrial fusion, fission, and cristae remodeling as key mediators of cellular function. Annual review of physiology. 2016;78:505–31. DOI: 10.1146/annurev-physiol-021115-105011.

[15] Mears JA, Lackner LL, Fang S, Ingerman E, Nunnari J, Hinshaw JE. Conformational changes in Dnm1 support a contractile mechanism for mitochondrial fission. Nature structural & molecular biology. 2011;18(1):20-6. DOI: 10.1038/nsmb.1949.

[16] Santel A, Fuller MT. Control of mitochondrial morphology by a human mitofusin. Journal of cell science. 2001;114(Pt 5):867–74.

[17] Burte F, Carelli V, Chinnery PF, Yu-Wai-Man P. Disturbed mitochondrial dynamics and neurodegenerative disorders. Nature reviews neurology. 2015;11(1):11–24. DOI: 10.1038/nrneurol.2014.228.

[18] Cai Q, Tammineni P. Alterations in mitochondrial quality control in Alzheimer's disease. Frontiers in cellular neuroscience. 2016;10:24. DOI: 10.3389/fncel.2016.00024.

[19] Wang X, Su B, Lee Hg, Li X, Perry G, Smith MA, et al. Impaired balance of mitochondrial fission and fusion in Alzheimer's disease. Journal of neuroscience. 2009;29(28):9090–103. DOI: 10.1523/jneurosci.1357-09.2009.

[20] Du H, Guo L, Yan S, Sosunov AA, McKhann GM, Yan SS. Early deficits in synaptic mitochondria in an Alzheimer's disease mouse model. Proceedings of the national academy of sciences of the United States of America. 2010;107(43):18670–5. DOI: 10.1073/pnas.1006586107.

[21] Wang X, Su B, Fujioka H, Zhu X. Dynamin-like protein 1 reduction underlies mitochondrial morphology and distribution abnormalities in fibroblasts from sporadic Alzheimer's disease patients. The American journal of pathology. 2008;173(2):470–82. DOI: 10.2353/ajpath.2008.071208.

[22] Quintanilla RA, Matthews-Roberson TA, Dolan PJ, Johnson GV. Caspase-cleaved tau expression induces mitochondrial dysfunction in immortalized cortical neurons: implications for the pathogenesis of Alzheimer disease. The journal of biological chemistry. 2009;284(28):18754–66. DOI: 10.1074/jbc.M808908200.

[23] Quintanilla RA, Dolan PJ, Jin YN, Johnson GV. Truncated tau and Abeta cooperatively impair mitochondria in primary neurons. Neurobiology of aging. 2012;33(3):619 e25–35. DOI: 10.1016/j.neurobiolaging.2011.02.007.

[24] Quintanilla RA, von Bernhardi R, Godoy JA, Inestrosa NC, Johnson GV. Phosphorylated tau potentiates Abeta-induced mitochondrial damage in mature neurons. Neurobiology of disease. 2014;71:260–9. DOI: 10.1016/j.nbd.2014.08.016.

[25] Manczak M, Calkins MJ, Reddy PH. Impaired mitochondrial dynamics and abnormal interaction of amyloid beta with mitochondrial protein Drp1 in neurons from patients with Alzheimer's disease: implications for neuronal damage. Human molecular genetics. 2011;20(13):2495–509. DOI: 10.1093/hmg/ddr139.

[26] Cho DH, Nakamura T, Fang J, Cieplak P, Godzik A, Gu Z, et al. S-nitrosylation of Drp1 mediates beta-amyloid-related mitochondrial fission and neuronal injury. Science. 2009;324(5923):102–5. DOI: 10.1126/science.1171091.

[27] Park J, Choi H, Min JS, Kim B, Lee SR, Yun JW, et al. Loss of mitofusin 2 links beta-amyloid-mediated mitochondrial fragmentation and Cdk5-induced oxidative stress in neuron cells. Journal of neurochemistry. 2015;132(6):687–702. DOI: 10.1111/jnc.12984.

[28] Manczak M, Reddy PH. Abnormal interaction between the mitochondrial fission protein Drp1 and hyperphosphorylated tau in Alzheimer's disease neurons: implica-

tions for mitochondrial dysfunction and neuronal damage. Human molecular genetics. 2012;21(11):2538–47. DOI: 10.1093/hmg/dds072.

[29] Ye X, Sun X, Starovoytov V, Cai Q. Parkin-mediated mitophagy in mutant hAPP neurons and Alzheimer's disease patient brains. Human molecular genetics. 2015;24(10):2938–51. DOI: 10.1093/hmg/ddv056.

[30] Nicholls DG, Budd SL. Mitochondria and neuronal survival. Physiological reviews. 2000;80(1):315–60. DOI.

[31] Calkins MJ, Manczak M, Mao P, Shirendeb U, Reddy PH. Impaired mitochondrial biogenesis, defective axonal transport of mitochondria, abnormal mitochondrial dynamics and synaptic degeneration in a mouse model of Alzheimer's disease. Human molecular genetics. 2011;20(23):4515–29. DOI: 10.1093/hmg/ddr381.

[32] Manczak M, Anekonda TS, Henson E, Park BS, Quinn J, Reddy PH. Mitochondria are a direct site of A beta accumulation in Alzheimer's disease neurons: implications for free radical generation and oxidative damage in disease progression. Human molecular genetics. 2006;15(9):1437–49. DOI: 10.1093/hmg/ddl066.

[33] Maruszak A, Zekanowski C. Mitochondrial dysfunction and Alzheimer's disease. Progress in neuro-psychopharmacology & biological psychiatry. 2011;35(2):320–30. DOI: 10.1016/j.pnpbp.2010.07.004.

[34] Chen Z, Zhong C. Oxidative stress in Alzheimer's disease. Neuroscience bulletin. 2014;30(2):271–81. DOI: 10.1007/s12264-013-1423-y.

[35] Eckert A, Schmitt K, Gotz J. Mitochondrial dysfunction—the beginning of the end in Alzheimer's disease? Separate and synergistic modes of tau and amyloid-beta toxicity. Alzheimer's research & therapy. 2011;3(2):15. DOI: 10.1186/alzrt74.

[36] Pagani L, Eckert A. Amyloid-beta interaction with mitochondria. International journal of Alzheimer's disease. 2011;2011:925050. DOI: 10.4061/2011/925050.

[37] Rhein V, Song X, Wiesner A, Ittner LM, Baysang G, Meier F, et al. Amyloid-beta and tau synergistically impair the oxidative phosphorylation system in triple transgenic Alzheimer's disease mice. Proceedings of the national academy of sciences of the United States of America. 2009;106(47):20057–62. DOI: 10.1073/pnas.0905529106.

[38] Leuner K, Schutt T, Kurz C, Eckert SH, Schiller C, Occhipinti A, et al. Mitochondrion-derived reactive oxygen species lead to enhanced amyloid beta formation. Antioxidants & redox signaling. 2012;16(12):1421–33. DOI: 10.1089/ars.2011.4173.

[39] Hauptmann S, Scherping I, Drose S, Brandt U, Schulz KL, Jendrach M, et al. Mitochondrial dysfunction: an early event in Alzheimer pathology accumulates with age in AD transgenic mice. Neurobiology of aging. 2009;30(10):1574–86. DOI: 10.1016/j.neurobiolaging.2007.12.005.

[40] Yao J, Irwin RW, Zhao L, Nilsen J, Hamilton RT, Brinton RD. Mitochondrial bioenergetic deficit precedes Alzheimer's pathology in female mouse model of Alzheimer's

disease. Proceedings of the national academy of sciences of the United States of America. 2009;106(34):14670–5. DOI: 10.1073/pnas.0903563106.

[41] Gillardon F, Rist W, Kussmaul L, Vogel J, Berg M, Danzer K, et al. Proteomic and functional alterations in brain mitochondria from Tg2576 mice occur before amyloid plaque deposition. Proteomics. 2007;7(4):605–16. DOI: 10.1002/pmic.200600728.

[42] Reddy PH, McWeeney S, Park BS, Manczak M, Gutala RV, Partovi D, et al. Gene expression profiles of transcripts in amyloid precursor protein transgenic mice: up-regulation of mitochondrial metabolism and apoptotic genes is an early cellular change in Alzheimer's disease. Human molecular genetics. 2004;13(12):1225–40. DOI: 10.1093/hmg/ddh140.

[43] Su B, Wang X, Bonda D, Perry G, Smith M, Zhu X. Abnormal mitochondrial dynamics—a novel therapeutic target for Alzheimer's disease? Molecular neurobiology. 2010;41(2-3):87–96. DOI: 10.1007/s12035-009-8095-7.

[44] Reddy PH, Tripathi R, Troung Q, Tirumala K, Reddy TP, Anekonda V, et al. Abnormal mitochondrial dynamics and synaptic degeneration as early events in Alzheimer's disease: implications to mitochondria-targeted antioxidant therapeutics. Biochimica et biophysica acta. 2012;1822(5):639–49. DOI: 10.1016/j.bbadis.2011.10.011.

[45] Wang ZX, Tan L, Yu JT. Axonal transport defects in Alzheimer's disease. Molecular neurobiology. 2015;51(3):1309–21. DOI: 10.1007/s12035-014-8810-x.

[46] Sheng ZH. Mitochondrial trafficking and anchoring in neurons: new insight and implications. The journal of cell biology. 2014;204(7):1087–98. DOI: 10.1083/jcb.201312123.

[47] Ohno N, Chiang H, Mahad DJ, Kidd GJ, Liu L, Ransohoff RM, et al. Mitochondrial immobilization mediated by syntaphilin facilitates survival of demyelinated axons. Proceedings of the national academy of sciences of the United States of America. 2014;111(27):9953–8. DOI: 10.1073/pnas.1401155111.

[48] Smith KD, Kallhoff V, Zheng H, Pautler RG. In vivo axonal transport rates decrease in a mouse model of Alzheimer's disease. Neuroimage. 2007;35(4):1401–8. DOI: 10.1016/j.neuroimage.2007.01.046.

[49] Vossel KA, Zhang K, Brodbeck J, Daub AC, Sharma P, Finkbeiner S, et al. Tau reduction prevents Abeta-induced defects in axonal transport. Science. 2010;330(6001):198. DOI: 10.1126/science.1194653.

[50] Vossel KA, Xu JC, Fomenko V, Miyamoto T, Suberbielle E, Knox JA, et al. Tau reduction prevents Abeta-induced axonal transport deficits by blocking activation of GSK3beta. The journal of cell biology. 2015;209(3):419-33. DOI: 10.1083/jcb.201407065.

[51] Kim TW, Tanzi RE. Presenilins and Alzheimer's disease. Current opinion in neurobiology. 1997;7(5):683–8.

[52] Guo Q, Fu W, Sopher BL, Miller MW, Ware CB, Martin GM, et al. Increased vulnerability of hippocampal neurons to excitotoxic necrosis in presenilin-1 mutant knock-in mice. Nature medicine. 1999;5(1):101–6. DOI: 10.1038/4789.

[53] Pigino G, Morfini G, Pelsman A, Mattson MP, Brady ST, Busciglio J. Alzheimer's presenilin 1 mutations impair kinesin-based axonal transport. The journal of neuroscience: the official journal of the Society for Neuroscience. 2003;23(11):4499–508.

[54] Magnani E, Fan J, Gasparini L, Golding M, Williams M, Schiavo G, et al. Interaction of tau protein with the dynactin complex. The EMBO journal. 2007;26(21):4546–54. DOI: 10.1038/sj.emboj.7601878.

[55] Allen B, Ingram E, Takao M, Smith MJ, Jakes R, Virdee K, et al. Abundant tau filaments and nonapoptotic neurodegeneration in transgenic mice expressing human P301S tau protein. The journal of neuroscience: the official journal of the society for neuroscience. 2002;22(21):9340–51.

[56] Onishi T, Matsumoto Y, Hattori M, Obayashi Y, Nakamura K, Yano T, et al. Early-onset cognitive deficits and axonal transport dysfunction in P301S mutant tau transgenic mice. Neuroscience research. 2014;80:76–85. DOI: 10.1016/j.neures.2013.12.006.

[57] Guo L, Du H, Yan S, Wu X, McKhann GM, Chen JX, et al. Cyclophilin D deficiency rescues axonal mitochondrial transport in Alzheimer's neurons. PloS one. 2013;8(1):e54914. DOI: 10.1371/journal.pone.0054914.

[58] Biasutto L, Azzolini M, Szabo I, Zoratti M. The mitochondrial permeability transition pore in AD 2016: an update. Biochimica et biophysica acta. 2016. DOI: 10.1016/j.bbamcr.2016.02.012.

[59] Chang DT, Reynolds IJ. Mitochondrial trafficking and morphology in healthy and injured neurons. Progress in neurobiology. 2006;80(5):241–68. DOI: 10.1016/j.pneurobio.2006.09.003.

[60] Engelhart MJ, Geerlings MI, Ruitenberg A, van Swieten JC, Hofman A, Witteman JC, et al. Dietary intake of antioxidants and risk of Alzheimer disease. JAMA. 2002;287(24): 3223–9.

[61] Kaduszkiewicz H, Zimmermann T, Beck-Bornholdt HP, van den Bussche H. Cholinesterase inhibitors for patients with Alzheimer's disease: systematic review of randomised clinical trials. BMJ. 2005;331(7512):321–7. DOI: 10.1136/bmj.331.7512.321.

[62] Kang JH, Ryoo NY, Shin DW, Trojanowski JQ, Shaw LM. Role of cerebrospinal fluid biomarkers in clinical trials for Alzheimer's disease modifying therapies. The Korean journal of physiology & pharmacology: official journal of the Korean physiological society and the Korean society of pharmacology. 2014;18(6):447–56. DOI: 10.4196/kjpp.2014.18.6.447.

[63] Suwa A, Nishida K, Utsunomiya K, Nonen S, Yoshimura M, Takekita Y, et al. Neuropsychological evaluation and cerebral blood flow effects of apolipoprotein E4 in

Alzheimer's disease patients after one year of treatment: an exploratory study. Dementia and geriatric cognitive disorders extra. 2015;5(3):414–23. DOI: 10.1159/000440714.

[64] Cummings J, Lai TJ, Hemrungrojn S, Mohandas E, Yun Kim S, Nair G, et al. Role of donepezil in the management of neuropsychiatric symptoms in Alzheimer's disease and dementia with Lewy bodies. CNS neuroscience & therapeutics. 2016;22(3):159–66. DOI: 10.1111/cns.12484.

[65] Kuzmickiene J, Kaubrys G. Cognitive results of CANTAB tests and their change due to the first dose of donepezil may predict treatment efficacy in Alzheimer disease. Medical science monitor: international medical journal of experimental and clinical research. 2015;21:3887–99.

[66] Kuzmickiene J, Kaubrys G. Selective ability of some CANTAB battery test measures to detect cognitive response to a single dose of donepezil in Alzheimer disease. Medical science monitor: international medical journal of experimental and clinical research. 2015;21:2572–82. DOI: 10.12659/MSM.895381.

[67] Francis PT, Palmer AM, Snape M, Wilcock GK. The cholinergic hypothesis of Alzheimer's disease: a review of progress. Journal of neurology, neurosurgery, and psychiatry. 1999;66(2):137–47.

[68] Blennow K, de Leon MJ, Zetterberg H. Alzheimer's disease. Lancet. 2006;368(9533):387–403. DOI: 10.1016/S0140-6736(06)69113-7.

[69] Danysz W, Parsons CG. Alzheimer's disease, beta-amyloid, glutamate, NMDA receptors and memantine—searching for the connections. British journal of pharmacology. 2012;167(2):324–52. DOI: 10.1111/j.1476-5381.2012.02057.x.

[70] Confaloni A, Tosto G, Tata AM. Promising therapies for Alzheimer's disease. Current pharmaceutical design. 2016;22(14):2050–2056.

[71] Nygaard HB, van Dyck CH, Strittmatter SM. Fyn kinase inhibition as a novel therapy for Alzheimer's disease. Alzheimer's research & therapy. 2014;6(1):8. DOI: 10.1186/alzrt238.

[72] Stone JG, Casadesus G, Gustaw-Rothenberg K, Siedlak SL, Wang X, Zhu X, et al. Frontiers in Alzheimer's disease therapeutics. Therapeutic advances in chronic disease. 2011;2(1):9–23. DOI: 10.1177/2040622310382817.

[73] Castellani RJ, Rolston RK, Smith MA. Alzheimer disease. Disease-a-month: DM. 2010;56(9):484–546. DOI: 10.1016/j.disamonth.2010.06.001.

[74] Wang X, Perez E, Liu R, Yan LJ, Mallet RT, Yang SH. Pyruvate protects mitochondria from oxidative stress in human neuroblastoma SK-N-SH cells. Brain research. 2007;1132(1):1–9. DOI: 10.1016/j.brainres.2006.11.032.

[75] Abdin AA, Sarhan NI. Intervention of mitochondrial dysfunction-oxidative stress-dependent apoptosis as a possible neuroprotective mechanism of alpha-lipoic acid

against rotenone-induced parkinsonism and L-dopa toxicity. Neuroscience research. 2011;71(4):387–95. DOI: 10.1016/j.neures.2011.08.008.

[76] Morais VA, Verstreken P, Roethig A, Smet J, Snellinx A, Vanbrabant M, et al. Parkinson's disease mutations in PINK1 result in decreased Complex I activity and deficient synaptic function. EMBO molecular medicine. 2009;1(2):99–111. DOI: 10.1002/emmm.200900006.

[77] Li XX, He GR, Mu X, Xu B, Tian S, Yu X, et al. Protective effects of baicalein against rotenone-induced neurotoxicity in PC12 cells and isolated rat brain mitochondria. European journal of pharmacology. 2012;674(2-3):227–33. DOI: 10.1016/j.ejphar.2011.09.181.

[78] Fernandez-Moriano C, Gonzalez-Burgos E, Gomez-Serranillos MP. Mitochondria-targeted protective compounds in Parkinson's and Alzheimer's diseases. Oxidative medicine and cellular longevity. 2015;2015:408927. DOI: 10.1155/2015/408927.

[79] Reddy PH. Role of mitochondria in neurodegenerative diseases: mitochondria as a therapeutic target in Alzheimer's disease. CNS spectrums. 2009;14(8 Suppl 7):8–13; discussion 6–8.

[80] Su B, Wang X, Zheng L, Perry G, Smith MA, Zhu X. Abnormal mitochondrial dynamics and neurodegenerative diseases. Biochimica et biophysica acta. 2010;1802(1):135–42. DOI: 10.1016/j.bbadis.2009.09.013.

[81] Zhu JY, Vereshchagina N, Sreekumar V, Burbulla LF, Costa AC, Daub KJ, et al. Knockdown of Hsc70-5/mortalin induces loss of synaptic mitochondria in a drosophila Parkinson's disease model. PloS one. 2013;8(12):e83714. DOI: 10.1371/journal.pone.0083714.

[82] Procaccio V, Bris C, Chao de la Barca JM, Oca F, Chevrollier A, Amati-Bonneau P, et al. Perspectives of drug-based neuroprotection targeting mitochondria. Revue neurologique. 2014;170(5):390–400. DOI: 10.1016/j.neurol.2014.03.005.

[83] Rappold PM, Cui M, Grima JC, Fan RZ, de Mesy-Bentley KL, Chen L, et al. Drp1 inhibition attenuates neurotoxicity and dopamine release deficits in vivo. Nature communications. 2014;5:5244. DOI: 10.1038/ncomms6244.

[84] Pritchard SM, Dolan PJ, Vitkus A, Johnson GV. The toxicity of tau in Alzheimer disease: turnover, targets and potential therapeutics. Journal of cell molecular medicine. 2011;15(8):1621–35. DOI: 10.1111/j.1582-4934.2011.01273.x.

[85] Ly CV, Verstreken P. Mitochondria at the synapse. The neuroscientist: a review journal bringing neurobiology, neurology and psychiatry. 2006;12(4):291–9. DOI: 10.1177/1073858406287661.

[86] Verstreken P, Ly CV, Venken KJ, Koh TW, Zhou Y, Bellen HJ. Synaptic mitochondria are critical for mobilization of reserve pool vesicles at drosophila neuromuscular junctions. Neuron. 2005;47(3):365–78. DOI: 10.1016/j.neuron.2005.06.018.

[87] Nakagawa T, Shimizu S, Watanabe T, Yamaguchi O, Otsu K, Yamagata H, et al. Cyclophilin D-dependent mitochondrial permeability transition regulates some necrotic but not apoptotic cell death. Nature. 2005;434(7033):652–8. DOI: 10.1038/nature03317.

[88] Calkins MJ, Manczak M, Reddy PH. Mitochondria-targeted antioxidant SS31 prevents amyloid beta-induced mitochondrial abnormalities and synaptic degeneration in Alzheimer's disease. Pharmaceuticals. 2012;5(10):1103–19. DOI: 10.3390/ph5101103.

[89] Harris H, Rubinsztein DC. Control of autophagy as a therapy for neurodegenerative disease. Nature reviews neurology. 2012;8(2):108–17. DOI: 10.1038/nrneurol.2011.200.

[90] Luo Y, Hoffer A, Hoffer B, Qi X. Mitochondria: a therapeutic target for Parkinson's disease? International journal of molecular sciences. 2015;16(9):20704–30. DOI: 10.3390/ijms160920704.

[91] Villanueva Paz M, Cotan D, Garrido-Maraver J, Cordero MD, Oropesa-Avila M, de La Mata M, et al. Targeting autophagy and mitophagy for mitochondrial diseases treatment. Expert opinion on therapeutic targets. 2016;20(4):487–500. DOI: 10.1517/14728222.2016.1101068.

[92] Jiang J, Jiang J, Zuo Y, Gu Z. Rapamycin protects the mitochondria against oxidative stress and apoptosis in a rat model of Parkinson's disease. International journal of molecular medicine. 2013;31(4):825–32. DOI: 10.3892/ijmm.2013.1280.

[93] Johri A, Calingasan NY, Hennessey TM, Sharma A, Yang L, Wille E, et al. Pharmacologic activation of mitochondrial biogenesis exerts widespread beneficial effects in a transgenic mouse model of Huntington's disease. Human molecular genetics. 2012;21(5):1124–37. DOI: 10.1093/hmg/ddr541.

[94] Quintanilla RA, Godoy JA, Alfaro I, Cabezas D, von Bernhardi R, Bronfman M, et al. Thiazolidinediones promote axonal growth through the activation of the JNK pathway. PloS one. 2013;8(5):e65140. DOI: 10.1371/journal.pone.0065140.

[95] Heneka MT, Reyes-Irisarri E, Hull M, Kummer MP. Impact and therapeutic potential of PPARs in Alzheimer's disease. Current neuropharmacology. 2011;9(4):643–50. DOI: 10.2174/157015911798376325.

[96] Perez MJ, Quintanilla RA. Therapeutic actions of the thiazolidinediones in Alzheimer's Disease. PPAR research. 2015;2015:957248. DOI: 10.1155/2015/957248.

[97] Toledo EM, Inestrosa NC. Activation of Wnt signaling by lithium and rosiglitazone reduced spatial memory impairment and neurodegeneration in brains of an APPswe/PSEN1DeltaE9 mouse model of Alzheimer's disease. Molecular psychiatry. 2010;15(3):272–85, 28. DOI: 10.1038/mp.2009.72.

[98] Baloh RH, Schmidt RE, Pestronk A, Milbrandt J. Altered axonal mitochondrial transport in the pathogenesis of Charcot-Marie-Tooth disease from mitofusin 2 mutations.

The journal of neuroscience: the official journal of the society for neuroscience. 2007;27(2):422–30. DOI: 10.1523/JNEUROSCI.4798-06.2007.

[99] Du H, Yan SS. Mitochondrial permeability transition pore in Alzheimer's disease: cyclophilin D and amyloid beta. Biochimica et biophysica acta. 2010;1802(1):198–204. DOI: 10.1016/j.bbadis.2009.07.005.

[100] Chaturvedi RK, Beal MF. Mitochondria targeted therapeutic approaches in Parkinson's and Huntington's diseases. Molecular and cellular neurosciences. 2013;55:101–14. DOI: 10.1016/j.mcn.2012.11.011.

[101] Yang Y, Jiang S, Yan J, Li Y, Xin Z, Lin Y, et al. An overview of the molecular mechanisms and novel roles of Nrf2 in neurodegenerative disorders. Cytokine growth factor Review. 2015;26(1):47–57. DOI: 10.1016/j.cytogfr.2014.09.002.

[102] Denzer I, Munch G, Friedland K. Modulation of mitochondrial dysfunction in neurodegenerative diseases via activation of nuclear factor erythroid-2-related factor 2 by food-derived compounds. Pharmacological research. 2016;103:80–94. DOI: 10.1016/j.phrs.2015.11.019.

[103] Dumont M, Kipiani K, Yu F, Wille E, Katz M, Calingasan NY, et al. Coenzyme Q10 decreases amyloid pathology and improves behavior in a transgenic mouse model of Alzheimer's disease. Journal of Alzheimer's disease: JAD. 2011;27(1):211–23. DOI: 10.3233/JAD-2011-110209.

[104] Feng Y, Wang X. Antioxidant therapies for Alzheimer's disease. Oxidative medicine and cellular longevity. 2012;2012:472932. DOI: 10.1155/2012/472932.

[105] McManus MJ, Murphy MP, Franklin JL. The mitochondria-targeted antioxidant MitoQ prevents loss of spatial memory retention and early neuropathology in a transgenic mouse model of Alzheimer's disease. The journal of neuroscience: the official journal of the society for neuroscience. 2011;31(44):15703–15. DOI: 10.1523/JNEUROSCI.0552-11.2011.

[106] Manczak M, Mao P, Calkins MJ, Cornea A, Reddy AP, Murphy MP, et al. Mitochondria-targeted antioxidants protect against amyloid-beta toxicity in Alzheimer's disease neurons. Journal of Alzheimer's disease: JAD. 2010;20 Suppl 2:S609–31. DOI: 10.3233/JAD-2010-100564.

[107] Gruber J, Stanick K, Krewenka C, Moldzio R, Patel A, Bohmdorfer S, et al. Tocopheramine succinate and tocopheryl succinate: mechanism of mitochondrial inhibition and superoxide radical production. Bioorganic & medicinal chemistry. 2014;22(2):684–91. DOI: 10.1016/j.bmc.2013.12.036.

[108] Solesio ME, Prime TA, Logan A, Murphy MP, Del Mar Arroyo-Jimenez M, Jordan J, et al. The mitochondria-targeted anti-oxidant MitoQ reduces aspects of mitochondrial fission in the 6-OHDA cell model of Parkinson's disease. Biochimica et biophysica acta. 2013;1832(1):174–82. DOI: 10.1016/j.bbadis.2012.07.009.

[109] Rao VK, Carlson EA, Yan SS. Mitochondrial permeability transition pore is a potential drug target for neurodegeneration. Biochimica et biophysica acta. 2014;1842(8):1267–72. DOI: 10.1016/j.bbadis.2013.09.003.

[110] Du H, Guo L, Zhang W, Rydzewska M, Yan S. Cyclophilin D deficiency improves mitochondrial function and learning/memory in aging Alzheimer disease mouse model. Neurobiology of aging. 2011;32(3):398–406. DOI: 10.1016/j.neurobiolaging.2009.03.003.

[111] Baines CP, Kaiser RA, Purcell NH, Blair NS, Osinska H, Hambleton MA, et al. Loss of cyclophilin D reveals a critical role for mitochondrial permeability transition in cell death. Nature. 2005;434(7033):658–62. DOI: 10.1038/nature03434.

[112] Basso M, Gelernter J, Yang J, MacAvoy MG, Varma P, Bronen RA, et al. Apolipoprotein E epsilon4 is associated with atrophy of the amygdala in Alzheimer's disease. Neurobiology of aging. 2006;27(10):1416–24. DOI: 10.1016/j.neurobiolaging.2005.08.002.

[113] Liu J, Wang Y, Zhuang Q, Chen M, Wang Y, Hou L, et al. Protective effects of cyclosporine A and hypothermia on neuronal mitochondria in a rat asphyxial cardiac arrest model. The American journal of emergency medicine. 2016;34(6):1080-5. DOI: 10.1016/j.ajem.2016.02.066.

[114] Valasani KR, Sun Q, Fang D, Zhang Z, Yu Q, Guo Y, et al. Identification of a small molecule cyclophilin D inhibitor for rescuing Abeta-mediated mitochondrial dysfunction. ACS medicinal chemistry letters. 2016;7(3):294-9. DOI: 10.1021/acsmedchemlett.5b00451.

[115] Joshi G, Gan KA, Johnson DA, Johnson JA. Increased Alzheimer's disease-like pathology in the APP/PS1DeltaE9 mouse model lacking Nrf2 through modulation of autophagy. Neurobiology of aging. 2015;36(2):664–79. DOI: 10.1016/j.neurobiolaging.2014.09.004.

[116] Ramsey CP, Glass CA, Montgomery MB, Lindl KA, Ritson GP, Chia LA, et al. Expression of Nrf2 in neurodegenerative diseases. Journal of neuropathology and experimental neurology. 2007;66(1):75–85. DOI: 10.1097/nen.0b013e31802d6da9.

[117] Kobayashi DT, Chen KS. Behavioral phenotypes of amyloid-based genetically modified mouse models of Alzheimer's disease. Genes, brain, and behavior. 2005;4(3):173–96. DOI: 10.1111/j.1601-183X.2005.00124.x.

[118] Dinkova-Kostova AT, Baird L, Holmstrom KM, Meyer CJ, Abramov AY. The spatiotemporal regulation of the Keap1-Nrf2 pathway and its importance in cellular bioenergetics. Biochemical society transactions. 2015;43(4):602–10. DOI: 10.1042/BST20150003.

[119] Kraft AD, Johnson DA, Johnson JA. Nuclear factor E2-related factor 2-dependent antioxidant response element activation by tert-butylhydroquinone and sulforaphane occurring preferentially in astrocytes conditions neurons against oxidative insult. The

journal of neuroscience: the official journal of the society for neuroscience. 2004;24(5): 1101–12. DOI: 10.1523/JNEUROSCI.3817-03.2004.

[120] Shih AY, Johnson DA, Wong G, Kraft AD, Jiang L, Erb H, et al. Coordinate regulation of glutathione biosynthesis and release by Nrf2-expressing glia potently protects neurons from oxidative stress. The journal of neuroscience: the official journal of the society for neuroscience. 2003;23(8):3394–406. DOI.

[121] Calkins MJ, Jakel RJ, Johnson DA, Chan K, Kan YW, Johnson JA. Protection from mitochondrial complex II inhibition in vitro and in vivo by Nrf2-mediated transcription. Proceedings of the national academy of sciences of the United States of America. 2005;102(1):244–9. DOI: 10.1073/pnas.0408487101.

[122] Komatsu M, Kurokawa H, Waguri S, Taguchi K, Kobayashi A, Ichimura Y, et al. The selective autophagy substrate p62 activates the stress responsive transcription factor Nrf2 through inactivation of Keap1. Nature cell biology. 2010;12(3):213–23. DOI: 10.1038/ncb2021.

[123] Alzheimer's A. 2015 Alzheimer's disease facts and figures. Alzheimer's & dementia: the journal of the Alzheimer's association. 2015;11(3):332–84.

[124] Hyman BT, Phelps CH, Beach TG, Bigio EH, Cairns NJ, Carrillo MC, et al. National Institute on Aging-Alzheimer's Association guidelines for the neuropathologic assessment of Alzheimer's disease. Alzheimer's & dementia: the journal of the Alzheimer's association. 2012;8(1):1–13. DOI: 10.1016/j.jalz.2011.10.007.

[125] Lanfranco RG, Manriquez-Navarro P, Avello LG, Canales-Johnson A. Early evaluation of Alzheimer's disease: biomarkers and neuropsychological tests. Revista medica de Chile. 2012;140(9):1191–200. DOI: 10.4067/S0034-98872012000900014.

[126] Khan TK, Alkon DL. Alzheimer's disease cerebrospinal fluid and neuroimaging biomarkers: diagnostic accuracy and relationship to drug efficacy. Journal of Alzheimer's disease : JAD. 2015;46(4):817–36. DOI: 10.3233/JAD-150238.

[127] Sancesario GM, Bernardini S. How many biomarkers to discriminate neurodegenerative dementia? Critical reviews in clinical laboratory sciences. 2015;52(6):314–26. DOI: 10.3109/10408363.2015.1051658.

[128] Khan TK, Alkon DL. Peripheral biomarkers of Alzheimer's disease. Journal of Alzheimer's disease: JAD. 2015;44(3):729–44. DOI: 10.3233/JAD-142262.

[129] Joachim CL, Mori H, Selkoe DJ. Amyloid beta-protein deposition in tissues other than brain in Alzheimer's disease. Nature. 1989;341(6239):226–30. DOI: 10.1038/341226a0.

[130] Soininen H, Syrjanen S, Heinonen O, Neittaanmaki H, Miettinen R, Paljarvi L, et al. Amyloid beta-protein deposition in skin of patients with dementia. Lancet. 1992;339(8787):245.

[131] Johnston JA, Cowburn RF, Norgren S, Wiehager B, Venizelos N, Winblad B, et al. Increased beta-amyloid release and levels of amyloid precursor protein (APP) in

fibroblast cell lines from family members with the Swedish Alzheimer's disease APP670/671 mutation. FEBS letters. 1994;354(3):274–8. DOI.

[132] Hampel H, Blennow K, Shaw LM, Hoessler YC, Zetterberg H, Trojanowski JQ. Total and phosphorylated tau protein as biological markers of Alzheimer's disease. Experimental gerontology. 2010;45(1):30–40. DOI: 10.1016/j.exger.2009.10.010.

[133] Wang T, Xiao S, Liu Y, Lin Z, Su N, Li X, et al. The efficacy of plasma biomarkers in early diagnosis of Alzheimer's disease. International journal of geriatric psychiatry. 2014;29(7):713–9. DOI: 10.1002/gps.4053.

[134] DuBoff B, Feany M, Gotz J. Why size matters—balancing mitochondrial dynamics in Alzheimer's disease. Trends in neurosciences. 2013;36(6):325–35. DOI: 10.1016/j.tins.2013.03.002.

[135] Veitinger M, Varga B, Guterres SB, Zellner M. Platelets, a reliable source for peripheral Alzheimer's disease biomarkers? Acta neuropathologica communications. 2014;2:65. DOI: 10.1186/2051-5960-2-65.

[136] Bush AI, Martins RN, Rumble B, Moir R, Fuller S, Milward E, et al. The amyloid precursor protein of Alzheimer's disease is released by human platelets. The journal of biological chemistry. 1990;265(26):15977–83.

[137] Neumann PJ, Araki SS, Arcelus A, Longo A, Papadopoulos G, Kosik KS, et al. Measuring Alzheimer's disease progression with transition probabilities: estimates from CERAD. Neurology. 2001;57(6):957–64.

[138] Mukaetova-Ladinska EB, Andras A, Milne J, Abdel-All Z, Borr I, Jaros E, et al. Synaptic proteins and choline acetyltransferase loss in visual cortex in dementia with Lewy bodies. Journal of neuropathology and experimental neurology. 2013;72(1):53–60. DOI: 10.1097/NEN.0b013e31827c5710.

[139] Forlenza OV, Torres CA, Talib LL, de Paula VJ, Joaquim HP, Diniz BS, et al. Increased platelet GSK3B activity in patients with mild cognitive impairment and Alzheimer's disease. Journal of psychiatric research. 2011;45(2):220–4. DOI: 10.1016/j.jpsychires.2010.06.002.

[140] Trimmer PA, Swerdlow RH, Parks JK, Keeney P, Bennett JP, Jr., Miller SW, et al. Abnormal mitochondrial morphology in sporadic Parkinson's and Alzheimer's disease cybrid cell lines. Experimental neurology. 2000;162(1):37–50. DOI: 10.1006/exnr.2000.7333.

[141] Wang S, Song J, Tan M, Albers KM, Jia J. Mitochondrial fission proteins in peripheral blood lymphocytes are potential biomarkers for Alzheimer's disease. European journal of neurology. 2012;19(7):1015–22. DOI: 10.1111/j.1468-1331.2012.03670.x.

[142] Dreses-Werringloer U, Lambert JC, Vingtdeux V, Zhao H, Vais H, Siebert A, et al. A polymorphism in CALHM1 influences Ca^{2+} homeostasis, Abeta levels, and Alzheimer's disease risk. Cell. 2008;133(7):1149–61. DOI: 10.1016/j.cell.2008.05.048.

[143] Zoumakis E, Kalantaridou SN, Chrousos GP. The "brain-skin connection": nerve growth factor-dependent pathways for stress-induced skin disorders. Journal of molecular medicine. 2007;85(12):1347–9. DOI: 10.1007/s00109-007-0270-6.

[144] Kalman S, Garbett KA, Janka Z, Mirnics K. Human dermal fibroblasts in psychiatry research. Neuroscience. 2016;320:105–21. DOI: 10.1016/j.neuroscience.2016.01.067.

[145] Mangialasche F, Polidori MC, Monastero R, Ercolani S, Camarda C, Cecchetti R, et al. Biomarkers of oxidative and nitrosative damage in Alzheimer's disease and mild cognitive impairment. Ageing research reviews. 2009;8(4):285–305. DOI: 10.1016/j.arr.2009.04.002.

[146] Butterfield DA, Perluigi M, Sultana R. Oxidative stress in Alzheimer's disease brain: new insights from redox proteomics. European journal of pharmacology. 2006;545(1):39–50. DOI: 10.1016/j.ejphar.2006.06.026.

[147] Mecocci P, MacGarvey U, Beal MF. Oxidative damage to mitochondrial DNA is increased in Alzheimer's disease. Annals of neurology. 1994;36(5):747–51. DOI: 10.1002/ana.410360510.

[148] Cervellati C, Wood PL, Romani A, Valacchi G, Squerzanti M, Sanz JM, et al. Oxidative challenge in Alzheimer's disease: state of knowledge and future needs. Journal of investigative medicine: the official publication of the American federation for clinical research. 2016;64(1):21–32. DOI: 10.1136/jim-2015-000017.

[149] Lunnon K, Ibrahim Z, Proitsi P, Lourdusamy A, Newhouse S, Sattlecker M, et al. Mitochondrial dysfunction and immune activation are detectable in early Alzheimer's disease blood. Journal of Alzheimer's disease: JAD. 2012;30(3):685–710. DOI: 10.3233/JAD-2012-111592.

[150] Lee TS, Goh L, Chong MS, Chua SM, Chen GB, Feng L, et al. Downregulation of TOMM40 expression in the blood of Alzheimer disease subjects compared with matched controls. Journal of psychiatric research. 2012;46(6):828–30. DOI: 10.1016/j.jpsychires.2012.03.006.

[151] Mota SI, Costa RO, Ferreira IL, Santana I, Caldeira GL, Padovano C, et al. Oxidative stress involving changes in Nrf2 and ER stress in early stages of Alzheimer's disease. Biochimica et biophysica acta. 2015;1852(7):1428–41. DOI: 10.1016/j.bbadis.2015.03.015.

[152] Vignini A, Nanetti L, Moroni C, Tanase L, Bartolini M, Luzzi S, et al. Modifications of platelet from Alzheimer disease patients: a possible relation between membrane properties and NO metabolites. Neurobiology of aging. 2007;28(7):987–94. DOI: 10.1016/j.neurobiolaging.2006.05.010.

[153] Vignini A, Morganti S, Salvolini E, Sartini D, Luzzi S, Fiorini R, et al. Amyloid precursor protein expression is enhanced in human platelets from subjects with Alzheimer's disease and Frontotemporal lobar degeneration: A real-time PCR study. Experimental gerontology. 2013. DOI: 10.1016/j.exger.2013.10.008.

[154] Cardoso SM, Proenca MT, Santos S, Santana I, Oliveira CR. Cytochrome c oxidase is decreased in Alzheimer's disease platelets. Neurobiology of aging. 2004;25(1):105–10.

[155] Bosetti F, Brizzi F, Barogi S, Mancuso M, Siciliano G, Tendi EA, et al. Cytochrome c oxidase and mitochondrial F1F0-ATPase (ATP synthase) activities in platelets and brain from patients with Alzheimer's disease. Neurobiology of aging. 2002;23(3):371–6.

[156] Mancuso M, Filosto M, Bosetti F, Ceravolo R, Rocchi A, Tognoni G, et al. Decreased platelet cytochrome c oxidase activity is accompanied by increased blood lactate concentration during exercise in patients with Alzheimer disease. Experimental neurology. 2003;182(2):421–6.

[157] Parker WD, Jr., Filley CM, Parks JK. Cytochrome oxidase deficiency in Alzheimer's disease. Neurology. 1990;40(8):1302–3.

[158] Valla J, Schneider L, Niedzielko T, Coon KD, Caselli R, Sabbagh MN, et al. Impaired platelet mitochondrial activity in Alzheimer's disease and mild cognitive impairment. Mitochondrion. 2006;6(6):323-30. DOI: 10.1016/j.mito.2006.10.004.

[159] Mosconi L, de Leon M, Murray J, E L, Lu J, Javier E, et al. Reduced mitochondria cytochrome oxidase activity in adult children of mothers with Alzheimer's disease. Journal of Alzheimer's disease : JAD. 2011;27(3):483–90. DOI: 10.3233/JAD-2011-110866.

[160] Sultana R, Mecocci P, Mangialasche F, Cecchetti R, Baglioni M, Butterfield DA. Increased protein and lipid oxidative damage in mitochondria isolated from lymphocytes from patients with Alzheimer's disease: insights into the role of oxidative stress in Alzheimer's disease and initial investigations into a potential biomarker for this dementing disorder. Journal of Alzheimer's disease : JAD. 2011;24(1):77–84. DOI: 10.3233/JAD-2011-101425.

[161] Maynard S, Hejl AM, Dinh TS, Keijzers G, Hansen AM, Desler C, et al. Defective mitochondrial respiration, altered dNTP pools and reduced AP endonuclease 1 activity in peripheral blood mononuclear cells of Alzheimer's disease patients. Aging. 2015;7(10):793–815.

[162] Ponce DP, Salech F, SanMartin CD, Silva M, Xiong C, Roe CM, et al. Increased susceptibility to oxidative death of lymphocytes from Alzheimer patients correlates with dementia severity. Current Alzheimer research. 2014;11(9):892–8.

[163] Behrens MI, Silva M, Salech F, Ponce DP, Merino D, Sinning M, et al. Inverse susceptibility to oxidative death of lymphocytes obtained from Alzheimer's patients and skin cancer survivors: increased apoptosis in Alzheimer's and reduced necrosis in cancer. The journals of gerontology series A, biological sciences and medical sciences. 2012;67(10):1036–40. DOI: 10.1093/gerona/glr258.

[164] Sultana R, Baglioni M, Cecchetti R, Cai J, Klein JB, Bastiani P, et al. Lymphocyte mitochondria: toward identification of peripheral biomarkers in the progression of

Alzheimer disease. Free radical biology & medicine. 2013;65:595–606. DOI: 10.1016/j.freeradbiomed.2013.08.001.

[165] Gray NE, Quinn JF. Alterations in mitochondrial number and function in Alzheimer's disease fibroblasts. Metabolic brain disease. 2015;30(5):1275–8. DOI: 10.1007/s11011-015-9667-z.

[166] Gibson G, Martins R, Blass J, Gandy S. Altered oxidation and signal transduction systems in fibroblasts from Alzheimer patients. Life sciences. 1996;59(5-6):477–89.

[167] Naderi J, Lopez C, Pandey S. Chronically increased oxidative stress in fibroblasts from Alzheimer's disease patients causes early senescence and renders resistance to apoptosis by oxidative stress. Mechanisms of ageing and development. 2006;127(1):25–35. DOI: 10.1016/j.mad.2005.08.006.

[168] Moreira PI, Harris PL, Zhu X, Santos MS, Oliveira CR, Smith MA, et al. Lipoic acid and N-acetyl cysteine decrease mitochondrial-related oxidative stress in Alzheimer disease patient fibroblasts. Journal of Alzheimer's disease : JAD. 2007;12(2):195–206.

[169] Cecchi C, Fiorillo C, Sorbi S, Latorraca S, Nacmias B, Bagnoli S, et al. Oxidative stress and reduced antioxidant defenses in peripheral cells from familial Alzheimer's patients. Free radical biology & medicine. 2002;33(10):1372–9.

[170] Richardson JS, Subbarao KV, Ang LC. On the possible role of iron-induced free radical peroxidation in neural degeneration in Alzheimer's disease. Annals of the New York academy of sciences. 1992;648:326–7.

[171] Ito E, Oka K, Etcheberrigaray R, Nelson TJ, McPhie DL, Tofel-Grehl B, et al. Internal Ca2+ mobilization is altered in fibroblasts from patients with Alzheimer disease. Proceedings of the national academy of sciences of the United States of America. 1994;91(2):534–8.

[172] Area-Gomez E, Del Carmen Lara Castillo M, Tambini MD, Guardia-Laguarta C, de Groof AJ, Madra M, et al. Upregulated function of mitochondria-associated ER membranes in Alzheimer disease. The EMBO journal. 2012;31(21):4106–23. DOI: 10.1038/emboj.2012.202.

[173] Hedskog L, Pinho CM, Filadi R, Ronnback A, Hertwig L, Wiehager B, et al. Modulation of the endoplasmic reticulum-mitochondria interface in Alzheimer's disease and related models. Proceedings of the national academy of sciences of the United States of America. 2013;110(19):7916–21. DOI: 10.1073/pnas.1300677110.

[174] Hossini AM, Megges M, Prigione A, Lichtner B, Toliat MR, Wruck W, et al. Induced pluripotent stem cell-derived neuronal cells from a sporadic Alzheimer's disease donor as a model for investigating AD-associated gene regulatory networks. BMC genomics. 2015;16:84. DOI: 10.1186/s12864-015-1262-5.

Chapter 15

The Impact of the Eye in Dementia: The Eye and its Role in Diagnosis and Follow-up

Elena Salobrar-García, Ana I. Ramírez, Rosa de Hoz,
Pilar Rojas, Juan J. Salazar, Blanca Rojas,
Raquel Yubero, Pedro Gil, Alberto Triviño and
José M. Ramírez

Additional information is available at the end of the chapter

http://dx.doi.org/10.5772/64490

Abstract

Over the last few decades, the importance of ophthalmic examination in neurodegenerative diseases of the CNS has reportedly increased. The retina is an extension of the CNS and thus should not be surprising to find abnormal results in both the test exploring visual processing and those examining the retina of patients with CNS degeneration. Current in vivo imaging techniques are allowing ophthalmologists to detect and quantify data consistent with the histopathological findings described in the retinas of Alzheimer's disease (AD) patients and may help to reveal unsuspected retinal and optic-nerve repercussions of other CNS diseases. In this chapter, we perform an analysis of the physiological changes in ocular and cerebral ageing. We analyse the ocular manifestations in CNS disorders such as stroke, AD and Parkinson's disease. In addition, the pathophysiology of both the eye and the visual pathway in AD are described. The value of the visual psychophysical tests in AD diagnosis is reviewed as well as the main findings of the optical coherence tomography as a contribution to the diagnosis and monitoring of the disease. Finally, we examine the association of two neurodegenerative diseases, AD and glaucoma, as mere coincidence or possible role in the progression of the neurodegeneration.

Keywords: neurodegenerative disease, Alzheimer, optical coherence tomography, contrast sensitivity test

1. Introduction

The eye is a special sensory organ, as the retina is an extension of the brain. Both brain and retina derive from the neural tube and consist of neurons and glial cells. As with the CNS, any insult to the retina and optic nerve cause anterograde and retrograde axon degeneration, myelin destruction, and scar formation. Chronic progressive retinal neurodegeneration is involved in the pathophysiology of ocular diseases [1] such as glaucoma, age-related macular degeneration (ARMD) and diabetic retinopathy (DR).

In the brain, neurodegeneration is a key event in disorders such as Parkinson's disease (PD) and Alzheimer's disease (AD). PD is a neurodegenerative disease of middle and old age; the origin of defect lies in the basal ganglia and it is characterised by deficiency of dopamine in the mid-brain area.

AD, the most common cause of dementia, afflicts 67 in 1000 people over the age of 65 and more than 26 million people worldwide, its prevalence and incidence increasing exponentially with age [2, 3]. In 2006, the worldwide prevalence of Alzheimer's was 26.6 million, and by 2050, the prevalence is expected to quadruple [3]. A chronic progressive degenerative neurological disorder affecting cognition and memory [4], AD is characterised by the formation of extracellular amyloid beta (Aβ) plaques and intracellular neurofibrillary tangles (made of hyperphosphorylated tau), primarily in the cerebral cortex [5, 6]. Currently, there is no definitive antemortem diagnosis for AD, and therefore new biomarkers for diagnosis are needed. It can be argued that improved methods of screening and early detection are essential to identify patients without cognitive impairment but with a high risk of developing AD. Thus, protocols for early treatment could be established to help slow the disease progression [7]. Over the last few decades, the importance of ophthalmic examination in neurodegenerative diseases of the CNS has reportedly increased. As mentioned above, the retina is an extension of the CNS and thus the impairment of ocular function in patients with CNS degeneration should not be surprising. In fact, both the test exploring visual processing/visual pathways and those examining the retina of such patients display abnormal results. Current in vivo imaging techniques are allowing ophthalmologists to detect and quantify data consistent with the histopathological findings described in the retinas of AD patients years ago [8] and may help to reveal unsuspected retinal and optic-nerve repercussions of other CNS diseases. Specifically, over the last decades, accurate tools for analysing the eye fundus such as optical coherence tomography (OCT) and laser polarimetry have been developed, opening new ways of examining the retina in vivo. The retinal nerve-fibre layer (RNFL) is composed of retinal ganglion-cell axons, which form the optic nerve. Decreased thickness of the RNFL can reflect retinal neuronal ganglion-cell death and axonal loss in the optic nerve [9, 10], and RNFL reportedly thins with ageing [11, 12]. Notably, some studies have shown that AD patients show greater RNFL thinning than is normal for their age [9, 10, 13–20]. In this context, Hinton et al. [8] were the first to show histopathological evidence of retinal ganglion-cell loss and optic-nerve degeneration in AD patients. These findings were later confirmed in several follow-up studies [21–24]. Indeed, axonal degeneration of the large M-cells in AD has been documented [22, 25, 26]. Nevertheless, other histopathological studies [27–33] have failed to confirm these findings, suggesting that methodological differences were responsible for the different results. In addition to the anatomical findings in AD, this disease can exert an impact on most aspects of visual processing, such as visual-field abnormalities [34–36], colour-perception deficits [37–40], pattern electroretinogram changes [26, 41, 42] and reduced contrast sensitivity (CS) [43–46]. Psychophysical investigations of CS in AD patients have demonstrated results consistent with the neuropathological evidence [47]. However, studies of CS in patients with AD have reported no AD-related deficits in spatial CS [48, 49], while others have found deficits at all spatial frequencies tested [40, 50].

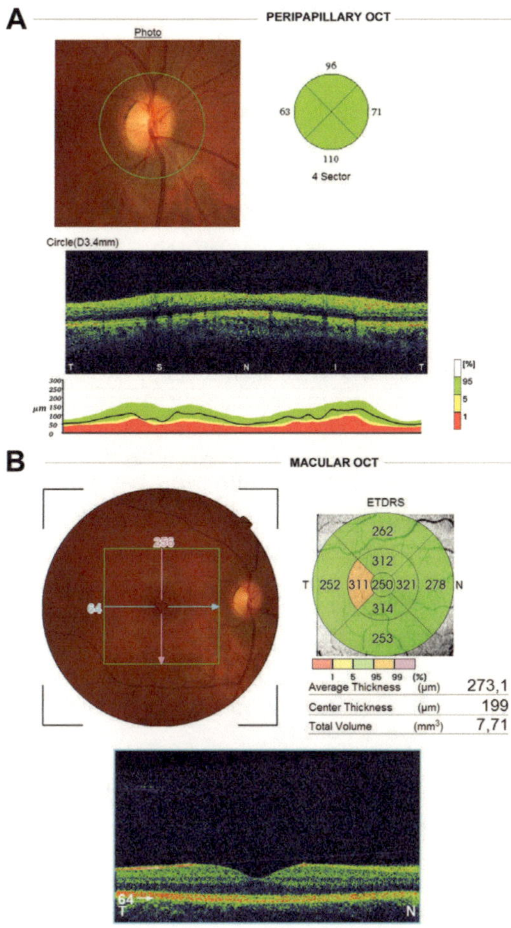

Figure 1. Retinal nerve fibre layer (RNFL) thickness analysis. Optical coherence tomography (OCT) study. (**A**) Peripapillary OCT. Upper left: peripapillary retinography with a green circle marking the retinal tissue considered for analysis. Upper right: diagram of the peripapillary quadrants analysed: temporal quadrant (316–45), superior quadrant (46–135), nasal quadrant (136–225), inferior quadrant (226–315). Bottom: retinal b-scan and diagram of thickness normality. (**B**) Macular OCT. Upper left: central retinography with a green square marking the retinal tissue considered for analysis. Upper right: diagram showing the concentric rings and quadrants considered for analysis of the macular RNFL thickness and measurements automatically provided by the analyser. Bottom: retinal b-scan of the macula. ETDRS: Early Treatment Diabetic Retinopathy Study (from Figure 1 of [19] with permission).

Diagnosis and follow-up of AD, especially the early-onset cases, become difficult, due to imprecise neuropsychological testing, sophisticated but expensive neuroimaging techniques, and invasive sampling of cerebrospinal fluid [31, 32]. OCT is a reliable noninvasive technique, routinely used in ophthalmology to visualise and quantify the layers of the retina. This technique enables quantitative cross-sectional imaging of the RNFL and macular volume. As a measure of neuronal degeneration, changes in longitudinal OCT measurements of the RNFL can act as a surrogate marker of axonal health. Thus, OCT could become an invaluable tool for measuring axonal loss, as a biomarker, in different neurological conditions [33, 51–61] (**Figure 1**).

In a review of a meta-analysis which investigates the role of OCT in detecting RNFL thinning in AD patients, it was found that the OCT is a well-suited paraclinical methodology to assess RNFL thickness in both AD and mild cognitive impairment (MCI) disorders [19]. Macular studies in AD using OCT have recently reported that mild AD patients with a high average score (23.3 ± 3.1) on the Mini-Mental State Examination (MMSE) had significantly reduced macular nerve-fibre-layer thickness with or without significant peripapillary involvement [19, 40, 62, 63]. OCT thus offers the clinician a fast, reliable, reproducible, noninvasive method to evaluate and monitor several neurological diseases [64].

2. Search strategy and selection criteria

A literature search was performed up to April 2016 using the MEDLINE database, PubMed and Google Scholar search services with the following key words and word combinations: dementia, Alzheimer's disease, ageing, vision, eye, physiopathology, visual pathway, visual psychophysical test, optical coherence tomography, glaucoma.

After filtering by author criteria, English or Spanish language, and the condition that they all addressed dementia and vision as the main theme, 325 articles were included after a full text review. All the abstracts were then carefully divided into subcategories covering topics including ageing and vision, visual pathway, physiopathology, visual psychophysical test, Alzheimer's and glaucoma.

This review covers systematic reviews, original articles and letters to the editor. We did not contact other authors for further articles inclusion.

3. Ageing and vision

The term 'ageing' refers to the process of morphofunctional changes that organisms experience as time goes by. That process can be analysed from two main perspectives. On the one hand, there is the view that takes into account the physiological changes that happen to any individual, regardless of life experiences. On the other hand, there is the perspective referring to pathological changes, unique in each individual and related to alterations on the organic balance [65]. The eye is not an exception to this process, and indeed the eye is one of the organs most affected by ageing.

3.1. Theories on ageing

Many theories and classifications have been proposed to explain human ageing, although a combination of several of them may explain the process. In 2013, in a review called 'The hallmarks of ageing' [66], the current theories were widely discussed and nine fundamental traits of ageing were described: genomic instability, telomere shortening, epigenetic changes, loss of proteostasis, deregulation of the detection of nutrients, mitochondrial dysfunction, cell ageing, depletion of stem cells, and altered intercellular communication. Additionally, it is clear that there are other environmental and behavioural factors that can contribute to this degradation process, such as, for instance, smoking and regular exposure to UV light.

3.2. The ageing eye

As the eye ages, some morphological, structural, and functional changes take place in both the eye itself and other extraocular structures. This process is generically referred to as 'eye ageing'.

3.2.1. Structural changes in the ageing eye

In the orbit and the adjacent tissue, there is a reduction of the adipose tissue with relative preservation of the nasal fat pad [67]. This generates eyeball sinking (enophthalmos).

The eyelids progressively lose their elastic properties, with an increase in palpebral skin laxity [68].

In the lacrimal gland, there is a proliferation of connective tissue and an atrophy of glandular elements resulting in a decrease in lacrimal tear production [69]. The lacrimal pathology in elderly patients involves different situations ranging from 'dry eye' to profuse lacrimation or epiphora. The result is an alteration in the lacrimal film with its corresponding discomfort and decline in visual acuity (VA).

The conjunctiva undergoes a decrease in density of dendritic cells due to ageing, as well as the degeneration of the subepithelial structures. There is an increase in conjunctival microcysts, indicating that the Goblet cell function is failing, since it has been demonstrated that the Goblet cell population does not decrease in number [70].

The ageing sclera shows hyaline plaques, fat deposits, and loss of aqueous content, hence provoking biomechanical changes due to greater rigidity [71, 72].

Refractively, the ageing cornea suffers a change in keratometry resulting in against-the-rule astigmatism. Ageing results in corneal degeneration with a progressive deposit of lipid material that provokes gerontoxon or arcus senilis. Some calcifications appear in the Bowman's membrane periphery while Descemet's membrane thickens. The cornea becomes more rigid and edematous, with a tendency to opacity, causing a sensitivity loss [72, 73]. There is also a reduction in the number of corneal endothelial cells, and hence the development of Fuchs endothelial dystrophy is common. This endothelial loss provokes a dysregulation in corneal homeostasis, which diminishes VA and even leads to blindness [72, 74].

The trabecular meshwork alters its shape due to the ageing process, changing from a wedge-shaped structure into a more rhomboidal one [72, 75]. The trabeculae thicken and an ultra-structural examination shows a change in the appearance of the extracellular materials [75]. There is a lower number of endothelial trabecular cells as well as of giant vacuoles and intracellular pores in Schelmm's canal [72]. Gonioscopy shows an increase in the trabecular meshwork pigmentation. All of these factors could result in greater resistance to the aqueous outflow, which may favour the onset of glaucoma [76].

The pupil tends to become smaller and the iris is less reactive. There are also more difficulties in terms of pharmacologic dilation of the pupil. Iris pigment is lost with ageing, resulting in iris transillumination in the slit-lamp examination, especially in the pupillary margin.

The changes in size and tone of the ciliary body, together with the loss of elasticity of the lens capsule and a packing in its fibres, weaken accommodative capacity, causing presbyopia [77].

With age, the lens tends to absorb more blue light (410 nm) due to the accumulation of yellow pigment caused by the oxidation of lens proteins [72]. This is called 'blue blindness' in the cataractogenic processes.

Clinical data from studies on the choroid, using OCT, show an inverse correlation between age and choroid volume [78]. Some histopathological studies have shown a negative correlation between age and choriocapillaris density [79]. Bruch's membrane is the structure that presents the most changes due to ageing, becoming thicker, with changes in the elastic fibres (calcification among others) and collagen [72]. The major proportion of thickening appears to be due to the deposits of lipids [80] and fibrillar and amorphous material [81]. The basal laminar deposits, material that accumulates between the Bruch's membrane and the retinal pigment epithelium (RPE), are located mainly in the macular area and occasionally appear as drusen [76, 82]. The aforementioned changes in Bruch's membrane lead to the appearance of waste accumulation in the overlying retina. The retinal pigment epithelium, which is vital for the integrity of the rods and cones, shows greater pleomorphism, a lower number of epithelial cells in the posterior pole, a loss of melanin content, an increase in lipofuscin, and a reduction of the cytoplasmic volume [72, 76, 82]. With age, photoreceptor density reduces in the retina [86]. An age-related loss of rods in the macula occurs with a decline in scotopic sensitivity [72]. In the astroglial plexus of the ganglion-cell layer and RNFL, the number of astrocytes significantly drops. These cells show stronger GFAP immunoreactivity, more cytoplasmic organelles, glial filaments and lipofuscin deposits [82]. As a result of the ageing process, the retinal-blood flow diminishes and macular microcirculation diminishes by an estimated 20% [83]. The number of retinal capillaries around the fovea falls and arteriosclerotic changes occur in retinal vessels [72].

In the optic nerve (ON), the number of ON axons reportedly declines [72, 84]. The connective tissue within the fibrovascular pial septae becomes more abundant. As a result, the exchange of nutrients between the capillaries and the nerve fibres is impaired [72]. With ageing, Corpora amylacea may be seen in the ON, appearing as accumulations of intracellular organelles (neurotubules, dense bodies, and mitochondria) in the axons [72].

In the vitreous humour, changes appear in the components of the collagen fibres and hyaluronic acid, causing vitreous floaters [85]. As a result of ageing, the vitreous attachment to the retina weakens, provoking posterior vitreous detachment. This may trigger a contraction at its base, leading to traction on the peripheral retina, which may result in retinal tears [72].

3.2.2. Functional changes in the ageing eye

Normal ageing implies changes in the functionality of the visual system, since there is less light transmission and scattering inside the eye. Also efficiency in phototransduction and photopigment regeneration declines. The quality of transmission and its synaptic processing in the retina and in the entire visual pathway diminishes [86]. Due to all these changes, vision is affected in different ways. The elderly population experiences significant refractive changes with age. Usually, a change of against-the-rule astigmatism takes place as a result of corneal flattening. Moreover, the spherical component becomes more hyperopic due to sclera rigidity, senile myosis and changes in the ageing lens, the latter resulting in a loss of the refractive capacity. The prevalence of oblique astigmatism and anisometropia also increase with age [87].

Visual acuity (VA) worsens with age for many reasons, the standard being a vision of 0.8. Regarding the ageing process, this reduction in near VA may be due to presbyopia or physiological loss of accommodation because of ciliary muscle-tone loss. Likewise, the changes in the lens can cause alterations in VA: late-onset myopia can appear, owing to the rigidity in the lens nucleus that is related to the senile cataract; also, early nuclear sclerosis can cause eye glare.

Contrast sensitivity (CS) undergoes small changes starting in childhood up until the age of 65. After that, the decline is more pronounced, especially in medium and high spatial frequencies. This decline in CS is due partially to the opacity in the media of the eye, which decreases depth perception [87, 88].

With age, the normal visual field (VF) is impaired due to a retraction. The blind spot size enlarges. Additionally, the reduction in the number of cones in the fovea causes a general decline in colour vision [76].

Old people experience trouble with light and dark adaptation and they are incapable of tolerating glare [76].

There are also age-related binocular problems that affect the neuromuscular mechanisms and the structures of the tissues adjacent to the eye. Patients suffer from accommodation-convergence problems and thus, they show greater exophoria in near vision. Vertical deviations and poor stereopsis are very frequent with ageing [89].

3.3. Brain ageing

The nervous system is particularly vulnerable to ageing due to the main cellular elements of this tissue are post-mitotic cells and thus their regeneration capacity is limited.

Age-related worsening of cognitive functions occurs both in humans and in animals. This is especially true for the functions related to executive capacities, attention processes, and the learning and storage of new information. Also, the senescent brain is capable of using functional strategies to compensate for functional and/or structural deficiencies. This brain plasticity observed in senescence can decrease or mask the clinical expression of brain ageing [90].

3.3.1. Structural changes in the brain

Research conducted a few years ago on anatomical brain changes seems to demonstrate a clear reduction in brain volume due to neuronal death [91]. The greatest part of this volume loss is the reduction of synaptic density [92] and volume of white matter in the frontal lobes [93]. Even so, the most recent studies indicate that age-related changes do not affect the brain globally. On the contrary, these changes would be highly limited to the dorsolateral prefrontal cortex and, to a lesser extent, to some subdivisions within the medial temporal lobe, such as the subiculum and the dentate gyrus [94]. It is believed that the age-related drop in cognitive skills is the consequence of a selective alteration in the corticocortical pathways that connect the temporal and frontal association areas to the corticostriatal pathways [93, 94].

Age-related microscopic changes include regional brain atrophy [93], axonal cortical dystrophy [95], lipofuscin accumulation [96], astrogliosis [91], neurofibrillary degeneration, senile plaques [97, 98] and scattered vascular or dystrophic focal changes in the white matter [99]. Many of these changes cannot be regarded as being specific to ageing. For instance, most cases of cortical atrophy could indicate an underlying degenerative brain [100] or vascular [101] disease. Changes in the periventricular white matter (leukoaraiosis or subcortical leukoencephalopathy) occur in patients with vascular risk factors, reflecting an insufficiency of the deep vessels of the brain secondary to a hypertensive, diabetic or multifactorial degenerative arteriopathy [102]. Perhaps the only brain change attributable to the passage of time is lipofuscin accumulation; this indicates oxidative stress and lipid peroxidation [96], as well as local synaptic loss [93, 94].

The vascular volume in the brain decreases, specifically the surface of the capillaries [103]. The blood-brain barrier is selective place for the exchange of nutrients between the blood and the brain parenchyma. With ageing, the molecular transport systems operating at this level are reduced. This has some metabolic consequences for the normal functioning of the nervous system [104].

One of the least known aspects in the ageing process is the role of the brain glial cells [105]. The glia is a group of CNS cells whose main function is to maintain the homeostasis of the neural environment (astrocytes), immunosurveillance (microglia) and the formation of myelin (oligodendrocytes).

It has been demonstrated that, in the ageing brain of experimental animals as well as humans, there is a proliferation of astrocytes which is called reactive gliosis. Its purpose is to mitigate the effects of the physiological age-related neuronal degeneration [106].

3.3.2. Cognitive functional changes

Age-related neuromorphological changes trigger cognitive alterations. Cognition is the set of brain activities that enable humans to be aware of themselves, of the others, and of the environment [107]. One of the most important features of cognitive ageing is memory loss. Learning and memory have their neurobiological origin in the hippocampus. The hippocampus is composed of a series of cell populations that establish certain very precise and well-organised synaptic pathways. The information received is processed and sent to the brain cortex for storage and for use in the long-term memory [108, 109]. Learning processes are based on neuroplasticity, whose neurophysiological basis is long-term potentiation. This is achieved by a proliferation of AMPA glutamate receptors as well as an increase in dendritic spine density in hippocampal postsynaptic neurons [110]. During the ageing process, a reduction may occur in the neural capacity to synthesise neurotransmitters involved in synapses [111]. The most common neurotransmitters are glutamate, GABA, acetylcholine and dopamine. Changes in the homeostatic levels of these neurotransmitters cause different pathologies that are accentuated during ageing [112]. For instance, the lowering of acetylcholine levels is one of the most striking features of AD [113].

4. The eye as an extension of the central nervous system

Given that the eye is an extension of the CNS, evidence is being sought to determine whether the retina is a window to the brain and whether eye research could improve our understanding of CNS disorders [114]. The retina is made up of specialised neuron layers that are interconnected via synapses. The light that enters the eye is captured by the photoreceptor cells in the outer retina, initiating a cascade of neural signals that finally reach the retinal ganglion cells (RGCs), whose axons form the ON. These axons project to the lateral geniculate nucleus (LGN) in the thalamus and to the superior colliculus (SC) in the midbrain, whose information is then transmitted to more specialised visual processing centres that provide a perception of the world [114, 115].

Most of the RGC axons come together to form the ON. After passing through the lamina cribrosa of the eye the ON is covered by a myelin sheath produced by the oligodendrocytes and surrounded by the three meningeal layers. As in the CNS, ON injury may result in anterograde and retrograde degeneration of the damaged axons, scarring, myelin destruction and creation of a neurotoxic environment involving oxidative stress, deprivation of neurotrophic factors, raised levels of excitotoxic neurotransmitters and abnormal aggregation of proteins and waste products. Such a hostile environment often provokes the death of the initially undamaged neighbouring neurons in a process called secondary degeneration [116–121].

Axonal regeneration after injury is limited both in the CNS and ON. In fact, most of our knowledge on axonal response to traumatic brain injury stems from studies of the ON [122–128]. The factors responsible for creating an environment that is non-permissive for axonal growth are the same by CNS and ON. The first discoveries of CNS axon regeneration in the presence of peripheral nerve grafts were performed in experimental models of ON transection and of spinal-cord injury [122, 123, 129]. We should underline that there are similar restrictive growth conditions in these two structures of the nervous system.

The eye, and especially the retina as a part of the CNS, must maintain regulated interactions with the immune system. In fact, the retina occupies a special immune site. The eyeball is made up of some unique physical structures and contains a set of surface molecules and cytokines responsible of some specialised immune responses, similar to those observed in the brain and the spinal cord [130, 131]. The eye possesses the blood-retinal barrier, whose structure, characteristics and mechanisms are similar to those of the blood-brain barrier. The anterior chamber of the eye contains the aqueous humour, a fluid with anti-inflammatory and immunoregulatory mediators. This fluid resembles the cerebrospinal fluid circulating around the brain and the spinal cord parenchyma [132, 133]. Besides the similarities with the CNS, the ocular immunoprivilege involves a unique phenomenon called 'anterior chamber associated immune deviation' (ACAID), wherein the antigen-presenting cells entering the anterior chamber capture the antigen and then migrate to the spleen. There the effector leukocytes become regulatory leukocytes. This process establishes a tightly regulated immune response towards ocular antigens [130]. The combination of the aforementioned mechanisms allows the eye to benefit from the immune defence machinery that would eliminate the risk of tissue damage due to uncontrolled inflammation [114].

4.1. Visual pathway

The visual information collected by the photoreceptors (rods, sensitive to contrast; and cones, sensitive to colour) goes through the inner plexiform layer of the retina (bipolar, horizontal and amacrine cells) to the RGC layer (midget, parasol and bistratified cells) [134]. The layout of these three different RGC types forms different receptive fields, which help in segregating and coding visual information [135]. Then, the RGC are projected through different pathways (parvocellular (P), magnocellular (M) and koniocellular (K)) to the sub-cortical region of the LGN and to the V1 cortical area [135–137]. The P-pathway receives colour and shape information from the midget cells. The K-pathway receives some blue-on/yellow-off opponent colour information from the bistratified cells. Finally, the M-pathway carries the luminance and motion data from the parasol cells. Thus, the visual information segregated in the V1 region is projected into the V2 region for processing [135, 138, 139]. The information about colour, orientation and spatial frequency continues ventrally through V2 and V4. This route continues to the infero-temporal cortex, where more-complex aspects of the visual processing of objects are carried out, such as face perception. Motion and location follow the dorsal pathway through V2 and V3. The V3 dorsal area seems to be specialised in the detection of global motion [140, 141]. The V5 is specialised in local movement [142]. The dorsal pathway continues to the posterior parietal cortex, where the complex aspects of spatial perception, e.g. details within a scene as an integrated perception are processed [141].

4.2. Ocular manifestations of CNS disorders

As mentioned above, the eye is an extension of the brain, and therefore it seems reasonable to look for some ocular manifestations of brain pathologies. In fact, in patients with CNS pathologies such as EP, multiple sclerosis (MS), amyotrophic lateral sclerosis, and AD, ophthalmological changes have been observed. Notably, many of these changes are not exclusive to a certain disease, highlighting the relationship between the retina and the brain. Likewise, in many of these CNS disorders the ocular symptoms precede the cerebral symptoms. Therefore, eye examinations could help in the early diagnosis of these CNS diseases.

4.2.1. Stroke

Prospective studies have shown that retinal microvascular abnormalities (formation of arteriovenous crossings, bleeding, and arteriolar narrowing) could predict the risk of cerebral ischemic changes and stroke [143–145]. In addition, the presence of a retinopathy with arteriovenous crossings has been linked to an increased risk of stroke, especially when these retinal abnormalities were associated with lesions in the cerebral white matter, a feature which is usually indicative of stroke [143, 145, 146]. Beyond these prospective studies, other research on the eyes in some animal models have shown that stroke is associated with functional impairment of the retina, including thinning of the retinal layers, reactive gliosis, increased expression of genes associated with cell damage, restricted oxygen supply, DNA fragmentation and ON neurodegeneration [147].

Ocular manifestations are to be expected in stroke, because the small vessels of the retina and the brain have similar embryological origins, anatomical characteristics and physiological properties [148, 149]. Some dysfunctions in the blood-brain and the blood-retinal barriers are suspected of playing a central role in the development of brain and retinal microangiopathy, respectively [131, 150, 151].

4.2.2. Multiple sclerosis (MS)

Visual impairment in MS is a major cause of disability. Visual loss is a symptom that occurs in up to 50% of patients with MS, resulting in some degree of visual impairment throughout the course of the disease for most cases [152–154].

It is not surprising that MS is related to eye disease, since the myelin components, which are essential in both the brain and the visual pathway, are the major autoimmune targets in MS. Visual defects are usually the result of axonal demyelination along the visual pathway [155]. It has been found that some internal areas of the retina, which are not associated with myelin, are also affected in MS. This suggests that the autoimmune response is also directed against other antigens in the eye [156].

Retrobulbar optic neuritis is an inflammatory optic neuropathy associated with demyelination and degeneration of the RGC. Diagnosed in 75% of patients with MS, this is often the first symptom of the disease [154, 155, 157]. It is important to highlight that visual deficits in MS also occur in patients without an optic neuritis diagnosis. Several studies have shown that, although the VA is not affected [158–160], there is a decrease in CS [158–160] and the RNFL thickness in MS patients in comparison with healthy individuals [160, 161]. RNFL thickening occurs in both the peripapillary [60, 160, 162, 163] and the macular area [54, 60]. Furthermore, RNFL thinning in MS patients directly correlates with the progression of neurological impairment and disease duration [160].

4.2.3. Parkinson's disease (PD)

PD is a chronic neurodegenerative disorder that is associated mainly with motor dysfunction, although it can also involve some non-motor symptoms, including visual deficits. These deficiencies may manifest as decreased CS [59, 163], impaired colour vision (the tritan axis is altered first) [57], and abnormal electrophysiological responses [57, 164]. The retinas of PD patients show photoreceptor and RGC dysfunction, morphological deterioration of the perifoveal dopaminergic plexus [165], and thinning of the RNFL [52, 53, 164, 166, 167]. According to the hypothesis that the disease results from a dopamine imbalance, it seems that visual deficits in PD could also be caused by dopamine depletion. In fact, some of the visual deficits experienced by PD patients can be improved by levodopa treatment [168].

4.2.4. Alzheimer's disease (AD)

The first abnormalities in the visual system for AD, observed in the 1970s, were regarded strictly as a dysfunction at the cortical level. Subsequent studies over the past 25 years have revealed that all parts of the visual system, including the ON and the retina, may be affected in AD. Some aspects of this involvement are still not well understood and are still the subject of recent research. Anatomical changes along the visual pathways and their corresponding functional changes have been detected and analysed by psychophysical procedures. AD can affect different aspects of the visual processing in line with the impact of the disease in the dorsal and ventral regions of the brain. Patients with dorsal-region damage suffer alterations in functions such as discrimination and angular-motion perception [169–172]. Those with damage in the ventral region show difficulty in discriminating faces, colours, and shapes [37, 173, 174].

5. Physiopathology of AD manifestations in the eye and the visual pathway

Changes in the visual system associated with AD have been the focus of the scientific community over many years, with some extensive reviews focus on different aspects of the problem [7, 47, 175–188]. All this evidence emphasises that visual changes may in medical practice help in the assessment of these patients and may even provide a predictive value potentially useful in diagnosis.

5.1. The lens

β-Amyloid deposits in the brain are a pathologic marker for AD. Amyloid β-peptides Aβ1–42 and Aβ1–40 have been identified in the human lens. Aβ1–40 was found in the aqueous humour, and its concentration is comparable to that found in the cerebral cortex and in the cerebrospinal fluid of AD patients [189]. On the one hand, it was recently discovered that there is an increase in β-amyloid deposits in the supranuclear lens fibres, which may be linked to the equatorial supranuclear cataracts more frequently found in these patients [1]. On the other hand, the study by Bei et al. determined that the measuring of the lens opacity was unlikely to provide a noninvasive measure of the risk of developing AD [190].

5.2. Retina

5.2.1. Retinal ganglion cells (RGCs)

The first histopathological studies on human-donor retinas of AD patients were made in the 1980s. Hinton et al. [8] examined four eyes from AD patients, finding a loss on the number of RGC, but a shortcoming of the study was that they did not provide numerical values in their results. However, Curcio et al. [27] found no significant difference in the number of RGC between the AD group and the age-matched controls. In the mid-1990s, Blanks et al. [23, 24] confirmed the initial observations of Hinton et al. These researchers compared the postmortem number of RGC from 12 retinas of nine patients with severe AD and 15 retinas from 12 age-matched controls. These studies found a 25% decrease in the number of RGC ($p < 0.001$) and an 82% increase in the astrocyte ratio per neuron in the retina ($p < 0.001$). However, a study with AD transgenic mice did not show a significant difference in the number of CGR compared to controls [191].

All the histopathological studies carried out so far involve a relatively small number of subjects. Therefore, it would be advisable to undertake more studies with larger numbers of subjects in order to verify the RGC decline in AD.

5.2.2. Vascularisation and retinal blood flow

Recent data suggest the vascular involvement of the retina in AD patients. Vascular changes in the retina are thought to share similar pathogenic mechanisms with cerebral vasculature [15, 192]. In fact, it is known that cerebral vascular insufficiency is one of the earliest pathological signs in the development of AD [193, 194].

Currently, there are few studies on vascularisation and retinal blood flow in AD. In 2007, Berisha et al. [15] studied the retinal vascularisation and blood flow in patients with AD. These researchers used Doppler laser in nine patients with probable mild ($n = 6$) and moderate AD ($n = 3$) plus eight age-matched controls. They detected a significant narrowing in the diameter of the retinal veins and decreased blood flow in AD patients, compared with controls. Mroczkowska et al. analysed the dynamic retinal vascularisation, noting that there were some signs of microvascular dysfunction that were correlated with the extent of cognitive impairment [195]. However, the study published by Tsai et al. found no differences either in the vascular structure or the calibre of retinal vessels in AD transgenic mice, compared to control animals [191].

5.2.3. Amyloid plaques, neurofibrillary tangles and vascular angiopathy

The first unsuccessful attempts to find amyloid plaques, neurofibrillary tangles or vascular retinal angiopathy in eyes of AD patients were performed in 1989 by Blanks et al. [21]. Although none of these typical AD signs were detected in the retina, their findings showed different levels of degeneration in RGC correlated with the degree of impairment of the patient.

In the last few years, β-amyloid deposits and hyperphosphorylated tau proteins have been detected in elderly retinas in a model of AD in double transgenic mice [196–198]. These β-amyloid plaques are distributed from the ganglion-cell layer to the inner plexiform layer. Some of these are also located in the outer nuclear layer, in the outer segments of the photoreceptors and in the ON [197]. These deposits, analysed with immunohistochemical techniques, are found to be accompanied by an increase in MCP-1+ immunoreactivity and F4/80+ in RGC layer. These results suggest that β-amyloid deposits cause neurodegeneration in the retina of these mice. This idea is further supported by the presence of TUNEL+ immunostaining in the RGC layer, so that there is some histological evidence of apoptosis in this layer [196]. In 2009, a β-amyloid vaccine was tested in the experimental mice model mentioned above, resulting in a lower number of retinal β-amyloid deposits. Nevertheless, there was a marked increase in retinal microvascular β-amyloid deposits as well as local neuroinflammation due to microglial infiltration and astrogliosis linked to a disorder in the organisation of the retina [197].

A postmortem study in human retinas showed for the first time the presence of β-amyloid plaques in AD patients [199]. Subsequently, other authors have confirmed the presence of β-amyloid deposits, which were more prevalent in perivascular and perimacular areas, both in AD patients and in those with mild cognitive impairment (MCI) [191, 200]. Campbell et al. recognised β-amyloid plaques in the retina by observing its polarisation properties and proposing it as a new diagnostic method [201].

5.3. Choroid

The latest improvement in OCT technology has enabled us to study the thickness of the choroid in vivo in patients with mild to moderate AD. A statistically significant generalised loss of foveal choroid thickness was found in these patients [191, 202, 203]. According to the authors, this choroidal thinning in AD may be associated with hypoperfusion and/or atrophic changes in this vascular layer. Several immunohistochemical studies in AD transgenic animals have reported a higher frequency of RPE hypertrophy and binucleated cells, but these changes were not seen in human retinas [191]. Previous studies have shown an Aβ accumulation in the choroidal vasculature in ageing mice and in a transgenic mouse model of AD [196, 204]. As happens in the brain, Aβ accumulation in the choroid may induce an inflammatory response and complement activation, which would lead to progressive vasoregression of the choroidal vasculature (and subsequent retinal neurodegeneration), through the same pathological cascade that has already been described in AD brains [191, 205–207].

5.4. The optic nerve

Hinton et al. [8] described widespread axonal degeneration of the optic nerves in 8 out of 10 AD patients that were analysed postmortem. In an additional study, a morphometric analysis of the ON suggested a predominant loss of magnocellular neurons that contribute large-calibre fibres. In a study published in 2005 by Syed et al. [208], some significant differences in axonal density were found by dyeing axon contours with toluidine blue, both in the central and in the peripheral areas of the ON. The analysis was performed on 12 AD patients, compared with 13 advanced-age control subjects. It should be pointed out that Syed's study found a decrease in smaller axons, with transversal section areas measuring less than 1.99 μm^2. Studies using magnetic resonance imaging (MRI) have found a statistically significant decrease in the ON volume in AD patients. However, this reduction does not correlate with brain volume [209].

Neurofibrillary tangles of tau protein have also been observed in ON [211], although this may not be specific for AD. Low-density lipoprotein receptor-related protein (LRP) is involved in the pathogenesis of AD by mediating the transport of amyloid-β (Aβ) out of the brain into the systemic circulation. Recently, Cuzzo et al. [210] found a decrease in the expression of LRP in the optic nerves of 11 patients with AD, compared to 10 control subjects. This would support the theory that LRP may play a role in the physiopathology of the optic neuropathy in AD. In the same study, the group of Cuzzo observed a decrease in neurofilament immunostaining in AD patients in comparison with control, thus confirming the previous findings by Hinton et al. [8]. Also, an increase in the receptor expression of advanced glycation end-products in the astrocytes near microvasculature has been reported in ON samples from AD patients [211].

Different studies have also pointed out some differences between the control group and the AD patients in the appearance of the ON head, both with red-free photography [13, 212, 213] and with scanning laser ophthalmoscope [214]. However, other studies failed to find such differences between AD patients and controls using the latter technique [31].

5.5. Lateral geniculate nucleus (LGN)

Scholtz et al. [215] noted a myelin loss and reduced function of neurons in the LGN in AD patients. The presence of β-amyloid plaques and neurofibrillary tangles of tau protein are also shown to be more abundant in the parvocellular than in the magnocellular layers of the LGN [218, 219]. On the contrary, a recent study found that tau pathology was scarce in the LGN and it did not differ significantly with age-matched control patients [216].

5.6. Other brain nuclei

5.6.1. Superior coliculus (SC)

The SC, sometimes referred to as the optic tectum, is a paired and laminated structure with a retinotopic organisation in the medium brain, which receives about 10% of RGC axons and is involved in the control of eye movements. Numerous amyloid plaques were found in the SC of AD patients [217]. Furthermore, subsequent studies identified abundant neuropathological neurofibrillary tangles [216, 218, 219] in this nucleus. These pathological changes in the SC may explain the problems of ocular motility frequently found in patients with AD [220].

5.6.2. Suprachiasmatic nucleus

The suprachiasmatic nucleus (SCN) is a paired structure formed by a group of neurons in the medial hypothalamus, above the optic chiasm, which receives direct RGC input through a retinal-hypothalamic tract [221]. In addition, it is a primary control centre of circadian rhythms by stimulating melatonin secretion by the pineal gland. It has been seen that there may be marked changes in the SCN in AD, such as decreases in the volume and number of cells (including specific neuronal subpopulations, such as vasopressin and neurotensin neurons) and the formation of neurofibrillary tangles [222–225]. These neuropathological findings may be correlated with the misalignment of the circadian rhythm in AD [226].

5.6.3. Pulvinar nuclei

Pulvinar nuclei, are a collection of nuclei located in the pulvinar thalamus, have reciprocal connections with association areas of the cerebral cortex, in the parietal, occipital and temporal lobes. They consist of several divisions that receive multiple inputs from the visual cortex subdivisions, from the SC and the retina (to a limited extent) [227]. This area is involved in visual attention and the control of eye movements.

Numerous amyloid plaques and some neuritic plaques (extracellular deposits within the brain grey matter which are a mixture between amyloid and death neuronal processes) were found along the various subdivisions of the pulvinar nuclei in nine AD patients compared with younger patients and age-matched controls [228]. This could explain the deterioration of visual attention in AD patients [174].

5.7. Visual cortex

The visual cortex is located in the occipital lobe. It comprises the striate cortex or V1 (primary visual cortex) and visual cortical extrastriate areas such as V2, V3, V4, V5, etc. (secondary visual cortex). Together, the primary and secondary visual cortex consists of a mosaic of several dozen visual areas occupying a large part of the cerebral cortex, approximately 20–25% in humans [229, 230].

In AD, the primary visual cortex is affected after the involvement of other cortical regions [231–233], except in a variant that manifests with early visual symptoms [234, 235]. Nevertheless, the accumulation of amyloid plaques and neurofibrillary tangles, the decrease in the number of neurons and capillary density, and the reduction of certain enzymes in V1 of AD patients are well documented [191, 233–236].

Although some preliminary studies claimed that there are minimal neurofibrillary tangles and amyloid plaques in primary and secondary visual cortex [237], subsequent studies have found abundant neurofibrillary tangles and plaques in the secondary visual cortex (mostly in the extrastriate 18 and 19 areas) [238, 239]. In both areas 17 and 18, the average neuronal density decreases to a similar degree (~30%) [240]. However, the difference between the two areas was the concentration of neurofibrillary tangles (2% of the neurons present tangles in area 17 vs. 10% in area 18) [240]. The reason for such discrepancy in neuronal loss could be related to the vulnerability of some neurons to the presence of neurofibrillary tangles or to the possibility of some cell loss unrelated to the degeneration of neurofibrillary tangles [47]. In addition to amyloid plaques and tangles, astrocytic gliosis was found in the primary visual cortex [241]. A likely associated dendritic pathology has also been observed in AD: dystrophic dendrites, loss of dendritic branches, and pathological alteration of dendritic spines [242, 243].

6. Visual psychophysical tests in Alzheimer's disease

To perform psychophysical tests in pathology such as AD can be a great challenge, because most of these tests require understanding and memorisation of the protocol for proper test performance. Therefore, without supervision by an experienced examiner, anomalies detected in testing may actually be the result of a failure to perform the task and not a visual deficit.

6.1. Visual acuity

The analysis of VA in AD patients was one of the most controversial tests. Although several studies claim that VA is not altered in this neurodegenerative condition [44, 48, 49, 239, 241, 244–246], other researchers find not only a decrease in VA [40, 247] (**Figure 2A**), but they also link this reduction to visual hallucinations when VA is severely decreased [248, 249]. A

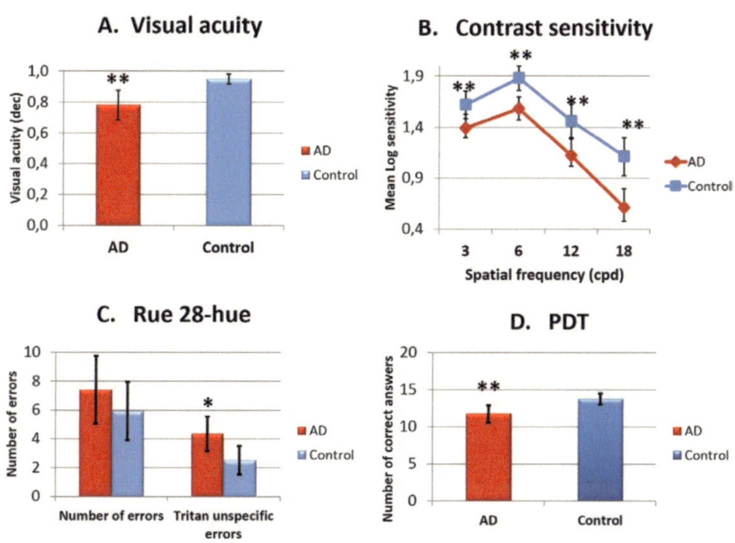

Figure 2. Mean data of the psychophysical tests. (**a**) Visual acuity, (**b**) contrast sensitivity, (**c**) desaturated Rue 28-hue colour test, and (**d**) perception digital test. Each bar represents the mean ± SD. $^{*}p < 0.05$ versus control. $^{**}p < 0.01$ versus control. Mann-Whitney *U* test (from **Figure 1** of [40] with permission).

correlation between the worsening in VA and the progression of AD has been described [250], together with a decline in AD patients and in AD patients with vascular dementia under low-luminosity conditions [44].

6.2. Colour vision

To perform the colour test in clinical practice in patients with AD is controversial because these patients have a naming deficit and therefore may have trouble verbalizing colours that they see or they might incorrectly name numbers or shapes. Despite this, some colour-vision tests do not require verbalisation, although they require concentration and memorisation of the task.

Some published studies which used Farsworth's test and Ishihara's test [251–253] found no differences in colour perception between the AD group and the control one. However, other authors found some tritan-axis defects, showing a correlation with the degree of dementia [37, 40, 238, 244] (**Figure 2C**). These data agree with the results of other authors [173, 240, 247, 254]. Pacheco et al., in their analysis with Ishihara test and PV-16, found impaired colour vision consisting of non-specific mistakes. Such responses were more prevalent in AD patients compared with controls, and were unrelated to the severity of the disease [38]. The disparity in the results may be due to the fact that each study used a different method for studying colour vision, so that comparisons of the results are difficult to interpret. Notably, Salamone et al. claimed that the problem of colour discrimination in AD patients is not purely cognitive but rather seems to be related to the damage of the structures responsible for colour perception [39].

6.3. Visual field

Like other psychophysical measures, automated perimetry requires considerable cooperation from the patient; therefore the reports on VF and AD are scarce and most are case reports. VF defects in AD vary from homonymous quadrantanopsia [255, 256] to non-hemianopic VF loss [239]. VF impairment in AD has been found both with manual perimetry [35] and with automated perimetry [34]. The latter showed a significant reduction in differential luminance sensitivity between AD and controls. This study additionally reported that AD patient underwent a diffuse sensitivity loss and, although VF defects involved the central field, deficits were more pronounced in the inferior field, appearing mostly as arcuate defects. They also found that the patients exhibited progressive VF loss 18 months after the initial examination.

6.4. Contrast sensitivity (CS)

CS tests evaluate the ability of the visual system to discriminate an object from the background in which it is located. This allows us to assess the integration of the information by the RGC and its cortical processing. The CS is measured by a threshold curve in which the spatial frequencies examined are depicted. High spatial frequencies examine the role of parvocellular cells, while low spatial frequencies represent the function of magnocellular cells.

The study of CS in AD has given rise to discrepancies in the results. Most reports have shown that CS function is affected in AD patients, the impairment ranging from a reduction in all spatial frequencies [26, 40, 43, 44, 245, 247, 251, 257–259], to a greater decline in high [26, 40, 258, 260] or low spatial frequencies [239, 244, 261, 262] (**Figure 2B**). By contrast, two studies found no differences between AD patients and controls [48, 246]. Such discrepancies in the results could be due to differences among the patients included in the studies as well as the CS test used [45]. Some CS tests are influenced by VA, such as the Regan chart, a low-contrast letter, and the Vistech VCTS 6500 whereas others are independent on VA, such as the Pelli-Robson test and the Freiburg test [45]. CS impairment in AD patients has consequences for daily functions and cognitive abilities, given that the spatial frequencies most affected appear to be those corresponding to macular function. An example of the importance of CS loss in AD patients is the capacity to predict the risk of falling [45].

6.5. Perception digital test (PDT)

The PDT is a quick, easy, and sensitive method recently developed for evaluating visual-perception disorders in mild AD patients [263]. The test aimed to assess the visual recognition of familiar situations, masked by geometric special effects that hinder perception. Each of the 15 sheets comprising the test shows the same picture at different positions in space. Special effects such as geometric effect (tile) or the effect of the frame 24/48 of MGI Photo Suite III program are used to distort the pictures. The test consists on a set of images that are shown to the patient to identify which one is properly oriented in space. Among the photographs are six common objects, five landscapes, two people, one letter, and one animal. The study of Rami et al. [263] showed that there were significant differences in PDT between mild-AD patients and control as well as a significant correlation with the MMSE. These results have been recently confirmed by Salobrar-García et al. [40] indicating that patients with mild AD had significantly more failures than controls and that there was a significant linear association with the MMSE [40] (**Figure 2D**).

6.6. Critical fusion frequency

The critical fusion frequency (CFF), also called temporal resolution, is a psychophysical threshold and in psychological terms is regarded as a measure of information-processing capacity [264]. It is defined as the frequency at which an intermittent light stimulus appears to be completely steady to the average human observer [265]. The CFF threshold is determined by the processing in the magnocellular pathway and frontal and parietal cortex [266]. In some studies the CFF appears normal in AD patients [244, 254, 267] with no retinocalcarine abnormality specific to AD patients [254]. By contrast, other authors found significantly lower CFF and descending scores compared with healthy elderly subjects [239, 264, 268].

6.7. Dark adaptation

Older adults have serious difficulty seeing under low illumination and at night, even in the absence of ocular disease. This fact can be attributed to delayed rhodopsin regeneration [269]. The study of Rizzo et al. showed that 7 of the 10 AD patients studied had a worse adaptation to darkness than did the control group of slightly younger patients [254].

6.8. Depth perception

The ability of the human eye to see in three dimensions and judge the distance of an object is called depth perception. Depth perception is grounded in both stereopsis and monocular cues. Because measuring monocular tracks is difficult, studies typically assess stereopsis. When an object is observed, each eye sees it from a slightly different angle. Those images are then sent back to the brain to be integrated into a single image, creating the 3D effect or stereopsis. Stereopsis relies mainly in the primary visual cortex. However, a more detailed analysis reveals that stereoscopic depth takes place in visual-association areas in the dorsal and ventral cortical pathways [270]. AD patients have been found to have abnormal depth perception in comparison with controls [238, 251, 254, 271, 272]. Disturbances in stereopsis, motion parallax and interpretation of static monocular cues may result from neuropathology in the AD visual cortex [272]. Other studies investigating stereopsis in AD were inconclusive [267] or found normal operation [171]. More recently, the link between worsening depth perception and AD has been demonstrated by means of functional magnetic resonance imaging (fMRI). The fMRI has revealed hypoactivation in the areas responsible for depth perception [273].

6.9. Motion perception

Motion perception is the process of deducing the speed and direction of different elements in a scene based on different sensory stimuli: visual, vestibular and proprioceptive. Visual sensory information for motion perception is based on retina [274], LGN [275] and primary and secondary visual cortex processing [276]. There is controversy in the reports on motion perception in AD patients, as some studies have found no differences in this regard [174, 246, 267] while others have identified several deficiencies in the motion perception [173, 277]. Specifically, patients with an early-stage of AD have great difficulty interpreting the movement of objects, a condition that worsens as the disease progresses [47]. The discrepancy of the results could be related to the test used, since some require discrimination of motion direction while others simply demand the recognition of the occurrence of motion.

6.10. Pupillary response to light

Pupillary response is controlled by a balance between the cholinergic and adrenergic innervation being influenced directly or indirectly by the input from the central and autonomic nervous system.

As an impairment of the cholinergic system is known to occur in dementia and AD [278], it would be expected for the pupillary light reflex to be affected in AD [279, 280]. The constriction at the onset of bright light relative to the resting amplitude was significantly reduced in AD compared with healthy age-matched older adults and young adults [279]. These findings point to the presence of a cholinergic deficit in AD patients [280, 281], as shown by the fact that pharmacological treatment with donepezil, an anticholinesterase agent, partially improves this deficit [280]. However, it is still a challenge to develop a pupillary-response-sensitivity test specific to clinical diagnosis of early AD.

In 1994, Scinto et al. reported that AD patients had hypersensitivity of the pupil dilation after diluted tropicamide instillation [282]. Since the publication of this work, numerous studies have been performed, with several results showing both negative [283–291] and positive results [281, 282, 292–297]. Some of these studies point to a lack of specificity to the pupil tropicamide test in AD [288, 298].

6.11. Ocular motility

For the proper coordination of eye movements the retina, the brain integration of the image, and the extraocular muscles need to be coordinated [299]. It has been reported that in post-mortem studies of AD patients, the oculomotor nuclei of the brain are affected [300, 301]. Boxer et al. reported that AD patients displayed reflexive visually guided saccade abnormalities, specifically, prominent increases in horizontal saccade latency [301].

6.12. The electroretinogram (ERG)

The electroretinogram (ERG) is a record of the bioelectrical response towards light stimuli. The three types used in daily practice are full-field ERG, pattern ERG (PERG) and multifocal ERG (mfERG). For clinical purposes, full-field ERG has been standardised so that the results of different researchers can be compared [302].

There is intense controversy with respect ERG impairment in AD patients. Some studies have found that the amplitude and latency of the retinal potentials did not differ between AD and control groups [29, 32, 254, 303, 304], indicating that the PERG may not be valuable in establishing an early diagnosis of AD [304]. In the study of Kergoat et al., amplitude and latency of ERG was not affected but there was a delay on the latency of the visual evoked potentials (VEP) [32]. Other studies have reported a significant amplitude reduction in AD patients [25, 26, 305] and postulated that this result is consistent with RGC dysfunction [26].

In PERG examination, increased implicit time of P50-wave and amplitude reduction in P50- and N95-waves were observed in AD patients [41, 42, 306], and this could reflect an impairment of the magnocellular stream [306]. In addition to PERG, Krasodomska et al. studied pattern VEP in patients with early stages of AD, and normal routine ophthalmological examination results. Their most prevalent findings were amplitude reduction in N95-wave and increased latency of P100-wave. Such results showed a dysfunction of RGC and optic nerve in early stages of AD [41]. The mfERG measures macular function [337], and a decrease in electrical activity has been found in the macula of AD patients [307].

6.13. Optical coherence tomography (OCT)

OCT is a non-invasive imaging technique that works in a similar way to ultrasound, except that it uses low-coherence light waves instead of sound waves. The light waves are used to take cross-section images of the retina. As OCT allows visualisation of the retinal layers, their thickness can be mapped and measured. In fact, this technique has already been established as the standard image model for retinal tests (**Figure 1**).

Currently, RNFL, RGC and inner layers of the retina are considered indirect biomarkers of the CNS, enabling the prediction of brain pathology in patients suffering from different neurological diseases [184, 308]. Since the development of OCT, this tool has been used to measure the thickness of the RNFL in different neurodegenerative pathologies. Despite that OCT was first developed in 1991 and commercially distributed in 1995, it was not until 2001 when a study was first published on the thickness of the RNFL in patients with AD [42].

During those first years, many studies appeared focusing on the peripapillary RNFL thickness in AD patients. In every study, a significant decrease in RNFL thickness was objectified in AD patients and compared with age-matched controls. These analyses were carried out by segmenting the measures of the peripapillary thickness according to the area (superior, inferior, nasal and temporal). Several studies showed a decrease in the peripapillary RNFL thickness in all areas [10, 14, 16, 18, 42, 309]; others found that the thinning occurred in the inferior and superior regions [17, 307, 310], while in still other studies this significant decrease appeared only in the superior peripapillary region [15, 213, 311–313]. Some studies reported a certain thinning in the RNFL associated with the progressive cognitive decline [203, 312, 314]. Some authors even suggest that the inferior peripapillary quadrants might be the area with most specificity and sensitivity regarding the detection of the cognitive decline in the initial stages of the AD [17]. However, Salobrar-García et al. [20] reported that their group of patients with mild AD showed no significant difference with respect to control subjects in terms of RNFL thickness of the peripapillary region (**Figure 3A**). These authors postulated that although no statistically significant differences in peripapillary RNFL were found between control and AD eyes, the increase in peripapillary thickness observed in mild-AD patients could be secondary to an inflammatory process that may represent an early stage of degeneration and could lead to progressive peripapillary fibre damage. The variability in peripapillary RNFL thickness reported in AD might be due to differences in disease progression among patients studied, since patients with greater involvement of the peripapillary region were those with a more advanced stage of AD.

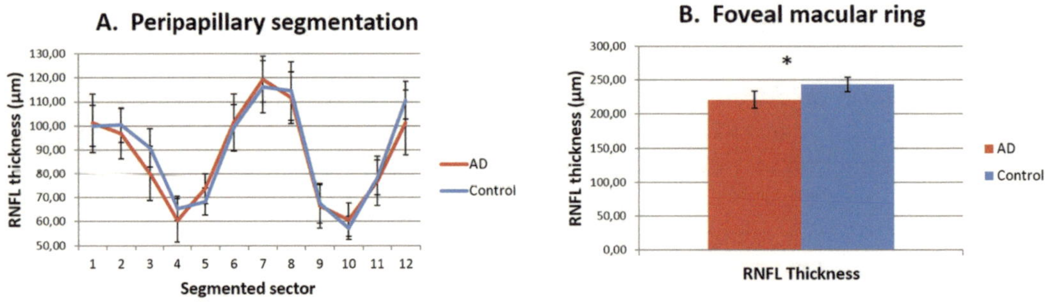

Figure 3. Mean data of RNFL thickness against eye quadrants assessed with optical coherence tomography (OCT). (**a**) Peripapillary segmentation retinal nerve fibre layer, (**b**) central macular ring (1 mm away from the fovea). *p value < 0.01 (modified from **Figure 2** [20] with permission).

Recently, some studies focusing on the analysis of patients with mild cognitive impairment (MCI) found a thinning of the peripapillary region [62, 314–316]. MCI patients also have a thinning in the macular ganglion cell-inner plexiform layer [317]. By contrast, Ascaso et al., reported an increase in the macular volume in MCI when compared to control subjects and AD patients [315]. These findings could be explained as an increase in the macular volume caused by a possible inflammation and gliosis prior to neuronal cell death.

Recently, studies in AD analysed the measurement of not only the peripapillary RNFL thickness but also the RNFL thickness in the macular region. They demonstrated a significant RNFL thinning in the macular region of AD patients compared with age-matched controls [14, 19, 62, 63, 307, 311, 315] (**Figure 3B**). A study carried out using the latest OCT technology, which allows an analysis of the different retinal layers separately, noted that the thickness reduction occurred in the inner layers of the retina (RNFL-RGC complex), whereas the outer layers were not affected [63, 203].

In the most incipient AD stages (mild AD), psychophysical tests having the greatest predictive value are reportedly the CS, VA, unspecific errors in tritan region and the PDT [40]. In addition, the macular RNFL thickness and total macular volume measured by OCT have highly significant sensitivity and specificity for differentiating mild AD patients from healthy subjects, the thickness of the inner upper macular RNFL seeming to have the highest diagnostic value in mild AD neurodegeneration. Probably, the first affected area of the retina in mild AD is the macular area, where, due to the arrangement of the multilayer bodies of the ganglion cells, the decrease is easier to detect [19, 20]. These observations highlight the importance of applying psychophysical tests and OCT in patients with incipient AD stages.

Due to the ageing population increasing, the incidence of neurodegenerative diseases such as AD is growing. As demonstrated by the results of the visual psychophysical test mentioned above, the eye gives us a valuable window for evaluating these neurodegenerations. Therefore, the inclusion of ophthalmological examination could become an important tool in early diagnosis and follow-up of these patients.

7. Alzheimer's disease and glaucoma

In the last decade, several studies have been made on some AD patients and experimental models of glaucoma. These studies have shown some significant similarities between the two pathologies [318–320]. Furthermore, in some clinical studies where the prevalence of primary open-angle glaucoma (POAG) in AD patients was studied, an increase was observed in the incidence rate of POAG in AD patients [321, 322]. Tamura et al. identified an increase in the prevalence of the ε 4 allele of the APOE in POAG patients, similar to those that occur in patients suffering from AD. This suggests that common mechanisms could contribute to both pathologies [322]. Lipton et al. [323] have postulated that treatment with memantine, a NMDA receptor blocker used in AD could help to slow the advance of glaucomatous neurodegeneration. This hypothesis is based on the fact that the apoptosis, mediated by excitotoxic cell death, is a factor in the physiopathology of many neurodegenerative diseases, including glaucoma.

This kind of excitotoxicity is caused by the excessive activation of NMDA glutamate receptors, at least partially. This excessive activity in the NMDA receptor entails an abnormally high influx of calcium ions in the neurons, which triggers multiple outcomes resulting in apoptosis. Thus, pharmacological blockage of NMDA receptor activity would prevent apoptosis related to excitotoxicity. However, the use of a neuroprotective drug (memantine) in patients with POAG gave discouraging results [324]. On the other hand, in a recent 12.7-year longitudinal study, no direct link was found between normotensive glaucoma and increase risk of developing dementia or AD, compared with the general population [325].

Whether or not glaucomatous optic neuropathy can be considered an ocular extension during Alzheimer's progression deserves further investigation.

Acknowledgements

This work was supported by the Ophthalmological Network OFTARED (RD12-0034/0002: Prevención, Detección Precoz y Tratamiento de la Patología Ocular Prevalente Degenerativa y Crónica) of the Institute of Health of Carlos III of the Spanish Ministry of Economy. This work has been funded by the PN I+D+i 2008–2011, by the ISCIII-Subdirección General de Redes y Centros de Investigación Cooperativa and by the European programme FEDER; grants to Elena Salobrar-Garcia are currently supported by a Predoctoral Fellowship (FPU) from the Spanish Ministry of Education, Culture and Sport. David Nesbitt corrected the English version of this work.

Author details

Elena Salobrar-García[1], Ana I. Ramírez[2], Rosa de Hoz[2], Pilar Rojas[3], Juan J. Salazar[2], Blanca Rojas[1], Raquel Yubero[4], Pedro Gil[4], Alberto Triviño[1] and José M. Ramírez[1*]

*Address all correspondence to: ramirezs@med.ucm.es

1 Ramon Castroviejo Institute of Ophthalmologic Research, School of Medicine, Complutense University of Madrid (UCM), Spain

2 Ramon Castroviejo Institute of Ophthalmologic Research, School of Optics and Optometry, Complutense University of Madrid (UCM), Spain

3 Service of Ophthalmology Hospital Gregorio Marañon, Ramon Castroviejo Institute of Ophthalmologic Research, Complutense University of Madrid (UCM), Spain

4 Service of Geriatrics, University Hospital Clinico San Carlos, Complutense University of Madrid (UCM), Spain

http://dx.doi.org/10.5772/64490

References

[1] Jindal V. Interconnection between brain and retinal neurodegenerations. Molecular Neurobiology. 2014; 51: 1–8.

[2] Hirtz D, Thurman D, Gwinn-Hardy K, Mohamed M, Chaudhuri A, Zalutsky R. How common are the "common" neurologic disorders? Neurology. 2007; 68: 326–337.

[3] Brookmeyer R, Johnson E, Ziegler-Graham K, Arrighi HM. Forecasting the global burden of Alzheimer's disease. Alzheimer's and Dementia. 2007; 3: 186–191.

[4] Blennow K, de Leon MJ, Zetterberg H. Alzheimer's disease. Lancet. 2006; 368: 387–403.

[5] Cummings JL, Cole G. Alzheimer disease. JAMA. 2002; 287: 2335–2338.

[6] Small BJ, Gagnon E, Robinson B. Early identification of cognitive deficits: preclinical Alzheimer's disease and mild cognitive impairment. Geriatrics. 2007; 62: 19–23.

[7] Ikram MK, Cheung CY, Wong TY, Chen CP. Retinal pathology as biomarker for cognitive impairment and Alzheimer's disease. Journal of Neurology, Neurosurgery & Psychiatry. 2012; 83: 917–922.

[8] Hinton DR, Sadun AA, Blanks JC, Miller CA. Optic-nerve degeneration in Alzheimer's disease. The New England Journal of Medicine. 1986; 315: 485–487.

[9] Varma R, Bazzaz S, Lai M. Optical tomography–measured retinal nerve fiber layer thickness in normal Latinos. Investigative Ophthalmology & Visual Science. 2003; 44: 3369–3373.

[10] Paquet C, Boissonnot M, Roger F, Dighiero P, Gil R, Hugon J. Abnormal retinal thickness in patients with mild cognitive impairment and Alzheimer's disease. Neuroscience Letters. 2007; 420: 97–99.

[11] Cohen MJ, Kaliner E, Frenkel S, Kogan M, Miron H, Blumenthal EZ. Morphometric analysis of human peripapillary retinal nerve fiber layer thickness. Investigative Ophthalmology & Visual Science. 2008; 49: 941–944.

[12] Bowd C, Zangwill LM, Blumenthal EZ, Vasile C, Boehm AG, Gokhale PA, et al. Imaging of the optic disc and retinal nerve fiber layer: the effects of age, optic disc area, refractive error, and gender. Journal of the Optical Society of America A, Optics, Image Science, and Vision. 2002; 19: 197–207.

[13] Hedges III TR, Galves RP, Speigelman D, Barbas NR, Peli E, Yardley CJ. Retinal nerve fiber layer abnormalities in Alzheimer's disease. Acta Ophthalmologica Scandinavica. 1996; 74: 271–275.

[14] Iseri PK, Altinas Ö, Tokay T, Yüksel N. Relationship between cognitive impairment and retinal morphological and visual functional abnormalities in Alzheimer disease. Journal of Neuro-ophthalmology. 2006; 26: 18–24.

[15] Berisha F, Feke GT, Trempe CL, McMeel JW, Schepens CL. Retinal abnormalities in early Alzheimer's disease. Investigative Ophthalmology & Visual Science. 2007; 48: 2285–2289.

[16] Valenti DA. Neuroimaging of retinal nerve fiber layer in AD using optical coherence tomography. Neurology. 2007; 69: 1060.

[17] Kesler A, Vakhapova V, Korczyn AD, Naftaliev E, Neudorfer M. Retinal thickness in patients with mild cognitive impairment and Alzheimer's disease. Clinical Neurology and Neurosurgery. 2011; 113: 523–526.

[18] Moreno-Ramos T, Benito-León J, Villarejo A, Bermejo-Pareja F. Retinal nerve fiber layer thinning in dementia associated with Parkinson's disease, dementia with Lewy bodies, and Alzheimer's disease. Journal of Alzheimer's Disease. 2013; 34: 659–664.

[19] Garcia-Martin ES, Rojas B, Ramirez AI, de Hoz R, Salazar JJ, Yubero R, et al. Macular thickness as a potential biomarker of mild Alzheimer's disease. Ophthalmology. 2014; 121: 1149–1151.

[20] Salobrar-Garcia E, Hoyas I, Leal M, de Hoz R, Rojas B, Ramirez AI, et al. Analysis of retinal peripapillary segmentation in early Alzheimer's disease patients. BioMed Research International. 2015; 2015: 636548.

[21] Blanks JC, Hinton DR, Sadun AA, Miller CA. Retinal ganglion cell degeneration in Alzheimer's disease. Brain Research. 1989; 501: 364–372.

[22] Sadun A, Bassi C. Optic nerve damage in Alzheimer's disease. Ophthalmology. 1990; 97: 9–17.

[23] Blanks JC, Torigoe Y, Hinton DR, Blanks RHI. Retinal pathology in Alzheimer's disease. I. Ganglion cell loss in foveal/parafoveal retina. Neurobiology of Aging. 1996; 17: 377–384.

[24] Blanks JC, Schmidt SY, Torigoe Y, Porrello KV, Hinton DR, Blanks RH. Retinal pathology in Alzheimer's disease. II. Regional neuron loss and glial changes in GCL. Neurobiology of Aging. 1996; 17: 385–395.

[25] Katz B, Rimmer S, Iragui V, Katzman R. Abnormal pattern electroretinogram in Alzheimer's disease: evidence for retinal ganglion cell degeneration? Annals of Neurology. 1989; 26: 221–225.

[26] Trick GL, Barris MC, Bickler-Bluth M. Abnormal pattern electroretinograms in patients with senile dementia of the Alzheimer type. Annals of Neurology. 1989; 26: 226–231.

[27] Curcio CA, Drucker DN. Retinal ganglion cells in Alzheimer's disease and aging. Annals of Neurology. 1993; 33: 248–257.

[28] Davies D, McCoubrie P, McDonald B, Jobst K. Myelinated axon number in the optic nerve is unaffected by Alzheimer's disease. British Journal of Ophthalmology. 1995; 79: 596–600.

[29] Justino L, Kergoat M, Bergman H, Chertkow H, Robillard A, Kergoat H. Neuroretinal function is normal in early dementia of the Alzheimer type. Neurobiology of Aging. 2001; 22: 691–695.

[30] Kergoat H, Kergoat MJ, Justino L, Robillard A, Bergman H, Chertkow H. Normal optic nerve head topography in the early stages of dementia of the Alzheimer type. Dementia and Geriatric Cognitive Disorders. 2001; 12: 359–363.

[31] Kergoat H, Kergoat M, Justino L, Chertkow H, Robillard A, Bergman H. An evaluation of the retinal nerve fiber layer thickness by scanning laser polarimetry in individuals with dementia of the Alzheimer type. Acta Ophthalmologica Scandinavica. 2001; 79: 187–191.

[32] Kergoat Hln, Kergoat M, Justino L, Chertkow H, Robillard A, Bergman H. Visual retinocortical function in dementia of the Alzheimer type. Gerontology. 2002; 48: 197–203.

[33] Petersen R, Stevens J, Ganguli M, Tangalos E, Cummings J, DeKosky S. Practice parameter: early detection of dementia: mild cognitive impairment (an evidence-based review). Report of the Quality Standards Subcommittee of the American Academy of Neurology. Neurology. 2001; 56: 1133–1142.

[34] Trick GL, Trick LR, Morris P, Wolf M. Visual field loss in senile dementia of the Alzheimer's type. Neurology. 1995; 45: 68–74.

[35] Steffes R, Thralow J. Visual field limitation in the patient with dementia of the Alzheimer's type. Journal of the American Geriatrics Society. 1987; 35:198–204.

[36] Risacher SL, WuDunn D, Pepin SM, MaGee TR, McDonald BC, Flashman LA, et al. Visual contrast sensitivity in Alzheimer's disease, mild cognitive impairment, and older adults with cognitive complaints. Neurobiology of Aging. 2013; 34: 1133–1144.

[37] Cronin-Golomb A, Sugiura R, Corkin S, Growdon JH. Incomplete achromatopsia in Alzheimer's disease. Neurobiology of Aging. 1993; 14: 471–477.

[38] Pache M, Smeets CH, Gasio PF, Savaskan E, Flammer J, Wirz-Justice A, et al. Colour vision deficiencies in Alzheimer's disease. Age and Ageing. 2003; 32: 422–426.

[39] Salamone G, Di Lorenzo C, Mosti S, Lupo F, Cravello L, Palmer K, et al. Color discrimination performance in patients with Alzheimer's disease. Dementia and Geriatric Cognitive Disorders. 2009; 27: 501–507.

[40] Salobrar-Garcia E, de Hoz R, Rojas B, Ramirez AI, Salazar JJ, Yubero R, et al. Ophthalmologic psychophysical tests support OCT findings in mild Alzheimer's disease. Journal of Ophthalmology. 2015; Article ID 736949.

[41] Krasodomska K, Lubiński W, Potemkowski A, Honczarenko K. Pattern electroretinogram (PERG) and pattern visual evoked potential (PVEP) in the early stages of Alzheimer's disease. Documenta Ophthalmologica. 2010; 121: 111–121.

[42] Parisi V, Restuccia R, Fattapposta F, Mina C, Bucci MG, Pierelli F. Morphological and functional retinal impairment in Alzheimer's disease patients. Clinical Neurophysiology. 2001; 112: 1860–1867.

[43] Cronin-Golomb A, Rizzo J, Corkin S, Growdon J. Visual function in Alzheimer's disease and normal aging. Annals of the New York Academy of Sciences. 1991; 640: 28–35.

[44] Lakshminarayanan V, Lagrave J, Kean ML, Dick M, Shankle R. Vision in dementia: contrast effects. Neurological Research. 1996; 18: 9–15.

[45] Neargarder SA, Stone ER, Cronin-Golomb A, Oross S. The impact of acuity on performance of four clinical measures of contrast sensitivity in Alzheimer's disease. The Journals of Gerontology Series B: Psychological Sciences and Social Sciences. 2003; 58: P54–P62.

[46] Valenti DA. Alzheimer's disease: visual system review. Optometry. 2010; 81: 12–21.

[47] Tzekov RT, Mullan M. Vision function abnormalities in Alzheimer's disease. Survey of Ophthalmology. 2013; 59: 414–433.

[48] Schlotterer G, Moscovitch M, Crapper-McLachlan D. Visual processing deficits as assessed by spatial frequency contrast sensitivity and backward masking in normal ageing and Alzheimer's disease. Brain: A Journal of Neurology. 1984; 107: 309–325.

[49] Wright CE, Drasdo N, Harding GF. Pathology of the optic nerve and visual association areas information given by the flash and pattern visual evoked potential, and the temporal and spatial contrast sensitivity function. Brain. 1987; 110: 107–120.

[50] Cronin-Golomb A, Corkin S, Growdon JH. Contrast sensitivity in Alzheimer's disease. Journal of the Optical Society of America A, Optics, Image Science, and Vision. 1987; 4: 7.

[51] Morris JC. Mild cognitive impairment and preclinical Alzheimer's disease. Geriatrics. 2005; Suppl: 9–14.

[52] Inzelberg R, Ramirez JA, Nisipeanu P, Ophir A. Retinal nerve fiber layer thinning in Parkinson disease. Vision Research. 2004; 44: 2793–2797.

[53] Altintas Ö, Iseri P, Özkan B, Çağlar Y. Correlation between retinal morphological and functional findings and clinical severity in Parkinson's disease. Documenta Ophthalmologica. 2008; 116: 137–146.

[54] Burkholder BM, Osborne B, Loguidice MJ, Bisker E, Frohman TC, Conger A, et al. Macular volume determined by optical coherence tomography as a measure of neuronal loss in multiple sclerosis. Archives of Neurology. 2009; 66: 1366–1372.

[55] Aaker GD, Myung JS, Ehrlich JR, Mohammed M, Henchcliffe C, Kiss S. Detection of retinal changes in Parkinson's disease with spectral-domain optical coherence tomography. Clinical Ophthalmology. 2010; 4: 1427–1432.

[56] Albert MS, DeKosky ST, Dickson D, Dubois B, Feldman HH, Fox NC, et al. The diagnosis of mild cognitive impairment due to Alzheimer's disease: Recommendations from the National Institute on Aging-Alzheimer's Association workgroups on diagnostic guidelines for Alzheimer's disease. Alzheimer's and Dementia. 2011; 7: 270–279.

[57] Bodis-Wollner I. Foveal vision is impaired in Parkinson's disease. Parkinsonism & Related Disorders. 2012; 19: 1–14.

[58] La Morgia C, Barboni P, Rizzo G, Carbonelli M, Savini G, Scaglione C, et al. Loss of temporal retinal nerve fibers in Parkinson disease: a mitochondrial pattern? European Journal of Neurology. 2012; 20: 198–201.

[59] Spund B, Ding Y, Liu T, Selesnick I, Glazman S, Shrier E, et al. Remodeling of the fovea in Parkinson disease. Journal of Neural Transmission. 2013; 120: 745–753.

[60] Tátrai E, Simó M, Iljicsov A, Németh J, DeBuc DC, Somfai GM. In vivo evaluation of retinal neurodegeneration in patients with multiple sclerosis. PLoS ONE. 2012; 7: e30922.

[61] Satue M, Garcia-Martin E, Fuertes I, Otin S, Alarcia R, Herrero R, et al. Use of Fourier-domain OCT to detect retinal nerve fiber layer degeneration in Parkinson's disease patients. Eye. 2013; 27: 507–514.

[62] Gao L, Liu Y, Li X, Bai Q, Liu P. Abnormal retinal nerve fiber layer thickness and macula lutea in patients with mild cognitive impairment and Alzheimer's disease. Archives of Gerontology and Geriatrics. 2015; 60: 162–167

[63] Marziani E, Pomati S, Ramolfo P, Cigada M, Giani A, Mariani C, et al. Evaluation of retinal nerve fiber layer and ganglion cell layer thickness in Alzheimer's disease using spectral-domain optical coherence tomography. Investigative Ophthalmology & Visual Science. 2013; 54: 5953–5958.

[64] Maldonado RS, Mettu P, El-Dairi M, Bhatti MT. The application of optical coherence tomography in neurologic diseases. Neurology: Clinical Practice. 2015; 5: 460–469.

[65] Millán Calenti JC. Gerontology and Geriatrics: assessment and intervention. Madrid; Médica Panamericana. 2010; 708.

[66] López-Otín C, Blasco MA, Partridge L, Serrano M, Kroemer G. The hallmarks of aging. Cell. 2013; 153: 1194–1217.

[67] Oh SR, Chokthaweesak W, Annunziata CC, Priel A, Korn BS, Kikkawa DO. Analysis of eyelid fat pad changes with aging. Ophthalmic Plastic & Reconstructive Surgery. 2011; 27: 348–351.

[68] Shore JW. Changes in lower eyelid resting position, movement, and tone with age. American Journal of Ophthalmology. 1985; 99: 415–423.

[69] Van Haeringen N. Aging and the lacrimal system. British Journal of Ophthalmology. 1997; 81: 824–826.

[70] Zhu W, Hong J, Zheng T, Le Q, Xu J, Sun X. Age-related changes of human conjunctiva on in vivo confocal microscopy. British Journal of Ophthalmology. 2010; 94: 1448–1453.

[71] Rada JA, Achen VR, Penugonda S, Schmidt RW, Mount BA. Proteoglycan composition in the human sclera during growth and aging. Investigative Ophthalmology & Visual Science. 2000; 41: 1639–1648.

[72] Grossniklaus HE, Nickerson JM, Edelhauser HF, Bergman LA, Berglin L. Anatomic alterations in aging and age-related diseases of the eye. Investigative Ophthalmology & Visual Science. 2013; 54: ORSF23–ORSF27.

[73] Faragher R, Mulholland B, Tuft S, Sandeman S, Khaw P. Aging and the cornea. British Journal of Ophthalmology. 1997; 81: 814–817.

[74] Gipson IK. Age-related changes and diseases of the ocular surface and cornea. Investigative Ophthalmology & Visual Science. 2013; 54: ORSF48–ORSF53.

[75] McMenamin PG, Lee WR, Aitken DA. Age-related changes in the human outflow apparatus. Ophthalmology. 1986; 93: 194–209.

[76] Salvi S, Akhtar S, Currie Z. Ageing changes in the eye. Postgraduate Medical Journal. 2006; 82: 581–587.

[77] Birren JE, Casperson RC, Botwinick J. Age changes in pupil size. Journal of Gerontology. 1950; 5: 216–221.

[78] Barteselli G, Chhablani J, El-Emam S, Wang H, Chuang J, Kozak I, et al. Choroidal volume variations with age, axial length, and sex in healthy subjects: a three-dimensional analysis. Ophthalmology. 2012;119: 2572–2578.

[79] Ramrattan RS, van der Schaft, Theo L, Mooy CM, De Bruijn W, Mulder P, De Jong P. Morphometric analysis of Bruch's membrane, the choriocapillaris, and the choroid in aging. Investigative Ophthalmology & Visual Science. 1994; 35: 2857–2864.

[80] Pauleikhoff D, Harper CA, Marshall J, Bird AC. Aging changes in Bruch's membrane: a histochemical and morphologic study. Ophthalmology. 1990; 97: 171–178.

[81] Newsome DA, Huh W, Green WR. Bruch's membrane age-related changes vary by region. Current Eye Research. 1987; 6: 1211–1221.

[82] Ramírez JM, Ramírez AI, Salazar JJ, de Hoz R, Triviño A. Changes of astrocytes in retinal ageing and age-related macular degeneration. Experimental Eye Research. 2001; 73: 601–615.

[83] Grunwald JE, Piltz J, Patel N, Bose S, Riva CE. Effect of aging on retinal macular microcirculation: a blue field simulation study. Investigative Ophthalmology & Visual Science. 1993; 34: 3609–3613.

[84] Moya FJ, Brigatti L, Caprioli J. Effect of aging on optic nerve appearance: a longitudinal study. British Journal of Ophthalmology. 1999; 83: 567–572.

[85] Sebag J. Ageing of the vitreous. Eye. 1987; 1: 254–262.

[86] Dagnelie G. Age-Related Psychophysical Changes and Low Vision. Investigative Ophthalmology & Visual Science. 2013; 54: ORSF88–ORSF93.

[87] Haegerstrom-Portnoy G, Schneck ME, Brabyn JA, Lott LA. Development of refractive errors into old age. Optometry & Vision Science. 2002; 79: 643–649.

[88] Derefeldt G, Lennerstrand G, Lundh B. Age variations in normal human contrast sensitivity. Acta Ophthalmologica. 1979; 57: 679–690.

[89] Leat SJ, Chan LL, Maharaj P, Hrynchak PK, Mittelstaedt A, Machan CM, et al. Binocular vision and eye movement disorders in older adults. Investigative Ophthalmology & Visual Science. 2013; 54: 3798–3805.

[90] Reuter-Lorenz PA. New visions of the aging mind and brain. Trends in Cognitive Sciences. 2002; 6: 394–400.

[91] Creasey H, Rapoport SI. The aging human brain. Annals of Neurology. 1985; 17: 2–10.

[92] Masliah E, Mallory M, Hansen L, DeTeresa R, Terry R. Quantitative synaptic alterations in the human neocortex during normal aging. Neurology. 1993; 43: 192.

[93] Hof PR, Morrison JH. The aging brain: morphomolecular senescence of cortical circuits. Trends in Neurosciences. 2004; 27: 607–613.

[94] Hedden T, Gabrieli JDE. Insights into the ageing mind: a view from cognitive neuroscience. Nature Reviews Neuroscience. 2004; 5: 87–96.

[95] Pappolla M, Omar R, Saran B. The "normal" brain." Abnormal ubiquitinilated deposits highlight an age-related protein change. American Journal of Pathology. 1989; 135: 585–591.

[96] Nakano M, Oenzil F, Mizuno T, Gotoh S. Age-related changes in the lipofuscin accumulation of brain and heart. Gerontology. 1995; 41: 69–80.

[97] Coria F, Moreno A, Rubio I, Garcia M, Morato E. The cellular pathology associated with Alzheimer β-amyloid deposits in non-demented aged individuals. Neuropathology and Applied Neurobiology. 1993; 19: 261–268.

[98] Morris JC, McKeel Jr D, Storandt M, Rubin E, Price J, Grant E, et al. Very mild Alzheimer's disease Informant-based clinical, psychometric, and pathologic distinction from normal aging. Neurology. 1991; 41: 469–478.

[99] Boone KB, Miller BL, Lesser IM, Mehringer CM, Hill-Gutierrez E, Goldberg MA, et al. Neuropsychological correlates of white-matter lesions in healthy elderly subjects: a threshold effect. Archives of Neurology. 1992; 49: 549–554.

[100] Zerfass R, Geiger-Kabisch C, Sattel H, Besthorn C, Hentschel F. Brain atrophy in normal ageing and Alzheimer's disease. Volumetric discrimination and clinical correlations. British Journal of Psychiatry. 1995; 167: 739–746.

[101] Reed BR, Eberling JL, Mungas D, Weiner M, Kramer JH, Jagust WJ. Effects of white matter lesions and lacunes on cortical function. Archives of Neurology. 2004; 61: 1545–1550.

[102] O'Brien JT, Erkinjuntti T, Reisberg B, Roman G, Sawada T, Pantoni L, et al. Vascular cognitive impairment. Lancet Neurology. 2003; 2: 89–98.

[103] Fratiglioni L, Mangialasche F, Qiu C. Brain aging: lessons from community studies. Nutrition Reviews. 2010; 68: S119–S127.

[104] Grammas P, Martinez J, Miller B. Cerebral microvascular endothelium and the pathogenesis of neurodegenerative diseases. Expert Reviews in Molecular Medicine. 2011; 13: e19.

[105] Mrak RE, Griffin S, Graham DI. Aging-associated changes in human brain. Journal of Neuropathology and Experimental Neurology. 1997; 56: 1269–1275.

[106] Li L, Lundkvist A, Andersson D, Wilhelmsson U, Nagai N, Pardo AC, et al. Protective role of reactive astrocytes in brain ischemia. Journal of Cerebral Blood Flow & Metabolism. 2007; 28: 468–481.

[107] Frith CD, Frith U. Implicit and explicit processes in social cognition. Neuron. 2008; 60: 503–510.

[108] Sander M, Bergersen LH, Storm-Mathisen J. Molecular approaches to understanding neural network plasticity and memory: the Kavli Prize Inaugural Symposium on Neuroscience. Neuroscience. 2009; 163: 965–976.

[109] Dámaso S, Viadero C. Normal and Pathological changes in aging brain. Revista Neuropsicología, Neuropsiquiatría y Neurociencias. 2012; 12: 21–36.

[110] Bliss TVP, Lømo T. Long-lasting potentiation of synaptic transmission in the dentate area of the anaesthetized rabbit following stimulation of the perforant path. Journal of Physiology. 1973; 232: 331–356.

[111] Alvarez VA, Sabatini BL. Anatomical and physiological plasticity of dendritic spines. Annual Review of Neuroscience. 2007; 30: 79–97.

[112] VanGuilder HD, Farley JA, Yan H, Van Kirk CA, Mitschelen M, Sonntag WE, et al. Hippocampal dysregulation of synaptic plasticity-associated proteins with age-related cognitive decline. Neurobiology of Disease. 2011; 43: 201–212.

[113] Schliebs R, Arendt T. The cholinergic system in aging and neuronal degeneration. Behavioural Brain Research. 2011; 221: 555–563.

[114] London A, Benhar I, Schwartz M. The retina as a window to the brain-from eye research to CNS disorders. Nature Reviews Neurology. 2013; 9: 44–53.

[115] Ramachandran VS. Encyclopedia of the Human Brain. Academic Press; 2002.

[116] Faden AI, Salzman S. Pharmacological strategies in CNS trauma. Trends in Pharmacological Sciences. 1992; 13: 29–35.

[117] Schwartz M, Belkin M, Yoles E, Solomon A. Potential treatment modalities for glaucomatous neuropathy: neuroprotection and neuroregeneration. Journal of Glaucoma. 1996; 5: 427–432.

[118] Crowe MJ, Bresnahan JC, Shuman SL, Masters JN, Crowe MS. Apoptosis and delayed degeneration after spinal cord injury in rats and monkeys. Nature Medicine. 1997; 3: 73–76.

[119] Yoles E, Schwartz M. Degeneration of spared axons following partial white matter lesion: implications for optic nerve neuropathies. Experimental Neurology. 1998; 153: 1–7.

[120] Levkovitch–Verbin H, Quigley HA, Kerrigan–Baumrind LA, D'Anna SA, Kerrigan D, Pease ME. Optic nerve transection in monkeys may result in secondary degeneration of retinal ganglion cells. Investigative Ophthalmology & Visual Science. 2001; 42: 975–982.

[121] Levkovitch-Verbin H, Quigley HA, Martin KR, Zack DJ, Pease ME, Valenta DF. A model to study differences between primary and secondary degeneration of retinal ganglion cells in rats by partial optic nerve transection. Investigative Ophthalmology & Visual Science. 2003; 44: 3388–3393.

[122] Vidal-Sanz M, Bray GM, Villegas-Perez M, Thanos S, Aguayo AJ. Axonal regeneration and synapse formation in the superior colliculus by retinal ganglion cells in the adult rat. Journal of Neuroscience. 1987; 7: 2894–2909.

[123] Villegas-Perez M, Vidal-Sanz M, Bray GM, Aguayo AJ. Influences of peripheral nerve grafts on the survival and regrowth of axotomized retinal ganglion cells in adult rats. Journal of Neuroscience. 1988; 8: 265–280.

[124] Keirstead S, Rasminsky M, Fukuda Y, Carter D, Aguayo A, Vidal-Sanz M. Electrophysiologic responses in hamster superior colliculus evoked by regenerating retinal axons. Science. 1989; 246: 255–257.

[125] Moalem G, Leibowitz–Amit R, Yoles E, Mor F, Cohen IR, Schwartz M. Autoimmune T cells protect neurons from secondary degeneration after central nervous system axotomy. Nature Medicine. 1999; 5: 49–55.

[126] Kipnis J, Yoles E, Porat Z, Cohen A, Mor F, Sela M, et al. T cell immunity to copolymer 1 confers neuroprotection on the damaged optic nerve: possible therapy for optic neuropathies. Proceedings of the National Academy of Sciences of the United States of America. 2000; 97: 7446–7451.

[127] Lingor P, Teusch N, Schwarz K, Mueller R, Mack H, Bähr M, et al. Inhibition of Rho kinase (ROCK) increases neurite outgrowth on chondroitin sulphate proteoglycan in

vitro and axonal regeneration in the adult optic nerve in vivo. Journal of Neurochemistry. 2007; 103: 181–189.

[128] Benowitz L, Yin Y. Rewiring the injured CNS: lessons from the optic nerve. Experimental Neurology. 2008; 209: 389–398.

[129] David S, Aguayo AJ. Axonal elongation into peripheral nervous system "bridges" after central nervous system injury in adult rats. Science. 1981; 214: 931–933.

[130] Streilein JW. Ocular immune privilege: therapeutic opportunities from an experiment of nature. Nature Reviews Immunology. 2003; 3: 879–889.

[131] Kaur C, Foulds W, Ling E. Blood–retinal barrier in hypoxic ischaemic conditions: basic concepts, clinical features and management. Progress in Retinal and Eye Research. 2008; 27: 622–647.

[132] Wilbanks GA, Wayne Streilein J. Fluids from immune privileged sites endow macrophages with the capacity to induce antigen-specific immune deviation via a mechanism involving transforming growth factor-β. European Journal of Immunology. 1992; 22: 1031–1036.

[133] Taylor A, Streilein J. Inhibition of antigen-stimulated effector T cells by human cerebrospinal fluid. Neuroimmunomodulation. 1996; 3: 112–118.

[134] Nassi JJ, Callaway EM. Parallel processing strategies of the primate visual system. Nature Reviews Neuroscience. 2009; 10: 360–372.

[135] Mandal PK, Joshi J, Saharan S. Visuospatial perception: an emerging biomarker for Alzheimer's disease. Journal of Alzheimer's Disease. 2012; 31: 117–135.

[136] Livingstone MS, Hubel DH. Psychophysical evidence for separate channels for the perception of form, color, movement, and depth. Journal of Neuroscience. 1987; 7: 3416–3468.

[137] Maunsell JH, Newsome WT. Visual processing in monkey extrastriate cortex. Annual Review of Neuroscience. 1987; 10: 363–401.

[138] Chatterjee S, Callaway EM. Parallel colour-opponent pathways to primary visual cortex. Nature. 2003; 426: 668–671.

[139] Roe AW, Ts'o DY. Visual topography in primate V2: multiple representation across functional stripes. The Journal of Neuroscience. 1995; 15: 3689–3715.

[140] Braddick OJ, O'Brien JM, Wattam-Bell J, Atkinson J, Hartley T, Turner R. Brain areas sensitive to coherent visual motion. Perception-London. 2001; 30: 61–72.

[141] Possin KL. Visual spatial cognition in neurodegenerative disease. Neurocase. 2010; 16: 466–487.

[142] Zeki S. The disunity of consciousness. Progress in Brain Research. 2007; 168: 11–268.

[143] Cheung N, Mosley T, Islam A, Kawasaki R, Sharrett AR, Klein R, et al. Retinal microvascular abnormalities and subclinical magnetic resonance imaging brain infarct: a prospective study. Brain. 2010; 133: 1987–1993.

[144] Wong TY, Klein R, Sharrett AR, Couper DJ, Klein BE, Liao D, et al. Cerebral white matter lesions, retinopathy, and incident clinical stroke. JAMA. 2002; 288: 67–74.

[145] Wong TY, Klein R, Couper DJ, Cooper LS, Shahar E, Hubbard LD, et al. Retinal microvascular abnormalities and incident stroke: the Atherosclerosis Risk in Communities Study. Lancet. 2001; 358: 1134–1140.

[146] Wong TY, Klein R, Klein BE, Tielsch JM, Hubbard L, Nieto FJ. Retinal microvascular abnormalities and their relationship with hypertension, cardiovascular disease, and mortality. Survey of Ophthalmology. 2001; 46: 59–80.

[147] Kalesnykas G, Tuulos T, Uusitalo H, Jolkkonen J. Neurodegeneration and cellular stress in the retina and optic nerve in rat cerebral ischemia and hypoperfusion models. Neuroscience. 2008; 155: 937–947.

[148] Patton N, Aslam T, MacGillivray T, Pattie A, Deary IJ, Dhillon B. Retinal vascular image analysis as a potential screening tool for cerebrovascular disease: a rationale based on homology between cerebral and retinal microvasculatures. Journal of Anatomy. 2005; 206: 319–348.

[149] Baker ML, Hand PJ, Wang JJ, Wong TY. Retinal signs and stroke: revisiting the link between the eye and brain. Stroke. 2008; 39: 1371–1379.

[150] London A, Itskovich E, Benhar I, Kalchenko V, Mack M, Jung S, et al. Neuroprotection and progenitor cell renewal in the injured adult murine retina requires healing monocyte-derived macrophages. Journal of Experimental Medicine. 2011; 208: 23–39.

[151] Wardlaw JM, Doubal F, Armitage P, Chappell F, Carpenter T, Muñoz Maniega S, et al. Lacunar stroke is associated with diffuse blood–brain barrier dysfunction. Annals of Neurology. 2009; 65: 194–202.

[152] Leibowitz U, Alter M. Optic nerve involvement and diplopia as initial manifestations of multiple sclerosis. Acta Neurologica Scandinavica. 1968; 44: 70–80.

[153] McDonald W, Barnes D. The ocular manifestations of multiple sclerosis. 1. Abnormalities of the afferent visual system. Journal of Neurology, Neurosurgery, and Psychiatry. 1992; 55: 747–752.

[154] Sørensen T, Frederiksen J, Brønnum-Hansen H, Petersen H. Optic neuritis as onset manifestation of multiple sclerosis: a nationwide, long-term survey. Neurology. 1999; 53: 473–473.

[155] Patel SJ, Lundy DC. Ocular manifestations of autoimmune disease. American Family Physician. 2002; 66: 991–998.

[156] Gundogan FC, Tas A, Erdem U, Sobaci G. Retinal pathology in multiple sclerosis: insight into the mechanisms of neuronal pathology. Brain: A Journal of Neurology. 2011; 134: 1–2 /e171.

[157] Ghezzi A, Martinelli V, Torri V, Zaffaroni M, Rodegher M, Comi G, et al. Long-term follow-up of isolated optic neuritis: the risk of developing multiple sclerosis, its outcome, and the prognostic role of paraclinical tests. Journal of Neurology. 1999; 246: 770–775.

[158] Regan D, Silver R, Murray TJ. Visual acuity and contrast sensitivity in multiple sclerosis – hidden visual loss: an auxiliary diagnostic test. Brain: A Journal of Neurology. 1977; 100: 563–579.

[159] Balcer L, Baier M, Cohen J, Kooijmans M, Sandrock A, Nano-Schiavi M, et al. Contrast letter acuity as a visual component for the Multiple Sclerosis Functional Composite. Neurology. 2003; 61: 1367–1373.

[160] Fischer P, Jungwirth S, Zehetmayer S, Weissgram S, Hoenigschnabl S, Gelpi E, et al. Conversion from subtypes of mild cognitive impairment to Alzheimer dementia. Neurology. 2007; 68: 288–291.

[161] Monteiro ML, Fernandes DB, Apóstolos-Pereira SL, Callegaro D. Quantification of retinal neural loss in patients with neuromyelitis optical and multiple sclerosis with or without optic neuritis using Fourier-domain optical coherence tomography. Investigative Ophthalmology & Visual Science. 2012; 53: 3959–3966.

[162] Frohman E, Costello F, Zivadinov R, Stuve O, Conger A, Winslow H, et al. Optical coherence tomography in multiple sclerosis. Lancet Neurology. 2006; 5: 853–863.

[163] Zaveri MS, Conger A, Salter A, Frohman TC, Galetta SL, Markowitz CE, et al. Retinal imaging by laser polarimetry and optical coherence tomography evidence of axonal degeneration in multiple sclerosis. Archives of Neurology. 2008; 65: 924–928.

[164] Adam CR, Shrier E, Ding Y, Glazman S, Bodis-Wollner I. Correlation of inner retinal thickness evaluated by spectral-domain optical coherence tomography and contrast sensitivity in Parkinson disease. Journal of Neuro-ophthalmology. 2013; 33: 137–142.

[165] Masson G, Mestre D, Blin O. Dopaminergic modulation of visual sensitivity in man. Fundamental & Clinical pharmacology. 1993; 7: 449–463.

[166] Moschos MM, Tagaris G, Markopoulos I, Margetis I, Tsapakis S, Kanakis M, et al. Morphologic changes and functional retinal impairment in patients with Parkinson disease without visual loss. European Journal of Ophthalmology. 2011; 21: 24–29.

[167] Yu J, Feng Y, Xiang Y, Huang J, Savini G, Parisi V, et al. Retinal nerve fiber layer thickness changes in Parkinson disease: a meta-analysis. PLoS One. 2014; 9: e85718.

http://dx.doi.org/10.5772/64490

[168] Onofrj M, Ghilardi M, Basciani M, Gambi D. Visual evoked potentials in parkinsonism and dopamine blockade reveal a stimulus-dependent dopamine function in humans. Journal of Neurology, Neurosurgery & Psychiatry. 1986; 49: 1150–1159.

[169] Mapstone M, Dickerson K, Duffy CJ. Distinct mechanisms of impairment in cognitive ageing and Alzheimer's disease. Brain : A Journal of Neurology. 2008; 131: 1618–1629.

[170] Prvulovic D, Hubl D, Sack A, Melillo L, Maurer K, Frölich L, et al. Functional imaging of visuospatial processing in Alzheimer's disease. NeuroImage. 2002; 17: 1403–1414.

[171] Rizzo M, Anderson SW, Dawson J, Nawrot M. Vision and cognition in Alzheimer's disease. Neuropsychologia. 2000; 38: 1157–1169.

[172] Tippett WJ, Black SE. Regional cerebral blood flow correlates of visuospatial tasks in Alzheimer's disease. Journal of the International Neuropsychological Society. 2008; 14: 1034–1045.

[173] Kurylo DD, Corkin S, Dolan RP, Rizzo JF, Parker SW, Growdon JH. Broad-band visual capacities are not selectively impaired in Alzheimer's disease. Neurobiology of Aging. 1994; 15: 305–311.

[174] Rizzo M, Anderson S, Dawson J, Myers R, Ball K. Visual attention impairments in Alzheimer's disease. Neurology. 2000; 54: 1954–1959.

[175] Holroyd S, Shepherd ML. Alzheimer's disease: a review for the ophthalmologist. Survey of Ophthalmology. 2001; 45: 516–524.

[176] Jackson GR, Owsley C. Visual dysfunction, neurodegenerative diseases, and aging. Neurologic Clinics. 2003; 21: 709–728.

[177] Cummings JL. Alzheimer's disease. The New England Journal of Medicine. 2004; 351: 56–67.

[178] Denise A. V. Alzheimer's disease: visual system review. Optometry. 2010; 81: 12–21.

[179] Frost S, Martins RN, Kanagasingam Y. Ocular biomarkers for early detection of Alzheimer's disease. Journal of Alzheimer's Disease. 2010; 22: 1–16.

[180] Kirby E, Bandelow S, Hogervorst E. Visual impairment in Alzheimer's disease: a critical review. Journal of Alzheimer's Disease. 2010; 21: 15–34.

[181] Chiu K, Chan T, Wu A, Leung IY, So K, Chang RC. Neurodegeneration of the retina in mouse models of Alzheimer's disease: what can we learn from the retina? Age. 2012; 34: 633–649.

[182] Chiu K, So K, Chang RC. Progressive neurodegeneration of retina in Alzheimer's disease—are β-amyloid peptide and tau new pathological factors in glaucoma? In: Rumelt S, editor. Glaucoma – basic and clinical aspects. InTech; 2013. p. 157–177.

[183] Sivak JM. The aging eye: common degenerative mechanisms between the Alzheimer's brain and retinal disease. Investigative Ophthalmology & Visual Science. 2013; 54: 871–880.

[184] Ong Y, Ong Y, Ikram MK, Chen CLH, Wong TY, Cheung CY. Potential applications of Spectral-Domain Optical Coherence Tomography (SD-OCT) in the study of Alzheimer's Disease. Proceedings of Singapore Healthcare. 2014; 23: 74–83.

[185] Dehabadi MH, Davis BM, Wong TK, Cordeiro MF. Retinal manifestations of Alzheimer's disease. Neurodegenerative Disease Management. 2014; 4: 241–252.

[186] Thomson KL, Yeo JM, Waddell B, Cameron JR, Pal S. A systematic review and meta-analysis of retinal nerve fiber layer change in dementia, using optical coherence tomography. Alzheimer's & Dementia: Diagnosis, Assessment & Disease Monitoring. 2015; 1: 136–143.

[187] Kopishinskaya S, Svetozarskiy S. Retinal optical coherence tomography in neurodegenerative diseases (review). Sovremennye Tehnologii v Medicine. 2015; 7: 116–123.

[188] Parnell M, Guo L, Abdi M, Cordeiro MF. Ocular manifestations of Alzheimer's disease in animal models. International Journal of Alzheimer's Disease. 2012; 2012: 786494.

[189] Goldstein LE, Muffat JA, Cherny RA, Moir RD, Ericsson MH, Huang X, et al. Cytosolic β-amyloid deposition and supranuclear cataracts in lenses from people with Alzheimer's disease. Lancet. 2003; 361: 1258–1265.

[190] Bei L, Shui Y, Bai F, Nelson SK, Van Stavern GP, Beebe DC. A test of lens opacity as an indicator of preclinical Alzheimer Disease. Experimental Eye Research. 2015; 140: 117–123.

[191] Tsai Y, Lu B, Ljubimov AV, Girman S, Ross-Cisneros FN, Sadun AA, et al. Ocular changes in TgF344-AD rat model of Alzheimer's disease. Investigative Ophthalmology & Visual Science. 2014; 55: 523–534.

[192] Frost S, Kanagasingam Y, Sohrabi H, Vignarajan J, Bourgeat P, Salvado O, et al. Retinal vascular biomarkers for early detection and monitoring of Alzheimer's disease. Translational Psychiatry. 2013; 3: e233.

[193] de la Torre JC. Alzheimer disease as a vascular disorder: nosological evidence. Stroke. 2002; 33: 1152–1162.

[194] Bell RD, Zlokovic BV. Neurovascular mechanisms and blood–brain barrier disorder in Alzheimer's disease. Acta Neuropathologica. 2009; 118: 103–113.

[195] Mroczkowska S, Benavente-Perez A, Patel S, Qin L, Bentham P, Gherghel D. Retinal vascular dysfunction relates to cognitive impairment in Alzheimer disease. Alzheimer Disease and Associated Disorders. 2014; 28: 366–367.

[196] Ning A, Cui J, To E, Ashe KH, Matsubara J. Amyloid-β deposits lead to retinal degeneration in a mouse model of Alzheimer disease. Investigative Ophthalmology & Visual Science. 2008; 49: 5136–5143.

[197] Liu B, Rasool S, Yang Z, Glabe CG, Schreiber SS, Ge J, et al. Amyloid-peptide vaccinations reduce β-amyloid plaques but exacerbate vascular deposition and inflammation in the retina of Alzheimer's transgenic mice. American Journal of Pathology. 2009; 175: 2099–2110.

[198] Gasparini L, Anthony Crowther R, Martin KR, Berg N, Coleman M, Goedert M, et al. Tau inclusions in retinal ganglion cells of human P301S tau transgenic mice: effects on axonal viability. Neurobiology of Aging. 2011; 32: 419–433.

[199] Koronyo-Hamaoui M, Koronyo Y, Ljubimov AV, Miller CA, Ko MK, Black KL, et al. Identification of amyloid plaques in retinas from Alzheimer's patients and noninvasive in vivo optical imaging of retinal plaques in a mouse model. NeuroImage. 2011; 54: S204–S217.

[200] Kayabasi U, Sergott R, Rispoli M. Retinal examination for the diagnosis of Alzheimer's disease. International Journal of Ophthalmic Pathology. 2014; 3: 4.

[201] Campbell MC, DeVries D, Emptage L, Cookson C, Kisilak M, Bueno J, Avila F. Polarization properties of amyloid beta in the retina of the eye as a biomarker of Alzheimer's disease. In Optics in the life sciences, OSA technical digest (online). Optical Society of America; 2015, paper BM3A.4.

[202] Gharbiya M, Trebbastoni A, Parisi F, Manganiello S, Cruciani F, D'Antonio F, et al. Choroidal thinning as a new finding in Alzheimer's disease: evidence from enhanced depth imaging spectral domain optical coherence tomography. Journal of Alzheimer's Disease. 2014; 40: 907–917.

[203] Bayhan HA, Aslan Bayhan S, Celikbilek A, Tanık N, Gürdal C. Evaluation of the chorioretinal thickness changes in Alzheimer's disease using spectral-domain optical coherence tomography. Clinical & Experimental Ophthalmology. 2014; 43: 145–151.

[204] Kam JH, Lenassi E, Jeffery G. Viewing ageing eyes: diverse sites of amyloid Beta accumulation in the ageing mouse retina and the up-regulation of macrophages. PLoS One. 2010; 5: e13127.

[205] Bailey TL, Rivara CB, Rocher AB, Hof PR. The nature and effects of cortical microvascular pathology in aging and Alzheimer's disease. Neurological Research. 2004; 26: 573–578.

[206] Marchesi VT. Alzheimer's dementia begins as a disease of small blood vessels, damaged by oxidative-induced inflammation and dysregulated amyloid metabolism: implications for early detection and therapy. FASEB. 2011; 25: 5–13.

[207] Miao J, Xu F, Davis J, Otte-Höller I, Verbeek MM, Van Nostrand WE. Cerebral microvascular amyloid β protein deposition induces vascular degeneration and neuroin-

flammation in transgenic mice expressing human vasculotropic mutant amyloid β precursor protein. American Journal of Pathology. 2005; 167: 505–515.

[208] Syed AB, Armstrong RA, Smith C. A quantitative analysis of optic nerve axons in elderly control subjects and patients with Alzheimer's disease. Folia Neuropatholica. 2005; 43: 1–6.

[209] Kusbeci T, Kusbeci OY, Mas NG, Karabekir HS, Yavas G, Yucel A. Stereological evaluation of the optic nerve volume in Alzheimer disease. Journal of Craniofacial Surgery. 2015; 26: 1683–1686.

[210] Cuzzo LM, Ross-Cisneros FN, Yee KM, Wang MY, Sadun AA. Low density lipoprotein receptor-related protein (LRP) is decreased in optic neuropathy of Alzheimer's disease. Journal of Neuro-ophthalmology. 2011; 31: 139–146.

[211] Wang MY, Ross-Cisneros FN, Aggarwal D, Liang C, Sadun AA. Receptor for advanced glycation end products is upregulated in optic neuropathy of Alzheimer's disease. Acta Neuropathologica. 2009; 118: 381–389.

[212] Tsai CS, Ritch R, Schwartz B, Lee SS, Miller NR, Chi T, et al. Optic nerve head and nerve fiber layer in Alzheimer's disease. Archives of Ophthalmology. 1991; 109: 199–204.

[213] Kromer R, Serbecic N, Hausner L, Aboul-enein F, Froelich L, Beutelspacher S. Detection of retinal nerve fiber layer defects in Alzheimer's disease using SD-OCT. Frontiers in Psychiatry. 2014; 5: 22.

[214] Danesh-Meyer H, Birch H, Ku JYF, Carroll S, Gamble G. Reduction of optic nerve fibers in patients with Alzheimer disease identified by laser imaging. Neurology. 2006; 67: 1852–1854.

[215] Scholtz C, Swettenham K, Brown A, Mann D. A histoquantitative study of the striate cortex and lateral geniculate body in normal, blind and demented subjects. Neuropathology and Applied Neurobiology. 1981; 7: 103–114.

[216] Dugger BN, Tu M, Murray ME, Dickson DW. Disease specificity and pathologic progression of tau pathology in brainstem nuclei of Alzheimer's disease and progressive supranuclear palsy. Neuroscience Letters. 2011; 491: 122–126.

[217] Iseki E, Matsushita M, Kosaka K, Kondo H, Ishii T, Amano N. Distribution and morphology of brain stem plaques in Alzheimer's disease. Acta Neuropathologica. 1989; 78: 131–136.

[218] Leuba G, Saini K. Pathology of subcortical visual centres in relation to cortical degeneration in Alzheimer's disease. Neuropathology and Applied Neurobiology. 1995; 21: 410–422.

[219] Parvizi J, Van Hoesen GW, Damasio A. The selective vulnerability of brainstem nuclei to Alzheimer's disease. Annals of Neurology. 2001; 49: 53–66.

[220] Katz B, Rimmer S. Ophthalmologic manifestations of Alzheimer's disease. Survey of Ophthalmology. 1989; 34: 31–43.

[221] Dai J, Vliet JVD, Swaab DF, Buijs RM. Human retinohypothalamic tract as revealed by in vitro postmortem tracing. Journal of Comparative Neurology. 1998; 397: 357–370.

[222] Swaab DF, Fliers E, Partiman T. The suprachiasmatic nucleus of the human brain in relation to sex, age and senile dementia. Brain Research. 1985; 342: 37–44.

[223] Goudsmit E, Hofman M, Fliers E, Swaab F. The supraoptic and paraventricular nuclei of the human hypothalamus in relation to sex, age and Alzheimer's disease. Neurobiology of Aging. 1990; 11: 529–536.

[224] Stopa EG, Volicer L, Kuo-Leblanc V, Harper D, Lathi D, Tate B, et al. Pathologic evaluation of the human suprachiasmatic nucleus in severe dementia. Journal of Neuropathology & Experimental Neurology. 1999; 58: 29–39.

[225] Harper DG, Stopa EG, Kuo-Leblanc V, McKee AC, Asayama K, Volicer L, et al. Dorsomedial SCN neuronal subpopulations subserve different functions in human dementia. Brain. 2008; 131: 1609–1617.

[226] Wu Y, Swaab DF. Disturbance and strategies for reactivation of the circadian rhythm system in aging and Alzheimer's disease. Sleep Medicine. 2007; 8: 623–636.

[227] Kaas JH, Lyon DC. Pulvinar contributions to the dorsal and ventral streams of visual processing in primates. Brain Research Reviews. 2007; 55: 285–296.

[228] Kuljis RO. Lesions in the pulvinar in patients with Alzheimer's disease. Journal of Neuropathology & Experimental Neurology. 1994; 53: 202–211.

[229] Braak H, Braak E. Neuropathological stageing of Alzheimer-related changes. Acta Neuropathologica. 1991; 82: 239–259.

[230] Braak H, Braak E. Evolution of neuronal changes in the course of Alzheimer's disease. In: Jellinger K, Fazekas F, Windisch M, editors. Ageing and Dementia. Vienna: Springer; 1998. p. 127–140.

[231] Dickerson BC, Bakkour A, Salat DH, Feczko E, Pacheco J, Greve DN, et al. The cortical signature of Alzheimer's disease: regionally specific cortical thinning relates to symptom severity in very mild to mild AD dementia and is detectable in asymptomatic amyloid-positive individuals. Cerebral Cortex. 2009; 19: 497–510.

[232] Hof PR, Bouras C, Constandinidis J, Morrison JH. Balit's syndrome in Alzheimer's disease: specific disruption of the occipito-parietal visual pathway. Brain Research. 1989; 493: 368–375.

[233] Hof PR, Morrison JH. Quantitative analysis of a vulnerable subset of pyramidal neurons in Alzheimer's disease. II. Primary and secondary visual cortex. Journal of Comparative Neurology. 1990; 301: 55–64.

[234] Buee L, Hof P, Bouras C, Delacourte A, Perl D, Morrison J, et al. Pathological alterations of the cerebral microvasculature in Alzheimer's disease and related dementing disorders. Acta Neuropathologica. 1994; 87: 469–480.

[235] Wong-Riley M, Antuono P, Ho K, Egan R, Hevner R, Liebl W, et al. Cytochrome oxidase in Alzheimer's disease: biochemical, histochemical, and immunohistochemical analyses of the visual and other systems. Vision Research. 1997; 37: 3593–3608.

[236] Leuba G, Saini K. Pathology of subcortical visual centres in relation to cortical degeneration in Alzheimer's disease. Neuropathology and Applied Neurobiology. 1995; 21: 410–422.

[237] Leuba G, Kraftsik R. Visual cortex in Alzheimer's disease: Occurrence of neuronal death and glial proliferation, and correlation with pathological hallmarks. Neurobiology of Aging. 1994; 15: 29–43.

[238] Cronin-Golomb A, Corkin S, Growdon JH. Visual dysfunction predicts cognitive deficits in Alzheimer's disease. Optometry & Vision Science. 1995; 72: 168–176.

[239] Levine DN, Lee JM, Fisher C. The visual variant of Alzheimer's disease A clinicopathologic case study. Neurology. 1993; 43: 305.

[240] Cohen J, Cronin-Golomb A, Growdon JH, Corkin S. Color vision deficits in Alzheimer's disease. Society for Neuroscience Abstracts. 1988; 14: 219.

[241] Martinelli V, Locatelli T, Comi G, Lia C, Alberoni M, Bressi S, et al. Pattern visual evoked potential mapping in Alzheimer's disease correlations with visuospatial impairment. Dementia and Geriatric Cognitive disorders. 1996; 7: 63–68.

[242] Baloyannis S. Dendritic pathology in Alzheimer's disease. Journal of the Neurological Sciences. 2009; 283: 153–157.

[243] Mavroudis IA, Fotiou DF, Manani MG, Njaou SN, Frangou D, Costa VG, et al. Dendritic pathology and spinal loss in the visual cortex in Alzheimer's disease: a Golgi study in pathology. International Journal of Neuroscience. 2011; 121: 347–354.

[244] Cronin-Golomb A, Corkin S, Rizzo JF, Cohen J, Growdon JH, Banks KS. Visual dysfunction in Alzheimer's disease: relation to normal aging. Annals of Neurology. 1991; 29: 41–52.

[245] Mendez MF, Tomsak RL, Remler B. Disorders of the visual system in Alzheimer's disease. Journal of Neuro-Ophthalmology. 1990; 10: 62–69.

[246] Rizzo M, Nawrot M. Perception of movement and shape in Alzheimer's disease. Brain. 1998; 121: 2259–2270.

[247] Sadun A, Borchert M, DeVita E, Hinton D, Bassi C. Assessment of visual impairment in patients with Alzheimer's disease. American Journal of Ophthalmology. 1987; 104: 113–120.

[248] Murgatroyd C, Prettyman R. An investigation of visual hallucinosis and visual sensory status in dementia. International Journal of Geriatric Psychiatry. 2001; 16: 709–713.

[249] Chapman FM, Dickinson J, McKeith I, Ballard C. Association among visual hallucinations, visual acuity, and specific eye pathologies in Alzheimer's disease: treatment implications. American Journal of Psychiatry. 1999; 156: 1983–1985.

[250] Uhlmann RF, Larson EB, Koepsell TD, Rees TS, Duckert LG. Visual impairment and cognitive dysfunction in Alzheimer's disease. Journal of General Internal Medicine. 1991; 6: 126–132.

[251] Bassi CJ, Solomon K, Young D. Vision in aging and dementia. Optometry & Vision Science. 1993; 70: 809–813.

[252] Wood S, Mortel KF, Hiscock M, Breitmeyer BG, Caroselli JS. Adaptive and maladaptive utilization of color cues by patients with mild to moderate Alzheimer's disease. Archives of Clinical Neuropsychology. 1997; 12: 483–489.

[253] Massoud F, Chertkow H, Whitehead V, Overbury O, Bergman H. Word-reading thresholds in Alzheimer disease and mild memory loss: a pilot study. Alzheimer Disease & Associated Disorders. 2002; 16: 31–39.

[254] Rizzo III JF, Cronin-Golomb A, Growdon JH, Corkin S, Rosen TJ, Sandberg MA, et al. Retinocalcarine function in Alzheimer's disease: a clinical and electrophysiological study. Archives of Neurology. 1992; 49: 93–101.

[255] Shuren J, Heilman KM. Visual field loss in Alzheimer's disease. Journal of the American Geriatrics Society. 1993; 41: 1114–1115.

[256] Whittaker K, Burdon M, Shah P. Visual field loss and Alzheimer's disease. Eye. 2002; 16: 206–208.

[257] Gilmore GC, Levy JA. Spatial contrast sensitivity in Alzheimer's disease: a comparison of two methods. Optometry & Vision Science. 1991; 68: 790–794.

[258] Gilmore GC, Whitehouse PJ. Contrast sensitivity in Alzheimer's disease: a 1-year longitudinal analysis. Optometry & Vision Science. 1995; 72: 83–91.

[259] Crow RW, Levin LB, LaBree L, Rubin R, Feldon SE. Sweep visual evoked potential evaluation of contrast sensitivity in Alzheimer's dementia. Investigative Ophthalmology & Visual science. 2003; 44: 875–878.

[260] Hutton JT, Morris JL, Elias JW, Poston JN. Contrast sensitivity dysfunction in Alzheimer's disease. Neurology. 1993; 43: 2328–2328.

[261] Baker D, Mendez M, Townsend J, Ilsen P, Bright D. Optometric management of patients with Alzheimer's disease. Journal of the American Optometric Association. 1997; 68: 483–494.

[262] Cronin-Golomb A, Gilmore GC, Neargarder S, Morrison SR, Laudate TM. Enhanced stimulus strength improves visual cognition in aging and Alzheimer's disease. Cortex. 2007; 43: 952–966.

[263] Rami L, Serradell M, Bosch B, Villar A, Molinuevo JL. Perception Digital Test (PDT) for the assessment of incipient visual disorder in initial Alzheimer's disease. Neurologia. 2007; 22: 342–347.

[264] Curran S, Wilson S, Musa S, Wattis J. Critical Flicker Fusion Threshold in patients with Alzheimer's disease and vascular dementia. International Journal of Geriatric Psychiatry. 2004; 19: 575–581.

[265] Valdés M, De Flores T. Psychobiology of stress. Barcelona: Martínez Roca; 1985.

[266] Carmel D, Lavie N, Rees G. Conscious awareness of flicker in humans involves frontal and parietal cortex. Current Biology. 2006; 16: 907–911.

[267] Mendola JD, Cronin-Golomb A, Corkin S, Growdon JH. Prevalence of visual deficits in Alzheimer's disease. Optometry and Vision Science. 1995; 72: 155–167.

[268] Curran S, Wattis J. Critical flicker fusion threshold: a potentially useful measure for the early detection of Alzheimer's disease. Human Psychopharmacology: Clinical and Experimental. 2000; 15: 103–112.

[269] Jackson GR, Owsley C, McGwin G. Aging and dark adaptation. Vision Research. 1999; 39: 3975–3982.

[270] Blake R, Wilson H. Binocular vision. Vision Research. 2011; 51: 754–770.

[271] Kiyosawa M, Bosley T, Chawluk J, Jamieson D, Schatz N, Savino P, et al. Alzheimer's disease with prominent visual symptoms. Clinical and metabolic evaluation. Ophthalmology. 1989; 96: 1077–1085; discussion 1085–1086.

[272] Mendez M, Chekrier M, Meadows R. Depth perception in Alzheimer's disease. Perceptual and Motor Skills. 1996; 83: 987–995.

[273] Thiyagesh SN, Farrow TF, Parks RW, Accosta-Mesa H, Young C, Wilkinson ID, et al. The neural basis of visuospatial perception in Alzheimer's disease and healthy elderly comparison subjects: an fMRI study. Psychiatry Research: Neuroimaging. 2009; 172: 109–116.

[274] Vaney DI, Sivyer B, Taylor WR. Direction selectivity in the retina: symmetry and asymmetry in structure and function. Nature Reviews Neuroscience. 2012; 13: 194–208.

[275] Chapman C, Hoag R, Giaschi D. The effect of disrupting the human magnocellular pathway on global motion perception. Vision Research. 2004; 44: 2551–2557.

[276] Skottun B. On the use of visual motion perception to assess magnocellular integrity. Journal of Integrative Neuroscience. 2011; 10: 15–32.

[277] Trick GL, Silverman SE. Visual sensitivity to motion age-related changes and deficits in senile dementia of the Alzheimer type. Neurology. 1991; 41: 1437–1437.

[278] Francis PT, Palmer AM, Snape M, Wilcock GK. The cholinergic hypothesis of Alzheimer's disease: a review of progress. Journal of Neurology, Neurosurgery & Psychiatry. 1999; 66: 137–147.

[279] Tales A, Troscianko T, Lush D, Haworth J, Wilcock G, Butler S. The pupillary light reflex in aging and Alzheimer's disease. Aging. 2001; 13: 473–478.

[280] Fotiou F, Fountoulakis K, Tsolaki M, Goulas A, Palikaras A. Changes in pupil reaction to light in Alzheimer's disease patients: a preliminary report. International Journal of Psychophysiology. 2000; 37: 111–120.

[281] Prettyman R, Bitsios P, Szabadi E. Altered pupillary size and darkness and light reflexes in Alzheimer's disease. Journal of Neurology, Neurosurgery & Psychiatry. 1997; 62: 665–668.

[282] Scinto LF, Daffner KR, Dressler D, Ransil BI, Rentz D, Weintraub S, et al. A potential noninvasive neurobiological test for Alzheimer's disease. Science. 1994; 266: 1051–1054.

[283] Ferrario E, Molaschi M, Villa L, Varetto O, Bogetto C, Nuzzi R. Is videopupillography useful in the diagnosis of Alzheimer's disease? Neurology. 1998; 50: 642–644.

[284] FitzSimon JS, Waring SC, Kokmen E, McLaren JW, Brubaker RF. Response of the pupil to tropicamide is not a reliable test for Alzheimer disease. Archives of Neurology. 1997; 54: 155–159.

[285] Fridh M, Havelius U, Elofsson G, Hindfelt B. The pupillary response to tropicamide in Alzheimer's disease. Acta Ophthalmologica Scandinavica. 1996; 74: 276–279.

[286] Graff-Radford NR, Lin SC, Brazis PW, Bolling JP, Liesegang TJ, Lucas JA, Uitti RJ, O'Brien PC. Tropicamide eyedrops cannot be used for reliable diagnosis of Alzheimer's disease. Mayo Clinic Proceedings. 1997; 72: 495–504.

[287] Growdon JH, Graefe K, Tennis M, Hayden D, Schoenfeld D, Wray SH. Pupil dilation to tropicamide is not specific for Alzheimer disease. Archives of Neurology. 1997; 54: 841–844.

[288] Kálmán J, Kanka A, Maglóczky E, Szóke A, Járdánházy T, Janka Z. Increased mydriatic response to tropicamide is a sign of cholinergic hypersensitivity but not specific to late-onset sporadic type of Alzheimer's dementia. Biological Psychiatry. 1997; 41: 909–911.

[289] Kurz A, Marquard R, Fremke S, Leipert K. Pupil dilation response to tropicamide: a biological test for Alzheimer's disease? Pharmacopsychiatry. 1997; 30: 12–15.

[290] Loupe DN, Newman NJ, Green RC, Lynn MJ, Williams KK, Geis TC, et al. Pupillary response to tropicamide in patients with Alzheimer disease. Ophthalmology. 1996; 103: 495–503.

[291] Treloar A, Assin M, MacDonald A. Pupillary response to topical tropicamide as a marker for Alzheimer's disease. British Journal of Clinical Pharmacology. 1996; 41: 256–257.

[292] Gómez-Tortosa E, Barrio A, Jiménez-Alfaro I. Pupil response to tropicamide in Alzheimer's disease and other neurodegenerative disorders. Acta Neurologica Scandinavica. 1996; 94: 104–109.

[293] Granholm E, Morris S, Galasko D, Shults C, Rogers E, Vukov B. Tropicamide effects on pupil size and pupillary light reflexes in Alzheimer's and Parkinson's disease. International Journal of Psychophysiology. 2003; 47: 95–115.

[294] Grünberger J, Linzmayer L, Walter H, Rainer M, Masching A, Pezawas L, et al. Receptor test (pupillary dilatation after application of 0.01% tropicamide solution) and determination of central nervous activation (Fourier analysis of pupillary oscillations) in patients with Alzheimer's disease. Neuropsychobiology. 1999; 40: 40–46.

[295] Hou R, Samuels E, Raisi M, Langley R, Szabadi E, Bradshaw C. Why patients with Alzheimer's disease may show increased sensitivity to tropicamide eye drops: role of locus coeruleus. Psychopharmacology. 2006; 184: 95–106.

[296] Iijima A, Haida M, Ishikawa N, Ueno A, Minamitani H, Shinohara Y. Re-evaluation of tropicamide in the pupillary response test for Alzheimer's disease. Neurobiology of Aging. 2003; 24: 789–796.

[297] Kaneyuki H, Mitsuno S, Nishida T, Yamada M. Enhanced miotic response to topical dilute pilocarpine in patients with Alzheimer's disease. Neurology. 1998; 50: 802–804.

[298] Reitner A, Baumgartner I, Thuile C, Dilmaghani R, Ergun E, Kaminsky S, et al. The mydriatic effect of tropicamide and its diagnostic use in Alzheimer's disease. Vision Research. 1997; 37: 165–168.

[299] Levin LA, Nilsson SFE, Ver Hoeve J, Wu S, Kaufman PL, Alm A. Adler's physiology of the eye. Elsevier Health Sciences; 2011. p. 796.

[300] Rüb U, Del Tredici K, Schultz C, Büttner-Ennever J, Braak H. The premotor region essential for rapid vertical eye movements shows early involvement in Alzheimer's disease-related cytoskeletal pathology. Vision research. 2001; 41: 2149–2156.

[301] Boxer AL, Garbutt S, Seeley WW, Jafari A, Heuer HW, Mirsky J, et al. Saccade abnormalities in autopsy-confirmed frontotemporal lobar degeneration and Alzheimer disease. Archives of Neurology. 2012; 69: 509.

[302] McCulloch DL, Marmor MF, Brigell MG, Hamilton R, Holder GE, Tzekov R, et al. ISCEV Standard for full-field clinical electroretinography (2015 update). Documenta Ophthalmologica. 2015; 130: 1–12.

[303] Strenn K, Dal-Bianco P, Weghaupt H, Koch G, Vass C, Gottlob I. Pattern electroretinogram and luminance electroretinogram in Alzheimer's disease. Journal of Neural Transmission Suppl. 1991; 33: 73–80

[304] Prager TC, Schweitzer FC, Peacock LW, Garcia CA. The effect of optical defocus on the pattern electroretinogram in normal subjects and patients with Alzheimer's disease. American Journal of Ophthalmology. 1993; 116: 363–369.

[305] Nesher R, Trick GL. The pattern electroretinogram in retinal and optic nerve disease. Documenta Ophthalmologica. 1991; 77: 225–235.

[306] Sartucci F, Borghetti D, Bocci T, Murri L, Orsini P, Porciatti V, et al. Dysfunction of the magnocellular stream in Alzheimer's disease evaluated by pattern electroretinograms and visual evoked potentials. Brain Research Bulletin. 2010; 82: 169–176.

[307] M Moschos M, Markopoulos I, Chatziralli I, Rouvas A, G Papageorgiou S, Ladas I, et al. Structural and functional impairment of the retina and optic nerve in Alzheimer's disease. Current Alzheimer Research. 2012; 9: 782–788.

[308] Simao LM. The contribution of optical coherence tomography in neurodegenerative diseases. Current Opinion in Ophthalmology. 2013; 24: 521–527.

[309] He XF, Liu YT, Peng C, Zhang F, Zhuang S, Zhang JS. Optical coherence tomography assessed retinal nerve fiber layer thickness in patients with Alzheimer's disease: a meta-analysis. International Journal of Ophthalmology. 2012; 5: 401–405.

[310] Lu Y, Li Z, Zhang X, Ming B, Jia J, Wang R, et al. Retinal nerve fiber layer structure abnormalities in early Alzheimer's disease: evidence in optical coherence tomography. Neuroscience Letters. 2010; 480: 69–72.

[311] Chi Y, Wang YH, Yang L. The investigation of retinal nerve fiber loss in Alzheimer's disease. Chinese Journal of Ophthalmology. 2010; 46: 134–139.

[312] Shen Y, Shi Z, Jia R, Zhu Y, Cheng Y, Feng W, et al. The attenuation of retinal nerve fiber layer thickness and cognitive deterioration. Frontiers in Cellular Neuroscience. 27 2013; 7: 142.

[313] Kirbas S, Turkyilmaz K, Anlar O, Tufekci A, Durmus M. Retinal nerve fiber layer thickness in patients with Alzheimer disease. Journal of Neuro-Ophthalmology. 2013; 33: 58–61.

[314] Oktem EO, Derle E, Kibaroglu S, Oktem C, Akkoyun I, Can U. The relationship between the degree of cognitive impairment and retinal nerve fiber layer thickness. Neurological Sciences. 2015; 36: 1141–1146.

[315] Ascaso FJ, Cruz N, Modrego PJ, Lopez-Anton R, Santabárbara J, Pascual LF, et al. Retinal alterations in mild cognitive impairment and Alzheimer's disease: an optical coherence tomography study. Journal of Neurology. 2014; 261: 1522–1530.

[316] Liu D, Zhang L, Li Z, Zhang X, Wu Y, Yang H, et al. Thinner changes of the retinal never fiber layer in patients with mild cognitive impairment and Alzheimer's disease. BMC Neurology. 2015; 15: 14.

[317] Cheung CY, Ong YT, Hilal S, Ikram MK, Low S, Ong YL, et al. Retinal ganglion cell analysis using high-definition optical coherence tomography in patients with mild cognitive impairment and Alzheimer's disease. Journal of Alzheimer's Disease. 2015; 45: 45–56.

[318] Vickers J. The cellular mechanism underlying neuronal degeneration in glaucoma: parallels with Alzheimer's disease. Australian and New Zealand Journal of Ophthalmology. 1997; 25: 105–109.

[319] McKinnon SJ. Glaucoma: ocular Alzheimer's disease. Frontiers in Bioscience. 2003; 8: s1140–s1156.

[320] Guo L, Duggan J, Cordeiro M. Alzheimers disease and retinal neurodegeneration. Current Alzheimer Research. 2010; 7: 3–14.

[321] Bayer A, Ferrari F, Erb C. High occurrence rate of glaucoma among patients with Alzheimer's disease. European Neurology. 2002; 47: 165–168.

[322] Tamura H, Kawakami H, Kanamoto T, Kato T, Yokoyama T, Sasaki K, et al. High frequency of open-angle glaucoma in Japanese patients with Alzheimer's disease. Journal of the Neurological Sciences. 2006; 246: 79–83.

[323] Lipton SA. Possible role for memantine in protecting retinal ganglion cells from glaucomatous damage. Survey of Ophthalmology. 2003; 48: S38–S46.

[324] Osborne NN. Recent clinical findings with memantine should not mean that the idea of neuroprotection in glaucoma is abandoned. Acta Ophthalmologica. 2009; 87: 450–454.

[325] Bach-Holm D, Kessing SV, Mogensen U, Forman JL, Andersen PK, Kessing LV. Normal tension glaucoma and Alzheimer disease: comorbidity? Acta Ophthalmologica. 2012; 90: 683–685.

Chapter 16

Caring for Individuals with Dementia on a Continuum: An Interdisciplinary Approach Between Music Therapy and Nursing

Kendra Ray, Ayelet Dassa, Jan Maier,
Renita Davis and Olayinka Ogunlade

Additional information is available at the end of the chapter

http://dx.doi.org/10.5772/00000

Abstract

Background: Music has long been used to ease symptoms of dementia. Several studies have shown the therapeutic benefits of music therapy to decrease symptoms of agitation in people with dementia (PWD). Other research has demonstrated that the use of music during caregiving can ease agitated behaviors. However, few studies have shown the clinical benefits of using translational research in practice between music therapists and certified nursing assistants.

Introduction: We recruited 28 nursing home residents who were diagnosed with moderate to severe dementia to determine the effects of music therapy and music in aid of caregiving on symptoms of agitation.

Methods: Participants were evaluated for agitation, then baseline assessments were completed 2 weeks apart. After the 2-week music therapy intervention, participants were evaluated immediately, 2 weeks post music therapy, and immediately following music in aid of caregiving.

Results: A repeated measures analysis of variance (ANOVA) found that after 2 weeks of music therapy, agitation was significantly reduced and symptoms continued to decline following music in aid of caregiving.

Conclusion: Results suggest that consideration for interdisciplinary use of music therapy and music in aid of caregiving should be considered to reduce and sustain symptoms of agitation in nursing home residents with dementia.

Keywords: dementia, caregiving, Alzheimer's disease, nursing, nonpharmacological, music therapy, interdisciplinary, agitation, music, brain, neuroscience

1. Introduction

Caring for people with dementia (PWD) has become a focal point of policy makers, researchers, and healthcare providers. With over 30 million people globally and five million people in the USA diagnosed with Alzheimer's disease and other types of dementia, the need for capable and effective caregiving is necessary [1]. Music therapy has been shown to decrease neuropsychiatric symptoms of dementia [2]. It is well known that music serves as a positive nonpharmacological intervention, and when used therapeutically has the effect to reduce agitation in people who are diagnosed with dementia [3].

Caregiver burden in nursing professionals who work in long-term care facilities is often associated with compassion fatigue, burnout, moral, and psychological distress [4–6]. Music therapists are equipped with therapeutic tools that may assist in making caregiving tasks easier. Research has shown that both music therapy and caregiver-initiated music-based interventions can reduce agitation in people with dementia [7–10]. Singing and rhythm-based interventions are two examples of therapeutic techniques that may be initiated to aid in triggering a memory, changing a mood, or moving toward a desired behavior. Paid caregivers, such as nursing professionals, may be able to assist people with dementia even without any musical skills or background.

The aims of this chapter are to provide evidence of the effectiveness of a music therapy intervention used to lower agitation symptoms in nursing home residents with moderate to severe dementia. We give examples of music in aid of caregiving that may help sustain or further reduce symptoms of agitation. We hope that this chapter may be used as a resource for practitioners and paid caregivers to broaden the scope of how music may be used collaboratively in institutional settings such as nursing homes, hospitals, and hospices.

2. Literature review

2.1. Music therapy and neurological disorders

The use of music therapy in treating mental and neurological disorders is on the rise. Over the past 60 years, music therapy has developed as a clinically applied treatment in various healthcare settings administered by trained professionals who have completed an approved music therapy program.

Bonde et al. [11] explained that the process of defining music therapy both as a profession and as a discipline can vary depending on the orientation and perspective of a particular group of practitioners, or different cultures. However, the process of defining music therapy can be reflected in the way the profession itself has emerged in different countries and through various traditions. In this way, one has to take into consideration three main factors: professional background of practitioners, needs of the clients, and approach used in treatment. Music therapy can be defined as a three-dimensional therapeutic interaction between a trained music therapist, the music, and a patient who meet to reach defined goals and objectives.

Alzheimer's disease and other types of dementia are among the disorders most commonly treated with music therapy [12]. Music therapy for individuals with dementia focuses on improved communication, memory, behavioral management, and facilitating interactive relationships with therapists and carers. Music is seen as a tool to achieve those goals, and the outcomes of music sessions are measured either quantitatively [13, 14] or qualitatively [15, 16]. Hence, in both the neuroscience and music therapy models, music is used instrumentally as an isolated material for impacting change.

The research on music therapy with PWD focuses on two main topics. One examines the effect of music therapy on an increase in desirable behaviors such as concentration span and degree of participation in an activity, and the other examines how music therapy affects the reduction of unwanted behaviors such as restlessness, anxiety, and depression [17].

Music has the power to unlock memories, to be a safe place, and offer solace for people with dementia [18]. The greatest challenge, arguably, in unraveling the myriad effects of music on the brain is the sheer complexity and interactivity of neural network stimulation observed in response to music. As early as 1984, case studies and anecdotal reports described people with dementia with severe cognitive deficits who could still play and/or sing with surprising skill [13, 19–21]. This led to the development of the preservation theory—that areas of the brain involved in the recall of music memories may be preserved from the progression of the disease. Using functional magnetic resonance imagings (fMRIs) in 2009, Janata [22] suggested a role of the dorsal medial prefrontal cortex, which is slower to atrophy in Alzheimer's disease, in connection with emotionally salient long-term memories. In a more recent study, researchers used fMRIs to identify specific brain regions where musical long-term memories seemed to be stored (in the caudal anterior cingulate and the ventral pre-supplemental motor area) in healthy adults. They then contrasted scans of these same regions of healthy older adult controls with people with mild-moderate Alzheimer's disease. The results strongly support the preservation of these regions in people with Alzheimer's disease [23]. This access allows music therapists to connect with PWD where other potential treatments may fail.

2.2. Using music therapy to address agitation with PWD

Neuropsychiatric symptoms, such as agitation, in dementia have been estimated to be between 80 and 90%, and more than 80% of these symptoms persist for at least 18 months [24]. In nursing homes, agitation may be prevalent in up to 20% of individuals diagnosed with dementia [25]. Agitation may interfere with the nursing staff's ability to provide care as it is one of the most difficult symptoms to manage [26].

Many studies have shown that music therapy should be considered as treatment for individuals with dementia who exhibit signs and symptoms of agitation [10, 27–29]. In a systematic review, Livingston et al. (2014) analyzed 33 randomized controlled trials and found that music therapy along with other types of nonpharmacological interventions decreases overall agitation [30]. In their randomized controlled trial, Ridder et al.'s [31] results showed that after 6 weeks of music therapy, agitation in individuals with dementia was significantly reduced, while in the control group agitation increased. Other authors [32] found similar results for nursing home residents with dementia who received music therapy for 6 weeks. In comparison with the control group, agitation was significantly reduced following music therapy and results were sustained for 1 month after the music therapy intervention.

2.3. Daily care for PWD

With the rising number of individuals diagnosed with dementia accompanied by neuropsychiatric symptoms such as agitation, the need for capable care staff is imminent. Nursing professionals are challenged with the difficulty of tasks associated with caregiving and the behaviors that often accompany a diagnosis of dementia. PWD experience problems with activities of daily living including bathing, dressing, and eventually decision making, which for over 60% of people with dementia leads to institutionalization for assistance with care [33].

Caregiver burden in nursing home staff who work in long-term care facilities is often associated with compassion fatigue, burnout, moral, and psychological distress. These caregivers may be at risk of burnout between 5 and 37% of the time. Outcomes from a focus group performed concluded that nurses who care for people with dementia want to alleviate their suffering and improve their quality of life and may feel strained due to inadequate resources for caregiving [34]. Two other studies indicated an increasing prevalence in psychological distress in care staff who work in nursing homes for people with dementia [5, 6].

2.4. The use of music by care staff

Music medicine involves passive listening of music (usually recorded) that is provided by a medical practitioner or a paid caregiver. The music used during the interaction may or may not be selected based either on the subject's musical preference. Music medicine or music in aid of caregiving (as referred to in this chapter) is different from music therapy in that there is no attempt to develop a therapeutic relationship and the interaction does not involve psychological processes [35].

A review of nonpharmacological interventions among PWD over the past two decades found that music can decrease resistance to treatment and care [3, 29]. Music helps to reduce symptoms of anxiety during activities that pose difficulties. Several studies have documented the effectiveness of the use of music by care staff for people with dementia. One study found that nursing personnel who used singing had a positive effect on the individuals with dementia, including improved posture, increased awareness of self and surroundings, motivation, and skills to perform daily tasks. The care staff who sang with residents benefited by developing mutuality and increased interactions more than those who only played background music [36, 37]. PWD showed better cooperation and fewer behaviors exhibiting resistance to care when singing and recorded music were used, compared to these activities without the use of music [36]. Other benefits that caregiver singing appeared to influence was communication, decreased levels of aggression, and disruptive screaming [36]. Gerdner [38] has created evidence-based guidelines for paid caregivers to use individualized music for people with dementia. Her techniques are often used by professional caregivers to lessen symptoms of agitation in people with dementia. Hammar et al. (2011) performed a study using a technique called Music Therapeutic Caregiving (MTC). The author compared patterns of behavior in participants whose caregiver used the MTC with patterns of behavior of participants whose caregiver performed care as usual [39]. She found that the caregivers who did not use the MTC experienced more episodes of aggression and resistance from their care recipients than those who did not. In other studies using MTC, this author reported that caregivers described a feeling of well-being, happy, and positive interactions with the person who they were caring for. The individuals with dementia demonstrated increased positive emotions and expressed pleasure and appeared more alert due to the MTC [39].

Nursing professionals who sing and play background music can have positive effects on people with dementia. Results from a randomized controlled trial found that regularly listening to music and singing familiar songs can benefit people with dementia cognitively, emotionally, and socially. In this study, researchers found that these musical activities led by the nurses, family caregivers, choral leaders, and music therapists helped to reduce psychological burden and that singing and listening to music can have positive effects for up to 6 months for people with early dementia [40].

Other researchers have described qualitatively and quantitatively how music can help to reduce agitation during caregiving [37, 41–43]. A review article found that carers for people with dementia played a significant role in decreasing agitation and in the work of music therapy for elders with dementia in nursing homes [44]. Choi et al. [45] found that music therapy was useful in not only reducing agitation in residents with dementia but also reducing irritability, distress, and anxiety in their caregivers. Numerous studies reported that caregivers who used a tape player or a CD player were effective in reducing agitation in clients diagnosed with dementia [46–48]. Using music during caregiving taps into memories, stimulates emotions, inspires, rewards engagement, and has an effect on individuals with dementia like no other treatment [49].

2.4.1. Training program for care staff: utilizing music in daily care

Since music is an accessible tool that is a part of most people's day-to-day life, main elements (recorded music, singing, and rhythm) can be used by music therapists to instruct and make it possible for care staff, even those without any musical experience, to employ it in their work with PWD. Minimizing restlessness is significant and contributes to the person with dementia's quality of life, and also improves the caregiver's ability to give optimal and safe care. Music's positive effect renders it useful for relaxation and for softening resistance, and thus alleviating the day-to-day life of the caregiver and the person with dementia.

2.5. Elements of music: Background music, singing, and rhythm

The various musical activities that can be used in a training program for caregivers serve as a therapeutic tool with an optimum impact. Following is a review of the literature addressing each of these musical tools in working with people with dementia.

2.5.1. *The effect of background music*

Studies examining musical interventions among PWD indicate that individually or culturally matched music significantly increases the music's positive effect on the person. Individually matched music was found to be the best and most effective way to reduce restlessness among Alzheimer's patients [48, 50]. The effect of culturally matched background music on the degree of the patients' restlessness was examined among the residents of a retirement home [51]. While listening to music, a marked reduction in restlessness characteristics was observed, such as less shouting, repetitive requests for attention, and so forth. Also, positive behaviors such as singing, drumming/tapping to the rhythm of the music, smiling, and others were observed. On the other hand, when music was not heard, the number of problematic behaviors increased and the number of positive behaviors decreased [51].

2.5.2. *The effect of singing*

Singing has a central place in music therapy with PWD. The literature shows that despite their memory loss, these patients continue to sing old songs, which remain intact in their memory for longer than songs learned at a later stage in their lives. Episodic/explicit memory for songs is not only for the melody and lyrics but also for the world of associations and personal memories that the songs evoke. In practice, the songs work like a stimulus to evoke multitude memories associated with the song [22, 52–54]. The songs stimulate and encourage conversation associated with the topic of the song. Music therapy groups that focus on singing have led to an improvement in the patients' conversational capabilities and to a lively discussion about the experience of singing in the group [55]. Singing thus provides PWD with a feeling of social belonging. Singing is comforting in that it is a familiar activity, whereas cognitive activity arouses difficulty and frustration. Singing provides respites of stimulation, awareness, a pleasant feeling, and an experience of success [52]. The feeling of success is important among PWD encountering difficulty and poor functioning, which generally lead to a damaged sense of self-worth and depression. A music therapy group that focuses on singing and evoking memories can alleviate the symptoms of depression among PWD [56]. Singing can also reduce the degree of restlessness among PWD. A decrease in problematic behavior stemming from restlessness is evident during participation in a singing-focused music therapy group [57].

2.5.3. *The effect of rhythm*

Rhythm has an effect on the movement system. The body reacts automatically to rhythmic musical stimulus. Even when the listener is not moving, rhythm stimulates activity in the premotor cortex as if priming the body for movement [2, 58–60]. Movement to music is a common phenomenon across cultures, and moving in time with the beat (entrainment) appears to be pleasurable [61–64]. Toe tapping, head nodding, and dance involve perception of rhythm and the beat, which can enable synchrony among individuals, whether playing, singing, or moving.

Music helps to boost physical activity and it also has a calming effect. A group of 18 participants with dementia who took part in exercise sessions with background music showed a reduction in restlessness signs after 4 weeks of activity (twice a week), compared to a group of 18 patients who did not receive the intervention, but only "regular treatment"[50].

Even though many studies have investigated the effectiveness of using music therapy and music-based activities for people with dementia, there lacks evidence of a study that describes collaborative efforts between music therapy and nursing for nursing home residents with dementia. This study was intended to examine whether music therapy could reduce agitation in nursing home residents with moderate to severe dementia and if the reduction in agitation could be sustained or further reduced through the facilitation of music to aid in caregiving by Certified Nursing Assistants (CNAs).

3. Methods

3.1. Participants

3.1.1. Certified nursing assistants (CNAs)

At MJHS, certified nursing assistants (CNAs) are responsible for providing direct care to nursing home residents. Their duties include but are not limited to dressing, feeding, toileting, bathing, and other activities of daily living. CNAs have the most frequent and most intimate contact with nursing home residents. They report directly to unit nurse supervisors and the director of nursing who oversee their assignments and duties. At the time of the study, two CNAs reported singing with residents but for pleasure instead of with the desire to decrease or alleviate agitation. Only one of the CNAs had a history of formal musical training prior to this study. Previously, she was employed as a school teacher, but had not used music during her caregiving. For this study, there were eight CNAs recruited at the Menorah Center for Nursing and Rehabilitation, six at Metropolitan Jewish Geriatric Center, and 10 at Shorefront Center for Nursing and Rehabilitation. The majority of the CNAs were Black Caribbean American, followed by Latino and Russian. All were female, aged between 35 and 60 and reported to have five or more years of experience working with nursing home residents diagnosed with dementia.

3.1.2. CNA training

The CNAs participated in a 3-day intensive training course. The purpose of the training was to educate CNAs to facilitate music in aid of caregiving activities appropriate for the participants that they provided care. Topics in the training included foundations of music, recognizing and identifying agitation, working with an iPod for music in aid of caregiving, selecting person-preferred music and music that may influence participant behavior, and preventing agitation through the use of recorded music with six protocols that are described below. CNAs were tested on music in aid of caregiving facilitation and on their ability to use an iPod in a mock-group setting at the end of the training. Video recordings of the CNAs' use of music in aid of caregiving with participants were used for training purposes as a reflective process with the music therapist and to determine if additional education was needed.

CNAs were assigned an iPod mini that was attached to their uniform. The iPod was loaded with personalized playlists created by the research music therapist. The CNAs were also given portable speakers that could be easily stored in their pockets until ready for use. Selections for each song in the playlists were created based on individualized preference and the success of observed reductions of agitation during music therapy groups. The music therapists created other general playlists that were loaded onto the iPod. These were meant to stimulate, relax, or prompt caregiving activities depending on the need of the resident. Some examples of the types of playlists included the following: sing-a-long, Russian classical, music-assisted bathing, energizing, Caribbean, etc., **Figure 1**. As needed, the music therapists created playlists for CNAs to use with residents when they were engaged in activities that triggered agitation such as bath/shower time [42].

Sing-a-long Playlist (24 minutes)

Song-Artist	Album
Side by Side Kate Smith	I'll Be Seeing You
You Are My Sunshine Rosemary Clooney	Learnin' the Blues
Hava Nagilah The Moshe Silberstein Ensemble and Chorus	The Music of Israel
Tumbalalaika Theodore Bikel	Yiddish Folk and Theatre
Quizas, Quizas, Quizas Celia Cruz	Cuba Bella
Michael Row the Boat Ashore Peter, Paul and Mary	Sing Along
Red River Valley Frank Corrales and Cisco Trio	Sing Along
Tzenah Tzenah The Neshoma Orchestra	Jewish Play Along
God Bless America Kate Smith	The Best of Kate Smith

Figure 1. Sample sing-a-long playlist. Source: Kendra Ray, Michael McGaughy, Scott Stuart, *Music Therapy: Keys to dementia care* (New York, MJHS) 34. Print [65].

There were six music in aid of caregiving protocols written by the research music therapists and used by the CNAs in this study. A detailed description of each of these protocols can be

http://dx.doi.org/10.5772/00000

found online at https://issuu.com/mjhs/docs/2013_dementia_workbook_lr_fnl_upt. All protocols used participants' individually preferred music based on a music therapy assessment and were created specifically for the nursing home residents who participated in this study. The developed protocols were singing, music and movement, music-assisted bath/shower, music-assisted wound care, music-assisted range of motion, and tonal protocol. A variety were created in order for the CNA to have a selection to choose from that would fit most appropriately when addressing agitation. Each protocol lists the following criteria to be considered before use: staff requirements, objectives, entrance and exit criteria, duration, safety considerations, facility/equipment required, and methods for facilitation.

Singing protocol uses live and/or recorded background music to facilitate a meaningful opportunity and to prevent or reduce verbal and/or physical agitation during activities of daily living. Music playlists or CNA lead singing should be used while providing care. Communication and singing are emphasized in this protocol.

Music and movement uses background music to engage residents to decrease symptoms of agitation, such as unexplained motor activity or verbalizations, until they decrease or are diminished. For this protocol, CNAs are asked to lead movements using sensory-stimulating items such as scarves or ribbons. Pre-recorded playlists were provided that stimulate slow to moderate movement.

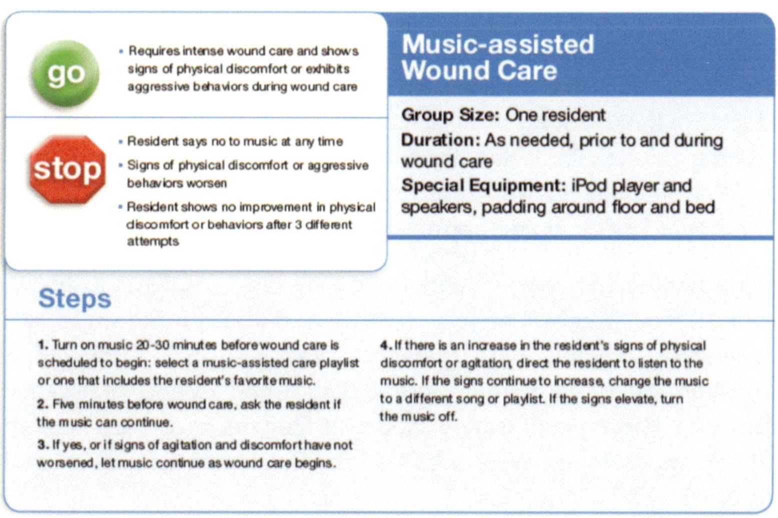

Figure 2. Abbreviated version of music-assisted wound care provided for CNAs and nursing staff. Source: Kendra Ray, Michael McGaughy, Scott Stuart, *Music Therapy: Keys to dementia care* (New York, MJHS) 70. Print [65].

Music-assisted bath/shower uses background music designed to decrease physical tension and aggressive behaviors often associated with bath time for nursing home residents with dementia. CNAs are encouraged to begin music during preparation of the bath/shower to reduce agitation and distract from anticipated stress. The selected music was customized with songs that have historically relaxed the resident. Communication, listening, and awareness of sensitivity to noise and temperature and other residents' preferences are emphasized.

For music-assisted wound care, staff are encouraged to play background music during preparation of wound care to distract the resident from anticipated stress or agitated behaviors. The music should continue to be played during and following the procedure to reach desired objectives that may include decreased discomfort, fewer or no aggressive behaviors toward nursing staff and less resistance to wound care. Instructions are demonstrated subsequently (**Figure 2**).

Music-assisted range of motion uses background music to motivate residents' involvement in motion exercises. The objectives are to decrease resistance to movement, and reduce episodes of agitation. CNAs are provided with songs of measured tempos that begin slowly and gradually increase in beats per minute as the playlist develops. Rhythm and movement are emphasized in this activity.

The tonal protocol is a music-based activity with an objective of reducing agitation and increasing socialization. Residents are encouraged to sing familiar songs and play tone bars as led by the CNA. Rhythm and movement are emphasized in this activity.

3.1.3. Residents

The CNAs and music therapists worked with a total of 28 adults between the ages of 59 and 101 whom assented to participate in this study. Legal representatives were contacted to obtain informed consent and video consent for each individual. This was part of a larger study [10] that was conducted in three Brooklyn-based nursing homes, part of the MJHS system, Menorah Center for Nursing and Rehabilitation, the former Shorefront Center for Nursing and Rehabilitation, and Metropolitan Jewish Geriatric Center. The New York University School of Medicine Institutional Review Board approved the protocol for this study.

Inclusion criteria required for participants to be long-term residents in the nursing home, informed consent from caregiver or legal guardian, mid-stage dementia as measured by Functional Assessment Staging for Alzheimer's Disease (FAST), stabilized comorbidities, auditory recognition with or without an assisted device, and absence of psychiatric disorders other than dementia. Participants were excluded if they declined participation, were being introduced to new medications, were admitted for short-term rehabilitation, had unstable comorbidities, or who had hearing loss that was uncorrectable.

Consented participants were mostly female ($n = 26$, 92.9%). The majority of participants were Caucasian ($n = 22$, 78.6%) followed by African American ($n = 4$, 14.3%). Their country of origins varied, but most were born in America ($n = 14$, 50%). Many of the participants were taking anti-anxiety ($n = 4$, 14.3%), antipsychotic ($n = 6$, 21.4%) medications, but the majority was not taking any psychotropic medications ($n = 15$, 53.6%). Participants had a documented diagnosis of dementia in their medical chart with varying types: mixed ($n = 12$, 42.9%), Alzheimer's disease ($n = 7$, 25%), unspecified/other ($n = 8$, 28.5%).

3.4. Study design

Convenience sampling was used for recruitment. Along with chart review, we received referrals for study participation from therapeutic recreation, social work and nursing departments.

3.4.1. Assessment

The Functional Assessment Staging for Alzheimer's Disease (FAST) was used to measure staging for dementia during screening process [66]. Participants who scored between 5 and 6 on the FAST were considered eligible for participation in this study. To the validity of this study, the tester did not contribute to the intervention and had no prior relationship with study participants.

3.4.2. Outcome measure

The outcome measure of the study was the Cohen-Mansfield Agitation Inventory [67]. This tool consists of 29 agitated behaviors and the score can range from 34 to 128. The Cohen-Mansfield Agitation Inventory has high inter-rater agreement rates for each behavior for nursing home residents [67]. Other researchers found that the test/retest reliability for this tool was moderate to good in nursing home residents (n = 105) who were evaluated for agitation [68].

3.4.3. Music therapy intervention

Participants in this study took part in music therapy three times a week for 2 weeks. The intervention was facilitated by two nationally board-certified music therapists who conducted music therapy assessments prior to the intervention to obtain historical, musical preferences. This information was gathered from the nursing home resident, his/her family member, recreation, or nursing staff members. Music selections for the music therapy sessions were tailored according to participants' individual preferences.

Music therapy was conducted in small groups of four to six participants in a private lounge in the nursing home where the participant lived. Each session lasted from 15 min to an hour depending on the tolerance of the participant. Musical expression was demonstrated through singing, music and movement, and tonal activities. The music therapists encouraged the residents to play a variety of rhythm instruments, djembe drums, and ocean drums. Movement was encouraged through the use of colorful scarves and ribbons. The music therapists used live music for the sessions and were self-accompanied by guitar and electronic keyboard. An in-depth description of the music therapy intervention including the songs chosen and common themes that occurred is described in our previous publication [10].

3.4.4. CNA music programming

Following the music therapy intervention, the music therapists trained CNAs to integrate music in aid of caregiving during their daily routine. The transformation design model was used to guide the training created for the CNAs [69]. The transformation design model is a framework specifically for music therapy treatment. The treatment design was created to make available scientific outcomes in clinical practice immediately [69]. The treatment design is directed by nonmusical outcomes with consideration for the nursing home residents' music and music activity preference. Steps to this model are illustrated in the following example:

1. *Gather information on nonmusical behavior*

CNA reports that resident gets agitated especially during morning care. The CNA informs the music therapist that the resident becomes agitated as soon as it is time to get dressed. The resident kicks and screams as the CNA attempts to dress her. The resident has been checked for signs and symptoms of pain or distress.

2. *Develop treatment goals and objectives*

Goal: Decrease agitation during morning care

Objectives: Decrease kicking and screaming.

3. *Design functional nonmusical activities*

Set a relaxing, musical environment for morning care activities.

4. *Design music activities*

Music therapist visits resident's room prior to morning care and sings resident's favorite songs with her. CNA joins in singing and initiates morning care and dressing resident. Music therapist exits when appropriate.

5. *Transfer outcomes to everyday setting*

Therapist creates a protocol for CNA to use that includes playing familiar music and singing lyrics of resident's favorite songs while dressing during morning care. Music therapist creates playlist on an iPod or a CD player of resident's preferred music based on positive outcomes observed during music therapy. Music therapist instructs CNA with resident's musical preferences to use with resident during morning care [69].

3.4.5. Analysis

IBM Statistical Package for Social Science (SPSS) Statistics software (version 21) was used to obtain frequencies, percentages, means and standard error, and confidence intervals for demographic information and repeated measures ANOVA analysis related to study participants.

A repeated measures ANOVA was conducted to analyze changes in Cohen-Mansfield Agitation Inventory scores for multiple data points. IBM SPSS Statistics software was used to perform the analysis. This method of analysis was chosen since each participant served as her/his own control and it enabled us to compare changes in agitation between multiple data points over time including the following: baseline 1 and baseline 2; baseline 1 and immediately following music therapy; after music therapy and 2 weeks post music therapy; immediately following music therapy and CNA facilitated music in aid of caregiving. This procedure helped to determine any changes in agitation that occurred during care as usual (between baseline 1 and baseline 2), following the music therapy intervention and following the CNA-initiated music activities.

4. Results

The goal of this study was to determine if music therapy could reduce agitation symptoms and if these changes could be sustained by music in aid of caregiving. A repeated measures ANOVA found that Cohen-Mansfield Agitation Inventory scores differed significantly between the various time points. The assumption of sphericity was met according to Mauchly's test of sphericity, x^2 (9) = 14.81, $p = 0.097$. Mauchly's test of sphericity demonstrated that the average agitation scores were significantly different between time frames F (4, 92) = 7.03, $p <$ 0.001, and that these changes can be seen visibly on a graph, **Table 1**, **Figure 3**.

Comparisons	**Mean score difference**	**Standard error**	**95% CI**	
			Lower bound	**Upper bound**
Baseline 1 vs Baseline 2	−3.33	3.77	−15.04	8.37
Post music therapy vs Baseline 1	−11.42*	2.86	−20.28	−2.55
2 weeks post music therapy vs post music therapy	1.71	2.70	−6.67	10.09
CNA MAC vs Baseline 1	−16.67*	4.03	−29.18	−4.15
CNA MAC vs post music therapy	−5.25	4.49	−19.19	8.69

*$p < 0.05$

Table 1. Bonferroni comparison of agitation scores at various time points.

Post hoc tests were performed using the Bonferroni adjustment for multiple comparisons. The results revealed that between first and second baseline, when participants were receiving care as usual, there were no significant differences in agitation scores (60.87 ± 23.00 vs 57.54 ± 24.17, $p = 1.0$). When post-music therapy scores were compared to baseline 1 scores, there was a significant difference in agitation (60.87 ± 23.00 vs 49.46 ± 21.92, $p = 0.006$) indicating that music therapy significantly contributed to reduced agitation. We measured agitation scores again 2 weeks post music therapy and found that there was a slight, but insignificant increase in agitation (49.46 ± 21.92 vs 51.17 ± 16.33, $p = 0.189$). The agitation scores declined again following CNA-initiated music in aid of caregiving activities (49.46 ± 15.25 vs 44.21 ± 15.25, $p = 0.605$), although these changes were not significant. The participants' agitation after music in aid of caregiving was significantly lower than the initial baseline scores (44.21 ± 15.25 vs 60.87 ± 23.00,

$p = 0.004$). These results suggest that routine care did not significantly affect agitation, but music therapy significantly decreased agitation symptoms. The effects of the music therapy intervention were not sustainable for 2 weeks post music therapy, but agitation declined again after music in aid of caregiving.

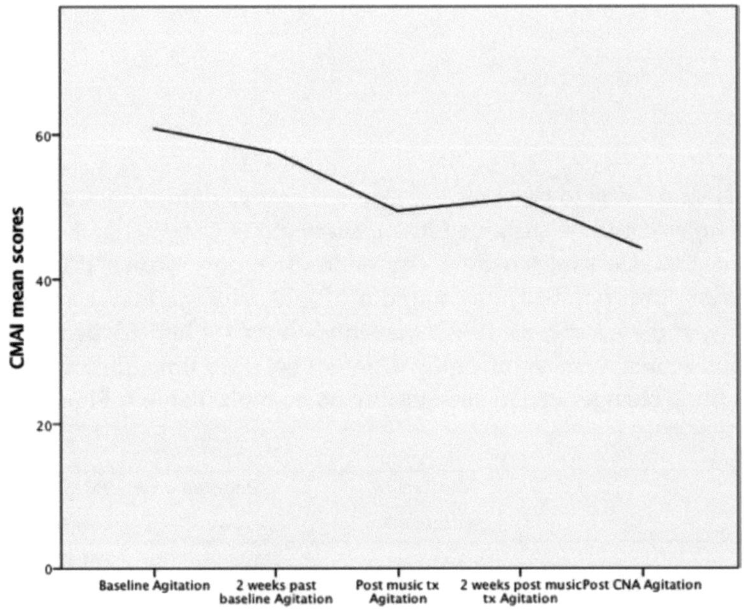

Figure 3. Changes in Cohen-Mansfield agitation scores over time.

5. Discussion and conclusion

Music therapy has been recommended as a nonpharmacological intervention to reduce behavioral symptoms related to dementia such as agitation [3, 29], though there is little research documenting the use of music as an interdisciplinary method between music therapists and nursing professionals. In the current study, we hypothesized that music therapy would reduce symptoms of agitation and that music in aid of caregiving facilitated by educated CNAs would sustain those results. We found that when compared to usual care, music therapy reduced agitation significantly, but following music therapy symptoms began to rise again slightly. When nursing home residents were introduced to music in aid of caregiving by the CNAs, agitation began to decline again. This evidence supports the initiative of researchers that nonpharmacological treatments such as music should be used to manage symptoms of agitation in PWD [70]. Because the majority of residents were taking medications to cope with agitation symptoms, our outcomes also suggest that music therapy followed by music in aid of caregiving should be considered as an interdisciplinary, yet complimentary treatment alongside pharmaceutical therapy.

Prior to the intervention, we observed that many of our residents exhibited symptoms of agitation that included spitting on staff members, cursing, and yelling. These behaviors led to CNAs spending much of their time trying to redirect and console residents using techniques that were often ineffective. The reduction of agitation scores that occurred following the music in aid of caregiving indicates that the education for the CNAs and provision of music-based tools were sufficient.

Our study followed the transformational design which presents the theory that nonmusical behaviors can be changed through the introduction of a music therapy treatment plan [69]. For this study, music therapy followed by CNA education and facilitation of music in aid of caregiving activities led to a decrease in agitation for most of our participants. The plan began with specific goals set by the music therapy researchers who used therapeutic techniques to reduce agitation. Next, music in aid of caregiving or "pleasant (musical) diversions from daily routines or struggles" [52] were used to assist in sustaining the goals set by the music therapists. These protocols (e.g., singing and music-assisted bathing) allowed for CNAs to practice skills that may have been effective during music therapy sessions [52]. From our observations, the results positively affected not only the PWD as evidenced by fewer symptoms but also the CNA who was providing care.

5.1. Conclusion

The tremendous need for nonpharmacological treatment in patients with dementia particularly highlights the importance of making music accessible as a simple and everyday tool that can help in these patients' care. The authors believe that music therapists should challenge this need and that specific training for caregivers at home or in institutions will help ease the burden of care and promote the well-being of both caregivers and people with dementia. Music therapists who work with people with dementia should expand their knowledge and expertise beyond the boundaries of the music therapy room. For that, we must differentiate between music therapy, which is performed by a professional and certified person and the use of music in aid of caregiving done by anyone who cares for people with dementia without the need for any musical background or skill. By promoting training programs in institution settings and at home, we can provide better care for those who need it.

A larger study is needed to test the effects of our intervention and provide evidence of its usefulness. We would like to propose that music in aid of caregiving is not only useful in nursing situations with CNAs but also may be beneficial for all nursing professionals to use to reduce resistance to care while giving medication and for wound care.

Because of the brain's ability to process music even in late stages of dementia [23], it may be beneficial for other healthcare practitioners besides nurses to consider adding music as a tool to aid them in their treatment. Presently, the protocols in this study have been adapted for work with home health aides, family caregivers, occupational and physical therapists, and social workers in multiple types of settings. It is currently being used in the United States, Israel, and Spain. Our future research includes work with a physiotherapist using music to aid with walking. This work will be based on a music therapy technique for patients with neurological problems that make use of rhythm to organize locomotion. Based on previous research with patients with Alzheimer's in which individuals required assistance with walking and inertia, we will test the rhythmic stimulus that may have a physiological effect and help to organize control over walking. This intervention may also reduce the need for multiple caregivers who assist the patient with walking [71].

In conclusion, the limits for the use of music in aid of caregiving are inexhaustible, but larger samples with more stringent designs are needed to confirm its worthiness. Since music is an accessible tool that is part of most people's day-to-day life, it is possible for even those without musical experience, to employ it in their work with a PWD. Minimizing restlessness is significant and contributes to the person with dementia's quality of life, and also improves caregiver's ability to give optimal and safe care. Music's positive effect renders it useful for relaxation and for softening resistance, and thus alleviating the day-to-day life of the caregiver and the person with dementia.

Author details

Kendra Ray[1,2*], Ayelet Dassa[3,4], Jan Maier[5], Renita Davis[6] and Olayinka Ogunlade[7]

*Address all correspondence to: kray@mjhs.org

1 MJHS, Menorah Center for Nursing and Rehabilitation, Brooklyn, NY, USA

2 Drexel University, Philadelphia, PA, USA

3 Bar-Ilan University, Ramat Gan, Israel

4 Alzheimer's Medical Center, Ramat Gan, Israel

5 Jemsong, LLC, Waltham, MA, USA

6 Troy University at Phenix City, AL, USA

7 Gemma Regis Center for Music Therapy, Lagos, Nigeria

References

[1] Prince M, Bryce R, Albanese E, Wimo A, Ribeiro W, Ferri CP. The global prevalence of dementia: a systematic review and metaanalysis. Alzheimer's & Dementia: The Journal of the Alzheimer's Association. 2013;9(1):63–75.e2.

[2] Patel AD, Iversen JR. The evolutionary neuroscience of musical beat perception: the action simulation for auditory prediction (ASAP) hypothesis. Frontiers in Systems Neuroscience. 2014;8:57.

[3] Ueda T, Suzukamo Y, Sato M, Izumi S. Effects of music therapy on behavioral and psychological symptoms of dementia: a systematic review and meta-analysis. Ageing Research Reviews. 2013;12(2):628–41.

[4] Albers G, Van den Block L, Stichele RV. The burden of caring for people with dementia at the end of life in nursing homes: a postdeath study among nursing staff. International Journal of Older People Nursing. 2014;9:106–17.

[5] Astrom S, Nilsson M, Norberg A, Winbald B. Empathy, experience of burnout and attitudes towards demented patients amoung nursing staff in geriatric care. Journal of Advanced Nursing. 1990;15:1236–44.

[6] Kuremyr D, Kihlgren M, Norberg A, Astrom S, Karlsson I. Emotional experiences, empathy and burnour among staff carring for demented patients at a collective living unit and a nursing home. Journal of Advanced Nursing. 1994;19:670–9.

[7] Garland K, Beer E, Eppingstall B, O'Connor DW. A comparison of two treatments of agitated behavior in nursing home residents with dementia: simulated family presence and preferred music. The American Journal of Geriatric Psychiatry: Official Journal of the American Association for Geriatric Psychiatry. 2007;15(6):514–21.

[8] Guetin S, Portet F, Picot MC, Pommie C, Messaoudi M, Djabelkir L, et al. Effect of music therapy on anxiety and depression in patients with Alzheimer's type dementia: randomised, controlled study. Dementia and Geriatric Cognitive Disorders. 2009;28(1): 36–46.

[9] Raglio A, Bellelli G, Traficante D, Gianotti M, Ubezio MC, Villani D, et al. Efficacy of music therapy in the treatment of behavioral and psychiatric symptoms of dementia. Alzheimer Disease and Associated Disorders. 2008;22(2):158–62.

[10] Ray KD, Mittelman MS. Music therapy: A nonpharmacological approach to the care of agitation and depressive symptoms for nursing home residents with dementia. Dementia. 2015.

[11] Wigram T, Pedersen N, Bonde LO. A Comprehensive Guide to Music Therapy: Theory, Clinical Practice and Training. London: Jessica Kingsley Publishers, Ltd; 29–35, 2002.

[12] Hara M. Music in dementia care: increased understanding through mixed research methods. Music and Arts in Action. 2011;3(2):34–58.

[13] Cuddy L, Duffin J. Music, memory, and Alzheimer's disease; Is music recognition spared in dementia, and how can it be assessed? Medical Hypotheses. 2005;64(2):229–35.

[14] Vink AC, Bruinsma MS, Scholter RJPM. Music therapy for people with dementia. The Cochrane Collaboration. 2011(4):1–50.

[15] Clair AA. The effect of singing on alert responses in persons with late stage dementia. Journal of Music Therapy. 1996;33:234–47.

[16] Simpson F. Creative music therapy: Last resort? In: Aldridge D, editor. Music Therapy for People with Dementia. London: Jessica Kingsley Publishers; 2000. p. 166–83.

[17] Music therapy in dementia treatment. Presentatoin to the 19th International Symposium on Research in Music Behavior; 2011; Barcelona, Spain.

[18] Clark CN, Warren JD. Music, memory and mechanisms in Alzheimer's disease. Brain: A Journal of Neurology. 2015;138(Pt 8):2122–5.

[19] Beatty WW, Winn P, Adams EW, Wilson DA, Prince JR, et al. Preserved cognitive skills in dementia of the Alzheimer's type. Archives of Neurology. 1994;51:1040–6.

[20] Beatty WW, Zavadil KD, Bailly R, Rixen G, et al. Preserved musical skill in a severely demented patient. International Journal of Clinical Neuropsychology. 1988;10(4):158–64.

[21] Sacks OW. Musicophillia. New York: Alfred A. Knopf; 2007.

[22] Janata P. The neural architecture of music-evoked autobiographical memories. Cerebral cortex (New York, NY: 1991). 2009;19(11):2579–94.

[23] Jacobsen JH, Stelzer J, Fritz TH, Chetelat G, La Joie R, Turner R. Why musical memory can be preserved in advanced Alzheimer's disease. Brain: A Journal of Neurology. 2015;138(Pt 8):2438–50.

[24] Steinberg M, Tschanz JT, Corcoran C, Steffens DC, Norton MC, Lyketsos CG, et al. The persistence of neuropsychiatric symptoms in dementia: the Cache County Study. International Journal of Geriatric Psychiatry. 2004;19(1):19–26.

[25] Morley JE. Dementia-related agitation. Journal of the American Medical Directors Association. 2011;12(9):611–2.e2.

[26] Faull C, Carter YH, Daniels L. Handbook of Palliative Care. MA: Blackwell Publishing; 2005.

[27] Cox E, Nowak M, Buettner P. Managing agitated behavior in people with Alzheimer's disease: the role of live music. The British Journal of Occupational Therapy. 2011;11:517–24.

[28] Raglio A, Bellelli G, Traficante D, Gianotti M, Ubezio MC, Gentile S, et al. Efficacy of music therapy treatment based on cycles of sessions: a randomised controlled trial. Aging & Mental Health. 2010;14(8):900–4.

[29] Patel B, Perera M, Pendleton J, Richman A, Majumdar B. Psychosocial interventions for dementia: from evidence to practice. Advances in Psychiatric Treatment. 2014;20:340–9.

[30] Livingston G, Kelly L, Lewis-Holmes E, Baio G, Morris S, Patel N, et al. Non-pharmacological interventions for agitation in dementia: systematic review of randomised

controlled trials. The British Journal of Psychiatry: The Journal of Mental Science. 2014;205(6):436–42.

[31] Ridder HM, Stige B, Qvale LG, Gold C. Individual music therapy for agitation in dementia: an exploratory randomized controlled trial. Aging & Mental Health. 2013;17(6):667–78.

[32] Lin Y, Chu H, Yang CY, Chen CH, Chen SG, Chang HJ, et al. Effectiveness of group music intervention against agitated behavior in elderly persons with dementia. International Journal of Geriatric Psychiatry. 2011;26(7):670–8.

[33] Rabins PV, Blass DM. In the Clinic. Dementia. Annals of Internal Medicine. 2014;161(3):ITC1; quiz ITC16.

[34] Edberg AK, Bird M, Richards DA, Woods R, Keeley P, Davis-Quarrell V. Strain in nursing care of people with dementia: nurses' experience in Australia, Sweden and United Kingdom. Aging & Mental Health. 2008;12(2):236–43.

[35] Dileo C. Effects of music and music therapy on medical patients: a meta-analysis of the research and implications for the future. Journal of the Society for Integrative Oncology. 2006;4(2):67–70.

[36] Gotell E, Brown S, Ekman SL. Influence of caregiver singing and background music on posture, movement, and sensory awareness in dementia care. International Psychogeriatrics/IPA. 2003;15(4):411–30.

[37] Gotell E, Brown S, Ekman SL. Caregiver singing and background music in dementia care. Western Journal of Nursing Research. 2002;24(2):195–216.

[38] Gerdner LA. Consumer version of evidence-based guidelines: Individualized music for elders with dementia. In: Titler M, editor. Series on Evidence-Based Practice for Older Adults. Iowa City, IA: The University of Iowa College of Nursing Gerontological Nursing Interventions Research Center; Research Dissemination Core; 2007.

[39] Hammar LM. Caregivers' Singing Facilitates Mutual Encounter: Implementation and Evaluation of Music Therapeutic Caregiving in Complex Dementia Care Situations. Karolinska Institute. Stockholm, Sweden; 2011.

[40] Sarkamo T, Tervaniemi M, Laitinen S, Numminen A, Kurki M, Johnson JK, et al. Cognitive, emotional, and social benefits of regular musical activities in early dementia: randomized controlled study. The Gerontologist. 2014;54(4):634-50 doi:10.1093/geront/gnt100.

[41] Hoeffer B, Talerico KA, Rasin J, Mitchell CM, Stewart BJ, McKenzie D, et al. Assisting cognitively impaired nursing home residents with bathing: effects of two bathing interventions on caregiving. The Gerontologist. 2006;46(4):524–32.

[42] Ray KD, Fitzsimmons S. Music-assisted bathing: making shower time easier for people with dementia. Journal of Gerontological Nursing. 2014;40(2):9–13.

[43] Thomas D, Heltman R, Alexander T. The effects of music on bathing cooperation for residents with dementia. Journal of Music Therapy. 1997;34(4):246–59.

[44] Wall M, Duffy A. The effects of music therapy for older people with dementia. British Journal of Nursing 2010;19(2):108–13.

[45] Choi AN, Lee MS, Cheong KJ, Lee JS. Effects of group music intervention on behavioral and psychological symptoms in patients with dementia: a pilot-controlled trial. The International Journal of Neuroscience. 2009;119(4):471–81.

[46] Cohen-Mansfield J, Werner P. Management of verbally disruptive behaviors in nursing home residents. The Journals of Gerontology Series A, Biological Sciences and Medical Sciences. 1997;52(6):M369–77.

[47] Gerdner LA, Swanson EA. Effects of individualized music on confused and agitated elderly patients. Archives of Psychiatric Nursing. 1993;7(5):284–91.

[48] Gerdner LA. Effects of individualized versus classical "relaxation" music on the frequency of agitation in elderly persons with Alzheimer's disease and related disorders. International Psychogeriatrics/IPA. 2000;12(1):49–65.

[49] Weeks S. Connecting through music with people with dementia: A guide for caregivers. Journal of Mental Health. 2011;20:503.

[50] Sung HC, Chang AM, Lee WL. A preferred music listening intervention to reduce anxiety in older adults with dementia in nursing homes. Journal of Clincal Nursing. 2010;19(7–8):1056–64.

[51] Ziv N, Granot A, Hai S, Dassa A, Haimov I. The effect of background stimulative music on behavior in Alzheimer's patients. Journal of Music Therapy. 2007;44(4):329–43.

[52] Clair AA, Memmott J. Therapeutic Uses of Music with Older Adults. Silver Spring, MD: American Music Therapy Association; 2008.

[53] Tomaino C. The role of music in the rehabilitation of persons with neurologic diseases. Music Therapy Today (online). 2002.

[54] Koelsch S. Music-evoked emotions: principles, brain correlates, and implications for therapy. Annals of the New York Academy of Science 2015;1337:193–201.

[55] Dassa A, Amir D. The role of singing familiar songs in encouraging conversation among people with middle to late stage Alzheimer's disease. Journal of Music Therapy. 2014;51(2):131–53.

[56] Ashida S. The effect of reminiscence music therapy sessions on changes in depressive symptoms in elderly persons with dementia. Journal of Music Therapy. 2000;37(3):170.

[57] Svansdottir HB, Snaedal J. Music therapy in moderate and severe dementia of Alzheimer's type: a case–control study. International Psychogeriatrics/IPA. 2006;18(4): 613–21.

[58] Kung SJ, Chen JL, Zatorre RJ, Penhune VB. Interacting cortical and basal ganglia networks underlying finding and tapping to the musical beat. Journal of Cognitive Neuroscience. 2013;25(3):401–20.

[59] Grahn JA, Brett M. Rhythm and beat perception in motor areas of the brain. Journal of Cognitive Neuroscience. 2007;19(5):893–906.

[60] Grahn JA, Rowe JB. Feeling the beat: premotor and striatal interactions in musicians and nonmusicians during beat perception. The Journal of Neuroscience: The Official Journal of the Society for Neuroscience. 2009;29(23):7540–8.

[61] Drake C, Penel A, Bigand E. Tapping in time with mechanically and expressively performed music. Music Perception. 2000;18:1–24.

[62] Nettl B. An ethnomusicologist contemplates universals in musical sound and musical culture. In: Wallin NL, Merker B, Brown S, editors. The Origins of Music. Cambridge, MA: MIT Press; 2000. p. 463–72.

[63] Brown S, Jordania J. Universals in the world's musics. Psychology of Music. 2013;41:229–48.

[64] Zatorre RJ, Salimpoor VN. From perception to pleasure: music and its neural substrates. Proceedings of the National Academy of Sciences of the United States of America. 2013;110(Suppl 2):10430–7.

[65] Ray KD, McGaughy M, Stuart S. Music Therapy: Keys to Dementia Care. New York, NY: MJHS; 2013.

[66] Sclan SG, Reisberg B. Functional assessment staging (FAST) in Alzheimer's disease: reliability, validity, and ordinality. International Psychogeriatrics/IPA. 1992;4(Suppl 1): 55–69.

[67] Cohen-Mansfield J, Marx MS, Rosenthal AS. A description of agitation in a nursing home. Journal of Gerontology: Medical Sciences. 1989;44(3):M77–M84.

[68] Zuidema SU, Buursema AL, Gerritsen MG, Oosterwal KC, Smits MM, Koopmans RT, et al. Assessing neuropsychiatric symptoms in nursing home patients with dementia: reliability and Reliable Change Index of the Neuropsychiatric Inventory and the Cohen-Mansfield Agitation Inventory. International Journal of Geriatric Psychiatry. 2011;26(2):127–34.

[69] Thaut M. Rhythm, Music, And the Brain: Scientific Foundations and Clinical Applications. New York, NY: Taylor & Francis; 2008.

[70] Herrman N, Gauthier S. Diagnosis and treatment of dementia: Management of severe Alzheimer's disease. Canadian Medical Association Journal. 2008;179(12):1279–87.

[71] Clair AA, O'Konski M. The effect of rhythmic audotiry stimulation (RAS) on gait characteristics of cadence, velocity, and stride length in persons with late stage dementia. Journal of Music Therapy. 2006;43(2):154–63.

Chapter 17

Behavior and Emotion in Dementia

Teresa Mayordomo Rodríguez, Alicia Sales Galán,
Rita Redondo Flores, Marta Torres Jordán and
Javier Bendicho Montes

Additional information is available at the end of the chapter

http://dx.doi.org/10.5772/64681

Abstract

During the course of disease, the patient and caregiver face emotional and behavioral problems that may occur. Therefore, it is important to knowing how emotions and the perception of them are modified and thus to know the impact they have on mood and behavior of the patient and caregiver. Publicizing the type of pathology, both emotional and behavioral levels, in a patient with dementia can help in the development of nonpharmacological interventions that could slow the symptoms and improve the quality of life of patients.

Keywords: reminiscence, autobiographical memory, behavior disorders, nonpharmacological therapies, dementia

1. Introduction

Given the impact of aging in today's society and the possible development of dementia throughout this stage of the life cycle; it is interesting to deal with this type of pathology. So far, studies have mainly focused on more cognitive and biological aspects, because its main symptom is a neurobiological origin. While in this disease, also changes in emotional and psychosocial part occur, which affects both the well-being of the largest and in its important work in dementia caregiver. This chapter describes the most effective methods, from the current literature by searching the database principals (scopus, science direct, psychology articles, etc.)., that could provide positive effects in emotions and psychological and behavioral symptoms. The keywords used for the search were aging, dementia, emotions, autobiographical memory, reminiscence, psychological and behavioral disorders, nonpharmacological interventions, etc. From these we selected those belonging to current and high-impact journals.

2. Emotions, aging, and dementia

Although the emotions have been studied for many years, a unanimous definition of this concept has not yet been reached. Emotions are physical responses controlled by the brain that make it possible to survive hostile environments and ensure the procreation of the species [1]. Emotions are actions expressed in the face, voice, or specific behaviors that tend to maintain the homeostasis of the organism [2]. In other words, and following other authors, the emotions are regulatory processes of action that arise in response to a trigger stimulus or identifiable object and activate estimative processes of the significance of these stimuli in relation to the goal pursued, producing changes in response systems, and different moods. Each emotion depends on a different neural network and produces specific corporal configurations that can be recognized in others [3].

We can distinguish between two main types of emotions; primary and secondary [4]. Primary emotions are considered innate and depend on the limbic system, especially the amygdala and anterior cingulated cortex. They are not culturally determined, but rather universal with a biological origin. The secondary emotions arise when the feeling is experienced, that is, when there is awareness of the emotions; they allow us to make connections between the stimuli, the situation, and the primary emotions. Secondary emotions are composed of the combination of primary emotions refined by experience, and they can give rise to possible emotional pathologies such as anxiety and depression.

For quite some time, aging has been studied on the basis of losses and gains, focusing the research above all on the cognitive part of the individual; however, it is well known that the noncognitive symptoms are disturbing to the families and caregivers of patients with dementia, and they can also seriously affect the well-being of the patients [5].

Following this line of thought, there is evidence that with age, one loses cognitive capacity. For example, it is more difficult to focus one's attention, and the memory begins to fail. This situation becomes more evident in the case of pathological aging framed within the field of cognitive impairment and dementia. However, with regard to the emotions, it is not clear to what degree their processing is affected by age or what these changes are, with contradictory results found regarding the perception of basic emotions by patients with dementia. In some cases, these patients show worse recognition of their emotions, whereas in other cases, no differences are found between patients with dementia and a group of healthy older people [6].

With regard to emotional processing in aging, this topic has been studied from two different and seemingly contradictory perspectives: the socio-cognitive approach to the emotions proposed and developed by Carstensen [7] and the neuropsychological approach, which relates certain brain areas to the processing of information with emotional content.

Both approaches study the emotions in aging, but obtaining different conclusions about the changes that occur in emotional processing. On the one hand, the sociocognitive component focuses on what people think or feel, basically studying this component and suggesting that it does not decline with age and even improves [7]. On the other hand, the neuropsychological approach, interested basically in the processing of the emotional content of stimuli, argues that in both normal and pathological aging, there is a change in the identification of the negative emotions produced by a deficit in certain cerebral areas. Therefore, the consequences of the physiological changes stemming from aging are related to their effects on people's affective lives [8].

It is well known that adequate emotional processing is fundamental for normal emotional development [9]. Alzheimer's disease (AD) has been widely studied with regard to the identification of emotions, given that the affective state declines progressively from the asymptomatic stage until the terminal phase. The patients no longer perceive their environment with the same emotional base as before the disease. It is possible that this new affective state is progressive and can be detected early, through a basic analysis of the deficits in emotional information processing that will evolve into a greater degree of cognitive and emotional impairment as the disease progresses [10].

Regarding emotional perception, in AD the deficit in emotional recognition could be due to the progressive atrophy of the amygdala, the anterior temporal cortex, and the orbital frontal cortex [11]. Their study consists of presenting faces showing the basic emotions to a sample of mild AD patients, who have to identify and indicate the name of the emotions. They repeated the task 3 years later. Their conclusions were that the recognition of emotional expression was affected as the disease progressed, and that this impairment was related to the degeneration of the cortical structures involved.

Other studies [12–14] indicate that patients with AD have an impaired capacity to process the facial expressions of emotion, probably due to the characteristic cognitive deterioration associated with the disease, especially in the attention and memory processes of the amygdala [11] and other brain structures that modulate emotional processing [15].

Taking the emotional process into account, some studies have pointed out that the depressive disorder is associated with a greater risk of developing cognitive alterations in aging [16] especially in AD [17]. Considering this relationship, some researchers have examined the temporal relationship between depression and AD in order to understand whether depression is simply a prodromic symptom of the disease that precedes the appearance of cognitive deficits, or whether a history of depression could be an independent risk factor for the development of the disease. Moreover, depression can occur in 30/40% of patients with AD [18], and it affects the clinical evolution of the disease. Many depressed people ignore positive information and focus on memories that support negative emotions, thus impeding the maintenance and achievement of psychological well-being or life satisfaction, while worsening the conservation of their identity in the present and, therefore, their quality of life.

However, people with AD can feel diverse emotions, even though they generally do not remember what sparked them [19]. Therefore, the emotions remain in the individual and, therefore, can be worked with as a way to improve the emotional well-being of patients with AD.

One of the aspects most linked to emotional well-being is the feeling of identity. People who have AD have limited access to the autobiographical memories related to identity maintenance, self-knowledge, and self-image.

Along these lines, the autobiographical memory (AM) plays a fundamental role in the construction and conservation of personal identity [20]. It is indispensable for maintaining a sense of continuity and understanding the self throughout the life cycle. In addition, it contributes to the development of daily activities such as social relationships, decision making, or problem solving [21].

Memories related to personal events from the past are much more complex and emotional than nonautobiographical memories, and they also contain more intimate information related to the self [22, 23]. Thus, they are more likely to be kept in the memory than nonautobiographical memories, even in pathological aging.

Therefore, autobiographical memories are an essential aspect in the progression of AD because they allow the preservation of the identity, which will contribute to the development of positive emotions or emotional well-being.

3. Autobiographical memory

3.1. Autobiographical memory: what it is and its main characteristics

Autobiographical memory (AM) is part of the episodic memory, as it deals with specific memories accompanied by a temporal and spatial context. However, the main characteristic that defines autobiographical knowledge and makes it distinctive is that the memories form part of a personal context because they are experiences the person had throughout the life cycle [24]. Generally, autobiographical memory consists of information about places, actions, people, objects, thoughts, and emotions. Some authors define it as the memory of our *self* (of our identity) in relation to the world and other people [22–25]. Thus, autobiographical memories, in addition to being situated in a specific time and place like any other memory, are also related to the individual; that is, the person experienced the past event to be remembered first-hand, and he/she is not only aware of the objective event, but also his or her own feelings, perceptions, and interpretations.

Although it is true that AM is based on episodic memory, there is also another much more generic and abstract type of autobiographical memory. AM involves two types of knowledge about oneself: episodic and semantic [26]. The episodic component consists of personal and specific events located in a specific place and time, and the semantic component stores general knowledge from the past, such as names, addresses, or general events [27–30].

These two components are associated with a different state of consciousness [31]: on the one hand, autonoetic consciousness, associated with the episodic component and, on the other,

http://dx.doi.org/10.5772/64681

noetic consciousness, associated with the semantic component [32, 33]. Autonoetic consciousness is defined as the feeling of re-experiencing or reliving a past event, in other words, subjectively traveling in time to our past. Not only is the event itself recalled, but sensory-perceptual details derived from the event are also recovered, that is, experiences that contain perceptual, affective, and temporal-spatial details. They give the memory a personal meaning that makes it form part of our identity and goes beyond mere knowledge. By contrast, noetic consciousness is the capacity to know or have certain information about the world or about our lives, without any contextual details.

Some studies [34–36] show the dissociation between aspects of the two types of consciousness in aging. As we age, we go from an autonoetic consciousness to a noetic consciousness. Therefore, with age, the semantic component of autobiographical memory increases, whereas the episodic component decreases.

Along the same lines, the AM forms part of the remote memory and, therefore, that its initial nature is episodic [37]. However, they propose that this information can gradually lose its contextual association and the details about a specific place and time, gradually acquiring semantic characteristics, with a generic and decontextualized organization like other semantic knowledge.

3.2. Localization of autobiographical memories

Regarding the temporal distribution of autobiographical memories throughout the life cycle, have been revealed a similar pattern of memory localization in older people [38, 39]. This irregular pattern is characterized by three key memory points: childhood amnesia, the reminiscence peak or *bump*, and the recency effect (see **Figure 1**).

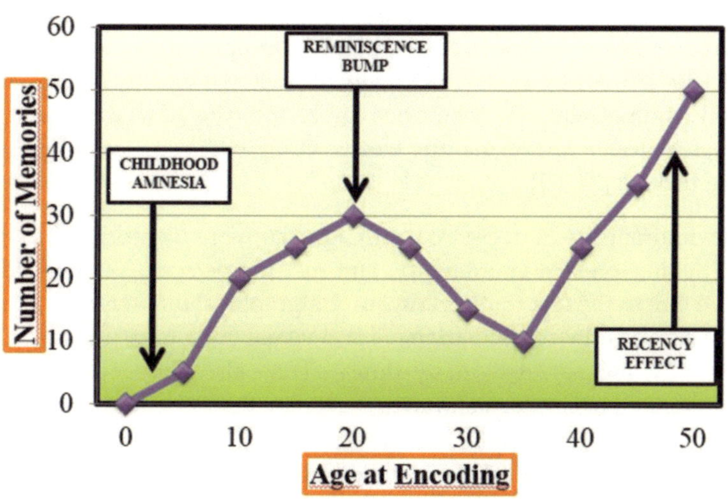

Figure 1. Localization of autobiographical memories.

3.2.1. Childhood amnesia

Memories from the first years of life are practically nonexistent, a phenomenon known as childhood amnesia. This absence of memories occurs because up to the age of 5, the brain structures that make it possible to codify and store memories are not fully developed. Everyone presents an almost complete absence of memories coming from the first years of life [40].

3.2.2. The reminiscence bump

From 10 to 30 years old, we have a large number of memories; in fact, it is the period in life that is remembered the most. Research shows that the memories most evoked by older people are those that took place during adolescence and early adulthood [41], which makes sense given that the majority of a person's relevant life events take place in this phase, such as the first love, first job, wedding, or in many cases, emigration to other places.

3.2.3. Recency effect

The last phenomenon presented on the autobiographical memory curve is the "recency effect". This effect involves events that took place in recent years, that is, a person's most recent memories. As time passes, the "recent" memories become "remote" and lose quality [42]. This fact can be observed in the figure, where, from the point of recency backward, the number of memories is lower as one tries to remember times further in the past.

3.3. Autobiographical memory during aging

Scientific research has pointed out that, as the years go by, the aging process affects memory in general. With regard to autobiographical memory, research reveals that there is deterioration in the episodic part of autobiographical memory in standard aging. Most studies have compared young subjects (about 35 years old) to older subjects [34, 43–47], but other studies have reported a progressive decline in episodic autobiographical memory, comparing healthy subjects aged 50–100 [35, 36, 45, 48, 49]. However, the fact that the loss of episodic details leads to a greater production of semantic memories can be interpreted as a process of **"semantization"** of autobiographical memory. In other words, the episodic memory is not lost, but instead it becomes semanticized [34, 35].

Nevertheless, even though AM decreases with age, there are memories that revive affective and perceptual details, present spontaneity, and mix the perspectives of field and observer [36]. This may be due to the fact that certain autobiographical memories are characterized by defining our identity, as they contain affective and visual imaginary aspects with a high level of practice (due to being narrated many times). They also have a high level of personal relevance and are linked to similar memories that share the same topic and accessibility [50].

3.4. Autobiographical memory decline in the course of Alzheimer-type dementia

Numerous studies have investigated the AM losses experienced by subjects with AD. Most studies agree that there is a deficit in this type of memory [37, 51–58], but there is disagreement

http://dx.doi.org/10.5772/64681

about the pattern of the deficit: which component is more deteriorated, the episodic or the semantic? Which memories show a greater degree of decline, the recent ones or the remote ones?

All the studies agree that in AD, the episodic component of AM is deteriorated [37, 48, 54, 55, 57, 59–61]. In other words, there are great difficulties in mentally reviving past events and phenomenological aspects such as visual images [48]. In this direction, it has been shown that patients with AD presented a worse capacity to recover specific autobiographical events [62], a deficit related to the lack of ability to mentally recover these events. This loss leads to the decontextualization or semantization of autobiographical memories, and a change in the ability to mentally recover events from the past. Thus, AD patients have a more general feeling of familiarity, expressed as the feeling of "having experienced this before".

In the case of semantic autobiographical knowledge, the conclusions do not coincide. On the one hand, some studies observe impairment in this type of autobiographical knowledge from the first stages of the disease [54, 57], while others point out that it is preserved until moderate phases of the disease [48, 63, 64].

3.5. Loss of identity

As mentioned above, AM is necessary for the development and maintenance of personal identity. Autobiographical memories contribute to the development of social relationships, decision making, or problem solving [21].

Patients with AD have limited access to memories that make up their self-awareness, self-knowledge, and self-image, leading to a compromised sense of identity. This problem has been evaluated in various studies, observing that poor autobiographical knowledge was significantly correlated with a weak sense of identity [54].

However, based on the fact that remote memories are better recalled than recent ones, at least until moderate phases of AD, certain personal memories would be expected to be relatively preserved in the memory. These memories probably come from the reminiscence bump stage, which includes the most important events that have defined their life stories. This stage is the one most studied in the literature, as it is the memory component most related to identity and, therefore, contains more self-defining memories and events with a high emotional charge and a strong impact on the sense of identity [22].

Along the same lines, many studies have investigated the effect of AD on self-defining memories. One of these studies pointed out that most of the autobiographical memories of participants with AD also came from their reminiscence bump. However, it has also been shown that the subjects with AD contribute fewer specific self-defining memories, compared to control subjects [45]. Therefore, self-defining memories, or memories that are highly relevant to one's self-image, seem to decline from moderate stages of AD, which can explain the reduced sense of identity that occurs in this disease. Even so, it should be mentioned that in AD the semantic component of autobiographical memory is maintained until moderate phases of the disease. Different studies have shown that the personal semantic memory contributes to numerous cognitive processes related to self-referential thinking, as a reflection of the self in the past, imagining the personal future, and maintaining one's self-identity [65]. In fact, the semantic AM supports the knowledge about personal traits, roles, thoughts, and beliefs, aspects related to self-referential thinking, which is highly conceptual and independent from the medial temporal lobe [65]. Therefore, semantic AM, which is relatively preserved in the initial and moderate stages of AD, can be used as an aid to improve self-identity and self-continuity, and to develop the self-referential cognition strategy.

3.6. Clinical rehabilitation of the autobiographical memory in AD

The objective of the clinical rehabilitation of the AM in AD is to recover, as much as possible, the inaccessible memories, or at least maintain the "pool" of autobiographical memories that are still available. There are different therapeutic strategies, one of which is reminiscence therapy.

This therapy focuses on the conscious recall of personal memories from one's life in order to report, think about, tell, or show something about our experiences from the past. Reminiscence was originally proposed by Butler [66], who has promoted it as a tool to improve well-being and reduce depressive symptoms in older adults. Since then, reminiscence has been widely applied in cognitive rehabilitation in aging, including in pathologies like AD.

4. Reminiscence therapy

Initially, reminiscence was developed for elderly people with normal aging to offer them a chance to remember and organize the most significant events in their lives [66]. However, the idea of using reminiscence therapy in people with dementia was introduced in 1979 [67].

Reminiscence, defined by Webster [68] as "the present recall and interpretation of life events experienced at some time in the past, generally in the distant past", is a way of maintaining the personal past and perpetuating the person's identity. It is a very complete technique because it uses stimulation, communication, socialization, and entertainment [69]. In addition, reminiscence involves the systematic recall of old memories: recalling personal events in all their depth, noises, smells, images, emotions, as a way of activating the personal past [70]. Thus, reminiscence can be described as the organized and systematic use of memories and recollections to awaken or strengthen identity and self-esteem.

Some definitions of reminiscence refer to recalling personally important memories from the past, a selective process in which the memories are events in the life of a person or group of people [71]. It is an organized, complex mental activity with an important purpose: to reawaken or strengthen identity and self-esteem, recoding them in scenarios and scenes, people, events, traumas, and topics based on autobiographical memory [72].

The definition of reminiscence in the field of dementias frequently appears in the literature and offers a more detailed description of the processes that intervene in it [73]. Reminiscence therapy includes the discussion of past activities, experiences, and events with another person or group of people, generally with the help of eliciting stimuli or indications [73].

Reminiscence has been shown to be a useful intervention in interdisciplinary work between the neuropsychologist and gerontologist, due to its low cost and because it allows the psychostimulation mainly of the language and memory functions. It establishes connections between the past, present, and future person, promoting sociability and openness to interpersonal relationships, confirming a sense of identity, and reinforcing feelings of self-esteem, personal worth, coherence, and continuity [74]. This intervention has commonly been used in people with cognitive impairment [75]. In fact, some authors [74, 76] show that people with dementia can benefit from this intervention to foment and/or strengthen their current relationships and maintain them over time, and protect themselves from isolation and withdrawal. In addition, others indicate an improvement in cognition, mood, and behavior in general, and a reduction in caregiver stress [73].

Before explaining the process of holding a reminiscence session for people with dementia and the benefits of doing so, it should be mentioned that Wong and Watt described six types of reminiscence [77], and in 2007 Cappeliez et al. [78] added two others, finally yielding eight types of reminiscence, defined in **Table 1**.

Integrative	Its main function is to try to give meaning to the person's relationship with his her past
Preparation for death	Which connotes a certain spirituality by facing the topic of death and the afterlife with a degree of serenity
Obsessive	In which certain individual problems are observed in integrating problematic past situations
Evasive or Escapist	In which the fantasy of some memories is used to "escape" from the individual s current situation
Instrumental	Takes advantage of the subject's previous experiences to resolve and deal with current problems
Transmitter	Where the person realizes that the reminiscence transmits to a younger generation some of the knowledge and lasting values he she acquired over time
Intimacy	Where the cognitive and emotional representations of important people in our lives who are no longer with us are recalled instead of their physical appearance
Narrative	Defined as the description of past events, in order to acquire biographical information, and for the pleasure of narrating them

Table 1. Types of reminiscence.

These eight types of reminiscence have been grouped in an integrated model through a triadic system [79] (see **Figure 2**). Therefore, the eight types of reminiscence are divided into three specific functions: the *self*, reminiscences of an interpersonal nature that seek coherence and meaning; *orientation,* in terms of recalling and sharing personal knowledge and experiences; and *social connectedness*, providing the basic elements for maintaining relationships, with an interpersonal and continuity nature, and proposing emotion management as a basic characteristic. Although the first two functions mainly refer to coping and the orientation, other authors point out that both involve the reactivation and strengthening of a feeling of personal competence or self-efficacy [79]. Therefore, there is a degree of overlapping between the function of guide and the *self*, especially in integrative reminiscence.

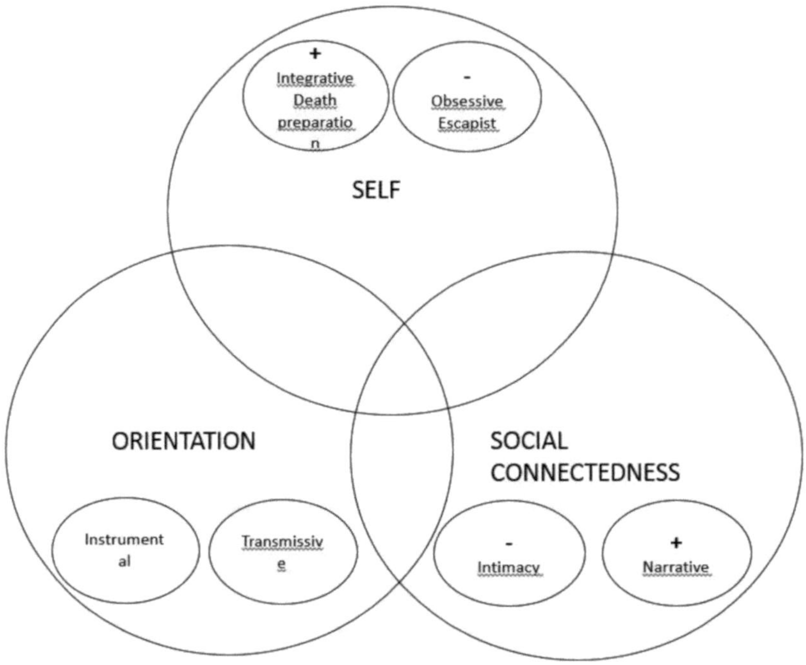

Figure 2. Triadic reminiscence system.

Using reminiscence with people with dementia is not the same as using this type of intervention with people who have no cognitive pathologies. It is necessary to make a series of changes or modifications [80]. The objectives of the sessions have to be flexible enough to adapt them to the participants and their cognitive ability. The materials used should be as close as possible to the participants to facilitate the evocation of the memory. The groups must be small, and the cognitive performance of the participants should be taken into account. It is important to obtain the participation of family members in preparing the sessions, or they can even participate in them. In this way, there is better knowledge about the participants' personal information, and they can refer to their own biography during the sessions and provide support when necessary. It is advisable and important to refrain from correcting memories that diverge from reality, as the main objective of the activity must be the emotional validation of the orientation, and not of the memory itself.

The intervention must be directed by a psychologist or professional trained in carrying out these types of programs. Normally, it will consist of 10 or 15 sessions lasting 60 min each, with one session per week. In each session, all the life stages will be worked on (childhood, youth, adulthood, and old age) through a specific topic. All the sessions must follow the same structure: at the beginning, the members of the group are welcomed and told what topic will be addressed. After that, two activities are performed using specific stimuli (music, images, objects, etc.) to evoke their memories and sayings and quotations related to the topic of the session. In both cases, participants perform a free-association exercise that consists of saying or writing the first word or expression the stimulus brings to mind; then open questions are formulated to facilitate the emergence of positive personal memories; finally, participants try to connect these memories with the present [81].

With regard to the results obtained from reminiscence therapy in people with dementia, various studies have shown their efficacy and effectiveness, especially in improving mood and reducing depressive symptoms, increasing life satisfaction, and reducing agitation behaviors [75, 82–85].

In the case of depressive symptomatology and self-esteem, some studies reveal the effectiveness of this type of therapy [86–91]. This therapy has been shown to have the main consequence of reducing depressive symptomatology, reducing feelings of desperation and loneliness, and increasing positive mood state. Moreover, if we take into account the relationship between this type of therapy and positive psychology, some authors [92] indicate that one of the most characteristic facets of reminiscence is its capacity to transform negative events into good results, as the intervention fosters the positive reevaluation of less favorable situations for the participants. Thus, the use of this type of intervention leads to positive results in improving the life satisfaction of people who participate in reminiscence sessions [83, 93, 94].

In addition to the improvement in mood, an increase has also been found in some of the dimensions of psychological well-being, self-acceptance, positive relations with others, autonomy, and control over the environment [71, 81, 87, 95, 96].

As described above, Alzheimer-type dementia is produced as a characteristic of the loss of consciousness of the self. Therefore, the increase in or maintenance of the self-acceptance dimension, as shown in the studies highlighted, could slow down the appearance of dependence in the person with this pathology and play a large role in the reconstruction of the self, approaching the idea of integrity developed by Erikson [97]. Regarding the dimension of positive relationships with others, authors highlight that there is an active interaction among the members of the group, making this therapy a stimulating, happy and integrating activity and establishing a connection among the participants that creates positive relationships [98]. This quality is achieved through the narrative contributions made by the group members throughout the sessions, as they help people with greater cognitive impairment and difficulty in evoking their memories to be able, for a few moments, to glimpse in their memory some hint of their past or a similar situation experienced and share it with the other members of the group. Finally, the application of this type of therapy has increased their independent thinking, the feeling of control and competence in managing the environment they deal with in daily life, and their ability to choose and create contexts adapted to their own needs.

With regard to the results obtained on autobiographical memory after reminiscence intervention and life review procedure, results suggest that people with dementia who attend reminiscence sessions improve their autobiographical memory [85, 99, 100], being observed improvements in recalling both facts and events, that is, in semantic memory and episodic memory.

Numerous studies [85, 101–103] have shown the benefits of this therapy, observing that elderly people with AD who had participated in a reminiscence program, compared to a control group that did not participate, showed an improvement in the amount of autobiographical memory, specifically semantic AM.

Therefore, reminiscence therapy is a useful intervention that has many benefits for both the healthy population and people with cognitive impairment. Specifically in the AD population, positive effects have been observed at the emotional, cognitive, and psychosocial levels.

However, and on the emotional plane, in addition to the changes mentioned, there is a broad range of emotional or psychological and behavioral impairment in AD that has to be treated in order to improve the quality of life of the patient and his/her family context.

5. Behavioral disorders in dementia

The psychological and behavioral symptoms of dementia (BPSD) are the most worrisome symptoms because they significantly affect the patient and his/her family or main caregivers. However, they are classically the symptoms that have received less attention. These are symptoms such as depression, anxiety, irritability, hallucinations, delirium, aggressiveness, etc. In fact, this symptomatology has a high degree of frequency and is present in at least 50–90% of patients [104, 105]. Nevertheless, there is great variability in the percentages published, which shows the difficulty of estimating their prevalence.

BPSD have great repercussions because they cause a lot of problems for the patient and his/her family and social environment. They represent one of the consequences of the disease that produce the greatest disability, and one of the greatest threats to coexistence and the daily life of the family. They hinder the patient's autonomy and lead to frequent medical visits and admissions in emergency services and healthcare institutions. They have a decisive influence because they reduce the patient's quality of life and his/her level of functional autonomy [106], which leads to a decided reduction in the quality of life of the caregivers, increasing their stress. Thus, the caregivers of people with dementia suffer the consequences of these types of symptoms the most. Therefore, these symptoms become an important source of depression and desperation in caregivers [107], producing a large number of consultations with General Practitioners and becoming one of the main reasons for the institutionalization of AD patients [108, 109].

It is important to highlight that there is great heterogeneity in the appearance of these behavioral symptoms, given that not all patients present the same alterations, and they will not always appear in the same stages of the disease or increase linearly as the disease progresses [110].

Throughout the literature, diverse nomenclatures have been established to refer to this symptomatology. However, in 1996 the International Psychogeriatric Association coined the term psychological and behavioral symptoms of dementia (BPSD) to refer to the alterations in

http://dx.doi.org/10.5772/64681

perceptions, mood, or behaviors that are often present in patients with dementia [111]. Specifically, they include a variety of manifestations, such as physical aggressiveness, shouting, restlessness, agitation, erratic wandering, hyperactivity, culturally inappropriate behaviors, sexual disinhibition, abuse, inappropriate language, following another person around, etc. [112]. Below, **Table 2** shows the main alterations.

Symptoms	Definition
Delirium	Irrational or false idea or thought that distances them from a true comprehension and perception of the surroundings
Hallucinations	False perceptions that can affect any perceptual sphere
Anxiety	Feelings of anticipator fear of a danger that they consider imminent
Apathy	Loss of motivation that affects the behaviors, emotions and cognition, manifested as behaviors of lack of initiative, indifference, and loss of interest
Emotional lability	Fluctuations and brusque changes in their feelings and emotional expressions
Anomalous motor behavior	Imperious need to move without any defined objective, often accompanied by anxiety, wandering, walking around, motor hyperactivity
Sleep disorder	Insomnia, hypersomnia or parasomnias
Appetite disorder	Capricious eating, compulsive eating, or lack of appetite
Aggressiveness	Behaviors of physical or verbal violence toward people or objects, manifested as great activity involving movements, shouting, and aggression
Depression	Sadness, anhedonia, feeling of being a burden, lack of hope …
Euphoria	Abnormally good or inappropriate humor
Apathy	Lack of interest, motivation, feeling, emotion or concern
Disinhibition	Lack of social tact in language, body language, and other behaviors
Irritability	Bad mood, quick, unjustified changes in mood, impatience, intolerance
Repeated vocalizations	Any bothersome sound or vocal expression that is not due to a change in the patient or the environment

Table 2. Main behavioral and psychological symptoms of dementia.

The evaluation and diagnosis of the BPSD is carried out through observation and interviews with the patient and his/her caregivers. In addition, instruments such as the Behavioral Pathology in Alzheimer's Disease Rating Scale (BEHAVE-AD) [113] and the neuropsychiatric inventory (NPI) [114] can be quite useful.

5.1. Main causes of behavioral disorders

Behavioral problems have different origins. Below, a classification of these origins is presented:

5.1.1. Medical causes that lead to behavioral problems

First, many medications can produce secondary effects and cause confusion and changes in the level of functioning. In this situation, it is important to prepare a report of the changes occurring in the person.

Second, the sensory deficits that usually occur and accompany aging can lead to vision or hearing problems that can cause behavioral problems. Thus, it is important to carry out periodic revisions to avoid these problems.

Third, comorbidity with other diseases such as urinary infection, pneumonia, gastrointestinal infection, etc. can produce symptoms such as fever, which in turn will aggravate the confusion in the person with dementia, possibly leading to behavioral problems.

Fourth, situations of dehydration, constipation and other physiological causes such as hunger, sleepiness, or physical discomfort (e.g., headache, dizziness, etc.) can produce a strong feeling of distress and cause the person to behave in an irregular way.

5.1.2. Causes related to the environment:

At times, certain aspects or stimuli in the environment can produce some uncertainty, stress, or confusion in the patient. For example, very large and/or untidy spaces, too much stimulation, or a lot of activity in the environment (music while talking, too many people around, etc.) can make the person with dementia react with anger or frustration. In addition, an excess or lack of decorative elements, furniture, and lighting (e.g., visual contrasts between the wall and the floor, too much furniture, mirrors, etc.) and unfamiliar environments can interfere with orientation, creating more confusion.

Finally, people with dementia need a set routine and daily structure because environments without routines and disorganized surroundings can give rise to certain behavioral disorders.

5.1.3. Causes related to the task:

Certain characteristics of the task can cause some problem situations, for example:

A complicated task: Sometimes we ask a person with dementia to do tasks that are too difficult, even though they seem simple to us. Examples would be getting dressed or bathing.

An unfamiliar task: People with dementia gradually lose the ability to learn new tasks. If they are asked to do something they have never done before, they will not be able to learn it, no matter how simple it is. For example, if an appliance is changed, they will be incapable of learning how it works.

http://dx.doi.org/10.5772/64681

Too many tasks to do: The person is no longer able to do two or three things, especially at the same time. They do not know how to organize themselves or the order in which to do things, and they leave things half done and start something else, etc.

5.1.4. Causes related to communication:

Another possible cause of these problems stems from the existence of comprehension and/or expression difficulties. Communication between the family and the person with dementia is extremely important and can be difficult. People with dementia often become angry or agitated because they do not understand what is expected of them, or they get frustrated because they cannot make themselves understood. These difficulties in communication and adaptation to their surroundings arise because there are hidden or unsatisfied needs, due to behavioral learning (reinforcement systems), greater vulnerability to the environment, or less adaptation to stressful situations.

When there are hidden or unsatisfied needs that have not been identified, they can cause inappropriate behavior. These needs are often not detected by caregivers, or they do not know how to respond to them (e.g., sensory deprivation, boredom, etc.). In a recent study, the number of unaddressed needs was the main factor associated with BPSD [115]. Among these needs, there are three main types: biological (lack of food, sleep, lighting, temperature, etc.); psychological (security, empathy, affect, etc.); and social (social company, boredom, respect, etc.). The most frequently detected needs were related to doing activities, company, and help with psychological distress [115].

Regarding behavioral learning, the environmental stimuli maintain, extinguish, or change a behavior, depending on the associated reinforcement. Thus, in the presence of an antecedent stimulus, a behavior is produced, which has a consequence. But if there is a change in the antecedent or the consequence, there is a direct change in the behavior. When referring to the consequences of a behavior, we can talk about different behavioral reinforcement systems. Depending on the reinforcement applied, we can cause a behavior to increase, remain the same, or disappear. However, often the behavior of the caregiver can be creating or maintaining the BPSD, given that they positively reinforce behaviors that should be eliminated, thus producing an increase in these behaviors. For example, a caregiver could be reinforcing an agitated behavior if he/she only pays attention to the person with dementia when he/she is restless or agitated. Other caregiver behaviors that can create or maintain BPSD are: paternalistic authoritarian or infantilizing treatment, ignoring the patient, imposing things or power struggles, or frequently asking the same thing so that the patient will remember it [116]. Therefore, we must eliminate the positive reinforcement of inappropriate behaviors and promote the positive reinforcement of appropriate ones. We can also establish the learning of new behaviors by generating new stimulus-response associations; for example, if we want the patient to learn a new behavior, we have to encourage it as a response to a stimulus and reinforce it positively every time it appears.

Finally, another reason for this type of disorder is the vulnerability to the environment or poor adaptation to stressful situations. This vulnerability arises because patients gradually lose their ability to adapt to their surroundings or cope with a situation of stress, perceiving the environment as stressful and threatening. When the environmental stimuli surpass their stress tolerance threshold, they can cause anxiety, and this can lead to inappropriate behaviors. Examples of some stressful factors would be loud or irritating noises, shouts, excess heat/cold, unknown places that can be perceived as threatening, etc. Thus, in this situation, we must try to adapt the environment to the person's needs.

5.2. Intervention in behavioral disorders

Nonpharmacological therapies, specifically behavioral interventions, are usually the treatment of choice for BPSD, and although there are few results in the literature supporting its efficacy, a set of actions have been identified that integrate psychosocial and medical perspectives and respond to a coordinated and established plan. However, when these types of disorders are more serious, behavioral intervention is combined with pharmacological treatment. In practice, professionals should at least know about the essential components of the care management plan, promoting interactions between the parties involved in an agile and comfortable way for the person with dementia and the caregiver.

The essential aspects of the care management plan are early diagnosis, specific pharmacological treatment, control over comorbidity, prevention and treatment of the BPSD, and the continuous guidance and support for the patient and caregiver [117].

Before making changes, it is necessary to make a general proposal to find out what we want to change. Therefore, first the behavior to be modified must be defined. The definition of the behavior must be carried out in a specific and concrete way. Thus, this proposal includes:

1. Identify the BPSD that should be modified and make the clearest and most concise definition possible in order to better delineate the problem. In this way, the best action strategy for this specific BPSD (it is better to address them one by one) can be identified.

2. In order to adequately define the BPSD, information has to be gathered about it: what time of day it appears, in what environment or context, who is present, how often it appears, etc.

3. Locate the antecedents or triggers and consequences of the behavior. There can be various triggers, and the more the interrelations among these factors are determined, the more successful the intervention will be. Regarding the consequences of the behavior, they allow us to establish the intensity of the problematic symptom or behavior, and in analyzing the consequences, the key to the triggers can often be found.

4. Realistic goals have to be set, beginning with small ones that are easy to achieve. A realistic goal does not involve making all the behavior problems disappear completely and forever. Goals have to be established in relative terms. The objective might be for the behavior to appear less frequently, be less intense, last less time, produce less discomfort in the patient, and/or be better tolerated by the caregiver. The changes are slow, and it takes time to begin to see them.

http://dx.doi.org/10.5772/64681

5. Establish the right strategy for the change. Every strategy requires the involvement of both people, caregiver and patient, and the achievement of the intervention objectives and goals.

6. Continuously evaluate and modify the objectives and strategies employed. They must be continuously reviewed to determine whether they are efficacious and to what degree, whether they are useful, or by contrast, ineffective or even counter-productive, which would mean redefining the action plan and see or detect where the problem is.

However, in order for a behavioral intervention to be successful, it is important to take into account the environment and the family setting, so that they remain constant and do not produce stress. In addition, this environment must continually be adapted to the patient's different needs and the evolution of the disease. However, it is also reasonable to imagine that other nonpharmacological therapies that have a special influence on the affective sphere (reminiscence, music therapy, leisure activities, etc.) also avoid the appearance of BPSD [81, 103, 118].

Nevertheless, and in spite of the consensus between professionals and scientific societies about the priority of nonpharmacological management, certain circumstances, such as the lack of human resources for the necessary care, make it necessary to use pharmacological treatment for the BPSD. In this case, treatment with cholinesterase inhibitors reduces the appearance of apathy, hallucinations, and motor hyperactivity [119, 120], while memantine prevents the appearance of agitation and aggressiveness [121].

Specifically, for intervention in the main BPSD:

Thought alterations, hallucinations and delirium: Avoid triggers, arguing about the truth or joking; do not reinforce or increase the content of the altered thinking; orient and distract the person toward other topics.

Aggressiveness: Review the existence of a possible depravation or a need that may be provoking it; promote autonomy and privacy (avoid robbing the patient of his/her dignity); approach the patient face-to-face calmly, warn, use nonverbal communication, explain, negotiate, reinforce, etc.

Depression: Identity the possible trigger and modify it (mourning, entering a nursing home, etc.); provide light, open, and pleasant spaces; stimulate social interaction; establish a plan for pleasant and enjoyable activities (strolls, workshops, etc.).

Anxiety: Reduce stimuli; continuous explanation of what is going to happen and predicting new situations; offer security verbally and nonverbally; avoid distractors, etc.

Euphoria: Do not imitate or reinforce the patient; do not trivialize, try to put him/her in the place of others. Correct or offer affection in a respectful way.

Apathy: Verbal or physical requests, propose, and persuade the patient to do pleasant or group activities, imitation, and modeling, stimuli with movement and an affective component (music, animals, etc.). The caregiver must understand and know how to manage this symptom.

Disinhibition: Study possible triggers (getting undressed because they are hot or because a label irritates their neck), respect without judging, avoid getting irritated or angry about behaviors, understand the behavior as part of the disease, correct them with tact, etc. In the case of inappropriate sexual behaviors, try to carry out stimulus control, allowing the behavior in certain places and for a certain time and impeding it in other situations (differential and selective reinforcements).

Irritability: Study a possible modification of the environment (noise, caregiver's treatment, social setting, etc.), accept the limitations, propose realistic, and alternative activities, etc.

Motor-ambulation hyperactivity: Make sure shoes are suitable, appropriate spaces, and establishing safety measures such as constant supervision, railings, good lighting, direction signals, signs, eliminate obstacles, black rugs, etc., offer objects to manipulate, do not create obstacles, etc.

Repeated vocalizations: Check basic needs with special attention to social isolation, lack or excess of stimuli, or pain; reinforce calm moments.

Sleep alterations: Balanced diet, brief naps, activity during the day, delay bedtime, avoid noise, etc.

Increase in appetite: Reduce or avoid exposure to food or substances.

Loss of appetite: Reinforce with aromas, flavors and presentation of food, dental hygiene and check-ups, conversation during meals, select favorite meals, etc.

Author details

Teresa Mayordomo Rodríguez[1*], Alicia Sales Galán[2], Rita Redondo Flores[2], Marta Torres Jordán[2] and Javier Bendicho Montes[2]

*Address all correspondence to: teresamayordomor@gmail.com

1 Catholic University of Valencia, Valencia, Spain

2 University of Valencia, Valencia, Spain

References

[1] LeDoux J, Bernal IM. The emotional brain. Buenos Aires: Ariel Planeta; 1999. doi: 10.1016/j.janxdis.2014.09.001.

[2] Damasio AR. Looking for Spinoza: neurobiology of emotion and feelings. 2005.

[3] Ochsner KN, Gross JJ. Cognitive emotion regulation insights from social cognitive and affective neuroscience. Curr Dir Psychol Sci. 2008;17:153–8. doi: 10.1111/j.1467-8721.2008.00566.x.

[4] Damasio, AR. Descartes' Error: reason of emotions. Andrés Bello; 1994.

[5] Sadowsky CH, Galvin JE. Guidelines for the management of cognitive and behavioral problems in dementia. J Am Board Fam Pract. 2013;25:350–66. doi: 10.3122/jabfm.2012.03.100183.

[6] Roudier M, Marcie P, Grancher AS, Tzortzis C, Starkstein S, Boller F. Discrimination of facial identity and of emotions in Alzheimer's disease. J Neurol Sci. 1998;154:151–58. doi: 10.1016/S0022-510X(97)00222-0.

[7] Carstensen LL, Charles ST. Emotion in the second half of life. Curr Dir Psychol Sci. 1998;7:144–9. doi: 10.1111/1467-8721.ep10836825.

[8] García-Rodríguez B, Fusari A, Ellgring H. Emotional processing of facial expressions in normal and pathological aging Rev Neurol. 2008;46:609–17. doi: 10.5579/rnl.2011.0078.

[9] Moreno C, Borod JC, Welkowitz J, Alpert M. The perception of facial emotion across the adult life span. Dev Neuropsychol. 1993;9:305–14. doi: 10.1080/87565649309540559.

[10] León FG, Hernández LM, Martínez JMA Meilán JJG. Emotional processing of facial expressions in normal and pathological aging. 2011;48:33–8. doi: 10.5538/1137-1242.2011.48.33.

[11] Lavenu I, Pasquier F. Perception of emotion on faces in frontotemporal dementia and Alzheimer's disease: a longitudinal study. Dement Geriatr Cogn Disord. 2004;19:37–41. doi: 10.1159/000080969.

[12] Allender J, Kaszniak AW. Processing of emotional cues in patients with dementia of the Alzheimer's type. Int J Neurosci. 1989;46:147–55. doi: 10.3109/00207458908986252.

[13] Bucks RS, Radford SA. Emotion processing in Alzheimer's disease. Aging Ment Health. 2004;8:222–32. doi: 10.1080/13607860410001669750.

[14] Hargrave R, Maddock RJ, Stone V. Impaired recognition of facial expressions of emotion in Alzheimer's disease. J Neuropsychiatry Clin Neurosci. 2002;14;64–71. doi: 10.1176/appi.neuropsych.14.1.64.

[15] Spoletini I, Marra C, Di Iulio F, Gianni W, Sancesario G, Giubilei F, Trequattrini A, Bria P, Caltagirone C, Spalletta G. Facial emotion recognition deficit in amnestic mild cognitive impairment and Alzheimer disease. Am J Geriatr Psychiatry. 2008;16:389–98. doi: 10.1097/JGP.0b013e318165dbce.

[16] Castaneda AE, Tuulio-Henriksson A, Marttunen M, Suvisaari J, Lönnqvist J. A review on cognitive impairments in depressive and anxiety disorders with a focus on young adults. J Affect Disord. 2008;106:1–27. doi: 10.1016/j.jad.2007.06.006.

[17] Ownby RL, Crocco E, Acevedo A, John V, Loewenstein D. Depression and risk for Alzheimer disease: systematic review, meta-analysis, and metaregression analysis. Arch Gen Psychiatry. 2006;63:530–38. doi: 10.1001/archpsyc.63.5.530.

[18] Starkstein SE, Jorge R, Mizrahi R, Robinson RG. The construct of minor and major depression in Alzheimer's disease. Am J Psychiatry. 2005;162:2086–93. doi: 10.1176/appi.ajp.162.11.2086.

[19] Guzmán-Vélez E, Feinstein JS, Tranel D. Feelings without memory in Alzheimer disease. Cogn Behav Neurol. 2014;27(3):117–29. doi: 10.1097/WNN.0000000000000020.

[20] Locke J. In Nidditch PH, editor. An essay concerning human understanding. Oxford: Clarendon Press; 1694/1979.

[21] Bluck S, Alea N, Habermas T, Rubin DC. A tale of three functions: the self–reported uses of autobiographical memory. Soc Cogn. 2005;23:91–117. doi: 10.1521/soco.23.1.91.59198.

[22] Conway MA, Singer JA, Tagini A. The self and autobiographical memory: correspondence and coherence. Soc Cogn. 2004; 22:491–529. doi: 10.1521/soco.22.5.491.50768.

[23] Conway MA. Memory and the self. J Mem Lang. 2005;53(4):594–28. doi: 10.1016/j.jml.2005.08.005.

[24] Brewer WF. What is autobiographical memory? In Rubin D, editor. Autobiographical memory. New York: Cambridge University Press; 1986. p. 25–49.

[25] Fivush R. The functions of event memory: some comments on Nelson and Barsalou. In Neisser U, Winograd E, editors. Remembering reconsidered: ecological and traditional approaches to memory. New York: Cambridge University Press; 1988. p. 277–282.

[26] Tulving E, Schacter DL, McLachlan DR, Moscovitch M. Priming of semantic autobiographical knowledge: a case study of retrograde amnesia. Brain Cogn. 1988;8:3–20. doi: 10.1016/0278-2626(88)90035-8.

[27] Baddeley A. What is autobiographical memory? In Theoretical perspectives on autobiographical memory. Netherlands: Springer; 1992. p. 13–29.

[28] Conway MA. Autobiographical knowledge and autobiographical memories. In Rubin DC, editor. Remembering our past: studies in autobiographical memory. Cambridge: Cambridge University Press; 1996. p. 67–93.

[29] Conway MA, Bekerian DA. Organization in autobiographical memory. Mem Cognition. 1987;15:119–32. doi: 10.1037/a0015633.

[30] Larsen SF. Personal context in autobiographical and narrative memories. In Conway MA, Rubin DC, Spinnler H, Wagenaar WA, editors. Theoretical perspectives on autobiographical memory. Netherlands: Springer; 1992. p. 53–71.

[31] Tulving E, Markowitsch HJ. Episodic and declarative memory: role of the hippocampus. Hippocampus. 1998;8:198–204.

[32] Piolino P, Desgranges B, Eustache F. Episodic autobiographical memory over the course of time: cognitive; neuropsychological and neuroimaging findings. Neuropsychologia. 2009;47:2314–29. doi: 10.3109/00207458908986252.

[33] Tulving E. Episodic memory: from mind to brain. Annu Rev Psychol. 2002;53:1–25. doi: 10.1146/annurev.psych.53.100901.135114.

[34] Levine B, Svoboda E, Hay JF, Winocur G. Moscovitch M. Aging and autobiographical memory: dissociating episodic from semantic retrieval. Psychol Aging. 2002;17:677–89. doi: 10.1037//0882-7974.17.4.677.

[35] Piolino P, Desgranges B, Benali K, Eustache F. Episodic and semantic remote autobiographical memory in aging. Memory. 2002; 10:239–57. doi: 10.1080/09658210143000353.

[36] Piolino P, Desgranges B, Clarys D, Guillery-Girard B, Taconnat L, Isingrini M, Eustache F. Autobiographical memory, autonoetic consciousness, and self-perspective in aging. Psychol Aging. 2006;21:510–25. doi: 10.1037/0882-7974.21.3.510.

[37] Greene JD, Hodges JR, Baddeley AD. Autobiographical memory and executive function in early dementia of Alzheimer type. Neuropsychologia. 1995;33:1647–70. doi: 10.1016/0028-3932(95)00046-1.

[38] Rubin DC, Wetzler SE, Nebes RD. Autobiographical memory across the adult lifespan. In Rubin DC, editor. Autobiographical memory. Cambridge, England: Cambridge University Press; 1986. p. 202–221.

[39] Harley K, Reese E. Origins of autobiographical memory. Dev Psychol. 1999;35:1338–48. doi: 10.1080/09658219408258955.

[40] Pillemer DB, White SH. Childhood events recalled by children and adults. Adv Child Dev Behav. 1989;21:297–340. doi: 10.1016/S0065-2407(08)60291-8.

[41] Rubin DC, Rahhal TA, Poon LW. Things learned in early adulthood are remembered best. Mem Cognition. 1998;26:3–19. doi: 10.3758/BF03211366.

[42] Ebbinghaus H. Memory: a contribution to experimental psychology. New York: Dover; 1964. doi: 10.5214/ans.0972.7531.200408.

[43] Addis DR, Wong AT, Schacter DL. Age-related changes in the episodic simulation of future events. Psychol Sci. 2008;19:33–41. doi: 10.1111/j.1467-9280.2008.02043.x.

[44] Bluck S, Levine LJ, Laulhere TM. Autobiographical remembering and hypermnesia: a comparison of older and younger adults. Psychol Aging. 1999;14:671–82. doi: 10.1037/0882-7974.14.4.671.

[45] Fromholt P, Mortensen DB, Torpdahl P, Bender L, Larsen P, Rubin DC. Life-narrative and word-cued autobiographical memories in centenarians: comparisons with 80-year-

old control, depressed, and dementia groups. Memory. 2003;11:81–88. doi: 10.1080/741938171.

[46] Piolino P, Coste C, Martinelli P, Macé AL, Quinette P, Guillery B, Belleville S. Reduced specificity of autobiographical memory and aging: the role of executive and feature binding functions of working memory. Neuropsychologia. 2010;48:429–40. doi: 10.1016/j.neuropsychologia.2009.09.035.

[47] St. Jacques PL, Levine B. Ageing and autobiographical memory for emotional and neutral events. Memory. 2007;15:129–44. doi: 10.1080/09658210601119762.

[48] Irish M, Hornberger M, Lah S, Miller L, Pengas G, Nestor PJ, Hodges, JR, Piguet O. Profiles of recent autobiographical memory retrieval in semantic dementia, behavioural-variant frontotemporal dementia, and Alzheimer's disease. Neuropsychologia. 2011;49(9):2694–702. doi: 10.1016/j.neuropsychologia.2011.05.017.

[49] Berna F, Schönknecht P, Seidl U, Toro P, Schröder J. Episodic autobiographical memory in normal aging and mild cognitive impairment: a population-based study. Psychiatry Res. 2012;200(2):807–12. doi: 10.1016/j.psychres.2012.03.022.

[50] Conway MA; Holmes A. Psychosocial stages and the accessibility of autobiographical memories across the life cycle. J Personal. 2004;72:461–80. doi: 10.1111/j.0022-3506.2004.00269.x.

[51] Greene JD, Hodges JR. Identification of famous faces and famous names in early Alzheimer's disease. Brain. 1996;119(1):111–28. doi: 0.1093/brain/119.1.111.

[52] Graham, KS, Hodges JR. Differentiating the roles of the hippocampus complex and the neocortex in long-term memory storage: evidence from the study of semantic dementia and Alzheimer's disease. Neuropsychology. 1997;11:77–89. doi: 10.1037//0894-4105.11.1.77.

[53] Dorrego MF, Sabe L, Cuerva AG, Kuzis G. Remote memory in Alzheimer's disease. J Neuropsychiatry Clin Neurosci. 1999;11(4):490–7. doi: 10.1176/jnp.11.4.490.

[54] Addis D, Tippett L. Memory of myself: autobiographical memory and identity in Alzheimer's disease. Memory. 2004:12(1):56–74. doi: 10.1080/09658210244000423.

[55] Hou CE, Miller BL, Kramer JH. Patterns of autobiographical memory loss in dementia. Int J Geriatr Psychiatry. 2005;20:809–15. doi: 10.1002/gps.1361.

[56] Ivanoiu A, Jm Sindic C. Cerebrospinal fluid TAU protein and amyloid β42 in mild cognitive impairment: prediction of progression to Alzheimer's disease and correlation with the neuropsychological examination. Neurocase. 2005;11:32–9. doi: 10.3233/JAD-2010-101203.

[57] Leyhe T, Muller S, Milian M, Eschweiler GW, Saur R. Impairment of episodic and semantic autobiographical memory in patients with mild cognitive impairment and

early Alzheimer's disease. Neuropsychologia. 2009;47:2464–69. doi: 10.1016/j.neuropsychologia.2009.04.018.

[58] Irish M, Lawlor BA, O'Mara SM, Coen RF. Exploring the recollective experience during autobiographical memory retrieval in amnestic mild cognitive impairment. J Int Neuropsychol Soc. 2010;16:546–55. doi: 10.1017/S1355617710000172.

[59] Greene JD, Hodges JR. The fractionation of remote memory. Brain. 1996;119(1):129–42. doi: 10.1093/brain/119.1.129.

[60] Ivanoiu A, Cooper JM, Shanks MF, Venneri A. Patterns of impairment in autobiographical memory in the degenerative dementias constrain models of memory. Neuropsychologia. 2006;44(10):1936–55. doi: 10.1016/j.neuropsychologia.2006.01.030.

[61] Meeter M, Eijsackers EV, Mulder JL. Retrograde amnesia for autobiographical memories and public events in mild and moderate Alzheimer's disease. J Clin Exp Neuropsychol. 2006;28:914–27. doi: 10.1037/neu0000117.

[62] Piolino P, Desgranges B, Belliard S, Matuszewski V, Lalevée C, De La Sayette, V, Eustache F. Autobiographical memory and autonoetic consciousness: triple dissociation in neurodegenerative diseases. Brain. 2003;126(10):2203–19. doi: 10.1093/brain/awg222.

[63] Murphy KJ, Troyer AK, Levine B, Moscovitch M. Episodic, but not semantic, autobiographical memory is reduced in amnestic mild cognitive impairment. Neuropsychologia. 2008;46(13):3116–23. doi: 10.1016/j.neuropsychologia.2008.07.004.

[64] Martinelli P, Anssens A, Sperduti M, Piolino P. The influence of normal aging and Alzheimer's disease in autobiographical memory highly related to the self. Neuropsychology. 2013;27:69–78. doi: 10.1037/a0030453.

[65] Grilli MD, Verfaellie M. Personal semantic memory: insights from neuropsychological research on amnesia. Neuropsychologia. 2014;61:56–64. doi: 10.1016/j.neuropsychologia.2014.06.012.

[66] Butler RN. The life review: an interpretation of reminiscence in the aged. Psychiatry. 1963;26:65–76. doi: 10.1521/00332747.1963.11023339.

[67] Kiermat J. The use of live review activity with confused nursing home residents. Am J Occup Ther. 1979;33:306–10.

[68] Webster JD. The reminiscence circumplex and autobiographical memory functions. Memory. 2003;11:203–15. doi: 10.1080/09658210244000379.

[69] Laborda-Soriano AA. Terapia ocupacional en una Unidad de Demencias Avanzadas (UDA). Rev Geriatr. 2002;18:40–9.

[70] Peña-Casanova, J. Cognitive intervention in Alzheimer's disease. Fundació La Caixa; 1999.

[71] Bohlmeijer E, Roemer M, Cuijpers P, Smit F. The effects of reminiscence on psychological well-being in older adults: a meta-analysis. Aging Ment Health. 2007;11:291–300. doi: 10.1080/13607860600963547.

[72] Lin YC, Dai YT. Hwang SL. The effect of reminiscence on the elderly population: a systematic review. Public Health Nurs. 2003;20:297–306. doi: 10.1046/j.1525-1446.2003.20407.x.

[73] Woods B, Spector A, Jones C, Orrell M. Davies S. Reminiscence therapy for dementia. Cochrane Database Syst Rev. 2005;2. doi: 10.1002/14651858.

[74] Gibson F. The past in the present: using reminiscence in health and social care. Health Professions Press; 2004. doi: 10.1111/j.1447-0748.2005.00240.x.

[75] Wang JJ. Group reminiscence therapy for cognitive and affective function of demented elderly in Taiwan. Int J Geriatr Psychiatry. 2007;22:1235–40. doi: 10.1002/gps.1236.

[76] Parker J. I remember that… Reminiscence groups with people with dementia: a valuable site for practice learning. Groupwork. 2006;16:7–28. doi: 10.1921/0951824X.16.1.7.1.

[77] Wong PT, Watt LM. What types of reminiscence are associated with successful aging?. Psychol Aging. 1991;6:272–9.

[78] Cappeliez P, Rivard V, Guindon S. Functions of reminiscence in later life: proposition of a model and applications. Eur Rev Appl Psychol. 2007;57:151–6. doi: 10.1016/j.erap.2005.02.014.

[79] Cappeliez P, O'Rourke N, Chaudhury H. Functions of reminiscence and mental health in later life. Aging Ment Health. 2005;9:295–301. doi: 10.1080/13607860500131427.

[80] Martínez T. Entrenar la Memoria e Intervenir en Reminiscencias (Memory training and intervene in reminiscences). Barcelona: Panamericana Editorial; 2012.

[81] Gonzalez J, Mayordomo T, Torres M, Sales A, Meléndez JC. Reminiscence and dementia: a therapeutic intervention. Int Psychogeriatr. 2015;27:1731–7. doi: 10.1017/S1041610215000344.

[82] Lai CK, Chi I, Kayser-Jones J. A randomized controlled trial of a specific reminiscence approach to promote the well-being of nursing home residents with dementia. Int Psychogeriatr. 2004;16:33–49. doi: 10.1017/S1041610204000055.

[83] Thadaka E, Kanagawa K. Effects of reminiscence group in elderly people with Alzheimer disease and vascular dementia in a community setting. Geriatr Gerontol Int. 2007;7:167–73. doi: 10.1111/j.1447-0594.2007.00381.x.

[84] Serrani Azcurra DJL. A reminiscence program intervention to improve the quality of life of long-term care residents with Alzheimer's disease: a randomized controlled trial. Rev Bras Psiquiatr. 2012;34:422–33. doi: 10.1016/j.rbp.2012.05.008.

[85] Woods RT, et al. REMCARE: reminiscence groups for people with dementia and their family caregivers—effectiveness and cost-effectiveness pragmatic multicentre randomised trial. Health Technol Assess. 2012;16:1–116. doi: 10.1371/journal.pone.0152843.

[86] Ashida S. The effect of reminiscence music therapy sessions on changes in depressive symptoms in elderly persons with dementia. J Music Ther. 2000;37(3):170–82. doi: 10.1093/jmt/37.3.170.

[87] Bohlmeijer E, Smit F, Cuijpers P. Effects of reminiscence and life review on late-life depression: a meta-analysis. Int J Geriatr Psychiatry. 2003;18:1088–94. doi: 10.1002/gps.1018.

[88] Chao SY, Liu HY, Wu CY, Jin SF, Chu TL, Huang TS, Clark MJ. The effects of group reminiscence therapy on depression, self esteem, and life satisfaction of elderly nursing home residents. J Nurs Res. 2006;14:36–45. doi: 10.1002/gps.2350.

[89] Hsieh HF, Wang JJ. Effect of reminiscence therapy on depression in older adults: a systematic review. Int J Nurs Stud. 2003;40:335–45. doi: 10.1016/S0020-7489(02)00101-3.

[90] Karimi H, Dolatshahee B, Momeni K, Khodabakhshi A, Rezaei M, Kamrani AA. Effectiveness of integrative and instrumental reminiscence therapies on depression symptoms reduction in institutionalized older adults: an empirical study. Aging Ment Health. 2010;14:881–7. doi: 10.1080/13607861003801037.

[91] Pinquart M, Forstmeier S. Effects of reminiscence interventions on psychosocial outcomes: a meta-analysis. Aging Ment Health. 2012;16:541–58. doi: 10.1080/13607863.2011.651434.

[92] Cappeliez P, O'Rourke N. Empirical validation of a model of reminiscence and health in later life. J Gerontol B Psychol Sci Soc Sci. 2006;61:237–44. doi: 10.1093/geronb/61.4.P237.

[93] Morgan S. The impact of a structured life review process on people with memory problems living in care homes [Doctoral dissertation]. Bangor: University of Wales; 2000.

[94] Claudia K, Lai Y, Chi I, Kayser-Jones J. A randomized controlled trial of a specific reminiscence approach to promote the well-being of nursing home residents with dementia. Int Psychogeriatr. 2004;16:33–49. doi: 10.1017/S1041610204000055.

[95] Arkoff, A, Meredith GM, Dubanoski JP. Gains in well-being achieved through retrospective-proactive life review by independent older women. J. Humanist. Psychol. 2004;44:204–14. doi: 10.1177/0022167804263065.

[96] Meléndez JC, Charco L, Mayordomo T, Sales A. Effects of a reminiscence program among institutionalized elderly adults. Psicothema. 2010;25:319–23. doi: 10.7334/psicothema2012.253.

[97] Erikson EH. Childhood and society (rev. ed.) New York: Norton; 1963.

[98] Brooker D, Duce L. Wellbeing and activity in dementia: a comparison of group reminiscence therapy, structured goal-directed group activity and unstructured time. Aging Ment Health. 2000;4:354–8. doi: 10.1080/713649967.

[99] Morgan S, Woods RT. Life review with people with dementia in care homes: a preliminary randomized controlled trial. Non-pharmacol Ther Dementia. 2010;1:43–60. doi: 10.1080/13607863.2013.837144.

[100] Subramaniam P, Woods B. The impact of individual reminiscence therapy for people with dementia: systematic review. Expert Rev Neurother. 2012;12:545–55. doi: 10.1586/ern.12.35.

[101] Subramaniam, Woods B, Whitaker C. Life review and life story books for people with mild to moderate dementia: a randomised controlled trial. Aging Ment Health. 2014;18(3):363–75. doi: 10.1080/13607863.2013.837144.

[102] Lalanne J, Gallarda T, Piolino P. "The Castle of Remembrance": new insights from a cognitive training programme for autobiographical memory in Alzheimer's disease. Neuropsychol Rehabil. 2015;25:254–82. doi: 10.1080/09602011.2014.949276.

[103] Melendez JC, Torres M, Redondo R, Mayordomo T, Sales A. Effectiveness of follow-up reminiscence therapy on autobiographical memory in pathological ageing. Int J Psychol. 2015. doi: 10.1002/ijop.12217.

[104] Steele C, Rovner B, Chase GA, Folstein M. Psychiatric symptoms and nursing home placement of patients with Alzheimer's disease. Am J Psychiatry. 1996;147:1049–51. doi: 10.1176/ajp.147.8.1049.

[105] Mega MS, Cummings JL, Fiorello T, Gornbein J. The spectrum of behavioral changes in Alzheimer's disease. Neurology. 1996;46:130–5. doi: 10.1212/WNL.46.1.130.

[106] Burgio L. Interventions for the behavioral complications of Alzheimer's disease: behavioral approaches. Psychogeriatrics. 1996;8:45–52.

[107] Cummings JL. Neuropsychiatric assessment and intervention in Alzheimer's disease. Int Psychogeriatr. 1996;8:25–30.

[108] Mohamed S, Rosenheck R, Lyketsos CG, Schneider LS. Caregiver burden in Alzheimer disease: cross-sectional and longitudinal patient correlates. Am J Geriatr Psychiatry. 2010;18:917–27. doi: 10.1097/JGP.0b013e3181d5745d.

[109] Steinberg M, Lyketsos CG. Trastornos psiquiátricos en personas con demencia. In Weiner MF, Lipton AM, editors. Manual de enfermedad de Alzheimer y otras demencias. Madrid: Panamericana; 2010. p. 263–81.

[110] Reisberg BM, Franssen E, Sclan S. Stage specific incidence of potentiallyremediable conductuales symptoms in aging and Alzheimer's disease: a study of 120 patients using the BEHAVE-AD. Bull Clin Neurosci. 1989;54:95–112.

[111] Finkel SI, Silva JC, Cohen G, Miller S, Sartorius N. Consensus statement: behavioral and psychological signs and symptoms of dementia: a consensus statement on current

knowledge and implications for research and treatment. Int Psychogeriatr. 1996;8:497–500. doi: 10.1002/(SICI)1099-1166(199711)12:11<1060::AID-GPS658>3.0.CO;2-M.

[112] Finkel, S. The significance of the behavioural and psychological symptoms of dementia. Clinician-macclesfield. 1998;16:33–42.

[113] Reisberg B, Borenstein J, Salob SP, Ferris SH, Franssen E, Georgotas A. Behavioral symptoms in Alzheimer's disease: phenomenology and treatment. J Clin Psychiatry. 1987;48:9–15. doi: 10.1159/000017198.

[114] Cummings JL, Mega M, Gray K, Rosenberg-Thompson S, Carusi DA, Gornbein J. The neuropsychiatric inventory: comprehensive assessment of psychopathology in dementia. Neurology. 1994;44:2308–14. doi: 10.1212/WNL.44.12.2308.

[115] Miranda-Castillo C, Woods B, Galboda K, Oomman S, Olojugba C, Orrell M. Unmet needs, quality of life and support networks of people with dementia living at home. Health Qual Life Outcomes. 2010;8:1–14. doi: 10.1186/1477-7525-8-132.

[116] Brodaty H, Donkin M. Family caregivers of people with dementia. Dialogues Clin Neurosci. 2009;11:217–28.

[117] Lyketsos CG, Colenda CC, Beck C, Blank K, Doraiswamy MP, Kalunian DA, Yaffe K. Position statement of the American Association for Geriatric Psychiatry regarding principles of care for patients with dementia resulting from Alzheimer disease. Am J Geriatr Psychiatry. 2006;14:561–73. doi: 10.1097/01.JGP.0000221334.65330.55.

[118] Guétin S, Portet F, Picot MC, Pommié C, Messaoudi M, Djabelkir L, et al. Effect of music therapy on anxiety and depression in patients with Alzheimer's type dementia: randomised, controlled study. Dement Geriatr Cogn Disord. 2009;28:36–46. doi: 10.1159/000229024.

[119] Berman K, Brodaty H, Withall A, Seeher K. Pharmacologic treatment of apathy in dementia. Am J Geriatr Psychiatry. 2012;2:104–22. doi: 10.1097/JGP.0b013e31822001a6.

[120] Waldemar G, Gauthier S, Jones R, Wilkinson D, Cummings J, Lopez O, et al. Effect of donepezil on emergence of apathy in mild to moderate Alzheimer's disease. Int J Geriatr Psychiatry. 2011;26:150–7. doi: 10.1002/gps.2507.

[121] Grossberg GT, Pejović V, Miller ML, Graham SM. Memantine therapy of behavioral symptoms in community-dwelling patients with moderate to severe Alzheimer's Disease. Dement Geriatr Cogn Disord. 2009;124:164–72. doi: 10.1159/000200013.

Chapter 18

Non-Pharmacological Approaches in the Treatment of Dementia

Grazia D'Onofrio, Daniele Sancarlo, Davide Seripa,
Francesco Ricciardi, Francesco Giuliani,
Francesco Panza and Antonio Greco

Additional information is available at the end of the chapter

http://dx.doi.org/Chapter DOI: 10.5772/64232

Abstract

Currently, a pharmacological disease-modifying treatment for dementia is not available, but different non-pharmacological approaches appear to be useful. In this chapter, we describe traditional treatments such as cognitive and emotion-oriented interventions, sensory and multi-sensory stimulation interventions and also potentially alternative interesting options such as behavioural therapy, animal-assisted therapy, home-adaptation therapy and assistive technologies to support patient with dementia. Many non-pharmacological treatments have reported benefits in multiple research studies, but there is a need for further Randomized controlled trials (RCTs) with an adequate sample size to improve the strength of evidence in order to apply these approaches.

Keywords: dementia, neuropsychiatric symptoms, activities of daily living, cognitive and emotion-oriented interventions, sensory and multi-sensory stimulation interventions

1. Introduction

Dementia is a term that describes disorders causing cognitive impairment capable to significantly affect functional status [1]. Worldwide, 46.8 million people have dementia, and every year, there are over 9.9 million new diagnosed cases [2], with a total global societal costs of US $ 604 billion in 2010 [2]. Alzheimer's disease (AD) is the most common form of dementia [3] and represents one of the major causes of disability, dependency, burden and stress of caregivers increasing institutionalization among older people worldwide [4].

This condition also leads to severe social consequences: decreased quality of life and well-being, increased family burdens and healthcare demand and longer term utilization of care facilities that generate very significant impacts on healthcare services demand and consequently costs [5]. The symptoms of dementia are grouped under three main headings: cognitive aspects, functional aspects and neuropsychiatric symptoms (NPSs). Dementia is a disease characterized by a cognitive decline involving one or more cognitive domains (memory and learning, executive function, language, complex attention, perceptual-motor, social cognition, etc.) [6]. The deficits must correspond to a decline from previous level of function and could be severe enough to interfere with daily functions and independence. Memory impairment is one of the main cognitive issues that contribute to the inability to live independently [4, 7, 8]. In the early stages of AD, it limits memory processes and reduces older people's autonomy in performing more complex daily activities, and it concurrently causes deterioration of emotional control, social behaviour and motivation [4, 6].

The functional aspects can be described in two broad classes: (1) basic activities of daily living or BADL [9, 10] and (2) instrumental activities of daily living or IADL [11]. BADLs are physical tasks essential to maintaining the independence and include the ability to go to the toilet, feed, dress, groom, bathe and ambulate. IADLs are activities typically more cognitively demanding than BADL and include the ability to successfully use the telephone, shop, prepare food, do the housekeeping and laundry, manage medications and finances and use transportation outside of the home (e.g., driving a car, using public transit or riding in a taxi). In the early stage of dementia, most patients are independent with BADL, but they begin to need help with some IADLs [12]. In the moderate phase, cooking, housework and shopping require direct assistance, and BADL require assistance for set-up and safety. Moreover, the presence of NPS could increase anger, frustration and difficulty in communicating needs [13]. As dementia enters the severe stage, independence is progressively lost and caregivers must offer consistent direct care with most if not all BADL [14–17].

NPS are common features of Alzheimer's disease (AD) [18, 19] and are one of the major risk factors for institutionalization [20]. NPS may be correlated to AD independently of cognitive impairment severity or emerge in the course of the illness being a significant cause of a more rapid cognitive decline [21]. It was found that over 80% of AD patients had NPS in the history of the illness [21, 22]. Four separate neuropsychiatric syndromes were identified: hyperactive, psychotic, affective and apathetic [19, 23]. In particular, agitation, euphoria, disinhibition, irritability and aberrant motor behaviour were defined as hyperactive syndrome; delusions, hallucinations and night-time disturbances as psychotic syndrome; depression and anxiety as affective syndrome, and apathy and eating abnormalities as apathetic syndrome.

Currently, there is no effective disease-modifying cure, and treatment is directed mainly to manage the symptoms of dementia [24].

http://dx.doi.org/Chapter DOI: 10.5772/64232

The limited efficacy of the drug therapy and the plasticity of the human brain are the two most important reasons that explain the growing interest in non-pharmacological intervention for dementia patients.

Several non-pharmacological treatments targeting cognitive, functional and neuropsychiatric aspects have been proposed for patients with dementia [25, 26].

This chapter describes the most used non-pharmacological treatment for dementia in according to the best-practice recommendations in the research literature [27–30] and the Standards for the Reporting of Diagnostic accuracy studies in dementia (STARDdem) [31].

2. Methods

A narrative review was performed using qualitative data and best-practice recommendations in the research literature [32, 33]. The searches were performed in the MEDLINE, PubMed, EMBASE, CINAHL and PsycINFO databases.

The search queries included 'dementia', 'non-pharmacological treatment' and 'cognitive rehabilitation', and were limited to English language articles.

The inclusion/exclusion criteria used for this review protocol are the following.

Inclusion criteria were as follows: (1) age ≥60 years, (2) diagnosis of dementia according to the criteria of the National Institute on Aging-Alzheimer's Association (NIAAA) [34], (3) use of non-pharmacological tools to treat the cognitive and functional impairment in dementia and (4) acceptable clinical measures of cognitive impairment, disability, quality of life and global clinical assessments.

Exclusion criteria were as follows: (1) no English editing (because we had no resources for translation) and (2) diagnosis of non-dementia.

Quality of study reporting was assessed using the Standards for the Reporting of Diagnostic accuracy studies in dementia (STARDdem) [35].

3. Cognitive and emotion-oriented interventions

Cognitive and emotion-oriented care approach seeks to improve cognitive, emotional and social functioning by supporting patients with dementia [36]. The treatments commonly used are reminiscence therapy, reality orientation therapy and validation therapy.

3.1. Reminiscence therapy

Reminiscence therapy is a common and widely diffused intervention in dementia care although based on a few high-quality and sufficiently robust studies. Two studies explored group reminiscence [37, 38]. A study evaluated effects on neuropsychiatric and cognitive symptoms [37]. Another reminiscence group intervention [38] evaluated effectiveness in preventing cognitive impairment progression and enhancing affective function. The results showed improvement in most variables including cognition and depression than controls.

3.2. Reality orientation therapy

Reality orientation (RO) is a technique of cognitive stimulation [39, 40]. It entails presenting the patient by continuous memory and orientation information associated with personal environment and issues. Several methods of implementing RO have been explained [40–42]. Throughout the treatment sessions, the patient is supported to talk about various arguments linked to his daily routine and recent events. Encouraging the patient to connect socially is a very significant component of the therapy [40, 42, 43]. Following the first publication of a review about RO, interest in the subject increased dramatically and most subsequent articles reported substantial benefits following the use of these strategies [40, 42, 44].

RO focuses on new cognitive stimulation strategies emerged in recent studies. The cognitive stimulation therapy (CST) is an example [40, 45]. Beyond the features assessed in RO, the CST is based also on multi-sensory stimulation and reminiscence [40, 44, 46].

Some reviews about RO confirmed earlier findings of substantial benefits and also identified existing and new areas where further work is required [39–41].

3.3. Validation therapy

The validation therapy (VT) was developed stages: to address the shortcomings of other approaches, such as RO, in approaching patients who have more advanced dementia. The VT was the result of an attempt to provide practical solutions for difficulties experienced by patients and caregivers.

Important characteristics of VT include: means of classifying behaviours, provision of simple, practical techniques that help restore dignity, provision of an empathic listener, respect and empathy for older adults with dementia and acceptance of the person's reality [47].

The way in which these rules are applied to provide specific interventions depends on the dementia severity categorized into mal orientation, time confusion, repetitive motion and vegetation. Each stage is recognized through defined cognitive and behavioural features and defined VT interventions address the various cognitive and neuropsychiatric characteristics showed by dementia people at each stage [47]. Various observational studies have indicated that the application of VT determine positive effects about amount and duration of interactions that participants are able to make during validation groups session [48, 49]. Though, other studies showed no significant effects of VT [50].

4. Sensory and multi-sensory stimulation interventions

Sensory stimulation and multi-sensory stimulation refer to a variety of techniques used to stimulate the senses in order to increase alertness and reduce agitation [51]. Sensory stimulation includes auditory, visual, olfactory, tactile, taste and kinaesthetic stimulation [52, 53]. Several studies examined sensorial and multi-sensorial interventions. In this chapter, seven therapy types were identified.

4.1. Art therapy

Art therapy is the therapeutic use of art making within a professional relationship. It has been suggested as a treatment for people with dementia as it has the potential to provide meaningful stimulation, improve social interaction and improve levels of self-esteem [54]. Activities such as drawing and painting are thought to provide individuals the opportunity for self-expression and the chance to exercise some choices in terms of the colours and themes of their creations.

4.2. Music therapy

Music therapy is defined as the clinical and evidence-based use of music interventions to accomplish individualized goals within a therapeutic relationship by a credentialed professional [55]. Two studies showed the effect of music on neuropsychiatric symptoms [56, 57]. It was tested a live-music intervention on decreasing anxiety and agitation [55]. Results showed no significant differences in anxiety and agitation. However, a study [56] showed a statistically significant decrease of the agitation in a group music-listening intervention.

4.3. Occupational therapy

The primary focus of occupational therapy (OT) is to improve patients' ability to perform activities of daily living, promote independence, reduce caregiver burden and ultimately improve quality of life.

OT offers interventions associated with awareness of self-care, leisure activities, occupational identity and productivity [58]. Studies showed an association between cognitive impairment and occupational performance [59, 60]. Therefore, patients with dementia can be assisted through OT trying to preserve an adequate performance level in BADL and IADL [61]. Furthermore, caregivers can adopt OT techniques, in the family or institution, to stimulate patient performing daily activities, preventing disruptive behaviour, wandering and aggression.

4.4. Aromatherapy

Aromatherapy is the fastest growing of all complementary therapies, in terms of public interest [62]. It aids interaction while providing a sensory experience. Aromatherapy appears to have several advantages over the pharmacological treatments used for dementia [63]. It seems to be well tolerated in comparison with sedative or neuroleptic medication [63]. The two essential oils used in aromatherapy for dementia patients are extracted from lavender and Melissa balm and could be administered in numerous methods such as bathing, inhalation, massage and topical application in cream [63]. Aromatherapy can be addressed to patients with several behaviours. Recent controlled trials showed significant reductions in agitation, with excellent compliance and tolerability [63–65].

4.5. Bright-light therapy

Bright light therapy (BLT) consists of exposure to daylight or specific wavelengths of light using polychromatic polarised light, laser, light-emitting diodes, fluorescence lamps, dichroic lamps or very bright, full-spectrum light. Four studies tested the effect of BLT on behavioural symptoms [66–69]. Two studies compared the effect of morning BLT and afternoon/evening BLT with normal light [66, 67]. Other studies compared one single type of BLT with usual light [66], and no differences were found between morning and evening. Limited evidence of reduction in agitation and aggression among those receiving BLT was found [67, 70].

4.6. Activity therapy

Activity therapy (AT) implicates recreation activities such as dance, sport and drama. It was found that physical exercise can have health benefits for dementia patients, reducing the number of falls and improving mental health, sleep [63, 70] and mood [71]. In addition, it was found that daytime exercise aided to decrease daytime agitation and night-time restlessness [63, 72]. Perrin described an interesting approach to dance therapy: he employed a form of dance known as 'jabadeo', which allows the patients to engage with each other in interactive movements [63, 73].

4.7. Snoezelen multi-sensory stimulation

Snoezelen is a multi-sensory setting for implementation of several sensory-based tools. Snoezelen offers sensory stimuli to primary senses of hearing, touch, sight, smell and taste, by the use of music, odour of essential oils, lighting effects and tactile surfaces [74]. Several studies define snoezelen approach as a support therapy for dementia patients [75]. The goals of such therapy are to promote positive behaviours and to reduce maladaptive behaviours [76, 77].

Over the past decade, the clinical application of Snoezelen has been extended from the field of learning disability to dementia care. Its use resides in providing a sensory environment that capitalizes on the residual sensorimotor abilities of dementia patients. Moreover, encouraging results were obtained in the area of promoting adaptive behaviours [78]. In practice, snoezelen capitalize on the residual sensorimotor abilities of dementia sufferers and present a few attentional and intellectual demands [76].

5. Other interventions

5.1. Behavioural therapy

Traditionally, behavioural therapy has been based on principles of conditioning and learning theory using strategies aimed at suppressing or eliminating challenging behaviours. More recently, positive programming methodologies [79] have used non-aversive methods in helping to develop more functional behaviours. Moniz-Cook suggests that behavioural analysis is often the starting point of most other forms of therapeutic intervention in this area

[80] and can be wholly consistent with person-centred care. Behavioural therapy requires a period of detailed assessment in which the triggers, behaviours and reinforcers are observed and their relationships made clear to the patient. The therapists use chart or diary to collect information about the behavioural symptoms, and interventions are based on an analysis of these findings.

For Emerson, planning an intervention should be focussed on three key features: identifying the individual's preferences; changing the context in which the behaviour occurs; and using reinforcement strategies and schedules that reduce the behaviour [63, 81].

A few studies showed the efficacy of behavioural in the context of dementia [63, 82]. There is some evidence of successful reductions in wandering, incontinence and other forms of stereotypical behaviours [83].

5.2. Animal-assisted therapy

Animal-assisted therapy (AAT) most commonly involves interaction between a patient and a trained animal, facilitated by a human handler, with a therapeutic goal such as providing relaxation and pleasure, or incorporating activities into physical therapy or rehabilitation. The therapeutic effect has been described by Baun and McCabe with reference to the stage of dementia and the positive effect on caregivers [84]. A review showed that AAT may ameliorate NPS in patients with dementia [85].

5.3. Home adaptation therapy

Home modifications for patients with dementia should promote safety for the patient and peace of mind for the caregiver. The modifications allow patients with dementia to receive ongoing care in the least restrictive environment possible and may be implemented as the need arises [86]. Home modifications for patients with dementia are associated with improved caregiver effectiveness and less caregiver upset [87].

5.4. Assistive technologies

In recent years, there have been significant innovations in the application of assistive technologies (ATs) to support healthcare for patients with dementia. These technologies can be used by the patients with dementia, by the caregivers, and can run automatically (the so-called 'ambient intelligence') [88].

AT applications have the potential to support aging in place for patients with dementia, and they range from internet-based information and support groups to robotic companions comprising also the use of smartphones to report symptoms [89–91].

Several studies describe the responses of caregivers and patients with dementia (PWD) to technology [92–94]. In general, the objective of AT is to allow people to remain more independent and reside at home safely [91–93]. In an another study, it was found that involving the patients with dementia in the process of developing technological applications enhanced usability and acceptability and contributed to a sense of empowerment [95].

6. Conclusion

Great efforts have been made to develop strategies to improve the quality of life of dementia patients. A shared feature is the need to work with systems (families, professional careers, organisations, etc.) [63]. Care staff and families are regularly integral to treatment strategies and are essential in obtaining reliable information and constructing appropriate interventions [63]. It is evident, therefore, that training of carers (both professional and family) is an important part of most treatment programmes. A study suggested that the most common interventions for psychological and behavioural symptoms of dementia were not necessarily specific therapies but working with carers to change the attitudes and behaviour of those in their care [96]. The field of dementia care is growing, with an increasing number of articles about psychosocial interventions [63]. Though, there is a fundamental limitation within the current literature that clearly requires addressing. A care plan that focused on non-pharmacological interventions is considered best practice as the first-line management of most NPS of dementia. They can significantly improve quality of life and satisfaction of patients with dementia and their caregivers.

Author details

Grazia D'Onofrio[1*], Daniele Sancarlo[1], Davide Seripa[1], Francesco Ricciardi[2], Francesco Giuliani[2], Francesco Panza[1,3,4] and Antonio Greco[1]

*Address all correspondence to: g.donofrio@operapadrepio.it and graziadonofrio@libero.it

1 Geriatric Unit & Laboratory of Gerontology and Geriatrics, Department of Medical Sciences, IRCCS 'Casa Sollievo della Sofferenza', San Giovanni Rotondo, Foggia, Italy

2 ICT, Innovation & Research Unit, IRCCS 'Casa Sollievo della Sofferenza', San Giovanni Rotondo, Foggia, Italy

3 Department of Clinical Research in Neurology, University of Bari Aldo Moro, 'Pia Fondazione Cardinale G. Panico', Tricase, Lecce, Italy

4 Neurodegenerative Disease Unit, Department of Basic Medicine, Neuroscience, and Sense Organs, University of Bari Aldo Moro, Bari, Italy

References

[1] D'Onofrio G, Sancarlo D, Addante F, Ciccone F, Cascavilla L, Paris F, Picco M, Nuzzaci C, Elia AC, Greco A, Chiarini R, Panza F, Pilotto A. Caregiver burden characterization

in patients with Alzheimer's disease or vascular dementia. Int J Geriatr Psychiatry. 2015;30(9):891–899.

[2] World Health Organization. Dementia: A Public Health Priority, 2012. Available from: http://whqlibdoc.who.int/publications/2012/978924156445 8_eng.pdf. Accessed May 31, 2015.

[3] Cummings JL. Alzheimer's disease. N Engl J Med. 2004;351:56–67.

[4] Schultz R, Williamson GH. A 2-year longitudinal study of depression among Alzheimer's caregivers. Psychol Aging. 1991;6:569–578.

[5] Seelye A, Schmitter-Edgecombe M, Das B, Cook DJ. Application of cognitive rehabilitation theory to the development of smart prompting technologies. IEEE Rev Biomed Eng. 2012;5:29–44.

[6] American Psychiatric Association. Diagnostic and Statistical Manual of Mental Disorders (DSM-5), 5th ed. Arlington: American Psychiatric Association, 2013.

[7] Grady C, Craik F. Changes in memory processing with age. Curr Opin Neurobiol. 2000;10(2):224–231.

[8] Schmitter EM, Woo E. Characterizing multiple memory deficits and their relation to everyday functioning in individuals with mild cognitive impairment. Neuropsychology. 2009;23(2):168–177.

[9] Katz S, Downs TD, Cash HR, Grotz RC. Progress in the development of an index of ADL. Gerontologist. 1970;10:20–30.

[10] Lawton MP. Aging and performance of home tasks. Hum Factors. 1990;32(5):527–536.

[11] Lawton MP, Brody EM. Assessment of older people: self-maintaining and instrumental activities of daily living. Gerontologist. 1969;9:179–186.

[12] Wattmo C, Wallin AK, Minthon L. Progression of mild Alzheimer's disease: knowledge and prediction models required for future treatment strategies. Alzheimer's Res Ther. 2013;5:44.

[13] Nowrangi MA, Lyketsos CG, Rosenberg PB. Principles and management of neuropsychiatric symptoms in Alzheimer's dementia. Alzheimer's Res Ther. 2015;7:12.

[14] Fraga FJ, Falk TH, Kanda PAM, Anghinah R. Characterizing Alzheimer's disease severity via resting-awake EEG amplitude modulation analysis. PLoS One. 2013;8(8):e72240.

[15] Futrell M, Melillo KD, Remington R, Schoenfelder DP. Wandering. J Gerontol Nurs. 2010;36(2):6–16.

[16] Eshkoor SA, Hamid TA, Nudin SSH, Mun CY. A research on functional status, environmental conditions, and risk of falls in dementia. Int J Alzheimer's Dis. 2014;2014:6.

[17] Volicer L, van der Steen JT. Outcome measures for dementia in the advanced stage and at the end of life. Adv Geriatr. 2014;2014:10.

[18] Mega MS, Cummings JL, Fiorello T, Gornbein J. The spectrum of behavioral changes in Alzheimer's disease. Neurology. 1996;46:130–135.

[19] Aalten P, Verhey FR, Boziki M, Bullock R, Byrne EJ, Camus V, Caputo M, Collins D, De Deyn PP, Elina K, Frisoni G, Girtler N, Holmes C, Hurt C, Marriott A, Mecocci P, Nobili F, Ousset PJ, Reynish E, Salmon E, Tsolaki M, Vellas B, Robert PH. Neuropsychiatric syndromes in dementia. Results from the European Alzheimer Disease Consortium: part I. Dement Geriatr Cogn Disord. 2007;24:457–463.

[20] Steele C, Rovner B, Chase GA, Folstein M. Psychiatric symptoms and nursing home placement of patients with Alzheimer's disease. Am J Psychiatry. 1990;147:1049–1051.

[21] Finkel SI, Costa E, Silva J, Cohen G, Miller S, Sartorius N. Behavioral and psychological signs and symptoms of dementia: a consensus statement on current knowledge and implications for research and treatment. Int Psychogeriatr. 1996;8:497–500.

[22] Lyketsos CG, Lopez O, Jones B, Fitzpatrick AL, Breitner J, DeKosky S. Prevalence of neuropsychiatric symptoms in dementia and mild cognitive impairment: results from the cardiovascular health study. JAMA. 2002;288:1475–1483.

[23] Aalten P, Verhey FR, Boziki M, Brugnolo A, Bullock R, Byrne EJ, Camus V, Caputo M, Collins D, De Deyn PP, Elina K, Frisoni G, Holmes C, Hurt C, Marriott A, Mecocci P, Nobili F, Ousset PJ, Reynish E, Salmon E, Tsolaki M, Vellas B, Robert PH. Consistency of neuropsychiatric syndromes across dementias: results from the European Alzheimer Disease Consortium: part II. Dement Geriatr Cogn Disord. 2008;25:1–8.

[24] Atri A. Effective pharmacological management of Alzheimer's disease. Am J Manag Care. 2011;17:S346–S355.

[25] Acevedo A, Loewenstein DA. Non pharmacological cognitive interventions in aging and dementia. J Geriatr Psychiatry Neurol. 2007;20:239–249.

[26] D'Onofrio G, Sancarlo D, Addante F, Ciccone F, Cascavilla L, Paris F, Elia AC, Nuzzaci C, Picoco M, Greco A, Panza F, Pilotto A. A pilot randomized controlled trial evaluating an integrated treatment of rivastigmine transdermal patch and cognitive stimulation in patients with Alzheimer's disease. Int J Geriatr Psychiatry. 2015;30(9):965–975.

[27] Dixon-Woods M, Agarwal S, Jones D, Young B, Sutton A. Synthesising qualitative and quantitative evidence: a review of possible methods. J Health Serv Res Policy. 2005;10:45–53.

[28] Hannes K, Macaitis K. A move to more systematic and transparent approaches in qualitative evidence synthesis: update on a review of published papers. Qual Res. 2012;12:402–442.

[29] Barnett-Page E, Thomas J. Methods for the synthesis of qualitative research: a critical review. BMC Med Res Methodol. 2009;9:59.

[30] Grant MJ, Booth A. A typology of reviews: an analysis of 14 review types and associated methodologies. Health Info Libr J. 2009;26:91–108.

[31] Noel-Storr AH, McCleery JM, Richard E, Ritchie CW, Flicker L, Cullum SJ, Davis D, Quinn TJ, Hyde C, Rutjes AW, Smailagic N, Marcus S, Black S, Blennow K, Brayne C, Fiorivanti M, Johnson JK, Köpke S, Schneider LS, Simmons A, Mattsson N, Zetterberg H, Bossuyt PM, Wilcock G, McShane R. Reporting standards for studies of diagnostic test accuracy in dementia: The STARDdem Initiative. Neurology. 2014;83(4):364–373.

[32] Collings AJ, Fauser CJMB. Balancing the strengths of systematic and narrative reviews. Hum Reprod Update. 2005;11(2):103–104.

[33] Dixon-Woods M, Agarwal S, Jones D, Young B, Sutton A. Synthesising qualitative and quantitative evidence: a review of possible methods. J Health Serv Res Policy. 2005;10:45–53.

[34] McKhann GM, Knopman DS, Chertkow H, Hyman BT, Jack CR Jr, Kawas CH, Klunk WE, Koroshetz WJ, Manly JJ, Mayeux R, Mohs RC, Morris JC, Rossor MN, Scheltens P, Carrillo MC, Thies B, Weintraub S, Phelps CH. The diagnosis of dementia due to Alzheimer's disease: recommendations from the National Institute on Aging-Alzheimer's Association workgroups on diagnostic guidelines for Alzheimer's disease. Alzheimers Dement. 2011;7:263–269.

[35] Noel-Storr AH, McCleery JM, Richard E, Ritchie CW, Flicker L, Cullum SJ, Davis D, Quinn TJ, Hyde C, Rutjes AW, Smailagic N, Marcus S, Black S, Blennow K, Brayne C, Fiorivanti M, Johnson JK, Köpke S, Schneider LS, Simmons A, Mattsson N, Zetterberg H, Bossuyt PM, Wilcock G, McShane R. Reporting standards for studies of diagnostic test accuracy in dementia: the STARDdem Initiative. Neurology. 2014;83(4):364–373.

[36] Finnema E, Dröes RM, Ribbe M, Tilburg WV. The effects of emotion-oriented approaches in the care for persons suffering from dementia: a review of the literature. Int J Geriatr Psychiatry. 2000;15:141–161.

[37] Ito T, Meguro K, Akanuma K, Ishii H, Mori E. A randomized controlled trial of the group reminiscence approach in patients with vascular dementia. Dement Geriatr Cogn. 2007;24:48–54.

[38] Wang J. Group reminiscence therapy for cognitive and affective function of demented elderly in Taiwan. Int J Geriatr Psychiatry. 2007;22:1235–1240.

[39] Choi J, Twamley EW. Cognitive rehabilitation therapies for Alzheimer's disease: a review of methods to improve treatment engagement and self-efficacy. Neuropshycol Rev. 2013;23(1):48–62.

[40] Camargo CH, Justus FF, Retzlaff G. The effectiveness of reality orientation in the treatment of Alzheimer's disease. Am J Alzheimers Dis Other Demen. 2015;30(5):527–532.

[41] Aguirre E, Woods RT, Spector A, Orrell M. Cognitive stimulation for dementia: a systematic review of the evidence of effectiveness from randomized controlled trials. Ageing Res Rev. 2013;12(1):253–262.

[42] Spector A, Orrell M, Woods B. Cognitive Stimulation Therapy (CST): effects on different areas of cognitive function for people with dementia. Int J Geriatr Psychiatry. 2010;25(12):1253–1258.

[43] Spector A, Davies S, Bob Woods, Orrell M. Reality orientation for dementia: a systematic review of the evidence of effectiveness from randomized controlled trials. Gerontologist. 2000;40(2):206–212.

[44] Spector A, Woods B, Orrell M. Cognitive stimulation for the treatment of Alzheimer's disease. Expert Rev Neurother. 2008;8(5):751–757.

[45] Breuil V, De Rotrou J, Forette F. Cognitive stimulation of patients with dementia: preliminary results. Int J Geriatr Psychiatry. 1994;9:211–217.

[46] Clare L, Woods RT. Cognitive training and cognitive rehabilitation for people with early-stage Alzheimer's disease: a review. Neuropsychol Rehabil. 2004;14(4):385–401.

[47] Feil N. Validation therapy. Geriatr Nurs. 1992;13:129–133.

[48] Babins LH. Conceptual analysis of validation therapy. Int J Aging Hum Dev. 1998;26:161–168.

[49] Deponte A, Missan R. Effectiveness of validation therapy (VT) in group: preliminary results. Arch Gerontol Geriatr. 2007;44:113–117.

[50] Scanland SG, Emershaw EL. Reality orientation and validation therapy: dementia, depression, and functional status. J Gerontol Nurs. 1993;19:7–11.

[51] Gammeltoft BC. Invisible Handicaps among Persons Suffering from Brain Injury. Høng: Forlaget FCT, Eligius; 2005.

[52] Vozzella S. Sensory stimulation in dementia care: why it is important and how to implement it. Top Geriatr Rehabil. 2007;23(2):102–113.

[53] Baker R, Bell S, Baker E, Gibson S. A randomized controlled trial of the effect of multisensory stimulation (MSS) for people with dementia. Br J Clin Psychol. 2001;40:81–96.

[54] Killick J, Allan K. The arts in dementia care: tapping a rich resource. J Dementia Care. 1999;7:35–38.

[55] American Music Therapy Association. What is music therapy? 2005. Available from: http://www.musictherapy.org/about/musictherapy/

[56] Cooke M, Moyle W, Shum D, Harrison S, Murfield J. A randomized controlled trial exploring the effect of music on quality of life and depression in older people with dementia. J Health Psychol. 2010;15:765–776.

[57] Lin Y, Chu H, Yang CY, Chen CH, Chen SG, Chang HJ, Hsieh CJ, Chou KR. Effectiveness of group music intervention against agitated behavior in elderly persons with dementia. Int J Geriatr Psychiatry. 2011;26:670–678.

[58] Whiteford G, Fossey E. Occupation: the essential nexus between philosophy, theory and practice. Aust Occup Ther J. 2002;49(1):1–2.

[59] Nygård L, Amberla K, Bernspång B, Almkvist O, Winblad B. The relationship between cognition and daily activities in cases of mild Alzheimer's disease. Scand J Occup Ther. 1998;5:160–166.

[60] Ohman A, Nygard L, Kottorp A. Occupational performance and awareness of disability in mild cognitive impairment or dementia. Scand J Occup Ther. 2011;18:133–142.

[61] Nygård L. Responses of persons with dementia to challenges in daily activities: A synthesis of findings from empirical studies. Am J Occup Ther. 2004;58:435–445.

[62] Burns A, Byrne J, Ballard C, Holmes C. Sensory stimulation in dementia. An effective option for managing behavioural problems. BMJ. 2002;325:1312–1313.

[63] Douglas S, James I, Ballard C. Non-pharmacological interventions in dementia. BJPsych Adv. 2004;10:171–177.

[64] Ballard CG, O'Brien J, Reichelt K, Perry EK. Aromatherapy as a safe and effective treatment for the management of agitation in severe dementia: the results of a double blind, placebo controlled trial. J Clin Psychiatry. 2002;63:553–558.

[65] Holmes C, Ballard C. Aromatherapy in dementia. Adv Psychiatr Treat. 2004;10(4):296–300.

[66] Lyketsos CG, Lindell VL, Baker A, Steele C. A randomized, controlled trial of bright light therapy for agitated behaviors in dementia patients residing in long-term care. Int J Geriatr Psychiatry. 1999;14:520–525.

[67] Ancoli-Israel S, Martin JL, Gehrman P, Shochat T, Corey-Bloom J, Marler M, Nolan S, Levi L. Effect of light on agitation in institutionalized patients with severe Alzheimer disease. Am J Geriatr Psychiatry. 2003;11:194–203.

[68] Dowling GA, Graf CL, Hubbard EM, Luxenberg JS. Light treatment for neuropsychiatric behaviors in Alzheimer's disease. West J Nurs Res. 2007;29:961–975.

[69] Burns A, Allen H, Tomenson B, Duignan D, Byrne J. Bright light therapy for agitation in dementia: a randomized controlled trial. Int Psychogeriatr. 2009;21:711–721.

[70] King A, Oman R, Brassington G, Bliwise DL, Haskell WL. Moderate intensity exercise and self-rated quality of sleep in older adults. A randomised controlled trial. JAMA. 1997;277:32–37.

[71] Young A, Dinan S. ABC of sports medicine. Fitness for older people. BMJ. 1994;309:331–334.

[72] Alessi C, Yoon E, Schnelle J, Al-Samarrai NR, Cruise PA. A randomised trial of a combined physical activity and environment intervention in nursing home residents: do sleep and agitation improve? J Am Geriatr Soc. 1999;47:784–791.

[73] Perrin T. Lifted into a world of rhythm and melody. J Dementia Care. 1998;6:22–24.

[74] Pinkney L. A comparison of the Snoezelen environment and a music relaxation group on the mood and behaviour of patients with senile dementia. Br J Occup Ther. 1997;60(5):209–218.

[75] Burns I, Cox H, Plant H. Leisure or therapeutics? Snoezelen and the care of older persons with dementia. Int J Nurs Pract. 2000;6:118–126.

[76] Baker R, Bell S, Baker E, Gibson S, Holloway J, Pearce R, Dowling Z, Thomas P, Assey J, Wareing LA. A randomized controlled trial of the effects of multi-sensory stimulation (MSS) for people with dementia. Br J Clin Psychol. 2001;40(1):81–96.

[77] Slevin E, McClelland A. Multisensory environments: are they therapeutic? A single subject evaluation of the clinical effectiveness of a multisensory environment. J Adv Nurs. 1999;8(1):48–56.

[78] Kovach CR. Sensoristasis and imbalance in persons with dementia. J Nurs Scholorsh. 2000;32(4):379–384.

[79] La Vigna G, Donnellan A. Alternative to Punishment: Solving Behaviour Problems with Non-aversive Strategies. New York: Irvington, 1986.

[80] Moniz-Cook E, Agar S, Silver M, Woods R, Wang M, Elston C, Win T. Can staff training reduce behavioural problems in residential care for the elderly mentally ill? Int J Geriatr Psychiatry. 1998;13:149–158.

[81] Emerson E, Thompson S, Reeves D, Henderson D, Robertson J. Descriptive analysis of multiple response topographies of challenging behaviour across two settings. Res Dev Disabil. 1995;16:301–329.

[82] Burgio L, Fisher S. Application of psychosocial interventions for treating behavioural and psychological symptoms of dementia. Int Psychogeriatr. 2000;12(1):351–358.

[83] Woods RT. Psychological Problems of Ageing. Chichester: John Wiley and Sons, 1999.

[84] Baun MM, McCabe BW. Companion animals and persons with dementia of the Alzheimer's type: therapeutic possibilities. Am Behav Sci. 2003;47:42–51.

[85] Filan SL, Llewellyn-Jones RH. Animal-assisted therapy for dementia: a review of the literature. Int Psychogeriatr. 2006;18(4):597–611.

[86] U.S. Department of Health and Human Services Public Health Service. National Institutes of Health, National Institute on Aging. Home safety for people with Alzheimer's disease. Available from: file:///C:/Documents%20and%20Settings/tir03222/Documenti/Downloads/home_safety_for_people_with_alzheimers_disease_2.pdf. Accessed May 31, 2015.

[87] Gitlin LN, Corcoran M, Winter L, Boyce A, Hauck WW. A randomized, controlled trial of a home environmental intervention: effect on efficacy and upset in caregivers and on daily function of persons with dementia. Gerontologist. 2001;41(1):4–14.

[88] Cook DJ, Augustob JC, Jakkulaa VR. Ambient intelligence: technologies, applications, and opportunities. Pervasive Mob Comput. 2009;5(4):277–298.

[89] Czaja SJ, Rubert MP. Telecommunications technology as an aid to family caregivers of persons with dementia. Psychosom Med. 2002;64:469–476.

[90] Powell J, Chiu T, Eysenbach G. A systematic review of networked technologies supporting carers of people with dementia. J Telemed Telecare. 2008;14(3):154–156.

[91] Steis M, Prabhu V, Kolanowski A, Kang Y, Bowles KH, Fick D, Evans L. Detection of delirium in community-dwelling persons with dementia. Online J Nurs Inform. 2012;16(1) Available at http://ojni.org/issues/?p=1274.

[92] Pot AM, Willemse BM, Horjus S. A pilot study on the use of tracking technology: feasibility, acceptability, and benefits for people in early stages of dementia and their informal caregivers. Aging Ment Health. 2012;16(1):127–134.

[93] Steele R, Lo A, Secombe C, Wong YK. Elderly persons' perception and acceptance of using wireless sensor networks to assist healthcare. Int J Med Inform. 2009;78(12):788–801.

[94] van Hoof J, Kort HS, Rutten PG, Duijnstee MS. Ageing-in-place with the use of ambient intelligence technology: perspectives of older users. Int J Med Inform. 2011;80(5):310–331.

[95] Span M, Hettinga M, Vernooij-Dassen M, Eefsting J, Smits C. Involving people with dementia in the development of supportive IT applications: a systematic review. Ageing Res Rev. 2013;12(2):535–551.

[96] Bird M, Llewellyn-Jones R, Smithers H, Korten A. Psychosocial Approaches to Challenging Behaviour in Dementia: A Controlled Trial. Report to the Commonwealth Department of Health and Ageing. Canberra: CDHA, 2002.

Chapter 19

Medication Management for People Living with Dementia: Development and Evaluation of a Multilingual Information Resource for Family Caregivers of People Living with Dementia

Robyn Gillespie, Pippa Burns, Lindsey Harrison, Amanda Baker, Khin Win, Victoria Traynor and Judy Mullan

Additional information is available at the end of the chapter

http://dx.doi.org/10.5772/64661

Abstract

The aim of this chapter is to describe the development and evaluation of an online multilingual information resource focused on medication management, targeting people living with dementia and their family caregivers. Maintaining effective medication management is important to allow ongoing quality of life within the community setting and avoiding medication-related preventable hospitalisations for the person living with dementia. Family caregivers are likely to assume the role of medication management on behalf of the person in their care as dementia progresses. Little training or information is available to family caregivers to assist them with this role. A pilot online information resource was developed and evaluated. Responding to the evaluation, this resource was improved, and a more extensive evaluation process was undertaken. The development and evaluation process are outlined with a view to guiding the development of similar resources, especially those targeting linguistically diverse family caregivers and those with dementia. This is especially important given that many older adults will migrate during their lifetime, often to a country where they are not familiar with the language or health services. Extra support is needed to assist older immigrants who are themselves at risk or are caring for someone with dementia.

Keywords: medication management, family caregiver, dementia, ethnic minority, computer-based education, readability, health literacy

1. Introduction

Effective medication management enables people living with dementia to avoid hospitalisations related to preventable medication errors and prolongs their ability to remain living within a community setting. This chapter describes the development and evaluation of a multilingual online information resource on medication management for family caregivers of people living with dementia (PLWD). The resource aims to improve medication management to enable PLWD to remain living at home, in their community for as long as possible. This resource is unique in that it targets not only caregivers within the general Australian community but also Italian and Macedonian immigrant caregivers who find themselves caring for someone with dementia in their host country, Australia. Qualitative research identified caregiver concerns regarding medication management and findings from a literature review were used to inform were used to inform the development of the information resource. The principle of universal access was incorporated into the website design, and the precautionary principle was applied in regard to health literacy when planning the content of the resource. The initial site evaluated, changes were made, and a refined site developed and further evaluated in light of our two guiding principles and the reported usefulness of the site to caregivers. Lessons learned from the development and evaluations of the information resource to assist caregivers and PLWD with medication management tasks are explained. The chapter aims to outline a toolkit of resources that can be used by other projects to develop and evaluate similar information resources.

2. Background

Many older adults are not ageing in their place of origin as mobility increases within and between countries. Increases in net migration in countries with high rates of immigration, such as Australia, will see their growing older population become more ethnically diverse over time [1]. In Australia, linguistically diverse caregivers comprise 33% of caregivers of PLWD living in a community setting [2]. Health literacy rates are known to be generally lower in immigrant populations, and they continue to have increased difficulties when accessing health services and information [3]. For example, findings from a qualitative Australian study of 25 non-English-speaking community living adults from the former Yugoslavia suggest that language barriers, different expectations about medicines and the healthcare system resulted in members of this community being more likely to experience medication management problems [4]. Based on this example and anecdotal evidence from other linguistically diverse groups, it is likely that this population group of family caregivers may require additional support to safely and effectively manage medications for their older relatives who are living with dementia.

Regardless of ethnicity, people living with a dementia often need to manage complex medication regimes. They may be prescribed one or more cognitive enhancing medications for the management of their dementia. This is especially the case for those who live in developed countries where early diagnosis and treatment are available [5]. These cognitive enhancing medications can be useful in managing some symptoms of early-stage dementia and delay institutional placement [6]. PLWD may also experience other age-related chronic co-morbidities such as diabetes, cardiovascular diseases, arthritis and osteoporosis [7]. As a result, it is common for older adults with dementia to also have a number of co-existing illnesses that may be partly or completely managed by the use of medication. Ongoing safe and effective medication use for the management of all co-morbidities is important for PLWD to avoid medication-related adverse events, prevent hospitalisation or placement into permanent institutionalised aged care and to maintain or improve their quality of life [8, 9].

Recent studies have documented the impact of dementia on a person's ability to safely and effectively manage medications [10–12]. The cognitive, social and physical losses associated with dementia compound to make ongoing independent medication management more difficult for PLWD [13, 14]. Cognitive losses may affect memory, attention, language, communication and decision making; all capabilities which are necessary to maintain autonomy regarding safe and effective medication management [10]. Cotrell et al's. [10] study of 47 caregiving/care recipient dyads indicated that 85% of PLWD relinquish some or all medication management tasks to their family caregivers over the course of their disease, compared to only 30% of older adults receiving caregiver assistance for other chronic illnesses. Similar results were found in a larger study by Thorpe et al. [12] of 566 dyads which found the majority of family caregivers will assume a medication management role throughout the progression of a dementia with 54% noting involvement at any stage of dementia and rates exceeding 90% in the later stages of the disease.

Specific medication management tasks carried out by a caregiver of a PLWD may include maintaining continuous supplies of medications, assisting with administration, making clinical judgements and communicating with healthcare providers and care recipients [15]. To be effective in their medication management role, caregivers need to not only be informed about what is prescribed but also be capable of asking relevant questions of healthcare professionals, be able to monitor medication adherence, be aware of and watch out for medication-related side effects. They also need to be able to grant or refuse consent for medication use or discontinuation if the PLWD is no longer capable of making this decision [16].

Medication management issues, including compliance concerns for PLWD may be resolved by involving a family caregiver in the medication management process where possible. This has been shown to be a somewhat effective approach in reducing the number of identified medication misadventures, especially if support from health professionals is given to caregivers in addition to the PLWD [17]. Ongoing access to information and support in their medication management role is necessary for caregivers in order to adjust to the changes which accompany the progression of disease in the PLWD [18]. However, findings from a number of studies indicate that there is a lack of information, training and support for family caregivers in their medication management role [15, 19, 20]. This lack of information was confirmed by our own search for paper based on online information material which found that no specific Australian resource was available that targeted caregivers of PLWD in their medication management role.

Given the importance of ongoing safe and effective medication management for PLWD, we sought to fill the knowledge gap we had identified. Funding was obtained to develop an information resource for family caregivers of people living with dementia from linguistically diverse backgrounds. This group of caregivers were targeted as being the most in need of an information resource as evidenced by the findings of an earlier Australian report on the experiences of managing medications at home of 12 older adults and 10 family caregivers from linguistically diverse backgrounds [21]. The report highlighted that this group of Australian caregivers faced additional language and literacy barriers, requiring information to be available in their own language but also in a variety of formats to increase accessibility for those with low literacy [21]. In targeting this group which may have the lowest literacy and as a result the lowest health literacy levels, we aimed to produce a resource that was useful and accessible to everyone.

The following sections outline the development and evaluation of this online pilot resource.

3. Online resource development

3.1. Phase 1 Pilot online resource

We aimed to develop a useful, easy to use, accessible, up-to-date and trustworthy resource that met the needs of our target group of caregivers and was also available for all caregivers and PLWD. In order to do this we first conducted a review of the literature and a qualitative research project involving participants from our target audience which included the generation of older European immigrants who arrived in Australia following the Second World War. This group is now entering old age and are at high risk of developing dementia. These immigrants were mainly from southern European countries and as such the most common languages spoken among our target group included Macedonian, Italian, Greek Spanish, Maltese, Polish, Dutch and Hungarian [22]. Their education levels are generally low in both their original language and in English, especially among the women [23].

3.2. Literature review

To build our own knowledge of this topic and investigate other related research, a review of the relevant literature from January 2000 to April 2013 was conducted. This revealed a lack of research investigating the medication management experience of family caregivers, especially those caring for PLWD [24]. Furthermore, previous research of general medication management for older adults included linguistically diverse family caregivers; however, sample sizes were generally small or results for linguistically diverse groups had not been analysed separately [24]. We viewed this as a significant gap in the literature given that linguistically diverse caregivers make up a significant proportion of the family caregiving population in many countries, that have high immigration rates, like Australia.

Despite the limited availability of previous research, the main findings of the review concluded that family caregivers received little or no training, information or support as they performed medication management tasks [24]. The role is complex, and this complexity increases as medication regimens become more complicated. For instance, family caregivers are often responsible for the supply and scheduling of multiple medications, the administration of medications via different formulations (e.g. oral, rectal, transdermal patches, inhalers, injection, creams and drops), the calculation of dosages, the monitoring of side effects and communication with multiple healthcare providers.

3.3. Qualitative study

3.3.1. Background

A qualitative study, including focus group discussions and one-on-one interviews, was conducted in order to understand the everyday medication management experiences of linguistically diverse family caregivers of PLWD living in the Illawarra region, a multicultural urban area south of Sydney, Australia, with a population of 450,000. One quarter of people resident in the area are born overseas and 14.5% report speaking a language other than English at home [25].

The research team worked in partnership with the local multicultural health services in order to make contact with linguistically diverse family caregivers of PLWD living in the Illawarra. Local community workers involved with the area's carer support groups noted that family caregivers experienced isolation, having little time available outside of their caregiving role, low English proficiency and limited transport options. It was also noted that dementia was viewed with considerable stigma by many linguistically diverse communities and family caregivers may not identify as caregivers, as the roles they take on are seen as a normal part of family responsibility [26]. This knowledge and the established relationships formed by the multicultural workers were invaluable to the research team.

3.3.2. Findings

A total of 29 participants from five different cultural groups participated in the three focus groups and seven semi-structure interviews which were conducted between July and October 2012 (see **Tables 1** and **2**). The majority of the focus group participants were spouse caregivers, while most of the individual interviews were conducted with adult child caregivers. The majority of the participants were female, with only three male caregivers included in the study. The dominance of female participants reflects the gendered nature of informal caregiving and is comparable with samples in other studies of family caregivers of older adults and people with dementia [11, 27, 28]. Further details of the methodology of this study and the major findings have been published elsewhere [29].

Nationality	Number of caregivers	Gender	Carer status
Italian	$n = 6$	All female	Spouse caregivers
Macedonian	$n = 11$	8 female/3 male	Spouse caregivers
Portuguese	$n = 5$	All female	4 spouse caregivers/1 adult child caregiver

Table 1. Focus groups.

Nationality	Number of caregivers	Gender	Carer status
Italian	$n = 2$	Female	Adult child caregivers
Greek	$n = 2$	Female	1 adult child/1 spouse caregiver
Dutch	$n = 1$	Female	Spouse caregiver
Croatian	$n = 1$	Female	Adult child caregiver
Macedonian	$n = 1$	Female	Adult child caregiver

Table 2. Semi-structured individual interviews.

Overall, the following key themes were identified from the qualitative data:

1. *Managing medication is a source of stress for family caregivers.*
2. *Medication management may be a point of familial conflict that needs to be carefully controlled.*
3. *Family support of this caregiving role is important.*
4. *Family caregivers believe that they would benefit from more sources of external information and support regarding medication management.*

Quotes to support these four key themes are provided below:

1. *Managing medication is a source of stress for family caregivers.*

   Caregivers reported stress resulting from their medication management role as they managed complex medication regimes. Sometimes these difficulties arose as an outcome of the progression of dementia:

   > "He would say "No, No! 'That's not the tablet I'm supposed to have now' or 'I had it before!' or 'that's the one I'm supposed to have later in the night" so I just ignored this for a while and we would start all over again"…".Sometimes I gave him the tablet and he would take a sip of water and then next minute I found it, that tablet, on the floor. He spat it out!"' (Greek spouse caregiver interview)

   Caregivers adopted various strategies to help them manage this stress. The most common was the use of blister packaged medications prepared weekly by a pharmacist.

   This strategy was not always failsafe:

   > "My friend, his wife she has a Webster (blister) pack and he was not there…. she took the whole pack at once and had to go to hospital". (Macedonian Focus Group)

   > "And there were occasions when he was taking hers. He took her medication (pack) instead of his!" (Greek adult child caregiver interview):

2. *Medication management may be a point of familial conflict that needs to be carefully controlled.*

Caregivers lost trust in their relative's ability to manage their medications autonomously when they observed medication errors being made. This often became a source of conflict as the PLWD hoped to maintain autonomy while the caregiver feared that medication errors could result in problems.

> We were finding too much on the floor, not only from hers but also from his. Oh it was just horrendous, it was just horrendous!….. "And when we got the Webster (blister) packs he was so angry with us. He said 'What do you think?! Do you think I can't look after my medications?!'" (Greek adult child caregiver interview)

Crushing medications was the most common strategy adopted by caregivers in order to avoid further conflict around medication administration.

> So we started hiding the medication in food, so we crushed it for example, put it in some yoghurt if it was breakfast time". (Italian adult child caregiver interview)

3. *Family support of this caregiving role is important.*

Many caregivers in our study noted that they shared medication management tasks such as picking up prescriptions or taking the PLWD to the doctor to have medication prescriptions written. The burden of medication administration was also shared with other family members:

> "Yes, and the girls (daughters) are here all the time, in and out and sometimes they would encourage him to take this and that". (Greek spouse caregiver interview)

4. *Family caregivers believe that they would benefit from more sources of external information and support regarding medication management.*

Caregivers noted a general lack of information and support available to them in their medication management role even though they spoke of contact with community pharmacists, general practitioners (GP), geriatricians and family caregiver support groups. Caregivers noted that pharmacists were more accessible sources of information than doctors.

> "You know we would go and ask the pharmacist when we were picking up the Webster (blister) pack, you know most of the time it was the pharmacist not the GP". (Macedonian adult child caregiver interview)

Some participants used internet sources for information to assist with their medication management role.

> "Two tablets were interfering with each other and it was my daughter who saw it in the computer and she told the doctor". (Portuguese Focus Group)

Overall, the caregivers suggested that they lacked information about common medication-related side effects such as constipation, resulting from the use of pain medication, as well as concerns relating to the use of multiple medications.

> "Mum's on 12 or 10 or something and it's just such a chemistry set inside a body and how it reacts with Mum is so different to how it might react to someone else and so how can they get it right? You know that's what I'm wondering and especially at Mum's stage where the dementia is; what we should really be worrying about, just to make her life more comfortable from now….. Does she really have to worry?…. If you stopped something like cholesterol medication or thyroid medication she'll drop dead tomorrow, I don't know? I don't want that. But all the other peripheral medications are they really necessary, you know are they really necessary?" (Italian adult child caregiver interview)

Spouse caregivers in particular faced additional challenges in managing medications resulting from language barriers and a lack of access to appropriate services.

> "I go to a chemist where there is a Portuguese girl. We understand each other. It's the other ones I can't understand a word. I like to go in when she is working but she only works one day a week". (Portuguese Focus Group)

3.4. Resource development

3.4.1. Background

Once we had gathered the information based on our aforementioned literature review and qualitative study, we used our findings to inform the content of a pilot version of the resource to enable initial evaluation. Clearly a comprehensive information resource was needed to address the many medication management issues and/or questions caregivers faced. We wanted to design something that would be accessible to all, even for those with limited literacy. We also wanted to provide reliable information that could be kept up to date and could be revisited as the needs of the caregiver(s) changed. For this reason, the research team decided to produce an online resource.

An online resource has the advantage of being available at all times of the day and can be bookmarked and revisited if information is forgotten or caregiving requirements change [30]. The internet allows both written and oral versions of the information to be presented, addressing potential literacy issues. It also enables different language versions to be added to the resource, overcoming language barriers. We acknowledged that some of the older spouse caregivers might not be able to access this resource as many older adults are not familiar with technology use [31]. However, we hoped that the resource would be accessed by the adult children of spouse caregivers or could be used as a resource during family caregiver support group meetings.

We were mindful of the fact that the health information we provided online needed to be both understandable and reliable. This is especially true when considering older people living with a dementia and their caregivers; as it is highly probable that they are less likely to have the time or ability to evaluate online health information. We sought to ensure the reliability of the content by basing the content on current research findings. Caregivers were referred to links for other reliable sites if they wanted further information.

We knew that in developing our resource we needed to address literacy and health literacy concerns. Approximately 44% of Australians have problems in understanding health information [32]. Poor health literacy is particularly prevalent amongst older adults especially those with limited education, low incomes and from linguistically diverse populations [33, 34]. In order to cater for those with low health literacy, we drew on current health literacy research [35–37] and guidelines for web design suited to older adult users [38, 39] to guide the content and design of the resource.

3.4.2. Addressing literacy concerns

Based on evidence that in order to improve health literacy, information needs to be written at a grade 8 or below level [36], health literacy guidelines [35, 37] were followed to improve the readability of our online resource. We used plain language, avoiding overly technical jargon wherever possible. Sentence structures were simplified, an active voice used and dot point lists used where appropriate. Simple visuals were included if they would aid understanding allowing for white space on the page to avoid clutter. Furthermore, an audio version of each page (both in English and Italian) was made to cater for those who might have a stronger command of the oral language, as opposed to written text available in both languages.

3.4.3. Addressing website accessibility

Working on this assumption that many of our site visitors would be older people and/or their adult children, we approached the web design process aiming to make the website universally accessible. Our pilot web design was informed by the SilverWeb guidelines [39], and the checklist for the development of senior friendly websites available at https://www.nlm.nih.gov/pubs/staffpubs/od/ocpl/agingchecklist.html [38]. A larger font size and a sans-serif font were used in the written text, while avoiding yellow, green and blue colours to accommodate declining visual acuity. Visual content was kept to a minimum, which meant that the resource included only text relevant images. Navigation buttons were large, and each page had prompts to click forward or return to previous pages. Menu tabs were organised to make it easy to locate relevant information and the need for scrolling on pages was avoided where possible.

3.4.4. Content of the online Phase 1 resource

The key messages of the site included recommendations to:

- Undertake regular medication checks and reviews with a pharmacist and/or doctor familiar with the PLWD.

- Use reputable sources of information about medication—general practitioner, pharmacist, or nurse.
- Actively find information about medications taken by the person with dementia, document these and keep an up-to-date list.

The site also described practical strategies to help the person with dementia to take the right medicines at the right time. It was hoped that these strategies would also reduce familial conflict and stress experienced by the caregivers in their medication management role. The main recommendation was to use blister packaged medications; regularly checking for their ongoing safe usage, and as suggested by Zedler et al. [40] to help improve medication adherence. Blister packs also offer benefits for the PLWD and their caregiver by allowing them to see which medications need to be taken when, and whether or not they have been taken appropriately. Given that many caregivers reported crushing medications in our qualitative study, a page was included to alert caregivers that not all medications are safe to crush. The online resource advises PLWD and/or their caregivers to ask their pharmacist or doctor before crushing any medications or to enquire about alternate formulations (e.g. liquid or transdermal patches) that would avoid the need to crush medications.

Finally, the online resource also provided additional information regarding other reputable websites, support groups, translation services and organisations which could help facilitate safe and effective medication management for PLWD.

3.5. Evaluation of Phase 1 pilot resource

3.5.1. Survey evaluation of the pilot resource

We aimed to evaluate the pilot website considering our two guiding design principles: the accessibility of the site and the accessibility of the content, especially for our target audience. An adapted version of the 'Quality checklist for reviewing health information' [41] was used to initially assess the resource. This checklist asks the user to review the content, usefulness, appeal, cultural relevance, readability, presentation, accessibility, credibility and need for improvement of the information resource. The checklist, only available in English, was completed by nine users of the pilot resource all of whom gave positive responses. The survey respondents also provided useful suggestions about additional information regarding specific medications, the need for other formats such as a DVD version of the resource, and translation of the resource in to other languages.

3.5.2. Support group evaluations of the pilot resource

Evaluation of the pilot site was also undertaken with caregivers from English and Italian support groups, who also suggested a DVD version of the resource, as evident in the following participant quote:

> "Not sure how well used the online resource will be for the older Italian carers who I suspect may not be well versed in using this sort of media however I think

having things online is the way to go in the future…..even using a DVD version would be hard for them". (Italian adult child caregiver)

Support group participants were positive about the resource, suggesting that the information on the site was well received, comprehensive and useful. They suggested including support group contact details on the site and were not in favour of 'pop-outs' for some of the visual components on the site.

4. Phase 2 resource refinement and current evaluation underway

Background: The original research group was expanded to include researchers with backgrounds in nursing, public health, education and technology. Further funding was obtained which enabled the translation of the resources into a third community language; Macedonian, and the migration of the site to WordPress (https://wordpress.com/). This change to hosting platform was made to facilitate future editing and updating through a what-you-see-is-what-you-get (WYSIWYG) content management system. The results of the initial pilot study were used to inform the second iteration of the website, which is currently available at: (www.dementiameds.com) (**Figure 1**).

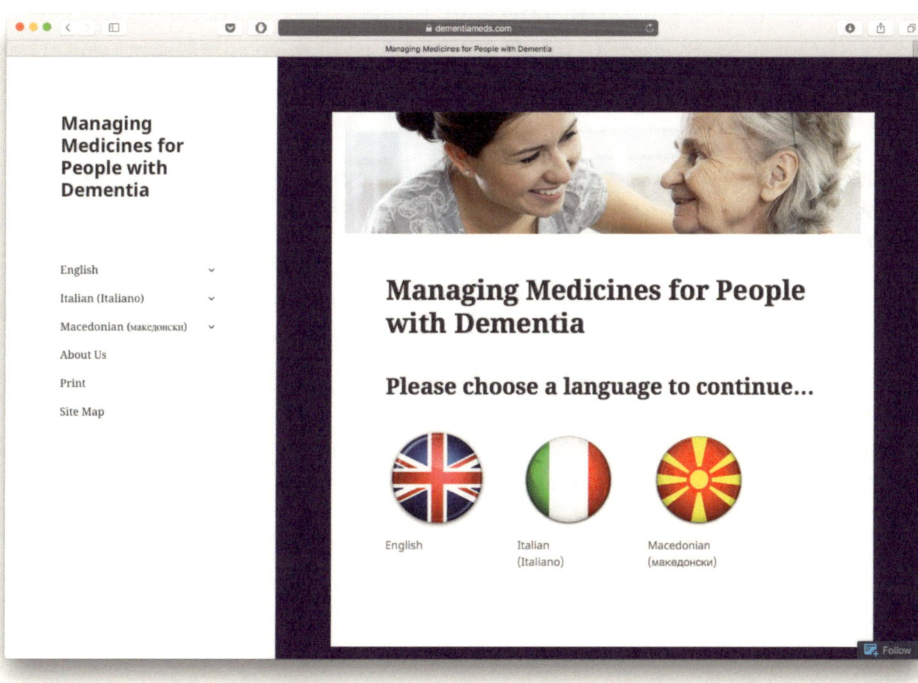

Figure 1. Managing medicines for people with dementia home page.

While the Managing Medicines site was designed to enable maximum accessibility for users, by utilising a larger font size and providing written information in an audio format, there remained the need to evaluate the site. This was completed using a mixture of methodologies, which incorporated readability, usability and server log data analysis.

4.1. Usability testing

Website users inherently rely on their previous internet experiences to inform their online behaviour. Nielsen[42] found that experienced users are faster at doing things on websites that they use often; they are, more confident at clicking and less afraid that they will break something, better at searching, using the mouse and scrolling. As such, usability testing was undertaken to ensure that the Managing Medicines for People with Dementia website met the needs of the end-users. Previous research has shown that usability testing with five participants can identify 85% of problems [42].

A convenience sample of ten participants (age range: 26–79 years of age; mean age 51.8 years) completed the usability testing. Participants were all family caregivers of PLWD, spoke English, had used the internet and were willing to be recorded during the usability testing process. Participants were also asked to complete a short demographic survey, which included questions on age, gender, language spoken at home, country of birth, computer and internet use. Participants were subsequently asked to think-aloud as they completed five set tasks. This allowed the researchers insight into their thought process, personal opinions and reactions to the website. The tasks were designed to mimic the actions that website visitors might have for example, "Please change the language settings from English to Italian", and goals e.g. "Please find the phone number for xxx".

The software program Morae Recorder (TechSmith, Okemos, Michigan) was used to conduct the usability testing. Morae records participant's interactions with the website in the form of visual, audio and mouse movements.

A number of small issues were identified through the usability testing. Most participants encountered difficulties when asked to find specific information. Participants suggested that a dedicated page be added to the site with contact details for support services. Currently, this information is embedded within the website. It was also observed that it would have been useful to have incorporated a short practice into the usability testing, to allow participants to become familiar with how Morae operates.

It should be noted that numerous variables affected task completion time, and the successful completion of tasks. Factors included the telling of personal stories, the presence of children during testing, and phones ringing. This supports the observations from another usability testing study with older adults[43].

Participants who reported over 10 hours internet usage per week were more likely to be successful in completing the tasks. It is likely that this difference was observed due to their increased familiarity with website navigation and increased internet skill level.

4.1.1. Method critique

While the use of dedicated usability software facilitated recording and analysis of sessions, it would be possible to undertake basic usability testing using traditional audio-visual recording methods and researcher notes. Ideally, usability testing should be undertaken by an expert. However, the use of the dedicated software enabled two research assistants to undertake the usability testing. Another possible method of testing would be a Cognitive Walk Through [43]. This involves an independent health researcher working their way through the website checking that the content is clear, uses plain English, and that the website had consistent formatting with images related to the text.

4.2. User research

In order to gain feedback from a larger number of site users, a site evaluation survey was compiled and made available using SurveyMonkey. Visitors to the site were asked to complete this online evaluation survey, through a message at the bottom of the left-hand side navigation bar. This message was visible on all site pages. The survey contained 26 items and was available for a four-month period in 2015. It included demographic questions as well as two previously validated tools: a modified version of the Perceived Health Web Site Usability Questionnaire for Older Adults (PHWSUQ) [44] and Chew's three screening questions for health literacy [45]. The evaluation was promoted through personal contacts and via articles in relevant state and national newsletters.

4.2.1. Method critique

While the use of SurveyMonkey allowed a large response rate, it was flawed in that the survey was only available in English, despite the site being promoted to people from Italian and Macedonian backgrounds. While this decision was made due to financial constraints, it is a significant limitation to the evaluation of the site. Further, the majority of respondents were healthcare workers and not the target audience of family caregivers of people living with a dementia. It is possible that healthcare workers are more comfortable using the internet and completing evaluation surveys. One of the strengths of this method was the ability to incorporate previously validated tools into the survey.

4.3. Web analytics

Google Analytics (https://www.google.com.au/analytics/) was used to track and report website traffic. This program can be easily configured to monitor a specific website and runs behind the scenes, collecting data and information about site visitors. Data on the number of unique site visits, visit duration and country of origin of the visitor were collected. Notably, many site visitors were from outside of Australia.

4.3.1. Method critique

One of the main benefits of Google Analytics is that it provides insight in to site users' behaviour and location, and is free to use.

4.4. Readability

Most health information and educational material on dementia are presented at high reading levels [33, 34, 46]. A recent review of online health information found that sites with information on dementia were the hardest to read when compared to 11 other health conditions [36].

The readability levels of the Managing Medicines for People with Dementia website were evaluated using six readability tools:

1. Flesch-Kincaid, readability statistics found in Microsoft Word, based on US school grade levels

2. Gunning Fog Index readability formula (http://gunning-fog-index.com/)

3. Simple Measure of Gobbledygook (SMOG - http://www.learningandwork.org.uk/misc/SMOG-calculator/smogcalc.php?redirectedfrom=niace)

4. Dale-Chall readability formula (http://www.readabilityformulas.com/free-dale-chall-test.php)

5. Italian Read-IT DyLan Text Tool v2.1.9 (http://www.ilc.cnr.it/dylanlab/apps/texttools/?tt_user=guest), and

6. Italian Readability Analyzer (http://labs.translated.net/text-readability/).

For each test, the text from the website was copied and pasted into the tool. We were unable to identify any tools that evaluated readability in Macedonian. Results of the readability tests indicated that the written content was somewhat difficult to understand. This result may be reflective of some of the medical terms used, for example "Alzheimer's" and may be improved by rewording the written content of each page to reduce the number of long sentences. It is recognised that reducing both sentence length and word count can improve upon the overall quality of the website [33]. However, it is worth noting that the information presented on the site is quite complex, which is why caregivers experience so many difficulties in managing the medications of their loved ones. Thus, it may not always be possible to avoid complex sentence structures or word use in medication management resources.

4.4.1. Method critique

Readability testing proved to be both quick and inexpensive to undertake as it did not require any specialist software. As with other studies, readability testing allowed the identification of content problems not found through usability testing alone [43]. The different readability tools produced different readability scores, which is reflective of the different criteria assessed and different formulae used to calculate the scores. Although the readability levels were found to be relatively high, it is worth noting that the information is also available on the website as an audio version in all three languages. This makes the information more accessible to people with stronger oral literacy skills.

A further Readability Analysis using VocabProfile Compleat (VPC) (http://www.lextutor.ca/vp/comp/) [47] was conducted as part of our site evaluation, to gain a better understanding of the readability for immigrants whose second language might be English. This tool is useful to analyse the text according to the most frequently used word families in the English language. VPC categorised all the words throughout the Managing Medicines for People with Dementia website into levels of the most common words used in English with 1000 words in each level: first (K-1 words), second (K-2), third (K-3.) thousand. The frequency scores show which words an immigrant is most likely to be exposed to. Those in the lower thousands would likely be known whereas those in the higher thousands, less so. The results of this analysis revealed that the majority of words fell within the first one thousand level (79.32%) and second thousand level (10.61%) categories overall, suggesting that the word choice throughout the site is accessible to English as a second language speakers.

This frequency information is important to consider because the greater the number of words that fall outside the first two categories (K 1-2), the greater the potential difficulty that second language speakers of English would likely experience in understanding the website, especially if they have limited proficiency in English. Ideally, websites imparting information to second language speakers should try to utilize words that make up at least 95% of the readers' receptive vocabulary. This figure was determined based on Hsueh-Chao and Nation's [48] description of optimal conditions for extensive reading within an English as a Second Language curriculum being 95–98% of known words and Nation's [49] argument that 98–99% is ideal.

4.5. Quality of information on health websites

Almost anyone can create a website and author content that can be accessed by the general public. It has been estimated that 30 million new websites are created every day, with the vast majority relating to health conditions [50]. As the number of people with easy access to the internet continues to rise, it is important that the information that they access be reliable, particularly in relation to health conditions.

A number of organisations have developed codes of ethics and evaluation instruments to determine the reliability and creditability of information on the internet. A third-party approach is often used to evaluate online health information, so that users can determine the quality of information, through displaying either a label, seal or logo on their website [51]. A number of such accreditation systems are available for medical and health websites. Credibility, relevance and accuracy are especially important for health websites where information can have a direct impact on the health and well-being of the site user.

Methods: Three website rating tools were used to assess the Managing Medicines for People with Dementia website for accessibility, quality and reliability.

1. Suitability Assessment of Materials (SAM http://aspiruslibrary.org/literacy/sam.pdf);
2. Health on the Net Checklist (HONcode - http://www.hon.ch/HONcode/Patients/);
3. Health-Related Website Evaluation Form [52].

The Suitability Assessment of Materials (SAM) instrument contains six sections: content, literacy demand, graphics, layout and type, learning stimulation and motivation and cultural appropriateness. The SAM rates factors affecting the difficulty of readability and the comprehension relative to understanding the meaning. For each factor, the materials were categorised and rated as not suitable (0), adequate (1) and superior (2) based on objective criteria.

The Health-Related Web Site Evaluation Form consists of 36 questions, covering: content, accuracy, author, currency, audience, navigation, external links and structure. The rating scale criteria were defined as poor (<75%), adequate (75–89%) and excellent (>90%).

The Health on the Net Foundation (HONcode) is a self-regulating non-government organisation with a set of principles adopted to standardise the creditability and reliability of health and medical information on the internet [51]. It was developed to provide a code of ethics for medical and health-related information on the internet, for three target audiences, the general public, health professionals and web publishers. It is suggested that if health information websites adhere to the HONcode, it will go a long way to ensuring that the health information provided to the public is both of good quality and reliable. The HONcode certification has eight principles: authority, complementary, confidentiality, attribution, justification, transparency, financial disclosure and advertising, which are assessed through 12 items.

4.5.1. Method critique

All of the instruments were found to be quick and easy to administer, and showed that the website provided reliable information and allowed the identification of some minor problems in the website design.

4.6. Future recommendations

It is important to plan to undertake assessment for usability, readability and accessibility levels when designing a website. Often this is an iterative, multimodal process. The Phase 2 evaluation highlighted the importance of involving end-users in the design of a health-information website. It showed that a combination of qualitative and quantitative methods can be effectively utilised to identify design and content problems. Further, the methodologies used were often simple to undertake and relatively cheap to conduct.

The results of the evaluation process will be used to inform the final design changes to the website. The site will subsequently be made available to national bodies within Australia, such as Alzheimer's Australia, for promotion. Further funding will be sought in order to translate information into other community languages.

5. Conclusion

Good management of the individual needs of the person with dementia may mean that they can live in the community setting for as long as possible. This includes attention to the safe and effective management of medications. Acknowledgement, information and support for caregivers in their medication management role are important, both for the ongoing care of the PLWD and to help prevent or reduce caregiver stress. Medication management support and information are especially needed by linguistically diverse caregivers.

The provision of accessible and reliable online information was found to be useful for caregivers of PLWD, including those from linguistically diverse backgrounds. It is important that resources are developed, evaluated and refined to ensure their content is accessible to a wide range of audience, including those with lower literacy levels. Following the precautionary principle, if the needs of low literacy groups are met, then a resource will be accessible to the widest audience. However, developing an online dementia-specific information resource to meet low literacy levels is problematic and requires attention to word choice and sentence length to improve readability. Uniquely, this resource incorporated additional languages, other than English, and oral versions of the content. This helped to address the specific literacy needs of the resource's target audience.

The research and development team recommend that further funding and research are urgently needed to meet the needs of those who are ageing in a host country, especially those with dementia. This is especially important given that many older adults will migrate during their lifetime, often to a country where they are not familiar with the language or health services.

Acknowledgements

The research team wishes to thank the Multicultural Health Service of the Illawarra and Shoalhaven Local Health District for their recognition of the importance of this study and the initial funding of the project.

Two summer scholarships were provided by the Illawarra Health and Medical Research Institute via the Bridgewater Family Trust to develop the initial pilot resource.

A Living Well Living Longer Global Challenges Grant was also received from the University of Wollongong to redesign the website and complete the evaluation stage.

We thank the Multicultural Health Workers who have assisted with the project giving helpful advice and making contact with study participants.

Finally, this work could not have been completed without the stories shared by the family caregivers of people living with dementia. We thank each one for their willingness to give of their time and talk about their experiences in their caring role.

The authors would like to acknowledge the work of Holly Gleeson, Rhett Thomas-Lee and Catherine Kostovski who undertook the: readability assessment, quality of information on health websites analysis and usability testing as part of their final year, undergraduate population health placement at the University of Wollongong.

Author details

Robyn Gillespie[1*], Pippa Burns[1], Lindsey Harrison[2], Amanda Baker[3], Khin Win[4], Victoria Traynor[5] and Judy Mullan[1]

*Address all correspondence to: rjg906@uowmail.edu.au

1 School of Medicine, University of Wollongong, Wollongong, Australia

2 School of Health and Society, University of Wollongong, Wollongong, Australia

3 School of Education, University of Wollongong, Wollongong, Australia

4 School of Computing and Information Technology, University of Wollongong, Wollongong, Australia

5 School of Nursing, University of Wollongong, Wollongong, Australia

References

[1] United Nations Population Division. International Migrant Stock: The 2008 Revision: United Nations; 2009 [05/06/2012] Available from: http://esa.un.org/migration/.

[2] Australian Institute of Health and Welfare. Dementia in Australia. Canberra 2012 [01/11/2012] Available from: http://www.aihw.gov.au/publication-detail/?id=10737422958

[3] CIRCA (Cultural and indigenous Research Centre, Australia): CALD Dementia Strategic Model: Literature Review, Report, Model. Sydney, Australia: NSW Department of Ageing, Disability and Homecare, 2008.

[4] Bajramovic F, Tett SE. Medication Management Reviews for People from the Former Yugoslavia Now Resident in Australia. Pharmacy World & Science. 2004; 26(5):271–6.

[5] Prince M, Wimo A, Guerchet M, Ali G, Wu Y, Prina M. World Alzheimer Report 2015. The Global Impact of Dementia. An Analysis of Prevalence, Incidence, Cost and Trends. London, England: Alzheimer's Disease International, 2015.

[6] Weimer DL, Sager MA. Early Identification and Treatment of Alzheimer's Disease: Social and Fiscal Outcomes. Alzheimer's & Dementia: the Journal of the Alzheimer's Association. 2009; 5(3):215–26.

[7] Prince MJ, Wu F, Guo Y, Robledo LMG, O'Donnell M, Sullivan R, et al. The Burden of Disease in Older People and Implications for Health Policy and Practice. The Lancet. 2015; 385(9967):549–62.

[8] Lau DT, Mercaldo ND, Harris AT, Trittschuh E, Shega J, Weintraub S. Polypharmacy and Potentially Inappropriate Medication Use among Community-Dwelling Elders with Dementia. Alzheimer Disease and Associated Disorders. 2010; 24(1):56.

[9] Maidment ID, Fox C, Boustani M, Katona C. Medication Management—the Missing Link in Dementia Interventions. International Journal of Geriatric Psychiatry. 2012; 27(5):439–42.

[10] Cotrell V, Wild K, Bader T. Medication Management and Adherence among Cognitively Impaired Older Adults. Journal of Gerontological Social Work. 2006; 47(3–4):31–46.

[11] Kaasalainen S, Dolovich L, Papaioannou A, Holbrook A, Lau E, Ploeg J, et al. The Process of Medication Management for Older Adults with Dementia. Journal of Nursing and Healthcare of Chronic Illness. 2011; 3(4):407–18.

[12] Thorpe JM, Thorpe CT, Kennelty KA, Gellad WF, Schulz R. The Impact of Family Caregivers on Potentially Inappropriate Medication Use in Noninstitutionalized Older Adults with Dementia. The American Journal of Geriatric Pharmacotherapy. 2012; 10(4):230–41.

[13] Reeve E, Simon Bell J, N Hilmer S. Barriers to Optimising Prescribing and Deprescribing in Older Adults with Dementia: A Narrative Review. Current Clinical Pharmacology. 2015; 10(3):168–77.

[14] Alsaeed D, Jamieson E, Gul MO, Smith FJ. Challenges to Optimal Medicines Use in People Living with Dementia and Their Caregivers: A Literature Review. International Journal of Pharmaceutics. 2015. Dec 22

[15] Smith F, Francis SA, Gray N, Denham M, Graffy J. A Multi-Centre Survey among Informal Carers Who Manage Medication for Older Care Recipients: Problems Experienced and Development of Services. Health & Social Care in the Community. 2003; 11(2):138–45.

[16] Brodaty H, Green A. Defining the Role of the Caregiver in Alzheimer's Disease Treatment. Drugs & Aging. 2002; 19(12): 891–898

[17] Lingler JH, Sereika SM, Amspaugh CM, Arida JA, Happ ME, Houze MP, et al. An Intervention to Maximize Medication Management by Caregivers of Persons with Memory Loss: Intervention Overview and Two-Month Outcomes. Geriatric Nursing. 2016; 37(3): 186–191

[18] Poland F, Mapes S, Pinnock H, Katona C, Sorensen S, Fox C, et al. Perspectives of Carers on Medication Management in Dementia: Lessons from Collaboratively Developing a Research Proposal. BMC Research Notes. 2014; Jul 21;7(1):463.

[19] Francis SA, Smith F, Gray N, Denham M. Partnerships between Older People and Their Carers in the Management of Medication. International Journal of Older People Nursing. 2006; 1(4):201–7.

[20] Reinhard SC, Choula R. Meeting the Needs of Diverse Family Caregivers. Washington DC: AARP Public Policy Institute, 2012 September 2012. Report No.69 [28/10/2012] Available from: http://www.ws6-md.aarp.org/content/dam/aarp/research/public_policy_institute/ltc/2012/meeting-needs-diverse-family-caregivers-insight-AARP-ppi-ltc.pdf

[21] Duane F, While, C., Beanland, C., Koch, S.,. Making Medicines Manageable: A Culturally and Linguistically Diverse Perspective. Royal District Nursing Service, 2011. [06/05/2012] Available from: http://www.rallyhealthcare.com.au/public/files/files/Making%20Medicines%20Manageable%20report%202011.pdf

[22] Broadley L, Mihajlovic M, Paschalidis-Chilas E, Perry A. Multicultural Health Profile, 2009. Multicultural Health Service, South Eastern Sydney Illawarra Health.; 2009. [04/03/2012] Available from http://www.sesiahs.health.nsw.gov.au/multicultural_health_service/Documents/MulticulturalHealthProfile2009.pdf

[23] Halilovic K. Post-War Portuguese Migration to the Illawarra. University of Wollongong, Australia Thesis Collection 2001.

[24] Gillespie R, Mullan J, Harrison L. Managing Medications: The Role of Informal Caregivers of Older Adults and People Living with Dementia. A Review of the literature. Journal of Clinical Nursing. 2014;23(23–24):3296–3308.

[25] Australian Bureau of Statistics. Population Projections, Australia, 2012(Base) to 2101 Canberra: ABS; 2013 [14/08/2014]. Available from: http://www.abs.gov.au/ausstats/abs@.nsf/Lookup/3222.0main+features52012%20%28base%29%20to%202101.

[26] Berisic M, Nesvadba N. Perceptions of Dementia in Ethnic Communities. Alzheimer's Australia Victoria, 2008. [05/07/2012] Available from: http://www.fightdementia.org.au/research-publications/cald-publications.aspx

[27] Travis SS, Bernard MA, McAuley WJ, Thornton M, Kole T. Development of the Family Caregiver Medication Administration Hassles Scale. The Gerontologist. 2003; 43(3): 360–8.

[28] Kao H-FS, Lynn MR. Use of the Measurement of Medication Administration Hassles with Mexican American Family Caregivers. Journal of Clinical Nursing. 2009; 18(18): 2596–603.

[29] Gillespie RJ, Harrison L, Mullan J. Medication Management Concerns of Ethnic Minority Family Caregivers of People Living with Dementia. Dementia. 2015; 14(1), pp47–62.

[30] Griffiths F, Lindenmeyer A, Powell J, Lowe P, Thorogood M. Why Are Health Care Interventions Delivered over the Internet? A Systematic Review of the Published Literature. Journal of Medical Internet Research. 2006; 8(2):e10.

[31] Eriksson-Backa K. The Role of Online Health Information in the Lives of Finns Aged 65 to 79 Years. International Journal of Networking and Virtual Organisations. 2013; 13(1):5–23.

[32] Australian Bureau of Statistics. 4228.0 – Programme for the International Assessment of Adult Competencies, Australia, 2011-12 Canberra, Australia: ABS; 2014 [19/04/2016] Available from: http://www.abs.gov.au/ausstats/abs@.nsf/Latestproducts/4228.0Main%20Features102011-12?opendocument&tabname=Summary&prodno=4228.0&issue=2011-12&num=&view=.

[33] Sabharwal S, Badarudeen S. Readability of Online Patient Education Materials from the AAOS Web Site. 2008:1245–50.

[34] Weih M, Reinhold A, Klein H, Kornhuber J. Unsuitable Readability Levels of Patient Information Pertaining to Dementia and Related Diseases : A Comparative Analysis. 2008 (June):1116–23.

[35] U.S. Department of Health and Human Services Centres for Disease Control and Prevention. Simply Put: A Guide to Creating Easy- to -Understand Materials. Atlanta Georgia 2009.

[36] Cheng C, Dunn M. Health Literacy and the Internet: A Study on the Readability of Australian Online Health Information. Australian and New Zealand Journal of Public Health. 2015; 39(4):309–14.

[37] DeWalt D, Callahan L, Hawk V, Broucksou K, Hink A, Rudd R, et al. Health Literacy Universal Precautions Toolkit.(Prepared by North Carolina Network Consortium, the Cecil G. Sheps Center for Health Services Research, the University of North Carolina at Chapel Hill, under Contract No. Hhsa290200710014. Ahrq Publication No. 10–0046–Ef). Rockville, MD: Agency for Healthcare Research and Quality. 2010.

[38] National Institute on Aging. Making Your Website Senior Friendly 2002 [28/01/2013] Available from: https://www.nlm.nih.gov/pubs/checklist.pdf.

[39] Zaphiris P, Kurniawan S, Ghiawadwala M. A Systematic Approach to the Development of Research-Based Web Design Guidelines for Older People. Universal Access in the Information Society. 2007;6(1):59–75.

[40] Zedler BK, Kakad P, Colilla S, Murrelle L, Shah NR. Does Packaging with a Calendar Feature Improve Adherence to Self-Administered Medication for Long-Term Use? A Systematic Review. Clinical Therapeutics. 2011; 33(1):62–73.

[41] Government of South Australia. Evaluating Health Information with Consumers. Sample Questions for Consumers. Children, Youth and Women's Health Service. 2006.

[42] Nielsen J. Why You Only Need to Test with 5 Users 2000 [29/04/2016] Available from: http://www.useit.com/alertbox/20000319.html.

[43] Burns P, Jones SC, Iverson D, Caputi P. Usability Testing of AsthmaWise with Older Adults. Computers Informatics Nursing. 2013; 31(5):219–26.

[44] Nahm E-S, Resnick B, Mills ME, editors. Development and Pilot-Testing of the Perceived Health Web Site Usability Questionnaire (PHWSUQ) for Older Adults 2006; Lansdale, PA, USA: IOS Press.

[45] Chew L, Griffin JM, Partin MR, Noorbaloochi S, Grill JP, Snyder A, et al. Validation of Screening Questions for Limited Health Literacy in a Large Va Outpatient Population. Journal of General Internal Medicine. 2008; 23(5):561–6.

[46] Walsh TM, Volsko Ta. Readability Assessment of Internet-Based Consumer Health Information. Respiratory Care. 2008; 53(10):1310–5.

[47] Cobb T. Compleat Lexical Tutor V.8 Université du Québec à Montréal; N.D. [19/04/2016]. Available from: http://www.lextutor.ca/.

[48] Hsueh-Chao MH, Nation P. Unknown Vocabulary Density and Reading Comprehension. Reading in a Foreign Language. 2000; 13(1):403–30.

[49] Nation I.S.P. Teaching Esl/Efl Reading and Writing. New York: Routledge; 2008.

[50] Usher W, Skinner J. Health Websites and Reliability Components. ACHPER Australia Healthy Lifestyles Journal. 2007; 55(4):31–6.

[51] Hanif F, Read JC, Goodacre Ja, Chaudhry A, Gibbs P. The Role of Quality Tools in Assessing Reliability of the Internet for Health Information. Informatics for Health & Social Care. 2009; 34(4):231–43.

[52] Teach L. Health-Related Website Evaluation Form Emory University, USA: Rollins School of Public Health; 1998 [29/04/2016] Available from: http://terpconnect.umd.edu/~kbedon/webeval3.html.

Chapter 20

Diabetes Mellitus and Depression as Risk Factors for Dementia: SADEM Study

Juárez-Cedillo Teresa, Hsiung Ging-Yuek,
Sepehry A. Amir, Beattie B. Lynn, Jacova Claudia and
Escobedo de la Peña Jorge

Additional information is available at the end of the chapter

http://dx.doi.org/10.5772/64678

Abstract

Aim: 3Evidence indicates that the comorbidity of dementia with diabetes and depression may affect most cognitive functions. Our chief interest was to examine the patterns of cognitive functioning in individuals diagnosed with dementia, diabetes, and depression as compared with dementia plus diabetes (DDM), or dementia plus depression (DD) and healthy controls.

Methods: We included 207 participants with dementia (age 60+), 83 with Alzheimer's disease (AD), 66 vascular dementia (VaD), and 58 mixed dementia (AD/VaD). The Mini-Mental State Examination (MMSE) was used for global neuropsychological assessment, and the Center for Epidemiologic Studies Depression Scale for symptoms of depression. Diabetes was confirmed by medical diagnosis. Results: Analysis showed differences in cognitive functioning among the groups with statistical significance. Notably, there was greater cognitive dysfunction in patients with diagnosis of dementia and depression than in controls, but the difference was reduced in patients with comorbid dementia diabetes. Subsequent comparisons indicated that vascular dementia with comorbid depression and diabetes presents significantly inferior cognitive performance than those with dementia alone or the control group.

Conclusions: These results suggest that dementia, when combined with depression or diabetes, adversely affects cognitive performance. These findings highlight the importance of identifying depression among diabetics and patients with dementia.

Keywords: dementia, depression, diabetes mellitus, cognitive function, Mexican population

1. Introduction

One of the most common neurological conditions that affect older adults is dementia[1]. In addition, public health reports in the United States show that one of the most frequent physical illnesses found in older adults is diabetes[2]. Dementia affects approximately 6–10% of people 65 years or older [1], and this prevalence rate increases with age. Neuropsychological impairment associated with dementia includes poor judgment, difficulty with calculation, and getting lost while driving [2]. Older patients with both dementia and depression typically show impairment in the domains of attention, memory, and psychomotor speed [3]. On the other hand, diabetes affects about 20% of people older than 65 years [4]. Patients treated for type II diabetes show cognitive deficits on brief cognitive screening [5], and subtle decrements in verbal memory and processing speed (mean difference in z scores -0.37 and -0.25 respectively) on in-depth cognitive testing. This suggests that diabetes is a significant risk factor for dementia [6]. Depression has been estimated to affect 1–5% of community-dwelling older adults [7]. Depression is common in dementia, with substantial variability in the reported base-rate ranging from 20 to 40% [4, 8, 9], and it is a probable risk factor for both vascular dementia (VaD) and Alzheimer's disease (AD) [10]. As for diabetes, the prevalence of depression is three times higher in these patients than in individuals free of diabetes (OR = 2.9, 95% CI 2.3–3.7) [10]. Diabetes and depression exhibit a closely linked bi-directional relationship: between 15 and 20% of people with diabetes will develop clinical depression, while depression is two to three times more common among people with diabetes compared to those without. Comorbid depression and diabetes have a 2.7-fold increased risk for dementia [11].

Taking these factors into account, our chief interest was to compare cognitive function in individuals diagnosed with dementia with comorbid diabetes and depressive symptoms, alone or combined, compared to those with dementia alone, and against healthy controls.

2. Methods

2.1. Subject

All subjects from that study come from the Study on Aging and Dementia in Mexico (SADEM). SADEM was a cross-sectional study conducted to determine the prevalence of MCI and dementia, between September 2009 and March 2010. Individuals age 60 years and older were invited into the study through a random sampling of the eligible population registered within 24 family medicine units from the Instituto Mexicano del Seguro Social (IMSS) encompassing all of Mexico City. All subjects were beneficiaries (users and non-users) of the IMSS. The inclusion criteria for SADEM were 1) community-dwelling individuals aged 60 years and older, living in Mexico City, 2) registered with IMSS; and 3) accepting to take part in the study through informed consent. We excluded individuals 1) resident in other states; 2) living in an institution; 3) altered mental status secondary to delirium; 4) died before study start; 5) currently taking antipsychotic medication (other psychotropic medications including antidepressants were allowed because of the potential negative impact of non-treatment on cognition); and 6) those who refused to participate or who after two attempted visits could not be located. All participants were assessed at doctor's office by a geriatric specialized in geriatric cognitive disorders. The diagnosis of dementia was performed during the study SADEM and was based on the DSM-IV. All subjects were clinically assessed. Final diagnoses were assigned by a consensus expert panel made up of neuropsychologists, neurologists, and geriatricians [12]. All subjects participating in the study, or their caregivers, gave signed informed consent. The research protocol was reviewed and approved by The National Commission of Scientific Research as well as by the IMSS Ethics Commission (registration number 2010-785-005).

In this way for 3D study, we included all patients diagnosed with dementia vascular, Alzheimer disease, or both, diagnosed during the study SADEM, both sexes. Subjects were excluded if they had a) problems with vision, b) poor auditory capacity, c) history of alcohol abuse, d) Parkinsonism or meningioma, and e) incomplete assessment scales or neurological examination. Finally, 330 patients were included and stratified into following groups: a) patients with only dementia: Alzheimer (AD), vascular (VaD) and mixed (MD) (1D†), b) patients with only depression (1D†), c) patients with only diabetes mellitus (1D†), d) patients with AD and diabetes mellitus (2D†), e) patients with AD and depression (2D†), f) patients with VaD and diabetes mellitus (2D†), g) patients with VaD and depression (2D†), h) patients with MD and diabetes mellitus (2D†), i) patients with MD and depression (2D†), j) patients with AD and diabetes mellitus and depression (3D†), k) patients with VaD and diabetes mellitus and depression (3D†), and l) patients with MD and diabetes mellitus and depression (3D†).

2.2. Dementia evaluation

Dementia case newly recognized was conducted in two steps. First all participants of SADEM study were screened with the Mini-Mental State Examination (MMSE) [13]. All participants with a cutoff ≤24 adjustment for educational level in an aging Mexican population were underwent a battery of neuropsychological measures and a standardized neurological examination. We used the Clinical Dementia Rating or CDR to quantify the severity of symptoms of dementia [14]. Complete details of the evaluation and diagnostic procedures have been described earlier [12]. The final diagnosis of dementia was determined by consensus expert panel review including neuropsychologists, neurologists, and geriatric physicians. Each diagnosis was based on based on the Diagnostic and Statistical Manual of Mental Disorders criteria for dementia [15], (DMS-IV-R) criteria for dementia. Once dementia was diagnosed, subjects were further grouped according to whether they met the National Institute for Neurological and Communicative Disorders and Stroke and the Alzheimer's Disease and Related Disorders Association (NINCDS-ADRDA) [16], and/or the National Institute of Neurological Disorders and Stroke Association Internationale Pour la Recherche et l'Enseignement en Neurosciences (NINDS-AIREN) criteria [17]. Diagnoses fell into three categories: a) probable Alzheimer's disease (AD), b) vascular dementia (VaD), and c) mixed type dementia (MD) and were ascertained using a two-step procedure: (1) diagnosis of dementia and (2) association of cognitive impairment to lesions of vascular of origin. The criteria for diagnosis of MD were that the course was suggestive of AD, and in addition, there were focal neurologic symptoms suggestive of ischemia. The presence of vascular risk factors alone, in a patient with otherwise clinically typical AD, was not enough to support a diagnosis of MD. Hence, patients suspected of MD were subjected to all procedures for diagnosis.

2.3. Control subjects

The control group consisted of 134 subjects healthy from the SADEM study, which did not meet MCI or dementia criteria, they had a CDR score of zero, and a memory test performance <1.5 standard deviations from the mean for age. There were no significant differences between controls and cases for age or years of education ($p > 0.01$).

2.4. Cognitive measure

Cognitive testing was performed on all the patients in whom MMSE [14] and was used to evaluate global cognitive performance. For the purpose of the present study, the 11 MMSE subtests and the global MMSE score were considered independently: *spatial orientation* (state, county, town, place, and floor=5 points), *temporal orientation* (year, season, month, day, and date=5 points), *immediate memory* (immediately repeating three words=3 points), *attention/concentration* (If the participants had education as serially subtracting 7, beginning with 100, or, alternatively, spelling the word world backward for the participants without education=5 points), *delayed recall* (recalling the previously repeated three words=3 points), *language* (naming two items=2 points), *verbal repetition* (repeating a phrase=1 points), *reading a sentence* (reading aloud and understanding a sentence=1 points), *writing a sentence* (1 points), *verbal comprehension* (following a three-step command=3 points), and *constructional praxis* (copying a design=1 points). [The MMSE is thoroughly familiar to any readership in geriatrics or neurology. You would only need to specify the above if you were intending to present subscores. That might be a good idea if you do not have access to the neuropsychological scores].

2.5. Depression

In addition to neuropsychological tests, depression symptoms were evaluated using the Center for Epidemiologic Studies Depression Scale (CES-D), a validated 20-item scale consisting of four factors: depressive affect, somatic complaints, positive affect, and interpersonal relations. Scores on the CES-D ranged from 0 to 60, where 0–15 is indicative of absence of depression, and scores of 16–60 are indicative of depressive symptomatology [18]. The presence of depression was corroborated with the self-reported treatment with antidepressants, selective serotonin reuptake inhibitors (SSRI—i.e., paroxetine, sertraline, fluoxetine, venlafaxine, citalopram), or tricyclic antidepressants at any time during the four-month preceding the interview.

2.6. Diabetes assessment

Diagnosis of diabetes mellitus was based on the patients' self-report to the question, "Are you taking medication for diabetes?" These diabetes diagnoses were then confirmed by blood glucose measurements, a fasting plasma glucose concentration >7.0 mmol/l (whole blood

>6.1 mmol/l) and hemoglobin A1c (HbA1c) (<48 mmol/mol (6.5%), and treatment. All patients in this study were receiving treatment for diabetes, and 90% of patients were taking sulfonylureas for controlling diabetes with the remaining 10% on insulin therapy.

2.7. Statistical analyses

We examined effects of dementia by type, depression, and diabetes by themselves. All comparisons were performed with MANOVAs that are being conducted using a Bonferroni correction of m [19], with dementia (AD, VaD, mixed), depression (yes/no), and diabetes mellitus (yes/no) as between-subject factors. The same MANOVAs models were then used within each diagnostic group (AD, VaD, MD). Main effects and statistically significant difference between groups were assessed by F-test [20]. Additionally, a complementary analysis to better interpret the results was carried-out using the standardized mean effect sizes (Hedges' g). Hedges' g is calculated on the basis of the standardized mean difference effect size, which uses the pooled within-groups SD but corrects for bias from small sample sizes. These effect sizes indicate the mean difference between two variables expressed in standard deviation units. Hedges' g is a conservative estimate of effect size, which typically is interpreted by Cohen's d guidelines (small effect=0.20, medium effect=0.50, large effect=0.80) [21]. A positive effect size indicates that the MMSE score in the control group was superior to the diagnostic groups, whereas a negative effect size indicates that the diagnostic groups outperformed the control.

3. Results

Table 1 presents the descriptive statistics (mean ± SD) of diagnostic groups. First of all, the MANOVA models revealed that the interaction effects were not significant on sex, age, and education ($p < 0.005$). When considering the main effect of the 2D† in the MMSE score, the MANOVAs demonstrated significant effect on diabetes mellitus and depression, AD-depression, and AD-diabetes mellitus, similarly MD-diabetes mellitus, ($p < 0.005$). With the complete model, we can identify significant differences between the means of the diagnostic groups (F: 39.36, p: 0.000, R2: 0.614), indicating significant differences between the three dementias and cognitive performance.

For each diagnostic groups, we measure cognitive functioning (MMSE total scores) by calculating the difference of mean. We then convert the difference to a standardized effect size by dividing it by the pooled standard deviation for the diagnostic groups. These results are shown in **Table 2**. The margin of error (for a 95% confidence interval) for each estimate is shown. For example, the global cognitive functioning measured in effect size from group AD-depression is -3.02 standard deviation. Because the margin of error for this estimate is 0.28, the lower bound of its 95% confidence interval is -3.54, and the upper bound is -2.46. The cognitive performance in **Table 2** exhibits a strikingly consistent pattern for combination of all three types of dementia with diabetes. Global cognitive functioning is largest in the groups with AD and then decline steadily into the groups with VaD and MD.

	MMSE				Ages			Education			Sex			
	n	Mean	SD	P of corrected model ages	Mean	SD	P	Mean	SD	P	Male (%)	Fe-male (%)	P	R2
Control group (0D †)	134	30.2	3.3	**0.00**	71.8	7.6	0.00	9.1	5.5	**0.00**	46.5	53.5	**0.00**	0.37
Group diabetes mellitus (1D †)	28	29.2	5.1	**0.00**	71.6	7.0	0.03	7.0	6.2	**0.00**	52.5	47.5	**0.00**	0.67
Group depression (1D †)	84	30.2	3.2	**0.00**	69.4	6.7	0.00	8.9	5.9	**0.00**	56.5	43.5	**0.00**	0.33
Group diabetes mellitus and depression (2D †)	10	28.7	6.7	**0.01**	67.8	8.1	0.01	6.9	6.2	0.35	45.6	54.4	**0.02**	0.72
Group AD * (1D †)	37	18.7	7.4	**0.03**	76.3	8.7	0.03	6.4	5.1	0.11	66.3	33.7	0.10	0.24
Group AD-depression (2D †)	25	18.7	5.3	**0.03**	78.2	8.9	0.03	5.8	5.1	0.68	75.0	25.0	0.07	0.35
Group AD-diabetes mellitus (2D †)	13	21.4	4.5	0.52	74.5	10.0	0.42	4.1	3.7	0.76	23.8	76.2	**0.00**	0.21
Group AD-diabetes and depression (3D †)	8	21.8	4.2	0.95	74.3	7.4	0.90	7.0	6.6	0.71	75.0	25.0	0.86	0.08
Group with VaD * (1D †)	24	21.5	4.2	0.48	76.0	8.5	0.24	6.7	6.6	0.89	55.2	44.8	0.41	0.12
Group VaD-Depression (2D †)	19	19.7	6.2	0.53	80.0	8.3	0.18	5.6	4.2	0.86	57.1	42.9	0.10	0.53
Group VaD-diabetes mellitus (2D †)	10	20.8	6.5	0.37	78.3	6.6	0.23	5.9	5.0	0.33	45.8	54.2	0.10	0.39
Group VaD-diabetes and depression (3D †)	14	20.8	6.0	0.46	76.7	7.9	0.41	6.6	6.5	0.30	57.1	42.9	0.88	0.22
Group MD * (1D †)	12	17.4	5.8	0.51	76.7	8.9	0.22	5.8	6.8	0.64	41.4	58.6	0.76	0.24
Group MD-depression (2D †)	7	15.3	7.7	0.47	77.3	9.8	0.22	9.7	6.0	0.48	21.1	78.9	0.30	0.39
Group MD-diabetes mellitus (2D †)	27	18.0	4.9	0.67	77.8	9.2	0.45	6.6	5.4	0.30	26.3	73.7	**0.01**	0.07
Group MD-diabetes and depression (3D †)	12	17.9	6.4	0.38	78.9	7.8	0.87	7.5	4.9	0.26	16.7	83.3	0.13	0.31

MANOVA (complete model): sum of squares = 14913.79, gl: 18, F: 39.36, p: 0.000, R2: 0.614.

MMSE: mini-mental state examination; 0D: group without "D", 1D group with one D, 2D group with 2D, 3D group with 3D; C-E: mean of control group—mean of group (0D or 1D or 2D or 3D).

*Dementia: Alzheimer (AD), vascular (VaD), and mixed (MD).

†D is dementia or diabetes mellitus or depression.

Table 1. Demographic characteristic of diagnostic groups.

http://dx.doi.org/10.5772/64678

Type of dementia	Mean difference (C–E)	p-Value for mean difference (2-tailed T-test)	95% confidence interval for effect size		Effect size	Bias corrected (Hedges)	Standard error of effect size estimate	95% confidence interval for effect size	
			Lower	Upper				Lower	Upper
Control group (0D †)									
Group diabetes (1D †)	-1.04	0.303	-2.55	-9.89	-0.28	-0.28	0.21	-0.69	0.13
Group depression (1D †)	-0.05	0.944	-0.94	0.85	-0.01	-0.01	0.14	-0.29	0.26
Group diabetes and depression (2D †)	-1.54	0.332	-3.89	0.81	-0.42	-0.42	0.33	-1.07	0.22
Group AD * (1D †)	-11.55	**0.000**	-13.20	-9.89	-2.56	-2.55	0.23	-3.00	-2.09
Group AD-depression (2D †)	-11.56	**0.000**	-13.21	-9.91	-3.02	-3.00	0.28	-3.54	-2.46
Group AD-diabetes (2D †)	-8.81	**0.000**	-11.78	-6.84	-2.57	-2.55	0.33	-3.19	-1.91
Group AD-diabetes and depression (3D †)	-8.43	**0.000**	-10.86	-6.01	-2.50	-2.49	0.39	-3.26	-1.72
Group with VaD * (1D †)	-8.78	**0.000**	-10.29	-7.26	-2.54	-2.52	0.26	-3.04	-2.01
Group VaD-depression (2D †)	-10.52	**0.000**	-12.35	-8.69	-2.78	-2.77	0.29	-3.34	-2.20
Group VaD-diabetes (2D †)	-12.20	**0.000**	-11.78	-7.11	-2.62	-2.60	0.36	-3.31	-1.89
Group VaD-diabetes and depression (3D †)	-9.48	**0.000**	-11.50	-7.47	-2.61	-2.60	0.32	-3.22	-1.97
Group MD * (1D †)	-13.78	**0.000**	-15.95	-11.61	-3.78	-3.76	0.37	-4.49	-3.03
Group MD-depression (2D †)	-14.97	**0.000**	-17.74	-12.10	-4.14	-4.11	0.46	-5.21	-3.21
Group MD-diabetes (2D †)	-12.20	**0.000**	-13.71	-10.69	-3.36	-3.34	0.28	-3.89	-2.79
Group MD-diabetes and depression (3D †)	-12.32	**0.000**	-14.49	-10.15	-3.38	-3.36	0.36	-4.07	-2.66

MMSE: mini-mental state examination; 0D: group without "D", 1D group with one D, 2D group with 2D, 3D group with 3D; C-E: mean of control group—mean of group (0D or 1D or 2D or 3D).

*Dementia: Alzheimer (AD), vascular (VaD), and mixed (MD).

†D is dementia or diabetes mellitus or depression.

Table 2. Mean and effect sizes of the MMSE by type of dementia.

We illustrate such cognitive performance gaps in **Figure 1**, which shows differences in terms of effect sizes, that is, the difference in mean scores divided by the standard deviation of scores for all groups. When comparing among the dementia groups, we observed that patients with AD presented better cognitive performance than patients with the diagnosis of VaD and MD, while patients with MD-depression had worse cognitive performance than patients with any type of dementias and diabetes and depression. Which confirms the finding that the worst cognitive performance is evident in the groups od MD and depression (**Figure 1**).

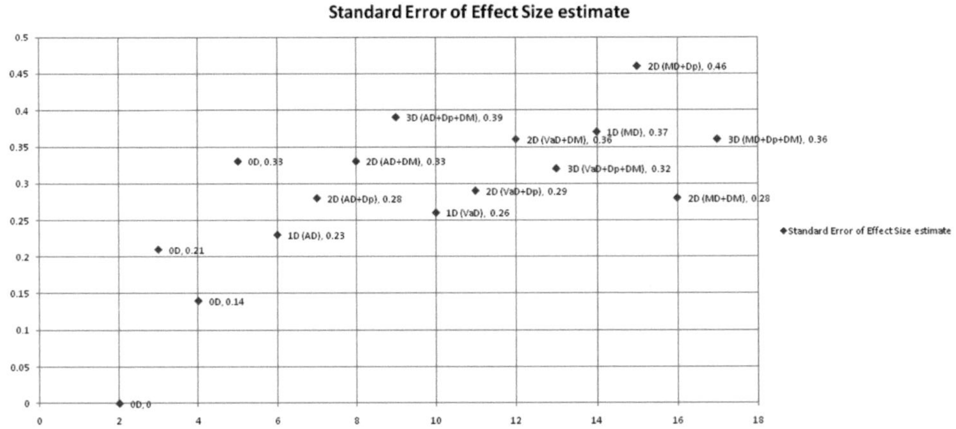

Figure 1. Hedges' g of the MMSE by type of dementia. Alzheimer (AD), vascular (VaD), and mixed (MD) and "#" is the number of "D" a group has (0 or 1 or 2 or 3), and the letter "D" is dementia or diabetes mellitus or depression.

4. Discussion

To our knowledge, this is the first study to attempt to examine the specific patterns of performance on measures of neuropsychological functioning among those with diagnosis of dementia with co-existing diabetes and depression. We found supporting evidence showing the variation in the neuropsychological functioning between individuals with 3Ds in contrast to dementia patients with either comorbid depression or diabetes. Overall, patients with dementia with coexisting diabetes and depression had greater cognitive impairment relative to dementia only, or healthy controls. There was a non-significant trend for cognitive scores of dementia and depression group to fall between the dementia with diabetes groups. These results illustrate the importance of controlling for depression and diabetes when diagnosing cognition. Some studies suggest that depression is a risk factor for dementia and depression treatment may be a causal factor for dementia [22]. Furthermore, depression may increase vulnerability to and/or exacerbate existing cognitive deficits [23]. Additionally, Ritchie et al. [24] examined the association between depression and diabetes and report that 36.8% of the patients with dementia have depression, while only 10.6% have diabetes. Similar reports [25] show that 23.7% of patients with dementia have dementia and depression. While the precise neurobiological mechanisms underlying depression and cognitive abnormalities in type 2 diabetes are unknown, both cognitive impairment and diabetes have been observed among older adults with major depression. In our study, patients with dementia and diabetes had lower scores on cognitive performance relative to healthy controls, which is consistent with previously reports in other populations.

Overall, type 2 diabetes has been associated with mild cognitive deficits, most frequently in the domains of verbal memory, processing speed, and to a lesser degree, executive functioning (see review) [5]. Another study suggests that there is a protector effect of insulin on surface plasma insulin receptors, although it is possible that the improvement of cognitive function is due to better glucose control rather than a direct effect on the neurons [27]. However, methodological and study design differences, such as variations in sampling, assessment instruments, degree of diabetes severity, and the presence of comorbid illnesses, have resulted in inconclusive results. Consistent with the literature on diabetes research, research examining the relationship between depression and cognitive functioning is filled with mixed results, as mentioned above. There is evidence suggesting that the pattern of cognitive impairment varies by depression subgroup or severity (e.g., major versus minor depression) [30, 31]. In general, depression has been linked with a range of declines in cognitive domains, including memory, executive functioning, attention, and psychomotor speed [32].

The present study differs from others in that previous studies typically relied only on self-report for depression with varying measurement instruments. In our study, we also corroborated our depression status with the medical prescription of any antidepressant.

The present study had several limitations. First, the specific treatments of the patients with diabetes were not verified, so that it is impossible to draw conclusions about the influence of diabetes treatment on cognitive impairment in this sample. Time with any of the conditions was not available, so the effect of short versus long term cannot be confirmed. In addition, other comorbidities, especially those affecting vascular, neuronal, or metabolic status, were not taken into account. The nature of the design does not allow for explanation of the mechanisms of the relationships observed. Another important limitation of this study is that we included only the MMSE, which is not a diagnostic instrument, to assess the cognitive function. We understand this test is widely used for its ability to follow cognitive changes over time [33]. Despite these limitations, with our large sample size, rigorous study design, and broad socioeconomic, and educational characteristics of our participants, we believe that it is possible to make valid inferences to the elderly population residing in Mexico City.

The patients with triple diagnoses of dementia, depression, and diabetes demonstrated greater cognitive dysfunction relative to those with double or single diagnosis of dementia. Additional research is needed to unravel this relationship, as to whether the cognitive impairment accrued in patients with DDD. These findings highlight the importance of identifying depression among diabetics and patients with dementia. Since depression is readily treatable, remission should lead to improved cognitive function and quality of life. The role of neuropsychology is expanding due to the increasing demand for differential diagnosis and to draw conclusions about patients' abilities to function independently. Further research is necessary to define and recognize patients with dementia with comorbid conditions.

Acknowledgements

This project was supported by grants from SSA/IMSS/ISSSTE-CONACYT (México) SALUD-2009-C01-114716 and the Fund for the Promotion of Health Research, Mexican Institute of Social Security, FIS/IMSS/PROT/G10/824. Authors state that there is no conflict of interest.

Author details

Juárez-Cedillo Teresa[1,2*], Hsiung Ging-Yuek[3,4], Sepehry A. Amir[3], Beattie B. Lynn[4,5], Jacova Claudia[3,4] and Escobedo de la Peña Jorge[1]

*Address all correspondence to: terezillo@yahoo.com.mx

1 Clinical Epidemiology Research Unit, Hospital General Regional 1, Dr Carlos McGregor, IMSS Mexican Institute of Social Security, Mexico City, Mexico

2 Faculty of High Studies (FES) Zaragoza, National Autonomous University of Mexico, Mexico City, Mexico

3 UBC Division of Neurology, Department of Medicine, Vancouver, B.C., Canada

4 UBC Hospital Clinic for Alzheimer Disease and Related Disorders, Vancouver, B.C., Canada

5 UBC Division of Geriatric Medicine, Department of Medicine, Vancouver, B.C., Canada

References

[1] Chapman DP, Williams SM, Strine TW, Anda RF, Moore MJ. Dementia and its implications for public health. Prev Chronic Dis 2006;3(2):A34. Available from: http://www.cdc.gov/pcd/issues/2006/apr/05_0167.htm.

[2] Grunblatt E, Zehetmayer S, Bartl J, Löffler C, Wichart I, Rainer MK, Jungwirth S, Bauer P, Danielczyk W, Tragl KH, Riederer P, Fischer P. Genetic risk factors and markers for Alzheimer's disease and/or depression in the VITA study. J Psychiatr Res 2009;43(3): 298–308. doi:10.1016/j.jpsychires.2008.05.008

[3] Mayberg HS, Keightley M, Mahurin RK. Neuropsychiatric aspects of mood and affective disorders. In Yudofsky SC & Hales RE (Eds.), Essentials of neuropsychiatry and clinical neurosciences. Washington, DC: American Psychiatric Publishing, Inc., 2004. pp. 489–517.

[4] National Institute of Mental Health Older Adults: Depression and Suicide Facts. [Internet]. 2007. Available from: www.nimh.nih.gov/publcat/elderlydepsuicide.cfm [accessed: 2014-01-22].

[5] Awad N, Gagnon M, Messier C. The relationship between impaired glucose tolerance, type 2 diabetes, and cognitive function. J Clin Exp Neuropsychol 2004;26(8):1044–1080. doi:10.1080/13803390490514875

[6] Hendrickx H, McEwen BS, Ouderaa F. Metabolism, mood and cognition in aging: the importance of lifestyle and dietary intervention. Neurobiol Aging 2005;26(1):1–5. doi: 10.1016/j.neurobiolaging.2005.10.005

[7] National Institute of Health. National Institute of Diabetes and Digestive and Kidney Diseases. [Internet]. 2016. Available from: http://www.nih.gov/about/almanac/organization/NIDDK.htm [accessed: 2014-01-25].

[8] Lyketsos CG, Lopez O, Jones B, Fitzpatrick AL, Breitner J, DeKosky S. Prevalence of neuropsychiatric symptoms in dementia and mild cognitive impairment: results from the cardiovascular health study. JAMA 2002;25(12):1475–1483. doi:10.1001/jama.288.12.1475.

[9] Berg D. Biomarkers for the early detection of Parkinson's and Alzheimer's disease. Neurodegener Dis 2008;5(3–4):133–136. doi:10.1159/000113682.

[10] Cankurtaran M, Yavuz BB, Cankurtaran ES, Halil M, Ulger Z, Ariogul S. Risk factors and type of dementia: vascular or Alzheimer? Arch Gerontol Geriatr 2008;47(1):25–34. doi:10.1016/j.archger.2007.06.005.

[11] Katon WJ, Lin EH, Von Korff M, Ciechanowski P, Ludman EJ, Young B, Peterson D, Rutter CM, McGregor M, McCulloch D. Collaborative care for patients with depression and chronic illnesses. N Engl J Med 2010;30(27):2611–2620. doi:10.1056/NEJMoa1003955.

[12] Juarez-Cedillo T, Sanchez-Arenas R, Sanchez-Garcia S, Garcia-Peña C, Hsiung GY, Sepehry AA, Beattie BL, Jacova C. Prevalence of mild cognitive impairment and its subtypes in the Mexican population. Dement Geriatr Cogn Disord 2012;43(5.6):271–281. doi:10.1159/000345251.

[13] Reyes de Beaman S, Peter E, Beaman PE, Garcia-Peña C, Villa MA, Heres J, Córdova A, Jagger C. Validation of a modified version of the mini-mental state examination (MMSE) in Spanish. Aging Neuropsychol Cognition 2004;11(1):1–11. doi:10.1076/anec.11.1.1.29366.

[14] Morris JC. The clinical dementia rating (CDR): current version and scoring rules. Neurology 1993;43(11):2412–2414. doi:10.1212/WNL.43.11.2412-a.

[15] American Psychiatric Association. Diagnostic and statistical manual of mental disorders: DSM-IV [Internet]. 4th ed. Washington, DC: American Psychiatric Association;

2000. Available from: http://www.psychiatryonline.com/DSMPDF/dsm-iv.pdf [accessed: 2014-01-22].

[16] McKhann G, Drachman D, Folstein M, Katzman R, Price D, Stadlan EM. Clinical diagnosis of Alzheimer's disease: report of the NINCDS-ADRDA Work Group under the auspices of Department of Health and Human Services Task Force on Alzheimer's Disease. Neurology 1984;34(7):939–944. doi:10.1212/WNL.34.7.939.

[17] Roman GC, Tatemichi TK, Erkinjuntti T, Cummings JL, Masdeu, JC, Garcia JH, Amaducci L, Orgogozo JM, Brun A, Hofman A, Moody DM, O'Brien, Yamaguchi T, Grafman J, Drayer BP, Bennett DA, Fisher M, Ogata J, Kokmen E, Bermejo F, Wolf PA, Gorelick PB, Bick KL, Pajeau AK, Bell MA, DeCarli C, Culebras MA, Korczyn AD, Bogousslavsky J, Hartmann A, Scheinberg P. Vascular dementia: Diagnostic criteria for research studies. Report of the ninds-airen international workshop. Neurology 1993;43(2):250–260. doi:10.1212/WNL.43.2.250.

[18] Jaccard J, Guilamo-Ramos V. Analysis of variance frameworks in clinical child and adolescent psychology: advanced issues and recommendations. J Clin Child Adolesc Psychol 2002;31(2):278–294. doi:10.1207/S15374424JCCP3102_13.

[19] Radloff LS. The CES-D Scale: a self-report depression scale for research in the general population. Appl Psychol Meas 1977;1(3):385–401. doi:10.1177/014662167700100306.

[20] Anderson RJ, Freedland KE, Clouse RE, Lustman PJ. The prevalence of comorbid depression in adults with diabetes: a meta-analysis. Diabetes Care 2001;24(6):1069–1078. doi:10.2337/diacare.24.6.1069

[21] Cohen J. Statistical power analysis for the behavioral sciences. 2nd ed. New Jersey: Lawrence Erlbaum, 1988.

[22] Jorm AF. Is depression a risk factor for dementia or cognitive decline? Gerontology 2000;46(4):219–227. doi:10.1159/000022163.

[23] Watari K, Letamendi A, Elderkin-Thompson V, Haroon E, Miller J, Darwin C, Kumar A. Cognitive function in adults with type 2 diabetes and major depression. Arch Clin Neuropsychol 2006;21(8):787–796. doi:10.1016/j.acn.2006.06.014.

[24] Ritchie K, Touchon J, Ledésert B. Progressive disability in senile dementia is accelerated in the presence of depression. Int J Geriatr Psychiatry 1998;13(7):459–461. doi:10.1002/(SICI)1099-1166(199807)13:7<459::AID-GPS796>3.0.CO;2-W.

[25] Weiner MF, Lipton AM. (Eds.). Clinical manual of Alzheimer disease and other dementias. Washington, DC: American Psychiatric Pub, 2012. Available from: http://samples.sainsburysebooks.co.uk/9781585629619_sample_131900.pd [accessed: 2014-02-05].

[26] Kumar A, Mintz J, Bilker W, Gottlieb G. Autonomous neurobiological pathways to late-life major depressive disorder: clinical and pathophysiological implications. Neuropsychopharmacology 2002;26(2):229–236. doi:10.1016/S0893-133X(01)00331-1.

[27] Domínguez RO, Marschoff ER, González SE, Repetto MG, Serra JA. Type 2 diabetes and/or its treatment leads to less cognitive impairment in Alzheimer's disease patients. Diabetes Res Clin Pract 2012;98(1):68–74. doi:10.1016/j.diabres.2012.05.013.

[28] Stewart R, Liolitsa D. Type 2 diabetes mellitus, cognitive impairment and dementia. Diabe Med 1999;16(2):93–122. doi:10.1046/j.1464-5491.1999.00027.x.

[29] Strachan MW, Frier BM, Deary IJ. Cognitive assessment in diabetes: The need for consensus. Diabet Med 1997;14(6):421–422. doi:10.1002/(SICI)1096-9136(199706)14:6<421::AID-DIA382>3.0.CO;2-F.

[30] Airaksinen E, Larsson M, Lundberg I, Forsell Y. Cognitive functions in depressive disorders: evidence from a population-based study. Psychol Med 2004;34(1):83–91. doi: 10.1017/S0033291703008559.

[31] Elderkin-Thompson V, Kumar A, Bilker WB, Dunkin JJ, Mintz J, Moberg PJ, Mesholam RI, Gur RE. Neuropsychological deficits among patients with late-onset minor and major depression. Arch Clin Neuropsychol 2003;18(5):529–549. doi:10.1016/S0887-6177(03)00022-2.

[32] Alexopoulos GS, Kiosses DN, Klimstra S, Kalayam B, Bruce ML. Clinical presentation of the "depression-executive dysfunction syndrome" of late life. Am J Geriatr Psychiatry 2002;10(1):98. doi:10.1097/00019442-200201000-00012.

[33] Crum RM, Anthony JC, Bassett SS, Folstein MF. Population-based norms for the mini-mental state examination by age and educational level. JAMA 1993;269(18):2386–2391. Available from: http://faculty.pepperdine.edu/shimels/Courses/Files/MMSE.pdf [accessed: 2016-01-13].

Chapter 21

Idiopathic Normal Pressure Hydrocephalus: An Overview of Pathophysiology, Clinical Features, Diagnosis and Treatment

Rubesh Gooriah and Ashok Raman

Additional information is available at the end of the chapter

http://dx.doi.org/10.5772/64198

Abstract

Normal pressure hydrocephalus is characterised by the triad of gait disturbance, dementia and urinary incontinence. Although our understanding of the condition has considerably improved since it was initially described over 50 years ago, its pathophysiology is still a matter of debate. We provide an overview of the current concepts in pathophysiology and discuss the clinical features, diagnosis and treatment of this cause of dementia.

Keywords: cerebrospinal fluid, cerebral blood flow, vascular compliance, CSF outflow resistance, neurodegeneration

1. Introduction

First described by Hakim and Adams [1] in 1965, normal pressure hydrocephalus (NPH) is a potentially reversible cause of dementia. It is a communicating hydrocephalus, which occurs as a result of impaired re-absorption of cerebrospinal fluid (CSF). This can be caused by a number of conditions including meningitis, trauma and subarachnoid haemorrhage. However, in a large number of cases, it is idiopathic (INPH). INPH is characterised clinically by the triad of gait disturbance, cognitive decline and urinary incontinence. Ventriculomegaly is observed on magnetic resonance imaging (MRI) or computed tomography (CT). However, the symptoms of INPH are non-specific and can occur in other conditions. Moreover, the classic triad is not always present. Varying combinations and degrees of each element of the triad are encountered in different patients and depending on the stage of the condition. INPH has an insidious onset and progresses gradually. Shunt surgery results in a positive response in as many as 84% in a European multicentre study [2]. Although the treatment is surgical, neurological input is important for the diagnosis and identification of suitable shunt candidates. In some countries, hydrocephalus is a purely surgical condition. However, like several authors, we believe that a multidisciplinary approach is essential for the optimal management of these patients. In our neuroscience centre, the management of INPH involves the neurologists, neurosurgeons and physiotherapists.

2. Methods

This review was prompted by the large number of publications on INPH. We searched the databases of Medline, Embase and the Cochrane Library for articles relating to INPH up to February 2016. We included review articles and research studies according to their relevance.

3. Epidemiology

It is difficult to accurately establish the incidence and prevalence of INPH because several cases are likely to be undiagnosed due to the non-specific nature of the symptoms. However, it is clear from epidemiological studies that the incidence increases with age. Tisell et al. [3] observed that one to two shunt operations per 100,000 inhabitants were being performed yearly for INPH. Brean and Eide [4] found that the prevalence was up to 181.7 per 100,000 people in the 70–79 years age group in Norway [4]. After randomly subjecting 497 individuals over the age of 65 to magnetic resonance imaging (MRI) of the brain, Tanaka et al. found a prevalence of 1.4% in that age group [5]. It is also estimated that up to 10% of patients with dementia may have INPH [6].

4. Pathophysiology

The CSF space is a dynamic pressure system. It is responsive to changes in CSF formation or reabsorption rates, arterial and venous flow, compliance of the intracranial structures and fluctuations in intracranial pressure (ICP). Around 500 ml of CSF is produced every day and the total volume of CSF at any one point is between 120 and 150 ml. The brain is unique in the sense that it is the only organ enclosed in a non-expansile box (i.e. the skull). According to the Monro-Kellie hypothesis, the total volume of the constituents in the cranium is fixed. Therefore, an increase in the volume of any of the constituents has to be matched by a decrease in the volume of another to avoid an increase in intracranial pressure. The volume of blood entering the brain varies with the cardiac cycle. There is a net intracranial inflow of blood during systole and a net outflow during diastole. Arterial supply to the brain is pulsatile whereas venous flow is less so, and this mismatch causes transient rises in pressure. The brain and other intracranial constituents can compensate for this in two ways. Firstly, the blood vessels have a degree of compliance which allows for a smoother influx of arterial blood. Secondly, CSF flows back and forth through the cerebral aqueduct in response to pulsatile blood flow, thereby maintaining intracranial pressure stable. However, in INPH, the intracranial constituents become less compliant [7]. A reduction in vascular compliance especially in the superior sagittal sinus has been found [8]. This can initially be countered by increased pulsatile CSF flow through the aqueduct. If this fails, the amplitude of arterial pulsatility increases during systole inducing large ICP pulsations ('water hammer' effect). These pulsations, in addition to causing venous damage in the periventricular region, displace the brain towards the skull [9]. Hydrocephalus occurs as a result of enlarging ventricles at the expense of a reduced subarachnoid space. This is secondary to increasing pressure within the ventricles directed towards the subarachnoid space. The pressure gradient arising between the ventricles and the subarachnoid space is termed 'transmantle pressure'. The transmantle pressure gradient has to be the only force which could cause such changes to the brain [9]. CSF spaces revert to normal following shunting, implying that the transmantle pressure gradient can be reduced or reversed. This pressure gradient also explains why, although there is increased intraventricular pressure, the measured opening pressure during a lumbar puncture is within normal limits. It also implies that 'normal pressure' in NPH is somewhat of a misnomer.

What triggers the initial reduction in compliance that results in INPH? Most theories on INPH attempt to explain the pathophysiology around the finding of reduced cerebral blood flow (CBF). There is a strong association between impaired CBF and INPH. Patients with INPH are more likely to have concomitant cerebrovascular disease [10]. MRI shows increased white matter changes (WMCs) [11] and this is further supported by neuropathological studies showing microvascular infarctions but also interstitial oedema, ependymal disruption, gliosis and neuronal degeneration [12, 13]. In addition, there is an association between high ICP and impaired cerebrovascular autoregulation [14]. Age-related atherosclerosis has been proposed as being responsible for the reduction in vascular compliance [15]. This would explain the association between NPH and vascular disease (VD). Bateman [8], on the other hand, proposes that increased transvenular resistance in the territory of the superior sagittal sinus is the initiating event in NPH. While some consider that CSF resorption occurs at the level of the arachnoid villi or arachnoid granulations, others believe that the majority of CSF resorption occurs through brain parenchyma at the levels of capillaries and veins [9, 16–18]. If the latter hypothesis is true, CSF resorption would be affected with increased transvenular resistance. Indeed, CSF resorption is unequivocally abnormal in INPH [19]. CSF outflow resistance or conductance (which is inversely proportional to resistance) has been investigated in a few studies [20–22] and found to be impaired. Early studies in animals and humans suggest that, in the initial stages, mounting CSF intraventricular pressure secondary to abnormal CSF flow causes ventricular dilatation [8]. It is therefore possible that CSF outflow disturbance, occurring secondary to reduced venous compliance, is directly related to the ventriculomegaly seen in INPH.

But why would venous resistance increase in an elderly patient? Bradley believes that deep white matter ischaemia is the triggering event [23]. Due to ischaemia, surrounding arterioles are already maximally dilated, and this would explain the loss of autoregulation [23]. When the arterioles are obstructed, venous collapse ensues, followed by impaired CSF drainage and ventricular enlargement [23]. The problem we have with this hypothesis is that if one wants a unifying theory with ischaemia as the initiating trigger, one would struggle to explain the appearance of NPH in disorders such as progressive supranuclear palsy (PSP), corticobasal degeneration (CBD) and Alzheimer's disease (AD). Periventricular white matter ischaemia is an uncommon finding especially in PSP and CBD. Yet, there has to be a final common pathway which results in hydrocephalus in all these conditions. We hypothesise that neurodegeneration has a role to play in INPH, at least in some cases. The following findings would support this:

- Of the 38 patients in two studies who were diagnosed with INPH, vascular changes (71%), AD (61%), PSP (2.6%) and CBD (2.6%) were the most frequent co-existing pathologies and none had specific neuropathological changes to suggest INPH as an entity [24, 25].
- Levels of tau protein in CSF, an index of neuronal degeneration, were found to be higher in patients with NPH compared to healthy controls [26] although phospho-tau181 was lower in INPH than in those with established AD [27].
- Midbrain atrophy is strongly associated with gait disturbance in NPH [28].
- Although the gait disturbance improves with shunting, the dementia seen in INPH often does not and it continues to progress, suggesting a difference in the aetiopathogenesis underlying these symptoms.
- Even if there is an initial response, overall the condition eventually progresses despite a functioning shunt in situ in the majority of cases. It is therefore possible that those who deteriorate quicker also have more rapid neurodegeneration (e.g. PSP) than those who deteriorate less rapidly (e.g. AD).

Finally, we take the opportunity to emphasise the possibility that INPH has different causes which form a pathophysiological continuum. This would not only explain the differences with shunt response and rates of progression but would also explain why a universal theory remains elusive. It would perhaps be more appropriate to refer to these conditions, where known, as VD-associated NPH, AD-associated NPH, etc.

5. Clinical features

5.1. Gait disturbance

Gait disturbance is usually the commonest and earliest symptom of INPH. Its onset is insidious over months and sometimes years. It is also the one that is most likely to respond to shunting. The gait impairment in NPH is frequently described as 'apraxic'. Other descriptors used are 'shuffling', 'magnetic' and 'broad-based'. Thompson [29] is in favour of the term 'frontal lobe ataxia' instead of gait apraxia, which is defined as an impairment of gait not attributed to motor or sensory deficits, although he acknowledges that this is based on observation rather than on firm evidence for this. Interestingly, some patients display normal ability to move the legs in a recumbent position while being practically unable to walk. This phenomenon indicates that the gait disturbance is due to a problem with locomotion rather than a pure motor dysfunction. There is no single feature that is pathognomonic of the gait disturbance in NPH. In mild cases, patients may display a broad-based gait but in more severe cases there is a reduction in stride length [30]. The feet appear clumsy and there is difficulty initiating foot movements. Patients are also slow to rise from a seated position. The gait is also characterised by reduced step height and a typical disturbance of the dynamic equilibrium [31]. About 30% of patients experience freezing of gait [31]. Patients tend to turn in multiple small steps. Postural instability and falls are common. The gait pattern in INPH is visibly different from that of Parkinson's disease [31]. A wider step, as well as increased foot angles, is uncharacteristic of Parkinson's disease but common in INPH. Upper limb movements are preserved. The reason is that the motor fibres controlling the upper extremities and face originate more laterally in the motor cortex and are subsequently subjected to less stretching due to hydrocephalus [32]. Upper motor neuron signs, such as spasticity and hyperreflexia, are unusual. Since the symptoms of INPH are symmetrical, any lateralising signs should raise suspicion of other disorders.

5.2. Dementia

The cognitive deficits in INPH are classically that of a subcortical dementia with predominantly frontal features [33–35] and are characterised by apathy, inattention, psychomotor retardation and poor executive function [36]. It is worth noting that the term 'dementia' is used to designate the cognitive impairment in INPH although some patients who present early may not have evidence of this or may not meet the criteria for dementia on cognitive testing. Saito et al. have shown that the deficits extend beyond executive function, attention and memory to visuoperceptual and visuospatial domains on neuropsychological testing [37]. There is substantial overlap between INPH and AD but frontal lobe dysfunction account for >50% of the cognitive deficit in INPH while memory impairment is responsible for >50% of the cognitive deficit in AD [37]. The degree of neuropsychological impairment in INPH has also been found to relate to the severity of other signs of INPH [38]. Those with vascular risk factors performed worse than those without [38]. Compared with Binswanger's disease, impairment of memory and visuospatial attention in NPH may be more pronounced [39].

5.3. Urinary incontinence

Urinary incontinence is often the last symptom to appear, although it is well established that each symptom can occur independently of the others [40]. Increased urinary urgency occurs earlier and is almost always present in INPH [40, 41]. Urinary incontinence is also very common in the elderly and therefore, on its own, lacks specificity. Fisher [40] considered it to be a frontal lobe incontinence as patients were indifferent regarding where and when to urinate. This correlates with the pattern of cognitive deficits mentioned earlier. Sakakibara et al. [42] have found that detrusor overactivity, seen in 95% of their cases, is fundamental to the appearance of urinary urgency, frequency and incontinence. Seventy-one per cent had voiding symptoms such as difficulties in initiating urination and poor flow [42]. Bladder dysfunction can improve after shunting suggesting that the symptoms are likely secondary to impaired cerebral control of bladder storage. The underlying mechanism for detrusor overactivity in patients with NPH appears to be related to reduced cerebral blood flow in the right frontal cortex, and to a lesser extent impaired basal ganglia function [43]. Reduced mobility could also be contributing to incontinence in these patients [43].

6. Investigations

6.1. Neuroimaging

The diagnosis of INPH in the right clinical context relies on the finding of hydrocephalus on brain imaging (**Figure 1A**). Hydrocephalus is not synonymous with ventriculomegaly. Although ventriculomegaly is commonly found in the elderly population, this does not imply the presence of NPH. In NPH, the ventriculomegaly is typically out of proportion to the amount of atrophy present. CT of the brain is a sensitive imaging modality to identify NPH but MRI provides additional information such as aqueductal stenosis, white matter changes or the presence of an underlying aetiology (e.g. AD). A coronal section reveals a narrow subarachnoid space surrounding the outer surface of the brain (hence the term 'tight convexity') and narrow medial cisterns. The cortical sulci at the vertex are effaced (**Figure 1B**), whereas the temporal horns are widened (**Figure 2A**). The third ventricle is often enlarged, whereas the fourth ventricle can be either dilated or normal. Therefore, a normal-sized fourth ventricle in the presence of enlarged lateral and third ventricles does not necessarily suggest aqueductal stenosis and is a finding consistent with NPH. Other imaging features of NPH are discussed below.

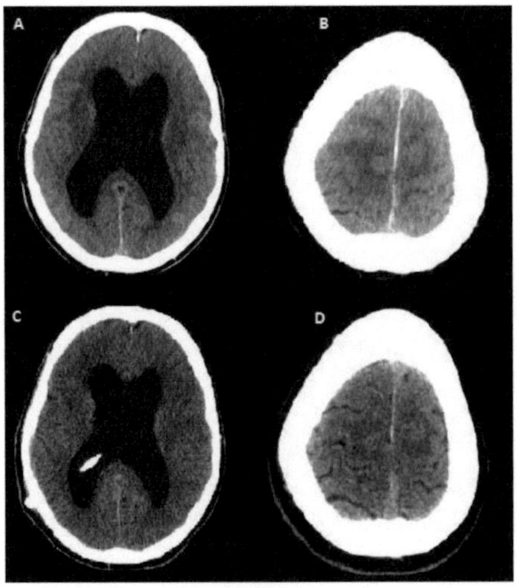

Figure 1. Ventriculomegaly and effacement of sulci at the vertex in a patient with INPH (**A** and **B**), with some post-operative improvement (**C** and **D**).

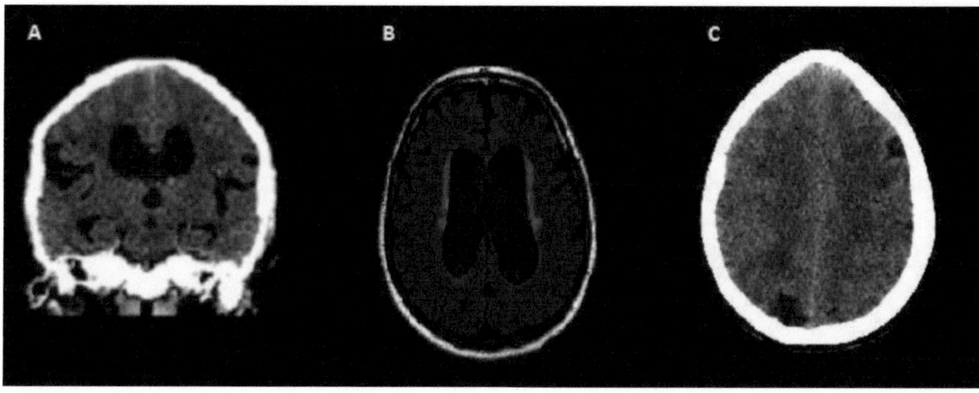

Figure 2. (A) Dilated Sylvian fissures and temporal horns. **(B)** Periventricular white matter hyperintensities on MRI. **(C)** Isolated dilated sulci.

6.1.1. Evan's index

An objective way of assessing whether the ventricles are enlarged is through the use of Evan's index. It is the ratio of the maximum width of the frontal horns of the lateral ventricles and the transverse inner diameter of the skull, measured at the same level on both axial CT and MRI images [44, 45]. A value above 0.30 is considered significant, although in our own experience, the higher the value, the more specific it is for NPH. Unfortunately, Evan's index is a crude marker of hydrocephalus and varies significantly depending on the location and angle of the slice [46]. It is therefore of limited value on its own.

6.1.2. Callosal angle

The concept of callosal angle with respect to NPH was first described on pneumoencephalogram by Benson et al. [47] and thereafter by Sjaastand and Nordvik [48]. The International guidelines mention an angle of greater than 40° as supportive of NPH [49]. However, using MRI, Ishii et al. [50] found that a callosal angle of less than 90°, measured on a coronal plane, which is perpendicular to the AC–PC plane on the posterior commissure plane, helped in differentiating INPH patients from AD and normally aged subjects. The narrow angle is caused by the elevation of dilated ventricles and compression due to dilated Sylvian fissures (**Figure 2A**). When combined with Evan's index of >0.3, INPH could be discriminated from AD with a sensitivity and specificity of 97 and 94%, respectively [50].

6.1.3. White matter changes (WMC)

INPH is known to be associated with deep white matter changes (DWMC) and smooth periventricular hyperintensity (PVH) [51] on MRI (**Figure 2B**). As discussed earlier, there is an element of cerebral hypoperfusion in INPH which is thought to contribute to the development of INPH. It is, however, unclear whether the WMC are cause or effect. Regardless of the underlying pathophysiological mechanisms implicated in NPH, there is consistent neuropathological evidence demonstrating the involvement of white matter. A diversity of pathological observations, such as direct mechanical compression of the periventricular white matter, ischaemic demyelination and infarction, have been noted in INPH [12, 13, 52]. Indeed, DWMC and subcortical infarctions are commonly seen in patients with Binswanger's disease, and these patients often have similar symptoms to those with INPH. Tullberg et al. [51] evaluated the diagnostic features of DWMC and PVH using MRI, and found that no MRI variable could reliably differentiate NPH from BD. One explanation for this result, put forward by the authors, is that NPH and BD are two disorders with similar pathophysiological mechanisms or that they form a pathophysiological continuum of increasing microangiopathy [51].

6.1.4. CSF flow void

As mentioned earlier, CSF flows back and forth the aqueduct during the cardiac cycle in response to arterial blood flow to the brain. This was initially observed as a flow void, consisting of a decreased MRI signal, mainly in the aqueduct on T2-weighted images of early MR scans in patients with communicating hydrocephalus [53–55]. CSF flow void can be observed in normal individuals, but it is more prominent in INPH [56]. Increased aqueductal CSF flow initially appeared to be predictive of a good response with shunting [55, 57, 58], but further studies have found poor correlation between the extent of CSF flow void and surgical outcome [56, 59].

6.2. CSF tap test

Patients with suspected INPH, based on clinical features and neuroimaging, should undergo a high-volume CSF tap to predict response with shunting. The rationale for a CSF tap is that it simulates the physiological effect of a shunt [45]. The patient is assessed pre- and post-CSF tap for gait and cognitive improvements. About 40–50 ml of CSF is usually removed. Gait is most likely to ameliorate following CSF tap; therefore, it is the best indicator of response. In our centre, we use the 10-m timed-walk test and Tinetti test to assess gait and balance before and after CSF removal. Our patients are also consented for video recordings as these can be useful to retrospectively assess patients especially when the improvement following CSF tap is not clear. It is common that some patients or their carers only notice an improvement a couple of days down the line. We therefore carry out follow-up telephone assessments in all our patients 3 days after they have undergone a CSF tap. This is quite a subjective measure for improvement. Nevertheless, it reduces the chances of missing potentially suitable candidates for shunt surgery. Unfortunately, although the CSF tap test has a high positive-predictive value for shunt success, it has a low sensitivity [60] and should not be used to exclude patients from shunt surgery. There are patients who do respond to shunt surgery after a negative tap test. The first edition of the Japanese guidelines advocated repeating the tap test if initially negative [61], but the more recent edition suggests that further investigation may be required [62]. Recently, Yamada et al. have shown that the timing of the CSF tap affects the accuracy of the test [63]. It should be carried out as soon as symptoms appear [63]. An external lumbar drain, which provides continuous drainage, has a similar predictive value to the CSF tap test, a higher sensitivity [64, 65], but a low negative-predictive value. It is important to note that this test is more invasive, and can give rise to complications such as radicular pain and meningitis.

7. Diagnostic guidelines

Different centres use different criteria for diagnosing INPH and recommending shunt surgery. The decision to shunt a patient with predominantly gait disturbance, typical imaging features and a positive CSF tap test is straightforward. However, the difficulty arises when patients do not show characteristic clinical features or do not show a definite improvement to CSF removal. The purpose of diagnostic guidelines in INPH is to identify those patients who are most likely to benefit from shunt surgery. Recently, the American Academy of Neurology has published its own practice guidelines [66]. However, the international [49] and Japanese [62] guidelines are probably the two most widely used and will be given further consideration in this chapter. Both have some similarities but also a few notable differences. The terms 'possible' and

Features	International guidelines	Japanese guidelines
Size of ventricles	Ventricular enlargement not entirely attributable to cerebral atrophy or congenital hydrocephalus (Evan's ratio >0.3 or equivalent)	Evan's ratio >0.3
Additional imaging features	No obvious obstruction to CSF flow	Dilated subarachnoid spaces in the Sylvian fissures and narrowed spaces over the high cerebral convexity and medial surface (DESH)
	And at least one of the following:	One or more elliptically dilated sulci over the medial surface and convexity in isolation* **(Figure 2C)**
	1. Enlargement of temporal horns not solely due to hippocampal atrophy	A callosal angle of less than 90° on coronal section perpendicular to the anterior commissure-posterior commissure plane*
	2. Callosal angle of 40° or more	
	3. Evidence of altered brain water content, including periventricular signal changes on CT and MRI not attributable to microvascular ischemic changes or demyelination	
	4. An aqueductal or fourth ventricular flow void on MRI	

DESH = disproportionately enlarged subarachnoid space hydrocephalus.

*These features are supportive but not essential for a diagnosis of possible INPH.

Table 1. Imaging features of INPH: comparing the international and Japanese guidelines.

'probable' INPH are employed in each, with diagnostic criteria based on clinical and imaging features. However, the Japanese guidelines use the term 'probable INPH' in those who improve following the removal of CSF. They also label those who respond to shunt surgery as having 'definite' INPH. The international guidelines make no mention of response to CSF removal or shunting in their diagnostic criteria. The neuroimaging criteria also differ. **Table 1** shows a comparison of the diagnostic neuroimaging features used in these guidelines.

8. Predictors of shunt efficacy

Apart from imaging findings and CSF tap test, there are other variables that can influence outcome after shunt surgery. Knowledge of these factors is important, and, when used in conjunction with diagnostic guidelines, can add weight to the decision-making process. Several factors have been associated with either good or poor outcomes. These are summarised in **Table 2**.

The presence of white matter changes is of unclear significance in predicting outcome. The absence of white matter and severe periventricular signals on T2-weighted imaging studies was associated with a good response to shunt placement [71]. The degree of periventricular and deep white matter lesions was shown to be inversely correlated with the degree of clinical improvement in 41 patients [72]. However, as mentioned earlier, Tullberg et al. [51] found that conventional MRI could not reliably differentiate between the causes of white matter changes and that the presence of DWMH or subcortical lacunar infarctions in NPH did not predict a poor outcome from shunt surgery [11]. These patients should not be denied surgery on the basis of these findings alone [11].

Features	Favourable outcome	Poor outcome
Clinical	Gait disturbance occurring before cognitive impairment	Dementia as the initial neurological sign
	Mild or moderate dementia	Severe dementia at presentation
	Shorter duration of symptoms	Dementia for more than 2 years [67, 68]
CSF measures	CSF outflow resistance of 18 mm Hg/ml/min or higher during lumbar constant flow infusion (boon 1998)	
	Occurrence of B-waves during 50% or more of the recording time during continuous ICP monitoring	
Pathological markers		AD pathology on cortical biopsy [69, 70]

Table 2. Factors influencing the outcome of shunt surgery.

9. Shunt surgery

Surgical diversion of CSF via a shunt is the standard intervention for INPH. This is based on the presumption that CSF diversion will reduce or normalise the transmantle pressure, thereby stabilising or improving symptoms. Ventriculoperitoneal shunts are most commonly used [73]. It is important to remember that not every patient with possible or probable INPH will be a candidate for shunt surgery. The risk-to-benefit ratio has to be assessed individually. The patient or family should understand that dementia is least likely to improve and that the mean chance of significant improvement is 30–50% [44]. Information about the risks of complications should also be explicit. Initial studies of shunting in INPH reported a low rate of significant long-term improvement, but a high rate of complications [74]. There is no definite consensus on how to best assess response to shunting. Also, there was no randomised control trial comparing the outcomes of shunting until 2011. This was a small study involving 14 patients who were randomised to open or closed shunts [75]. Those who initially had their shunts ligated after surgery had their shunts opened after 3 months. Those with open shunts experienced an improvement in motor and psychometric scores (30 and 23% increase, respectively) at 3 months, whereas those with ligated shunts were unchanged. This group, however, improved following opening of the shunts at 3 months, with an increase in motor and psychometric scores of 28 and 18%, respectively. A systematic review concluded that long-term response was 29% [76]. However, results of more recent studies show a significantly higher rate of 80–90% [2, 77]. It is clear that a general consensus is required to standardise the measurement of outcomes following shunting.

9.1. Complications

In their systematic review, Hebb et al. [76] also found a mean complication rate of 38%. Potential complications include infection, seizures, abdominal problems (peritonitis, perforation, volvulus and ascites), shunt failure or blockage, shunt over-drainage and intracranial haemorrhage. Shunt over-drainage is the commonest complication in the first year occurring in about one-third of patients [76, 78]. Complication rates can differ between centres. The Eu-iNPH study revealed a complication rate of 28% [2], while Poca et al. [77] found a complication rate of less than 12% in a prospective study involving 236 patients.

9.2. Follow-up

Follow-up after surgery helps to identify patients who are unchanged or worse, and those who can be helped by further adjustments or shunt revision. Repeat brain imaging is routinely undertaken in the immediate aftermath of surgery, but when performed further down the line, it can also identify a subdural haemorrhage in those who are over-drained. If this is the case, a higher opening pressure should be targeted. Conversely, a retrospective study found that in those with no substantial improvement and in whom under-drainage is suspected, selecting a lower pressure can improve the outcome [79].

10. Conclusions

INPH is probably more common that we realise. Due to its reversibility, it is imperative that not only neurologists but other physicians, in particular geriatricians, are more aware of this condition. Although significant progress has been made in our understanding of this condition, a unifying theory explaining its pathophysiology is still awaited. Numerous pathophysiological changes have been noted, but it remains unclear which is the cause, effect or epiphenomenon. Given that patients with INPH have pathologies such as VD, AD and PSP, among others, we therefore regard INPH as a multi-aetiological disorder. For similar reasons, we feel that the role of neurodegeneration should be explored further. Treatment with shunting remains the gold standard. Unfortunately, too often, the condition eventually progresses.

Author details

Rubesh Gooriah* and Ashok Raman

*Address all correspondence to: rubesh@doctors.org.uk

Department of Neurology, Hull Royal Infirmary, Hull, United Kingdom

References

[1] Hakim S, Adams RD: The special clinical problem of symptomatic hydrocephalus with normal cerebrospinal fluid pressure. Observations on cerebrospinal fluid hydrodynamics. J Neurol Sci. 1965;2:307–27.

[2] Klinge P, Hellstrom P, Tans J, et al: One-year outcome in the European multicentre study on iNPH. Acta Neurol Scand. 2012;126:145–53.

[3] Tisell M, Hoglund M, Wikkelso C: National and regional incidence of surgery for adult hydrocephalus in Sweden. Acta Neurol Scand. 2005;112:72–5.

[4] Brean A, Eide PK: Prevalence of probable idiopathic normal pressure hydrocephalus in a Norwegian population. Acta Neurol Scand. 2008;118:48–53.

[5] Tanaka N, Yamaguchi S, Ishikawa H, Ishii H, Megura K: Prevalence of possible idiopathic normal-pressure hydrocephalus in Japan: the Osaki-Tajiri project. Neuroepidemiology 2009;32:171–5.

[6] Spetzler RF: Normal pressure hydrocephalus. Barrow Q. 2003;19:1.

[7] Mase M, Yamada K, Banno T, et al: Quantitative analysis of CSF flow dynamics using MRI in normal pressure hydrocephalus. Acta Neurochir Suppl (Wein). 1998;71:350–3.

[8] Bateman G: Vascular compliance in normal pressure hydrocephalus. Am J Neuroradiol. 2000;21:1574–85.

[9] Greitz D, Greitz T, Hindmarsh T: A new view on the CSF-circulation with the potential for pharmacological treatment of childhood hydrocephalus. Acta Paediatr. 1997;86:125–32.

[10] Krauss, JK, Droste DW et al: Cerebrospinal fluid shunting in idiopathic normal-pressure hydrocephalus of the elderly: effect of periventricular and deep white matter lesions. Neurosurgery 1996;39(2):292–300.

[11] Tullberg M, Jensen C, Ekholm S, Wikkelso C: Normal pressure hydrocephalus: vascular white matter changes on MR images must not exclude patients from shunt surgery. AJNR Am J Neuroradiol. 2001;22:1665–73.

[12] Akai K, Uchigasaki S, et al: Normal pressure hydrocephalus. Neuropathological study. Acta Pathol Jpn. 1987;37(1):97–110.

[13] Del Bigio MR: Neuropathological changes caused by hydrocephalus. Acta Neuropathol. 1993;85(6):573–85.

[14] Haubrich C, Czosnyka Z, et al: Is there a direct link between cerebrovascular activity and cerebrospinal fluid pressure-volume compensation? Stroke. 2007;38(10): 2677–80.

[15] Grünewald RA: Normal pressure hydrocephalus: pathophysiology. Pract Neurol. 2006;6:264–6.

[16] Castro ME, Portnoy HD, Maesaka J: Elevated cortical venous pressure in hydrocephalus. Neurosurgery. 1991;29:232–8.

[17] Penar PL, Lakin WD, Yu J: Normal pressure hydrocephalus: an analysis of aetiology and response to shunting based on mathematical modelling. Neurol Res. 1995;17:83–8.

[18] Portnoy HD, Branch C, Castro ME: The relationship of intracranial venous pressure to hydrocephalus. Childs Nerv Syst. 1994;10:29–35.

[19] Boon AJ, Tans JT, Delwel EJ, Egeler-Peerdeman SM, Hanlo PW, Wurzer JA, et al: Does CSF outflow resistance predict the response to shunting in patients with normal pressure hydrocephalus? Acta Neurochir Suppl. 1998;71:331–3.

[20] Boon AJ, Tans JT, Delwel EJ, et al: Dutch normal pressure hydrocephalus study: prediction of outcome after shunting by resistance to outflow of cerebrospinal fluid. J Neurosurg. 1997;87:687–93.

[21] Malm J, Kristensen B, Karlsson T, et al: The predictive value of cerebrospinal fluid dynamic tests in patients with the idiopathic adult hydrocephalus syndrome. Arch Neurol. 1995;52:783–9.

[22] Borgesen SE, Gjerris F: The predictive value of conductance to outflow of CSF in normal pressure hydrocephalus. Brain. 1982;105:65–86.

[23] Bradley WG: Normal pressure hydrocephalus: new concepts on etiology and diagnosis. AJNR Am J Neuroradiol. 2000;21:1586–90.

[24] Cabral D, Beach TG, Vedders L, Sue LI, Jacobson S, Myers K, Sabbagh MN: Frequency of Alzheimer's disease pathology at autopsy in patients with clinical normal pressure hydrocephalus. Alzheimers Dement. 2011;7(5):509–13.

[25] Leinonen V, et al: Post-mortem findings in 10 patients with presumed normal-pressure hydrocephalus and review of the literature. Neuropathol Appl Neurobiol. 2012;38(1): 72–86.

[26] Kudo T, Mima T, Hashimoto R, Nakao K, Morihara T, et al: Tau protein is a potential biological marker for normal pressure hydrocephalus. Psychiatry Clin Neurosci. 2000;54:199–202.

[27] Tsai A, Malek-Ahmadi M, Kahlon V, Sabbagh NM: Differences in cerebrospinal fluid biomarkers between clinically diagnosed idiopathic normal pressure hydrocephalus and Alzheimer's disease. J Alzheimers Dis Parkinsonism. 2014;4(4): 1000150.

[28] Lee PH, Yong SW, Ahn YH, Huh K: Correlation of midbrain diameter and gait disturbance in patients with idiopathic normal pressure hydrocephalus. J Neurol. 2005;252:958–63.

[29] Thompson PD: Frontal lobe ataxia. Handb Clin Neurol. 2012;103:619–22.

[30] Knutsson E, Lying-Tunell U: Gait apraxia in normal pressure hydrocephalus: patterns of movement and muscle activation. Neurology. 1985;35:155–60.

[31] Stolze H, Kuhtz-Buschbeck JP, Drücke H, et al: Comparative analysis of the gait disorder of normal pressure hydrocephalus and Parkinson's disease. J Neurol Neurosurg Psychiatr. 2001;70:289.

[32] Scharre DW: Normal pressure hydrocephalus: measure twice, shunt once. Neurology 2011;77:1110–1.

[33] Gustafson L, Hagberg B: Recovery of hydrocephalic dementia after shunt operation. J Neurol Neurosug Psychiatr. 1978;41:940–7.

[34] Thomsen AM, Borgeson SE, Bruhn P, et al: Prognosis of dementia in normal pressure hydrocephalus after a shunt operation. Ann Neurol. 1986;20:304–10.

[35] Iddon JL, Pickard JD, Cross JJ, Griffiths PD, Czosnyka M, Sahakian BJ: Specific patterns of cognitive impairment in patients with idiopathic normal pressure hydrocephalus and Alzheimer's disease: a pilot study. J Neurol Neurosurg Psychiatr. 1999;67:723–32.

[36] Ogino A, Kazui H, Miyoshi N, Hashimoto M, Ohkawa S, Tokunaga H, Ikejiri Y, Takeda M: Cognitive impairment in patients with idiopathic normal pressure hydrocephalus. Dement Geriatr Cogn Disord. 2006;21:113–9.

[37] Saito M, Nishio Y, Kanno S, et al: Cognitive profile of idiopathic normal pressure hydrocephalus. Dement Geriatr Cogn Dis Extra. 2011;1:202–11.

[38] Hellström P, Edsbagge M, Archer T, Tisell M, Tullberg M, Wikkelsø C: The neuropsychology of patients with clinically diagnosed idiopathic normal pressure hydrocephalus. Neurosurgery. 2007;61:1219–26.

[39] Kazui H: Cognitive impairment in patients with idiopathic normal pressure hydrocephalus. Brain Nerve. 2008;60(3):225–31.

[40] Fisher CM: Hydrocephalus as a cause of disturbances of gait in the elderly. Neurology 1982;32:1358–63.

[41] Bret P, Chazal J: L'hydrocéphalie chronique de l'adulte. Neurochirurgie. 1990;36: [Suppl]1–159.

[42] Sakakibara R, Kanda T, Sekido T, et al: Mechanism of bladder dysfunction in idiopathic normal pressure hydrocephalus. Neurourol Urodyn. 2008;27:507–10.

[43] Sakakibara R, Uchiyama T, Kanda T, Uchida Y, Kishi M, Hattori T: Urinary dysfunction in idiopathic normal pressure hydrocephalus. Brain Nerve. 2008;3:233–9.

[44] Vanneste JA: Diagnosis and management of normal-pressure hydrocephalus. J Neurol. 2000;247:5–14.

[45] Williams MA, Relkin NR: Diagnosis and management of idiopathic normal-pressure hydrocephalus. Neurol Clin Pract. 2013;3:375–85.

[46] Toma AK, Holl E, Kitchen ND et al: Evans' index revisited: the need for an alternative in normal pressure hydrocephalus. Neurosurgery. 2011;68 (4):939–44.

[47] Benson DF, LeMay M, Patten DH, Rubens AB: Diagnosis of normal-pressure hydrocephalus. N Engl J Med. 1970;283:609–15.

[48] Sjaastad O, Nordvik A: The corpus callosal angle in the diagnosis of cerebral ventricular enlargement. Acta Neurol Scand. 1973;49:396–406.

[49] Relkin N, Marmarou A, Klinge P, et al: Diagnosing idiopathic normal-pressure hydrocephalus. Neurosurgery. 2005;57(3):S4–16.

[50] Ishii K, Soma T, Shimada K, Oda H, Terashima A, Kawasaki R: Automatic volumetry of the cerebrospinal fluid space in idiopathic normal pressure hydrocephalus. Dement Geriatr Cogn Dis Extra. 2013;3(1):489–96.

[51] Tullberg M, Hultin L, Ekholm S, Mansson JE, Fredman P, Wikkelso C: White matter changes in normal pressure hydrocephalus and Binswanger disease: specificity,

predictive value and correlations to axonal degeneration and demyelination. Acta Neurol Scand. 2002;105:417–26.

[52] Di Rocco C, Di Trapani G, Maira G, Bentivoglio M, Macchi G, Rossi GF: Anatomo-clinical correlations in normotensive hydrocephalus. Reports on three cases. J Neurol Sci. 1977:33:437–52.

[53] Sherman JL, Citrin CM, Gangarosa RE, Bowen BJ: The MR appearance of CSF flow in patients with ventriculomegaly. AJNR Am J Neuroradiol. 1986;7:1025–31.

[54] Bradley WG, Kortman KE, Burgoyne B: Flowing cerebrospinal fluid in normal and hydrocephalic states: appearance on MR images. Radiology. 1986;159:611–6.

[55] Bradley WG Jr, Whittemore AR, Kortman KE, et al: Marked cerebrospinal fluid void: indicator of successful shunt in patients with suspected normal-pressure hydrocephalus. Radiology. 1991;178:459–66.

[56] Krauss JK, Regel JP, Vach W, Jungling FD, Droste DW, Wakhloo AK: Flow void of cerebrospinal fluid in idiopathic normal pressure hydrocephalus of the elderly: can it predict outcome after shunting? Neurosurgery 1997;40:67–73.

[57] Gideon P, Stahlberg F, Thomsen C, Gjerris F, Sørensen PS, Henriksen O: Cerebrospinal fluid flow and production in patients with normal pressure hydrocephalus studied by MRI. Neuroradiology. 1994;36:210–5.

[58] Bradley WG Jr, Scalzo D, Queralt J, Nitz WN, Atkinson DJ, Wong P: Normal-pressure hydrocephalus: evaluation with cerebrospinal fluid flow measurements at MR imaging. Radiology. 1996;198:523–9.

[59] Hakim R, Black PM: Correlation between lumboventricular perfusion and MRI-CSF flow studies in idiopathic normal pressure hydrocephalus. Surg Neurol. 1998;49:14–19.

[60] Wikkelsø C, Hellström P, Klinge PM, Tans JT; European iNPH Multicentre Study Group: The European iNPH Multicentre Study on the predictive values of resistance to CSF outflow and the CSF Tap Test in patients with idiopathic normal pressure hydrocephalus. J Neurol Neurosurg Psychiatr. 2013;84:562–8.

[61] Ishikawa M, Hashimoto M, Kuwana N, Mori E, Miyae H, Wachi A, et al: Guidelines for management of idiopathic normal pressure hydrocephalus. Neurol Med Chir (Tokyo). 2008;48:S1–23.

[62] Mori E, Ishikawa M, Kato T, et al: Japanese Society of Normal Pressure Hydrocephalus. Guidelines for management of idiopathic normal pressure hydrocephalus: second edition. Neurol Med Chir (Tokyo). 2012;52:775–809.

[63] Yamada S, Ishikawa M, Miyajima M, Atsuchi M, Kimura T, Kazui H, Mori E: Disease duration: the key to accurate CSF tap test in iNPH. Acta Neurol Scand. 2016. doi: 10.1111/ane.12580

[64] Walchenbach R, Geiger E, Thomeer RT, et al: The value of temporary external lumbar CSF drainage in predicting the outcome of shunting on normal pressure hydrocephalus. J Neurol Neurosurg Psychiatr. 2002;72:503–6.

[65] Woodworth GF, McGirt MJ, Williams MA, Rigamonti D: Cerebrospinal fluid drainage and dynamics in the diagnosis of normal pressure hydrocephalus. Neurosurgery 2009;64:919–25.

[66] Halperin JJ, Kurlan R, Schwalb JM, Cusimano MD, Gronseth G, Gloss D: Practice guideline: idiopathic normal pressure hydrocephalus: response to shunting and predictors of response: report of the guideline development, dissemination, and implementation subcommittee of the American academy of neurology. Neurology. 2015;85:2063–71.

[67] Petersen RC, Mokri B, Laws ER Jr: Surgical treatment of idiopathic hydrocephalus in elderly patients. Neurology. 1985;35(3):307.

[68] Marmarou A, Young HF, Aygok GA, Sawauchi S, Tsuji O, Yamamoto T, Dunbar J: Diagnosis and management of idiopathic normal-pressure hydrocephalus: a prospective study in 151 patients. J Neurosurg. 2005;102(6):987.

[69] Hamilton R, Patel S, Lee EB, Jackson EM, Lopinto J, Arnold SE, Clark CM, Basil A, Shaw LM, Xie SX, Grady MS, Trojanowski JQ: Lack of shunt response in suspected idiopathic normal pressure hydrocephalus with Alzheimer disease pathology. Ann Neurol. 2010;68(4):535.

[70] Savolainen S, Hurskainen H, Paljarvi L, Alafuzoff I, Vapalahti M: Five year outcome of normal pressure hydrocephalus with or without a shunt: predictive value of the clinical signs, neuropsychological evaluation and infusion test. Acta Neurochir. 2002;144:515–23.

[71] Jack CR Jr, Mokri B, Laws ER Jr, Houser OW, Baker HL Jr, Petersen RC: MR findings in normal-pressure hydrocephalus: significance and comparison with other forms of dementia. J Comput Assist Tomogr. 1987;11:923–31.

[72] Krauss JK, Droste DW, Vach W, Regel JP, Orszagh M, Borremans JJ, Tietz A, Seeger W: Cerebrospinal fluid shunting in idiopathic normal-pressure hydrocephalus of the elderly: effect of periventricular and deep white matter lesions. Neurosurgery 1996;39:292–9.

[73] Bergsneider M, Black PM, Klinge P, Marmarou A, Relkin N: Surgical management of idiopathic normal-pressure hydrocephalus. Neurosurgery 2005;57(3 suppl):S29–39.

[74] Stein SC, Burnett MG, Sonnad SS: Shunts in normal-pressure hydrocephalus: do we place too many or too few? J Neurosurg. 2006;105:815–22.

[75] Tisell M, Tullberg M, Hellstrom P, Edsbagge M, Hogfeldt M, Wikkelso C: Shunt surgery in patients with hydrocephalus and white matter changes. J Neurosurg. 2011;114:1432–8.

[76] Hebb AO, Cusimano MD: Idiopathic normal pressure hydrocephalus: a systematic review of diagnosis and outcome. Neurosurgery. 2001;49(5):1166.

[77] Poca MA, Solana E, et al: Idiopathic normal pressure: results of a prospective cohort of 236 shunted patients. Acta Neurochir. 2012;114:247–53.

[78] Khan QU, Wharen RE, Grewal SS, Thomas CS, Deen HG Jr, Reimer R, Van Gerpen JA, Crook JE, Graff-Radford NR: Overdrainage shunt complications in idiopathic normal-pressure hydrocephalus and lumbar puncture opening pressure. J Neurosurg. 2013;119(6):1498–502.

[79] Zemack G, Romner B: Adjustable valves in normal-pressure hydrocephalus: a retrospective study of 218 patients. Neurosurgery. 2002;51(6):1392–400.